The Spine

A Radiological Text and Atlas

The Spine

A Radiological Text and Atlas

BERNARD S. EPSTEIN, M.D.

*Clinical Professor of Radiology, The Albert
Einstein College of Medicine, New York;
Director, Department of Radiology, The Long
Island Jewish Hospital, New Hyde Park,
New York; Radiologist-in-Chief, The Long
Island Jewish Hospital – Queens Hospital
Center Affiliation, New York*

THIRD EDITION

1251 Illustrations on 482 Figures

Lea & Febiger

PHILADELPHIA · 1969

Published in Great Britain by
Henry Kimpton, London

Library of Congress Catalog Card No. 68:18865

Printed in the United States of America

To My Wife

Preface

THIS book has been extensively revised. While the text maintains the same order of presentation, much has been rewritten. The illustrations have been increased by use of new material covering patients who have been under our observation in the last five years. Of the 388 illustrations in the second edition, only 158 have been retained, and 324 new ones have been added, including studies of anatomic preparations which were made to show areas of interest in better detail than before. The sections on myelography, discal herniations, tumors, spondylotic changes, hematologic and vascular disorders have been augmented in the light of new technics and advances in our understanding of the anatomy and physiology of the spine. Cineradiography, cinemyelography, angiography, the extension of positive contrast myelography to the investigation of the upper cervical spinal canal and the posterior cranial fossa, and the recurrent interest in gas myelography all have been sources of additional information. I have found that myelography is facilitated greatly by the addition of the syphon technic for removal of Pantopaque. The fact that in most patients this can be accomplished quickly and without pain, and that in many, all or almost all of the contrast material can be removed, has made it possible to utilize larger quantities when desirable. With the advent of these newer modalities, in addition to myelography, the radiologist who undertakes examination of the spine has to be able to perform such specialized examinations as aortic angiography, brachial and carotid angiography and in certain cases, selective angiography. Cineradiography and cinemyelography offer opportunities for increasing the scope of radiological examination which challenge the imagination. The fact that movement can be recorded and recalled presents an opportunity for further investigation. From a practical viewpoint, cinemyelography has practically eliminated the statement about "I saw thus and so," because a rerun of the film makes that unnecessary.

The clinical material on which this work is based was seen together with a group of co-workers who were interested, perceptive and skilled. My brother, Dr. Joseph A. Epstein, attending neurological surgeon to the Hospital, operated on almost every patient cited here. The privilege of working with him over the past years is one which I deeply appreciate. The correlations between the clinical, radiological, operative and pathological data were facilitated by the close cooperation of Dr. Leroy Lavine, attending orthopedist, Dr. Morton Nathanson, attending neurologist, and Dr. James Berkman, Director of the Department of Laboratories. Their colleagues, Drs. Robert Carras, Norbert Platt, Martin Green and Robert Mones have been most helpful as well. The publishers have, as before, extended all possible help, for which I am most grateful.

BERNARD S. EPSTEIN

New Hyde Park, New York

Contents

5. Neoplasms of the Vertebral Column

9.   Diseases of the Hematopoietic, Collagen and Reticuloendothelial Systems

10.   Vascular Disorders

The Spine
A Radiological Text and Atlas

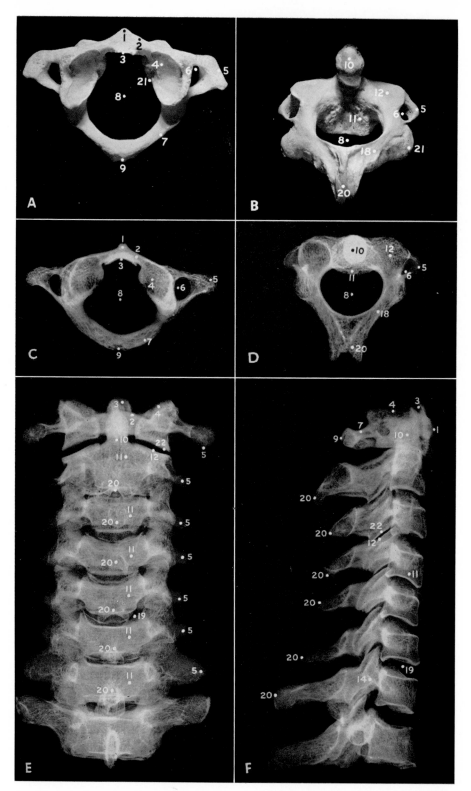

Fig. 1. Photographs and radiographs of various aspects of dried specimens of the *cervical vertebrae*, that demonstrate their anatomy (1st thoracic vertebra also shows in Fig. 1*E* and *F* and Fig. 2*C*).

A, Photograph of superior aspect of atlas. *B*, Photograph of superior aspect of axis. *C*, Supero-inferior radiograph of atlas. *D*, Supero-inferior radiograph of axis. *E*, Anteroposterior radiograph of articulated vertebrae. *F*, Lateral radiograph of articulated vertebrae.

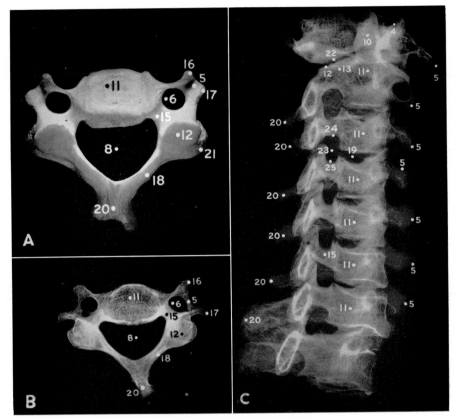

Fig. 2. *A*, Photograph of superior aspect of fourth cervical vertebra. *B*, Supero-inferior radiograph of 4th cervical vertebra. *C*, Oblique radiograph of articulated cervical vertebrae.

LEGEND FOR FIGURES 1 AND 2

1. Anterior tubercle of atlas
   (*tuberculum anterius atlantis*)
2. Anterior arch of atlas
   (*arcus anterior atlantis*)
3. Articular facet for odontoid process of axis
   (*fovea dentis*)
4. Superior articular facet of atlas
   (*fovea articularis superior atlantis*)
5. Transverse process
   (*processus transversus*)
6. Transverse foramen
   (*foramen transversarium*)
7. Posterior arch of atlas
   (*arcus posterior atlantis*)
8. Vertebral foramen
   (*foramen vertebrale*)
9. Posterior tubercle of atlas
   (*tuberculum posterius atlantis*)
10. Odontoid process of axis
    (*dens epistropheus*)
11. Body of vertebra
    (*corpus vertebrae*)
12. Superior articular facet
    (*facies articularis superior*)
13. Superior articular process
    (*processus articularis superior*)
14. Lateral mass
    (*massa lateralis*)
15. Pedicle of vertebral arch
    (*radix arcus vertebrae*)
16. Anterior tubercle of cervical vertebrae
    (*tuberculum anterius vertebrarum cervicalium*)
17. Posterior tubercle of cervical vertebrae
    (*tuberculum posterius vertebrarum cervicalium*)
18. Lamina of vertebral arch
    (*lamina arcus vertebrae*)
19. Intervertebral disc space
20. Spinous process
    (*processus spinosus*)
21. Inferior articular process
    (*processus articularis inferior*)
22. Inferior articular facet
    (*facies articularis inferior*)
23. Intervertebral foramen
    (*foramen intervertebrale*)
24. Superior vertebral notch
    (*incisura vertebralis superior*)
25. Inferior vertebral notch
    (*incisura vertebralis inferior*)

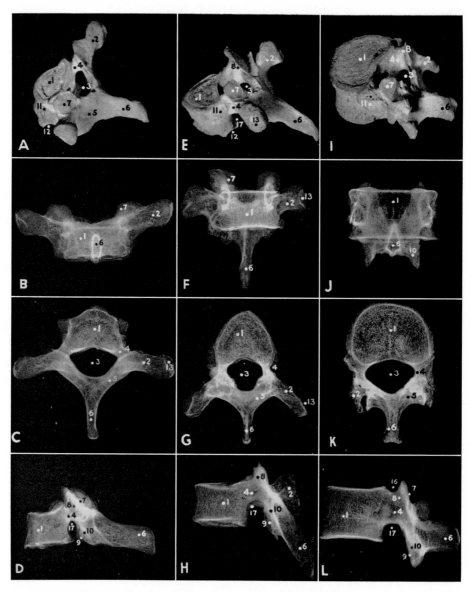

Fig. 3. Photographs and radiographs of thoracic vertebrae, that illustrate their anatomical details.

1st thoracic vertebra. A, photograph; B, anteroposterior radiograph; C, supero-inferior radiograph; D, lateral radiograph.

5th thoracic vertebra. E, photograph; F, anteroposterior radiograph; G, supero-inferior radiograph; H, lateral radiograph.

12th thoracic vertebra. I, photograph; J, anteroposterior radiograph; K, supero-inferior radiograph; L, lateral radiograph.

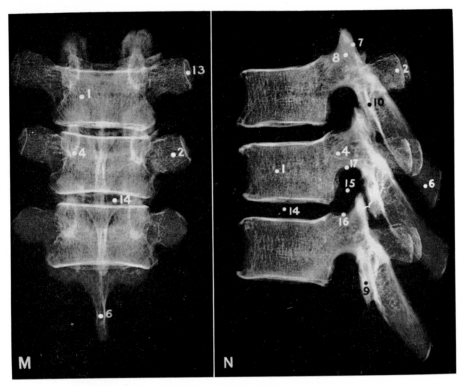

FIG. 3. (*Continued*)   6th, 7th, and 8th thoracic vertebrae, articulated.
M, anteroposterior radiograph; *N*, lateral radiograph.

LEGEND FOR FIGURE 3

1. Body of vertebra
   (*corpus vertebrae*)
2. Transverse process
   (*processus transversus*)
3. Vertebral foramen
   (*foramen vertebrale*)
4. Pedicle of vertebral arch
   (*radix arcus vertebrae*)
5. Lamina of vertebral arch
   (*lamina arcus vertebrae*)
6. Spinous process
   (*processus spinosus*)
7. Superior articular facet
   (*facies articularis superior*)
8. Superior articular process
   (*processus articularis superior*)
9. Inferior articular facet
   (*facies articularis inferior*)

10. Inferior articular process
    (*processus articularis inferior*)
11. Superior costal facet
    (*fovea costalis superior*)
12. Inferior costal facet
    (*fovea costalis inferior*)
13. Costal facet for tubercle of rib
    (*fovea costalis transversalis*)
14. Intervertebral disc space
15. Intervertebral foramen
    (*foramen intervertebrale*)
16. Superior vertebral notch
    (*incisura vertebralis superior*)
17. Inferior vertebral notch
    (*incisura vertebralis inferior*)
18. Intervertebral articulation
    (*Bracket is used in illustration
    to indicate articulation*)

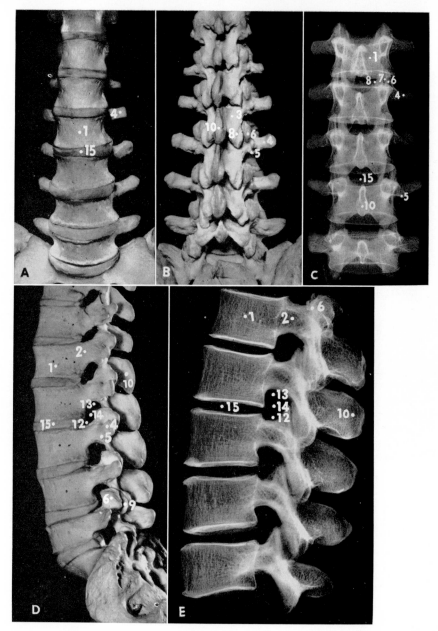

Fig. 4. Photographs and radiographs of dried specimens of articulated lumbar vertebrae, that illustrate their anatomic details.

A, Photograph of anterior aspect; *B*, photograph of posterior aspect; *C*, anteroposterior radiograph; *D*, photograph of lateral aspect; *E*, lateral radiograph.

LEGEND FOR FIGURES 4 AND 5

1. Body of vertebra
   (*corpus vertebrae*)
2. Root (pedicle) of vertebral arch
   (*radix arcus vertebrae*)
3. Lamina of vertebral arch
   (*lamina arcus vertebrae*)
4. Transverse process
   (*processus transversus*)
5. Accessory process
   (*processus accessorius*)
6. Superior articular process
   (*processus articularis superior*)
7. Superior articular facet
   (*facies articularis superior*)

8. Inferior articular process
   (*processus articularis inferior*)
9. Inferior articular facet
   (*facies articularis inferior*)
10. Spinous process
    (*processus spinosus*)
11. Vertebral foramen
    (*foramen vertebrale*)
12. Superior vertebral notch
    (*incisura vertebralis superior*)
13. Inferior vertebral notch
    (*incisura vertebralis inferior*)
14. Intervertebral foramen
    (*foramen intervertebrale*)
15. Intervertebral disc space

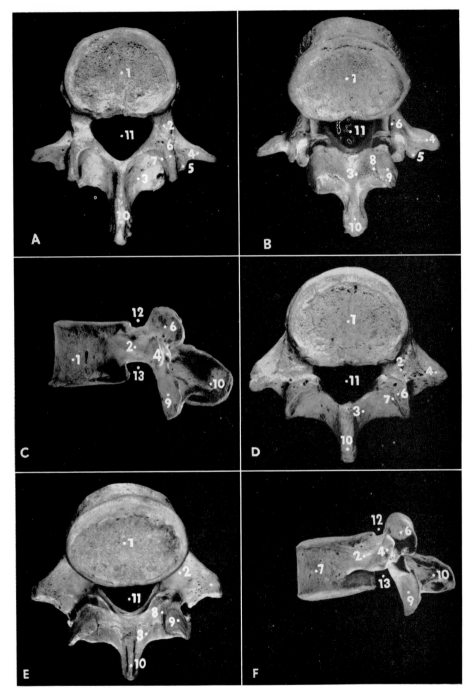

Fig. 5. Photographs of dried specimens of lumbar vertebrae, that illustrate their anatomic details.

3rd lumbar vertebra: *A*, superior aspect; *B*, inferior aspect; *C*, lateral aspect.

5th lumbar vertebra: *D*, superior aspect; *E*, inferior aspect; *F*, lateral aspect.

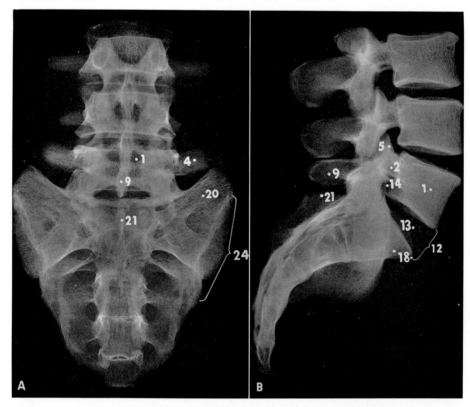

FIG. 6.   Radiographs of articulated lumbar vertebrae and sacrum.
A, anteroposterior radiograph; *B*, lateral radiograph.

LEGEND FOR FIGURES 6 AND 7

5TH LUMBAR VERTEBRA

 1. Body of vertebra
    (*corpus vertebrae*)
 2. Root of vertebral arch
    (*radix arcus vertebrae*)
 3. Lamina of vertebral arch
    (*lamina arcus vertebrae*)
 4. Transverse process
    (*processus transversus*)
 5. Superior articular process
    (*processus articularis superior*)
 6. Superior articular facet
    (*facies articularis superior*)
 7. Inferior articular process
    (*processus articularis inferior*)
 8. Inferior articular facet
    (*facies articularis inferior*)
 9. Spinous process
    (*processus spinosus*)
10. Superior vertebral notch
    (*incisura vertebralis superior*)
11. Inferior vertebral notch
    (*incisura vertebralis inferior*)

LUMBOSACRAL JUNCTION

12. Articulation for the vertebral bodies
    (*Bracket is used in illustration
    to indicate articulation*)

13. Intervertebral disc
    (*space*)
14. Intervertebral foramen
    (*foramen intervertebrale*)
15. Articulation for the vertebral arches
    (*Bracket is used in illustration
    to indicate articulation*)

1ST SACRAL VERTEBRA

16. Base
    (*basis ossis sacri*)
17. Body of vertebra
    (*corpus vertebrae*)
18. Promontory
    (*promontorium*)
19. Sacral canal
    (*canalis sacralis*)
20. Lateral mass
    (*pars lateralis*)
21. Spinous process
    (*processus spinosus*)
22. Superior articular process
    (*processus articularis superior*)
23. Superior articular facet
    (*facies articularis superior*)
24. Iliac articular surface
    (*facies auricularis*)
25. Anterior sacral foramen
    (*foramen sacralis anterior*)
26. Posterior sacral foramen
    (*foramen sacralis posterior*)

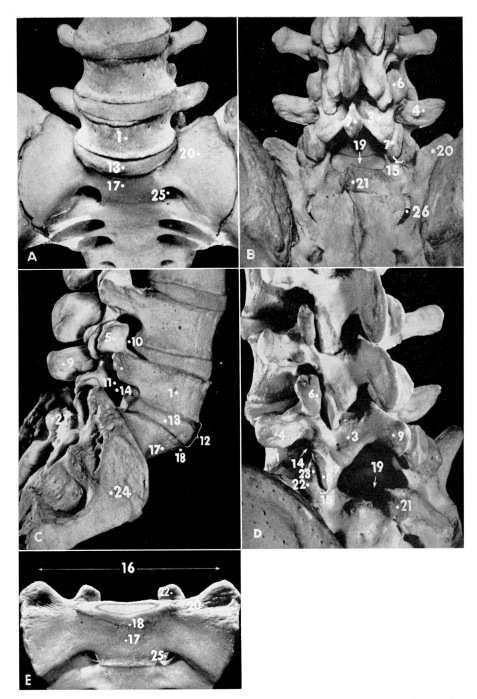

Fig. 7. Photographs and radiographs of dried specimens of articulated lumbar vertebrae and sacrum, illustrating the anatomy of these structures and the lumbosacral junction.

A, photograph of anterior aspect; B, photograph of posterior aspect; C, photograph of lateral aspect; D, photograph of lateroposterior aspect; E, photograph of anterior aspect of superior portion of sacrum.

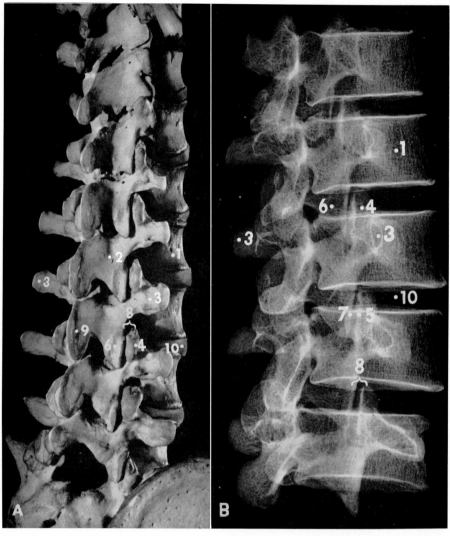

Fig. 8.   Photograph and radiograph of dried specimens of articulated lumbar vertebrae:
A, photograph of lateroposterior aspect; *B*, lateroposterior radiograph.

LEGEND FOR FIGURE 8

1. Body of vertebrae
   (*corpus vertebrae*)
2. Lamina of vertebral arch
   (*lamina arcus vertebrae*)
3. Transverse process
   (*processus transversus*)
4. Superior articular process
   (*processus articularis superior*)
5. Superior articular facet
   (*facies articularis superior*)

6. Inferior articular process
   (*processus articularis inferior*)
7. Inferior articular facet
   (*facies articularis inferior*)
8. Intervertebral articulation
   (*Bracket is used in illustration
   to indicate articulation*)
9. Spinous process
   (*processus spinosus*)
10. Intervertebral disc space

* Figs. 1 to 8.   From Radiography and Clinical Photography, William S. Cornwell, Editor; with permission of Eastman Kodak Company.

1

Normal Spine

Embryologic Considerations

FOLLOWING fertilization of the ovum, the male and female pronuclei unite into a new segmentation nucleus, which then divides into two cells, beginning the growth of the fetus. Passing through the morula stage, an outer layer of cells, the trophoblast, and an inner cluster, the inner cell mass, evolve. Secretion of fluid by the trophoblast into the morula results in the blastocyst, a vesicle formed by the trophoblast and to which the inner cell mass is attached. At about the 8th day after fertilization the blastocyst becomes imbedded in the endometrium, and is completely covered over by the 12th day. The trophoblast combines with the mesoderm, forming the chorion, the protecting coat which relates the fetus to the maternal nutritional and excretory resources.

During this time the inner cell mass enlarges, developing into the outer ectodermal and inner entodermal layers. These rapidly separate, the ectoderm forming the amnion and its contained amniotic cavity, while the entoderm constitutes the yolk sac protruding into the blastocyst. The embryo itself develops from the germ disc, that portion of the ectoderm and entoderm which remain in apposition. The extraembryonal mesodermal layer evolving from cells migrating from the borders of this disc form a loose network of cellular processes stretching across the blastocyst cavity, and occupy the space between the trophoblast and yolk sac. The entire embryo then becomes suspended in the chorionic cavity by the mesodermal primitive body stalk.

Further growth of the embryo proceeds from the embryonic disc. A primitive groove appears in the midline, beneath which the rapidly growing primitive streak develops. These cells later form the definitive mesoderm, part of which migrates to the cephalic end of the embryo, where it comes in contact with the primitive node of Hensen, another cluster of mesodermal cells. The notochord develops from Hensen's node as a medially situated rod. At the end of 2 weeks the embryo is about 1.5 mm long, somewhat oval in shape, and the three germ layers are well differentiated. Cephalic to Hensen's node thickened, rounded edges of ectoderm appear as the neural folds on either side of the notochord and prochordal plate, evolving into the neural groove. Further growth converts the groove into a tube. The cephalic end, which grows more rapidly, expands to form the brain. The caudal portion develops as the spinal cord.

By the 3rd week the cephalic end of the embryo is marked by prominence of the neural plate. Thereafter the paraxial bar, the mesodermal column on either side of the notochord, becomes segmented into triangular-shaped symmetrically disposed somites, situated so that their bases are medial and apices lateral in position (Fig. 9). From these the skeletal, muscular and nervous systems arise. The somites first appear at the cephalic end and progress caudally.

11

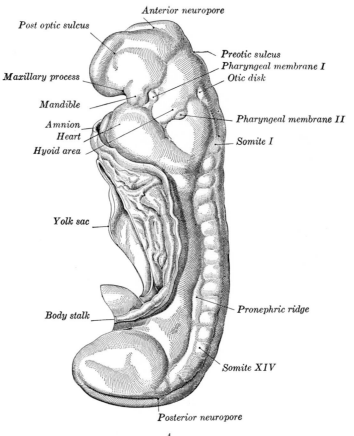

Anterior neuropore

Post optic sulcus

Preotic sulcus

Pharyngeal membrane I

Otic disk

Maxillary process

Mandible

Pharyngeal membrane II

Amnion

Heart

Somite I

Hyoid area

Yolk sac

Pronephric ridge

Body stalk

Somite XIV

Posterior neuropore

A

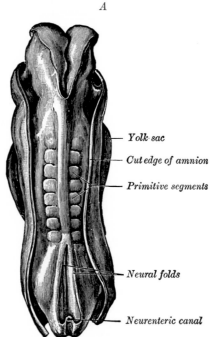

Yolk sac

Cut edge of amnion

Primitive segments

Neural folds

Neurenteric canal

B

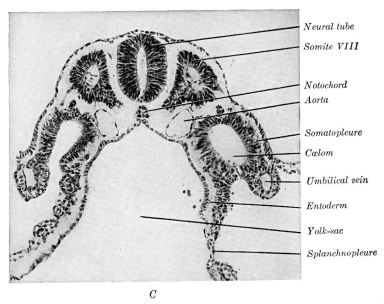

Neural tube

Somite VIII

Notochord

Aorta

Somatopleure

Cœlom

Umbilical vein

Entoderm

Yolk-sac

Splanchnopleure

C

Fig. 9. *A*, Lateral view of a 14-somite human embryo. × 50. *B*, Dorsum of human embryo, 2.11 mm in length. *C*, Transverse section through somite VIII (primitive segments of 14-somite human embryo). (*Gray's Anatomy*, Lea & Febiger.)

Each has a cavity called the myocele, which soon fills with proliferating cells. The coelomic cavity appears lateral to these, with somatopleure dorsally and splancho-pleure ventrally (Fig. 9). At the junction of the lateral mesoderm and somites a strand of cells, termed the intermediate cell mass, later forms the genitourinary system.

The vertebral column evolves around the notochord. Lying on the ventral aspect of the neural tube, it extends from the caudal extremity to the midbrain. In the 15-mm fetus its cephalic end passes through the basisphenoid to the pharyngeal surface, and reenters the sphenoid to terminate at the dorsum sellae (Fig. 10). The primitive vertebral segments are separated from each other by intersegmental septae. Each segment differentiates into three groups of cells. The cutis-plate, or dermatome, forms on the dorsolateral aspect of the myocele, and forms the skin. The muscle-plate, or myotome, situated on the medial side of the myocele, forms the muscles of the segment. From the core of the myocele, next to the noto-chord, arises the sclerotome, the sclerotog-enous layer of cells which rapidly proliferate to surround the notochord and neural tube with a continuous mesodermal sheath termed the membranous vertebral column. The sclerotome divides into cranial and caudal parts by a transverse fissure, the sclerotomic fissure, which is transient and soon vanishes. The original somite can be identified in these two portions, the anterior aspect formed by loosely arranged cells while the posterior half is more compact (Fig. 11*A*, *B*). Between these the intervertebral disc is formed, in the vicinity of the sclerotomic fissure. Cells from the denser posterior mass grow into the spaces between the myotomes of the adjacent and caudal segments, extending dorsally and ventrally. The dorsal segments form the neural arches, while the ventral segments extend into the body wall as the transverse processes. The vertebral bodies are formed by fusion of the caudally placed dense segment of one sclerotome and the anterior portion of the next caudal sclerotome. The vertebrae alternate in position with the myotomes. Muscles arising from one myotome are related thus to two skeletal

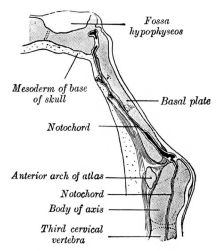

FIG. 10.   Sagittal section of cephalic end of notochord.   (*Gray's Anatomy*, Lea & Febiger.)

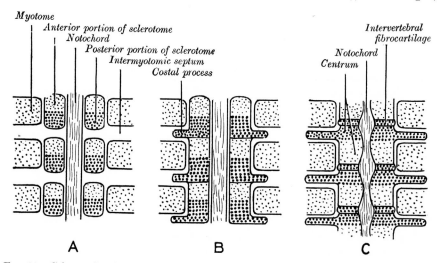

FIG. 11.   Scheme showing the manner in which each vertebral centrum is developed from
portions of two adjacent segments.   (*Gray's Anatomy*, Lea & Febiger.)

elements and the interposed intervertebral
disc (Fig. 11C).   The annulus fibrosus forms
from the peripheral portions of the primitive
discs.   The intersegmental arteries, which
arise from the primitive aorta, appear very
early just caudal to the dense zone of mesenchymal cells, and finally are placed in the
midportion of the vertebral bodies.

This "membranous vertebral column" is
succeeded at about the 4th week of fetal
life by the cartilaginous vertebral column.
Two cartilaginous centers separated by the
ventrodorsal extension of the perichordal

sheath appear on either side of the notochord, and rapidly extend around it, thereby
forming the bodies of the cartilaginous vertebrae.   The perichordal sheath quickly disappears at this stage.   Second pairs of
cartilaginous foci appear in the lateral parts
of the vertebral arch, grow backward on
either side of the neural tube to form the
cartilaginous vertebral arch, and still separate cartilaginous centers appear for each
costal arch.

The notochord, which remains unchanged
as a solid cord of uniform size during the

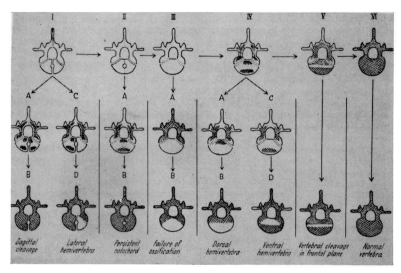

FIG. 12. Stages in vertebral development. Variations and anomalies in second and third rows. Ossification indicated by cross-hatching (after Junghanns). (From Schmorl, G. and Junghanns, H., Die gesunde und die kranke Wirbelsäule in Röntgenbild und Klinik, 4. Auflage, Thieme, Stuttgart, 1957.)

mesenchymal period, is progressively compressed into the regions of the dense intervertebral discs. This is attributed to the increased pressure prevailing during the rapid enlargement of the cartilaginous bodies. The dense mesenchymal anlage of the annulus fibrosus becomes markedly reduced during chondrification of the bodies, but the outermost rim of the disc separating the cartilaginous bodies persists.

By the 7th to 8th week of gestation, the cartilaginous cells in the centers of the vertebral bodies become surrounded by an interstitial matrix. During this stage the anterior and posterior longitudinal spinal ligaments develop. The anterior longitudinal ligament is firmly attached to the cartilaginous vertebral bodies. The posterior longitudinal ligament is attached to the intervertebral disc tissue, but is not as closely attached to the posterior surfaces of the vertebrae.

As chondrification proceeds, the notochordal cells are progressively squeezed out from the vertebral bodies and displaced into the intervertebral discs. Here they become enclosed by a dense rim of cells which have not undergone chondrification and which

form the annulus fibrosus. During this period, some mucoid degeneration and proliferation occurs in the notochordal cells, which then form the nucleus pulposus. During this migration of notochordal tissue the annulus fibrosus becomes larger. The perichordal sheath itself remains in the center of the respective cartilaginous vertebrae and is represented by a mucoid streak.

At the 9th week of fetal life anterior and posterior indentations into the cartilaginous body are produced by periosteal vessels. Soon after this the cartilage is invaded by these vessels, which produce ventral and dorsally situated blood lakes. Early in embryologic development, ossification centers are formed dorsally and ventrally in the vertebral body, separated by cartilaginous septae which soon disappear. Ossification proceeds rapidly and is well seen by the time the embryo reaches 3 months of age.

The early centers of ossification of the vertebral bodies lie dorsally and ventrally. They do not correspond with the centers of chondrification of the cartilaginous stage. the latter being situated to the left and right of the ventrodorsal extension of the perichordal sheath. The anterior and posterior centers fuse early and form one large center of ossification for the vertebral body. The first centers appear in the lower thoracic and upper lumbar regions and rapidly extend cranially, less rapidly caudally. As the dorsal blood lakes and the center of ossification enlarge, it displaces the mucoid streak ventrally, eventually destroying this structure. Occasionally some remnants of the mucoid streak remain in the vertebral body. The then-formed centrally situated body nucleus gives off capillary vessels which resorb the surrounding cartilage in a stellate manner.

At approximately the 5th to 6th month of fetal life, the ossification center has divided the cartilaginous body into two thick cartilaginous plates which show endochondral ossification towards the intervertebral disc sides. Anteriorly and posteriorly, large osseous channels delineate the entrance of the vertebral vessels. Along the anterior and lateral periphery of the vertebral bodies, horseshoe-shaped cartilaginous plates appear which represent the ring apophyses. Later these form the anlage of the bony ring apophyses which appear in adolescent life. This cartilaginous ring is the seat of some of the fibers of the anterior and lateral aspects of the annulus fibrosus, which later are incorporated as Sharpey's fibers at the time of ossification. The posterior margin of the cartilaginous plate and the annulus fibrosus is not involved in this arrangement.

Ossification of the bodies of the vertebrae does not extend to the bony structures of the entire vertebral body. The posterolateral portions of the vertebral body are ossified by extensions from the vertebral arch centers. During the first few years of life, therefore, the vertebral bodies show two synchondroses termed "neurocentral synchondroses," (Fig. 13B).

Ossification of the vertebral arches begins at approximately the 8th week of fetal life, appearing first in the upper cervical vertebrae, and gradually extending down the spinal column. Each lateral half of the vertebral arch originates from a separate center of ossification, and the vertebral body originates from a third center of ossification (Fig. 13A).

The rami of the lumbar neural arches unite during the 1st year of life, followed by similar changes in the neural arches of the thoracic and cervical regions. The neurocentral synchondroses of the cervical vertebrae are joined to the arches on either side at about the 3rd year of life, and similar union in the lower lumbar vertebrae is not complete until about the 6th year. The tips of the transverse spinal processes remain cartilaginous in the years before puberty. At about the 16th year secondary centers appear at the tips of the transverse processes, the tips of the spinous processes, and at the upper and lower surfaces of the vertebral body (Fig. 13B, F).

The development of the atlas and axis is rather different from the other cervical segments. The atlas usually ossifies from three centers, one for each lateral mass, which appear at about the 7th week of fetal life, and one for the anterior arch which may be seen soon after birth in about 20 per cent of cases on neck roentgenograms. These two lateral bony masses are separated by a cartilaginous bar, in which a third center of ossification appears at about the end of the 1st year of life in the other 80 per cent (Tompsett and Donaldson, 1941) (Fig. 13D).

The axis, or epistropheus, ossifies from five primary and two secondary centers. The body of the second cervical vertebra and its neural arch ossifies in much the same manner as the other vertebrae, namely from a single center for the body at about the 4th or 5th month and centers for each lateral half of the vertebral arch at about the 2nd month of gestation. The odontoid process is formed by an upthrust cartilaginous projection from the body of the vertebra. At about the 6th month of fetal life two laterally situated centers of ossification appear in the base of this process. At birth these unite into a single column at the apex of which a cleft remains, for which a separate center of ossification appears at about 2 years of age.

A cartilaginous plate separates the base of the odontoid process from the body of the second cervical vertebra. This gradually becomes ossified, and disappears at or somewhat before adolescence, at which time the apical tip of the dens also unites. Ossification involves the circumference of the odontoid process, so that cartilaginous material may persist in its center until late in life (Fig. 13E). The first two cervical vertebrae develop in an atypical manner. The odontoid process of the axis is formed by what

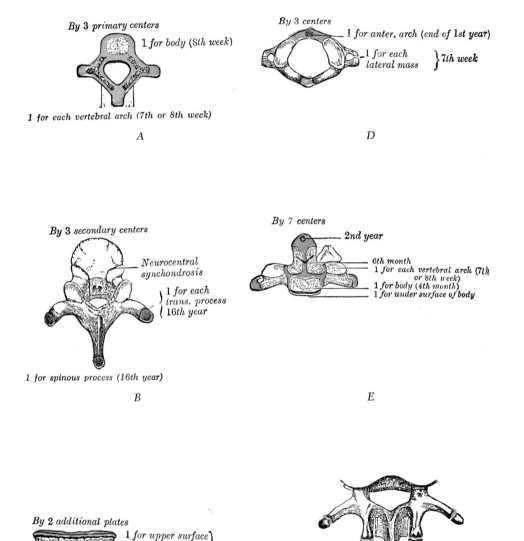

FIG. 13. *A,* Ossification of vertebra at 8 weeks. Three primary centers. *B,* Secondary centers at transverse and spinous processes at 16th year. *C,* Apophyseal plates at upper and under surfaces. *D,* Ossification of atlas. *E,* Ossification of axis. *F,* Two additional centers for mamillary processes. (*Gray's Anatomy,* Lea & Febiger.)

should be the body of the atlas, so that the atlas has an anterior arch rather than a body.

The anterior part of each transverse process of the cervical vertebrae is a costal process fused to the true transverse process, and hence is elongated. The lumbar transverse processes are also considerably elongated because of similarly fused costal and transverse processes. The transverse processes of the 7th cervical vertebra sometimes possess a secondary center of ossification from which false ribs form if they do not unite with the true transverse processes. Separate centers of ossification for the transverse processes of the fourth, fifth and sixth cervical vertebrae have also been observed.

Two additional centers of ossification are present in the lumbar vertebrae. These correspond to the mammillary processes, small prominences on the posterolateral aspects of the superior articular processes (Fig. 13F). The transverse processes of the first lumbar vertebra sometimes develop from separate centers of ossification. If these do not eventually unite with the vertebral body, a so-called lumbar rib results. This rather uncommon anomaly may cause some confusion in identification of vertebral segments, but this can be resolved by counting the vertebrae from the atlas down.

Ossification of the sacral vertebrae proceeds from a primary center and two epiphyseal plates, one for the superior and the other for the inferior surface. Each vertebral arch of the sacrum is ossified from two centers. Lateral to the anterior sacral foramina are two additional centers of ossification for each of the upper three sacral vertebrae. Ossification of the central part of the bodies of the upper three sacral vertebrae appears at about the 9th week of fetal life, and between the 6th and 8th month for the 4th and 5th sacral vertebrae. The costal centers for the lateral parts of the sacral vertebrae appear at about the 6th to 8th month of life at about the time ossification of the vertebral arches appears. During infancy, the sacral vertebrae are separated from each other by intervertebral fibro-

cartilages. The lowermost two unite at about the 18th year of life, and union proceeds gradually so that by adult life the entire sacrum is firmly united. The sites of these intervertebral fibrocartilages are visible on sagittal sections of specimens of the sacrum. They can be identified on anteroposterior tilt-up roentgenograms as horizontally placed, spindle-shaped radiolucent areas, sometimes containing small calcific deposits, lying most often at the junctions of the bodies of the first and second sacral segments. Occasionally intervertebral fibrocartilages are seen also between the second and third sacral segments, but these usually are smaller than the one above. The vertebral arches unite with the bodies of the lower sacral vertebrae at about 2 years, and the upper segments at about 6 years. Epiphyseal plates for the superior and inferior aspects of the vertebral bodies appear at about 16 years, and epiphyses appear on the lateral aspects of the sacrum between the 18th and 20th years (Fig. 14).

Each coccygeal segment ossifies from a single center. The first appears between the 1st and 4th year of life, the second at the 5th to 10th year, the third between the 10th and 15th year and the fourth between the 14th and 20th year. Sometimes the segments fuse with one another, and then are identified only by a thin radiolucent line between them. The first coccygeal segment has rudimentary transverse processes and cornua that represent parts of the superior articular processes and the pedicles. The other coccygeal segments are merely rudimentary vertebral bodies.

The vascular supply of the intervertebral discs is of considerable interest, especially in the consideration of pathological changes which occur in these structures. Very early in fetal development blood vessels extend to the intervertebral discs, and then regress equally rapidly. At about the 3rd month of gestation, vessels parallel to the notochord appear. Others derived from the periosteum penetrate into the cartilaginous plates without entering the central zone of ossification

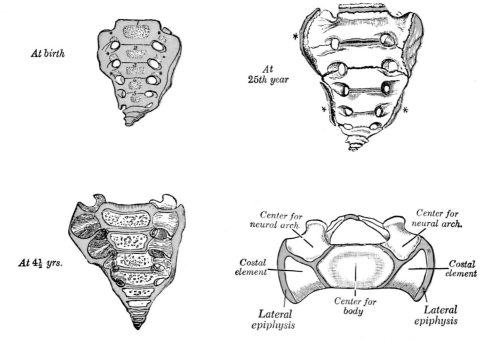

At birth

At 25th year

At 4½ yrs.

Center for neural arch.

Center for neural arch.

Costal element

Costal element

Lateral epiphysis

Center for body

Lateral epiphysis

Fig. 14. Ossification of sacrum. (*Gray's Anatomy*, Lea & Febiger.)

of the vertebral bodies. These vessels enter the intervertebral cartilages at regular intervals along the rims of the vertebral bodies, and run in the direction of the nucleus pulposus. These radially placed vessels are responsible for the dentate appearance of the epiphyseal plates of growing vertebrae and the deep indentations which are sometimes seen in the vertebral bodies of growing children. Zones of calcification with numerous foci of ossification may develop along these vessels, and later in life these fuse to form the ring apophyses. Still other vessels emerge from the vertebral body and penetrate into the cartilaginous plates directly, forming anastomotic arcades with those coming from the periosteum. Regression and thinning of the vascular supply to the intervertebral disc begins shortly after birth and continues progressively, so that by the age of 18 to 25 years most of the vessels have practically disappeared. Where these vessels have penetrated cartilaginous plates some gaps appear in the chondrification of the cartilaginous plates. At the time of complete degeneration of the vessels these chondrification cups may be replaced by scar tissue, and sometimes, by calcification. This may result in areas of diminished resistance to the increased turgor of the semisolid intervertebral disc substance, important particularly if the disc should be subjected to increased pressure. Through these points of reduced resistance nuclear prolapse occurs, forming Schmorl's nodes. The nucleus pulposus receives no direct vascular supply.

The only source of nutrition for the intervertebral discs is by diffusion through the cartilaginous plates from the cancellous vertebral bodies. The intervertebral discs present maximal elasticity at about the 25th to 30th year of life. Following this, the discs are subjected to gradual attrition and strains which produce chemical and hydropic alterations of cartilage.

The nucleus pulposus of the intervertebral disc is derived from the notochord. Soon after the notochordal cells are squeezed into the disc, the nucleus pulposus grows more rapidly than the annulus fibrosus. The notochordal cells proliferate in local expansions in the discal centers, while those in the vertebral bodies disappear. At about 6 months the discal notochordal cells begin to degenerate, and clump together to form a mucoid core surrounded by fibrous tissue and hyaline cartilage. Collagenous fibers extend into this gelatinous mucoid structure from the adjacent fibrocartilaginous capsule. In the primitive disc the nucleus pulposus is centrally situated, and the fibroblasts peripheral to it participate actively in the formation of the annulus fibrosus. The outer fibrous zone of the intervertebral disc is differentiated from the hyaline or precartilaginous inner zone. Notochordal cells can be demonstrated in the nucleus pulposus until adolescent life, and sometimes later. The nucleus pulposus remains centrally situated in the cervical and thoracic regions, while in the lumbar discs it is somewhat more posterior. The fibrocartilaginous annulus fibrosus is heaviest anteriorly and laterally, but its posterior aspect is weaker. Following avascularization of the disc which occurs progressively until the 3rd decade of life, the nucleus pulposus gradually is replaced by fibrous tissue, losing its gelatinous consistency. The question of innervation of the annulus fibrosus still is under discussion. There is some clinical evidence that these structures have a nerve supply. Recent studies have demonstrated nerve endings in the outer portion of the annulus fibrosus of a type associated with pain or pressure perception (Hirsch, Ingelmark and Miller, 1963).

The vascular tree which nourishes the vertebral column and its contents is virtually in its finished form at about the 7th month of gestation. In the cervical region the blood supply to the vertebrae, the spinal ligaments, the cord and the meninges is derived from branches of the vertebral, the ascending cervical, deep cervical and occipital arteries. In the thoracic region the arteries originate from dorsal branches of the intercostal arteries, and in the lumbar region from posterior branches of the lumbar arteries. The spinal arteries enter the canal through the intervertebral foramina, and divide into three main branches. The posterior and anterior branches both divide in the epidural fat into ascending and descending branches. These anastomose with similar branches from spinal arteries above and below to supply the vertebral column. The vertebral arches are supplied by posterior branches, one on either side of the midline. The ascending and descending anterior branches pass between the posterior longitudinal ligament and the bone, converging towards the middle of the dorsal surfaces of the vertebral bodies, entering the bone on the posterior surfaces of the respective vertebral bodies through varisized foramina. Adjacent to these are concomitant large vertebral veins. Other veins emerge from the anterolateral and anterior aspects of the vertebral bodies.

The venous trunks of the spine drain the vertebrae, the meninges and the adjacent musculature. These complex and profusely anastomosing veins are without valves or accompanying arteries. The plexuses surround the spine as four large longitudinal trunks. The anterior pair are situated on the posterior surfaces of the vertebral bodies, and the posterior pair are located in front of the vertebral arches and the ligamenta flava on either side of the midline. These communicate with the posterior external spinal plexus of veins by channels passing through the ligaments. A series of venous rings joins the anterior and the posterior internal plexuses. The internal and the external plexuses anastomose freely, terminating in the intervertebral veins which accompany the spinal nerves through the intervertebral foramina. The largest veins emerge through the perforations on the posterior aspect of the vertebral bodies, but some also pass through openings in the anterior and anterolateral aspects. The vertebral veins and the lumbo-azygos veins constitute the two systems which unite the inferior and superior vena cavae. Under normal conditions, in an individual with an open caval system, the direction of flow is quite variable and fluctuates with changes in pressure in the two systems. With vena caval obstruction a considerable increase in flow through the vertebral venous system takes place with consequent changes in pressure and direction.

Meningeal nerves enter the intervertebral foramina and are directed upwards and downwards in the spinal canal. These nerves contain fibers derived from the sympathetic trunks and from the spinal nerves. They supply the blood vessels, the inner aspect of the ligamenta flava, and terminate on the posterior longitudinal ligament and the annulus fibrosus. Posterior rami from the spinal nerves supply the synovial joints and the posterior vertebral ligaments. Medial branches of the posterior rami supply the outer aspect of the ligamenta flava and the supraspinous and the interspinous ligaments.

References

Abrams, H. L.: The Vertebral and Azygous Venous System, and Some Variations in Systemic Venous Return, Radiology, *69*, 508, 1957.

Albala, M. M., Barrick, C. W. and Jenkinson, E. L.: Vertebral Trans-Skeletal Phlebography, Radiology, *67*, 229, 1956.

Bardeen, C. R.: Studies of the Development of the Human Skeleton, Am. J. Anat., *4*, 265, 1905.

Batson, O. V.: Vertebral Vein System as a Mechanism for the Spread of Metastases. Am. J. Roentgenol., *48*, 715, 1942.

————: The Vertebral Vein System, Am. J. Roentgenol., *78*, 195, 1957.

Campbell, J. B.: Congenital Anomalies of the Neural Axis, Am. J. Surg., *75*, 231, 1948.

Cohen, J., Currarino, G. and Neuhauser, E. B. D.: A Significant Variant in the Ossification Centers of the Vertebral Bodies, Am. J. Roentgenol., *76*, 469, 1956.

Gray, H.: *Anatomy of the Human Body*, 28th ed., edited by C. M. Goss, Philadelphia, Lea & Febiger, 1966.

Harris, H. A.: Clinical Anatomy of the Veins, Brain, *64*, 291, 1941.

Hirsch, C., Ingelmark, B-E. and Miller, M.: The Anatomical Basis for Low Back Pain. Acta orthop. scandinav., *33*, 1, 1963.

Hollinshead, W. H.: Anatomy of the Spine, J. Bone & Joint Surg., *47-A*, 209, 1965.

Knuttson, F.: Die frontale Wirbelkörperspalte, Acta radiol., *21*, 597, 1940.

Lossen, H.: Chorda dorsalis im Röntgenbild, Anat. Anz., *73*, 168, 1931.

Mutch, J. and Walmsley, R.: The Aetiology of Cleft Vertebral Arch in Spondylolisthesis, Lancet, *1*, 74, 1956.

Noback, C. R. and Robertson, G. C.: Sequence of Appearance of Ossification Centers in the Human Skeleton During the First Five Prenatal Months, Am. J. Anat., *89*, 1, 1951.

Patten, B. M.: *Human Embryology*, 2nd ed., New York, McGraw-Hill Book Co., 1953.

Rowe, G. C. and Roche, M. B.: The Etiology of Separate Neural Arch, J. Bone & Joint Surg., *35-A*, 102, 1953.

Schinz, H. R. and Tondury, G.: Zur Entwicklung der menschlichen Wirbelsäule; die Frühossifikation der Wirbelkörper, Fortschr. a. d. Geb. d. Röntgenstrahlen, *66*, 253, 1942.

Schmorl, G. and Junghanns, H.: *Die gesunde und die kranke Wirbelsäule in Röntgenbild und Klinik*, 4. Auflage, Thieme, Stuttgart, 1957.

Sensenig, E. C.: The Early Development of the Human Vertebral Column, Carnegie Contrib. to Embryology, publication 583, *33*, 21, 1949.

Tomsett, A. C., Jr. and Donaldson, S. W.: The Anterior Tubercle of the First Cervical Vertebra and the Hyoid Bone; Their Occurrence in Newborn Infants, Am. J. Roentgenol., *65*, 582, 1941.

Tori, G.: The Radiologic Demonstration of the Azygos and other Thoraco-Abdominal Veins in the Living, Brit. J. Radiol., *27*, 16, 1954.

Walmsley, R.: Anatomy and Development. In *Modern Trends in Diseases of the Vertebral Column*. Edited by R. Nassim and H. J. Burrows, New York, Paul B. Hoeber, Inc., 1959.

Wiley, A. M. and Trueta, J.: The Vascular Anatomy of the Spine and its Relationship to Pyogenic Vertebral Osteomyelitis, J. Bone & Joint Surg., *41-B*, 796, 1959.

Functional Aspects of the Architecture of the Vertebral Column

The human spine is composed of 33 vertebrae, 7 cervical, 12 dorsal, 5 lumbar, the sacrum consisting of 5 segments and the coccyx with 4 or 5 segments. Counting the sacroiliac joints, the posterior intervertebral joints and the costovertebral joints, there are 97 diarthroses associated with the spine, each with its separate capsule and synovial system. All are paired, except the joint between the atlas and the dens.

The first and second cervical vertebrae are attached to the skull by strong ligamentous connections. The occipital condyles articulate with the superior articular surfaces of the lateral masses of the atlas in an arrangement which permits a nodding motion of the head. The joint cavities of this articulation communicate with the joint between the dens, the anterior arch and transverse ligaments of the atlas. This pivotal joint and the condyloid joints between the atlas and the axis permit nodding and rotary motions of the skull. The atlantooccipital joint permits flexion and extension, while the more complex atlantoaxial articulation affords flexion, extension, rotation, vertical approximation and lateral gliding movement as well. Flexion and extension of about 15 degrees occurs in both the atlantoaxial and the atlantooccipital joints. With tilting of the head sharply the articular surfaces of the atlantoaxial joint can shift laterally for 2 or 3 mm, a change which should not be confused with atlantoaxial dislocation. There is a close relationship between the anterior arch of the atlas and the dens. Widening of this space over 3 mm is important in the evaluation of atlantoaxial dislocations (Fig. 15).

There is no intervertebral disc between the first and second cervical vertebrae, the first disc occurring between the second and the third cervical vertebrae. Successive intervertebral discs increase slightly and progressively in size down to the lumbosacral articulation. Between the bodies of the first and the second sacral vertebrae one may frequently observe the remnants of an intervertebral disc. A similar structure is found less often between the second and the third sacral segments. The remainder of the sacrum usually is firmly fused into one mass. The coccyx articulates with the sacrum, and its various segments usually are separated from each other by intervening discs of cartilage. However, fusion of one or more of the coccygeal segments is not at all uncommon. When one transverse process of the first coccygeal segment fails to fuse with the sacrum above it, while the opposite side does unite, and the coccyx is tilted towards the ununited side, a bony defect representing the open inferior sacral notch appears.

The ribs, which are attached to the vertebral column by strong ligamentous bands, present two articulations with the vertebral column; one between the heads of the ribs with the bodies of the vertebrae and the other between the necks and tubercles of the ribs with the corresponding transverse processes. These joints are of the gliding or arthrodial type. The first, tenth, eleventh and twelfth ribs each articulate with a single vertebra. The remaining ribs articulate with the vertebrae above and beneath by two demi-facets in the posteroanterior and posterosuperior aspects of the vertebral bodies for the respective rib articulations.

The cervical vertebrae are the smallest of the true vertebrae, and are easily identified by their contours and the presence of a foramen in each transverse process. The first vertebral body is ring-like, and is made up of two lateral masses connected by an anterior and a posterior arch. The outer surface of the anterior arch is convex and presents a small protuberance in its midportion. This is called the anterior tubercle and serves for the attachment of the longus colli muscles. The inner aspect of the anterior arch is concave, smooth, and provides a receptacle for the odontoid process of the axis. The posterior arch of the atlas presents a more convex and wider configuration. Its mid-portion is tipped by a small process, the posterior tubercle, which corresponds to a rudimentary spinous process. Occasionally the posterior arch fails to unite, so that the ring is incomplete in the midportion of the dorsal aspect (Fig. 16B). In its anterior and superior portion, a groove for the vertebral artery and the first cervical nerve may be identified. Its transverse processes present rounded distal tips, and are broader, heavier and longer than the transverse processes of the other cervical vertebrae, except for the seventh. The basal portions of the transverse processes are perforated by the foramina transversaria for the passage of the vertebral arteries and veins.

The lateral masses of the first cervical vertebra are rather heavy, and present superiorly concave oval articular surfaces for the occipital condyles. These surfaces sometimes are slightly constricted in their medial portions. The inferior surfaces of the lateral masses bear the inferior articular facets which articulate with the axis beneath. These articular facets are circular in form, flat or slightly convex, and are directed downward and medially. Their structure is such as to permit rotary movement of the head. A rather heavy ligament passes between small tubercles along the medial margin of each superior facet. This divides the vertebral foramen into two compartments, one for the odontoid process and the other for the spinal cord and its membranes. The vertebral canal at this level is quite large, and almost pentagonal in contour, sufficient to permit some lateral displace-

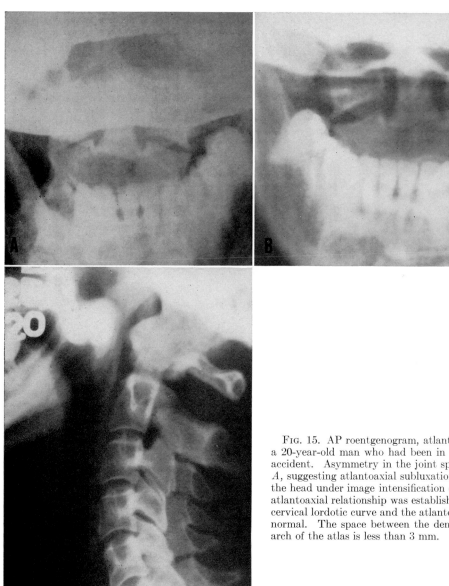

Fig. 15. AP roentgenogram, atlantoaxial joint in a 20-year-old man who had been in an automobile accident. Asymmetry in the joint space is present, *A*, suggesting atlantoaxial subluxation. On moving the head under image intensification control normal atlantoaxial relationship was established, *B*. *C*, The cervical lordotic curve and the atlantoaxial joint are normal. The space between the dens and anterior arch of the atlas is less than 3 mm.

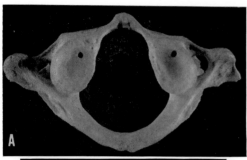

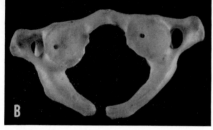

FIG. 16. Normal first cervical vertebra seen from above with intact anterior and posterior arches, *A*. A specimen with an unfused dorsal arch, *B*.

ment of the atlas without compressing the spinal cord (Fig. 16).

The second cervical vertebra, the axis or epistropheus, is characterized by the presence of the odontoid process which extends upward from the superior surface of its body. The articular surfaces of the lateral aspects of the body of the second cervical vertebra lie rather horizontally, and present rounded, slightly convex articular surfaces directed laterally and upwards to support the corresponding surfaces of the inferior aspects of the body of the first cervical vertebra. The transverse processes of the second cervical vertebra are considerably smaller than those of the first, and are penetrated by a foramen transversarium on each side. The spinous process and the heavy lamina of the second cervical vertebra are inclined downward and posteriorly. The tip of the spinous process of the second cervical vertebra usually protrudes beyond the others, and often is bifid (Fig. 1).

A constriction, or neck, exists at the junction of the odontoid process and the body of the second cervical vertebra until about the 4th to 6th year of life. This may

be seen as a radiolucent band between the dens and the subjacent vertebral body. The anterior aspect of the dens is in fairly close proximity to the apposing articular surface of the anterior arch of the first cervical vertebra. Radiologically a space of 1 to 3 mm between these two structures may be demonstrated.

The anterior aspect of the body of the second cervical vertebra slopes slightly anteriorly. It terminates in a lip inclined downward, following the contour of the rounded, sloping anterosuperior aspect of the body of the third cervical vertebra.

The seventh cervical vertebra is distinguished from the other cervical segments by the presence of a distinctive elongated heavy spinous process which terminates in a tubercle into which the nuchal ligament inserts. The transverse processes of the seventh cervical segment are somewhat more prominent than the others. The foramen transversarium in this segment is smaller than those in the remaining cervical vertebra, or may be absent (Fig. 17*A*).

The remaining cervical vertebrae are fairly similar to each other. The bodies are quadrilateral in configuration, with rather curved angles. The anterosuperior aspects recess slightly in front of the more prominent anteroinferior aspects of the suprajacent vertebral bodies. The articular facets are inclined more obliquely proceeding downward. The laminae are practically overlapping and are heavy. The spinous processes are small but increase in size proceeding from the third to the seventh cervical vertebrae. Their tips may be bifid, or terminate in a bulbous or flattened fashion. The transverse processes are about even in size, and each is perforated by a foramen transversarium (Fig 2).

The vertebral arteries arise from the first part of the subclavian arteries and pass behind the common carotid arteries for about 3 cm to enter the right and left foramen transversarium of the sixth cervical vertebra. Then they thread the foramina transversaria of the upper 6 cervical vertebrae, situated in front of the cervical nerve roots of the second to sixth segments. Not infrequently the vertebral arteries are asymmetric in size, the right being smaller than the left. At each level a branch vessel extends along the nerve roots to enter the spinal canal and supply the plexus surrounding the cord. Many small branches also extend to the adjacent muscles of the neck, and anastomose with branches of the external carotid artery. The size of the vessels traversing the foramina is quite variable.

On reaching the foramen transversarium of the atlas, each vertebral artery follows a tortuous course, directed posteriorly behind the lateral mass of the atlas. It then lies in a groove on the upper surface of the posterior arch of the atlas, and is directed into the cranium passing through the dura mater, situated obliquely in front of the medulla oblongata and the pons. Here the two vertebral arteries join to form the basilar artery. Emerging from the inner aspects of the lower third of each vertebral artery within the skull are two small branches directed downwards and medially. These unite to form the uppermost portion of the anterior spinal artery, which extends caudad on the anterior aspect of the cord in the midline (Fig. 31). Other vessels originating close by are the posterior inferior cerebellar artery, the small vessels to the medulla oblongata and the posterior spinal arteries.

The vertebral arteries are accompanied by sympathetic nerves which pass through the intervertebral foramina in front of the nerve roots. These are known as the posterior cervical sympathetic plexus, and accompany the vertebral arteries cephalad to enter the foramen magnum and then extend along the basilar artery to the circle of Willis. The vertebral arteries also are surrounded by a plexus of veins which unite to form the vertebral vein in the lower part of the neck.

The first and second cervical vertebral foramina present characteristic differences, being large and quite rounded. This permits adequate space for the medulla oblon-

gata and the upper cervical spinal cord during the wide range of motion which occurs here. The lowermost 5 cervical vertebrae normally present a rather rounded triangular configuration. However, a wide range of variation in the configuration of these structures exists (Fig. 17A). Of great importance from the viewpoint of possible compromise of the spinal cord is sagittal narrowing of the cervical spinal canal. This usually is accompanied by constriction of the lateral recesses of the canal and shortening of the pedicles, with consequent elongation and flattening of the intervertebral foramina. This finds its greatest expression in patients with achondroplasia, and also is observed in otherwise normal people but with lesser intensity. As a consequence of changes in the configuration of the intervertebral foramina, the available space for the emerging nerve roots becomes limited, so that these structures are likely to be subjected to pressure and trauma in the presence of spondylotic bony overgrowth or discal herniations.

In the neutral position the cervical spine assumes a moderate lordotic curve. With flexion the bodies move anteriorly, particularly in the upper cervical region. Such forward slipping is sometimes confused with subluxation, a situation not infrequently reported erroneously in infants and children. With forward flexion the superior articular facets move anteriorly, while in extension they shift posteriorly so that a range of motion of about 3 or 4 mm is observed (Fig. 18).

Considerable disagreement often occurs in the evaluation of a cervical vertebral column which presents a straight or moderately convex appearance. Much of this positional alteration is incident to muscle imbalance, as occurs with torticollis. Limitation of motion also is presumed sometimes to indicate injury to the cervical vertebrae, but only too often no evidence of bony abnormality is made out, even on detailed examinations (Fig. 19). The presence of muscular or ligamentous injury influences the align-

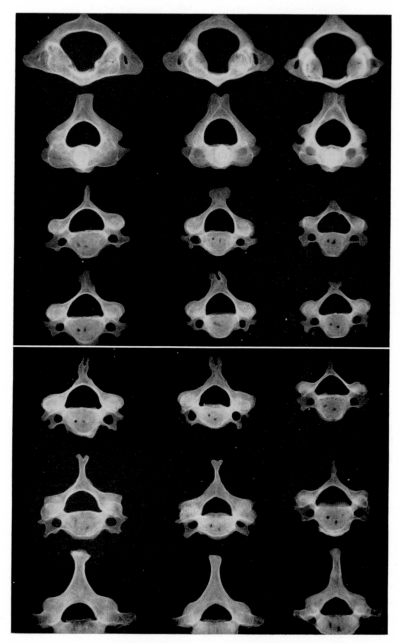

Fig. 17A. See legend, page 28.

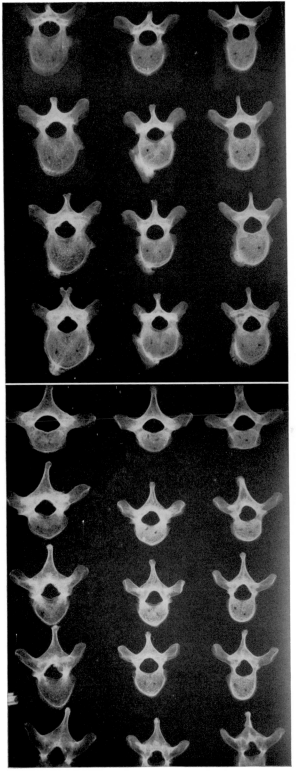

FIG. 17*B*. See legend, page 28.

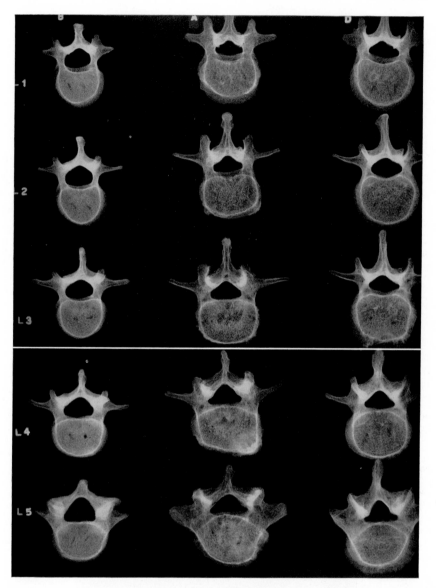

FIG. 17C

FIG. 17. *A,* Three normal cervical spine specimens in the craniocaudad position. Note the variations in the spinal foramina, transverse processes and foramina transversaria. *B,* The thoracic spine, same specimens. *C,* The lumbar spine, same specimens.

ment of the cervical vertebrae, and these can be painful and long-lasting without necessarily bringing into consideration the presence of a demonstrable fracture.

The question of dislocation also is one which often goes unsettled. Indeed, the definition of subluxation itself arouses controversy. Insofar as evaluating the align-

ment of the cervical spinal column from roentgenograms alone, one is well advised to also observe the patient before coming to a conclusion. It has often been noted that patients consciously or unconsciously restrict movement of the neck when requested to perform flexion and extension maneuvers by technicians, and that the same patient

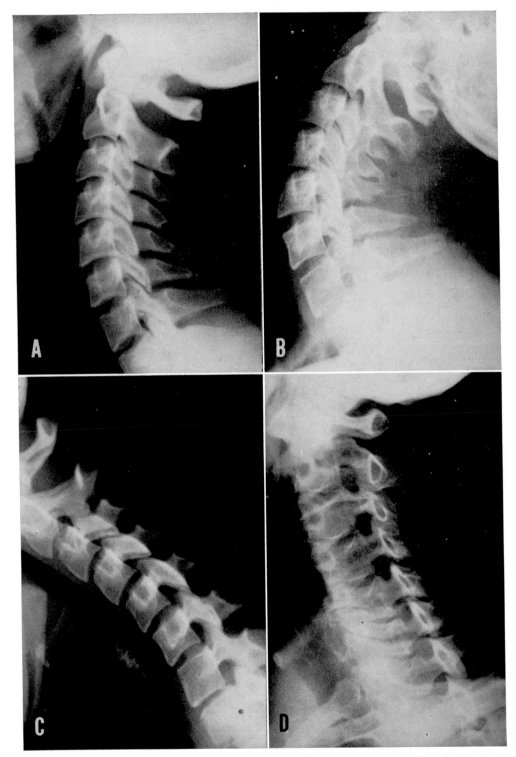

Fig. 18. *A*, Normal cervical lordotic curve in neutral position. *B*, In extension the spinous processes are approximated. Note the movement of the laminae and the changed configuration of the posterior aspect of the intervertebral discs. *C*, In forward flexion the spinous process tips separate and the articular facets permit a gliding movement. *D*, In the oblique projection the intervertebral foramina are visible. The right anterior oblique visualizes the right foramina and left articular facets.

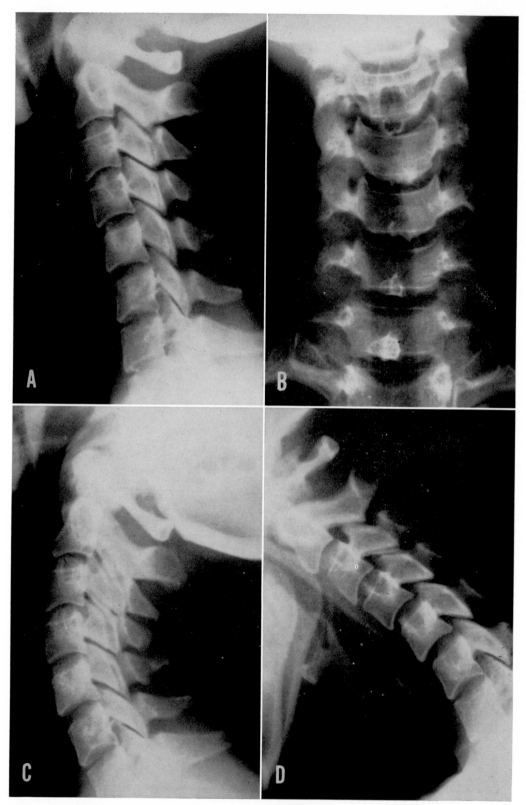

Fig. 19. *A*, Straightened cervical curve following automobile accident, with mild pain but no restriction of motion. *B*, Normal alignment in AP view. *C*, In extension the curve is mildly convex anteriorly, and in flexion, *D*, no malalignment is visible. Oblique roentgenograms were also normal. Probable muscle spasm.

will have a much wider range of movement when asked to go through the range of motion, as for a cineradiographic recording of head and neck movement. Even with such a record, interpretation of the radiologic changes can be difficult and arouse heated discussion.

The thoracic vertebrae are larger than the cervical vertebrae and smaller than the lumbar vertebrae. They increase progressively in size from the first to the twelfth vertebrae respectively, and can be recognized by facets on their sides for articulation with the rib heads. Articular facets are present on the transverse processes of all except the eleventh and twelfth segments. The pedicles and laminae of the upper thoracic vertebrae are directed downward and posteriorly, and practically overlap one another. In the lower thoracic spine the extent of imbrication of the pedicles and laminae is less marked than in the upper region. The spinous processes are heavy. Those of the upper thoracic spine are directed obliquely and rather sharply downward. The spinous processes become more vertical in position proceeding downwards. The transverse processes arise from the neural arches behind the superior articular processes of pedicles. They are directed laterally and backward, and each terminates in a blunt round tip. On their anterior aspects are the small articular surfaces for the rib tubercles.

The first, ninth, tenth, eleventh and twelfth dorsal vertebrae vary from the others in several respects. On either side of the body of the first thoracic vertebra is an articular facet for the first rib, while on its inferior portion a demi-facet for the costal articular process of the second rib can be seen. The transverse processes of the first dorsal vertebra are quite long. The body resembles a cervical vertebra, being quadrilateral and lipped on its antero-inferior and anterosuperior portions. The ninth dorsal vertebra has a demi-facet on its superoposterior aspect only. The tenth, eleventh and twelfth dorsal vertebrae present one entire facet corresponding to the articular heads of the respective ribs. The transverse processes of these three vertebral segments are rather variable, but usually are short and present no articular facets (Fig. 3).

The spinal foramina in the thoracic vertebrae are transitional at their upper and lower segments, resembling the lower cervical and upper lumbar vertebrae respectively. In the midthoracic region the spinal foramina are round. The lowermost 2 or 3 vertebrae present a triangular foraminal configuration, much like that seen in the upper 2 lumbar vertebrae (Fig. 17B).

The lumbar vertebrae are the heaviest of the spinal column, and are distinguished from the others by the absence of foramina transversaria or facets on the side of the body as well as by their distinctive size. As a rule, the vertebral bodies are wider from side to side than from before backward, and are a little thicker in front than behind. The pedicles are directed backward from the upper part of the vertebral body, so that the inferior vertebral notches are of considerable depth. The pedicles and laminae are dense and strong. The vertebral foramina present a triangular configuration and are larger than those in the thoracic spine but smaller than those in the cervical region. The spinous processes are thick, broad, somewhat quadrilateral and project downward and backward. These end in rough uneven borders which sometimes are notched. The superior and inferior articular processes of the neural arches are well defined, projecting upward and downward respectively from the junctions of the pedicles and laminae. The transverse processes vary in size; the first, second and fourth being somewhat shorter than the third. The fifth transverse processes are variable. In the first, second and third lumbar vertebrae, the transverse processes arise from the junctions of the pedicles and laminae, but in the fourth and fifth lumbar vertebrae they are set rather forward and originate from the pedicles and posterior portions of the bodies. The transverse processes are considered homologous with the ribs (Fig. 4).

Congenital variations in the configuration and dimensions of the lumbar spinal foramina are frequent. As with the cervical vertebrae, congenital narrowing of the canal carries with it the possibility of aggravated effects of spurs and discal extrusions (Fig. 17C). The dimensions of the spinal canal increase rapidly from birth up to 5 years of age, and then more slowly between 4 and 10 years. The canal then is fully formed. This corresponds with the time when the neurocentral synchondroses fuse, during the third to sixth years of life. The growth of the vertebral arches determines the development of the canal, as does the horizontal growth of the body with its consequent effect on the size and position of the pedicles.

The fifth lumbar vertebra is subject to many structural variations. The most common configuration is one in which the body is deeper in front than behind. Its transverse processes, as a rule, are heavier than those of the suprajacent vertebrae, and in the completely normal subject present rather bulbous tips which do not articulate with sacrum or iliac bones. The articular facets between the fifth lumbar and the first sacral vertebrae are very variable. The true vertical placement of the articular facets which is seen particularly well between the second and third and fourth lumbar vertebrae is quite uncommon in the lumbosacral region. In many these articular facets are coronally placed, while in others the articular facets are obliquely situated. Asymmetry between the articular facets on the right and left sides is not uncommon. The clinical significance of these variations in the apophyseal joints between the fourth and fifth lumbar and the fifth lumbar and first sacral vertebrae will be considered.

The neural arch of the fifth lumbar vertebra is often subject to congenital variations. Much discussion about the significance of incomplete fusion of the neural arches of the fifth lumbar vertebra has taken place. Occa-

sionally similar changes occur in the fourth and to a lesser degree in the neural arches of the other lumbar vertebrae.

The normal sacrum is composed of 5 fused vertebral bodies. It is wedge-shaped, with its apex directed downwards. Seen laterally, the sacrum is tilted dorsally, and is convex posteriorly. The degree of dorsal tilting is greater in females than in males. Occasionally, the first sacral segment is incompletely fused, referred to as lumbarization of the first sacral segment. In other instances fusion of the body of the fifth lumbar vertebra with that of the sacrum gives rise to 6 sacral segments, designated as sacralization of the fifth lumbar vertebra (Fig. 20). To either side of the midline, on the dorsal and ventral aspects, are the paired sacral foramina. Between them are transverse lines separating the sacral vertebral bodies. These are not visible on the dorsal aspect of the sacrum, and appear on the lateral studies only on the anterior surface of the bone. As a rule, 4 sacral spinous processes can be identified. Beneath the distal one and between the fourth anterior sacral foramina the inverted U-shaped sacral cornua can be seen, between which the sacral hiatus can be identified. The 4 anterior sacral foramina are irregularly circular in configuration. Their dorsal aspects are somewhat smaller than their anterior fellows. They diminish in size from above downward (Fig. 20). Beneath the fourth sacral foramen a notch corresponding to the fifth sacral foramen is sometimes present.

The coccyx articulates with the apex of the sacrum, which presents a small, oval flat surface formed by the body of the fifth sacral vertebra. The dorsal aspect of the first coccygeal segment presents two upward processes, the coccygeal cornua. The coccygeal segments represent rudimentary vertebrae, only the the bodies being present. These decrease in size from above downward and terminate in a small, somewhat oval flat bone. The first and second, and the second and third coccygeal vertebrae are usually united by a layer of fibrocartilage.

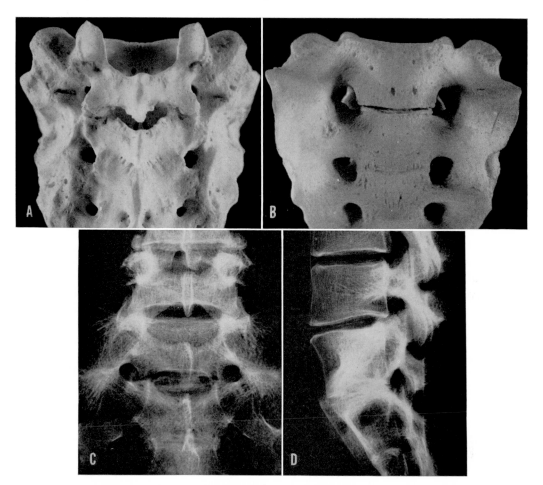

FIG. 20. *A*, PA photograph of specimen with fusion of the fifth lumbar vertebral transverse processes to the sacrum (transitional vertebra). *B*, AP view of the same specimen. *C*, AP roentgenogram reveals the rudimentary intervertebral disc between the transitional 5th lumbar and the first sacral segment, sacralized fifth lumbar vertebra. *D*, Lateral roentgenogram, same specimen.

The third, fourth and fifth segments often are fused. Considerable variation in the configuration and position of the coccygeal segments is frequent.

The spinal apophyseal joints are true arthrodial articulations, with articular cartilages and synovial linings. They are enveloped in loose articular capsules which permit the surfaces to glide one on the other. The cervical facets stand at right angles to the sagittal plane, and are quite flat. The thoracic facets are rotated anteriorly, forming an angle of about 70 degrees with the sagittal plane, and also are planar in configuration. The lumbar facets are heavier,

are rotated backwards to an angle of about 45 degrees, and present a somewhat cylindrically curved articular surface.

In the cervical spine flexion, extension and lateral flexion are freely accomplished, and some rotation also can be obtained. However, most of the rotation of the head takes place at the atlantoaxial articulations. Movement of the thoracic spine is limited by the thoracic cage. Flexion, extension and lateral bending are possible, as well as some degree of rotation. In the lumbar region rotation is limited to about 5 degrees, but flexion and extension are facilitated by the sagittal alignment of the apophyseal joints.

The lumbosacral joint permits rotary motion of varying extent. The alignment and positioning of these articular surfaces are quite variable, as is the range of motion in different individuals. The stress on the lumbosacral joint is greater than on those of the upper lumbar articulations, so that the pedicles, laminae and transverse processes of the fifth lumbar vertebra usually are heavier than those above.

Twenty-three intervertebral discs unite the vertebral bodies from the second cervical to the first sacral segments inclusive, forming a series of amphiarthrodial or slightly movable joints. No intervertebral disc is present between the cranium, the first and the second cervical vertebrae. In adult life the intervertebral discs are avascular and are composed of a surrounding annulus fibrosus made up of hyaline fibrocartilage enclosing the nucleus pulposus, a semigelatinous ovoid tissue whose function is principally that of maintaining the elasticity and bending abilities of the spinal column (Fig. 21). It has been estimated that approximately one-fourth of the length of the vertebral column is made up of the intervertebral fibrocartilages. The sizes of the intervertebral discs correspond to those of the intervening vertebrae, so that the upper cervical discs are small, while those in the lower lumbar spine are correspondingly large.

The configuration of the intervertebral discs contributes to the alignment of the vertebral column. The cervical discs are wedge-shaped, and are responsible for the usual cervical lordotic curve. Those in the thoracic region are a little more prominent posteriorly than anteriorly, but do not particularly affect the usual dorsal kyphotic curve. In the lumbar region the discs again affect the lumbar lordotic curve, being considerably heavier anteriorly, especially at the lumbosacral articulation. Measurements of intradiscal pressures in the lower lumbar spine were made by Nachemson and Morris (1964), who reported values of from 10 to 15 kg/cm^2 in seated patients, while in the standing position the pressures were about 30 per cent less, and about 50 per cent less in the reclining position. It was found that the lower lumbar discs support loads of as much as 100 to 175 kg when the subject is seated, but only 90 to 120 kg when erect. They regarded their data as helping to explain relief of pain when standing or reclining, the pain which occurs during the Valsalva

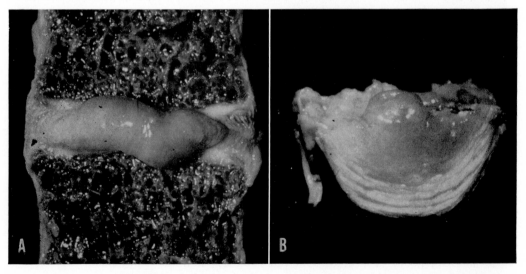

Fig. 21. A, Normal bulging cut nucleus pulposus, 14-year-old boy. B, Same specimen cut horizontally to show laminar formation of the annulus fibrosus.

maneuver, and the codfish vertebra appearance of osteoporotic spines with relatively normal discs.

Each disc is separated from the cancellous bone of the vertebral body by a plate of hyaline cartilage which in the child fits over the body of the vertebra as an epiphysis. Growth of the vertebra takes place at these epiphyseal plates.

The heights of the vertebral bodies are affected by the normal stresses of weight bearing during growth. In the absence of normal stresses an increase in the height of the vertebral bodies becomes manifest, as observed in children who never walk, or in patients with conditions such as amyotonia congenita or myelomeningocele. Such changes in height constitute a reversible phenomenon during growth, so that if normal stresses and pressures return the involved vertebrae resume their normal proportions (Gooding and Neuhauser, 1965).

The configuration of the vertebrae also vary somewhat in different races. Davis (1960) pointed out that while many similarities are present in the spines of Europeans and Africans, the strains imposed on the cervical vertebrae in, for example, Nigerian women who carry heavy weights on their heads, result in bony changes in the atlas and axis. A change in the range of motion in flexion and extension also occurs.

At about the age of 6 years, a ring apophysis appears as a narrow cartilaginous round structure lying on the rims of the cephalic and caudal surfaces of the respective vertebrae (Fig. 22). These take no part in longitudinal growth, and represent an apophysis

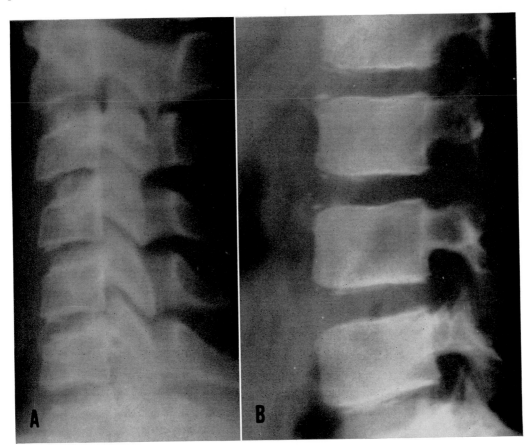

FIG. 22. A, Normal cervical spine in a 13-year-old boy with ring apophyses overlying anterior aspect of the vertebral bodies. B, Same patient, lumbar ring apophyses.

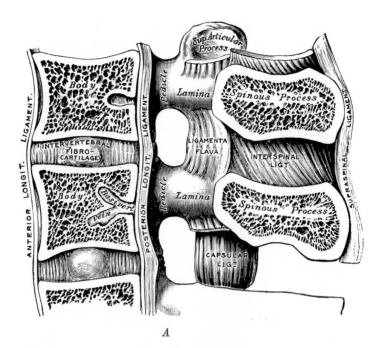

A

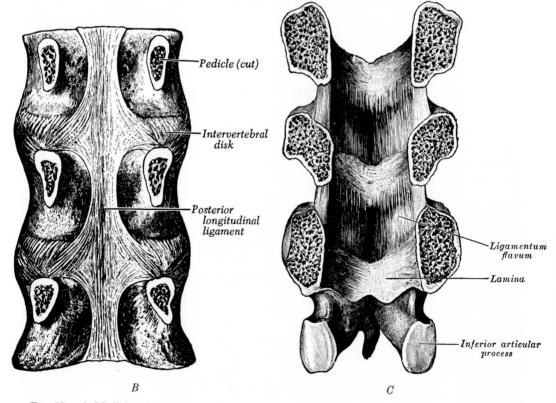

B   C

FIG. 23.   *A*, Medial sagittal section of two lumbar vertebrae and their ligaments.   *B*, Posterior longitudinal ligament of the lumbar vertebrae.   *C*, Anterior aspect of the lumbar ligamenta flava.   (*Gray's Anatomy*, Lea & Febiger.)

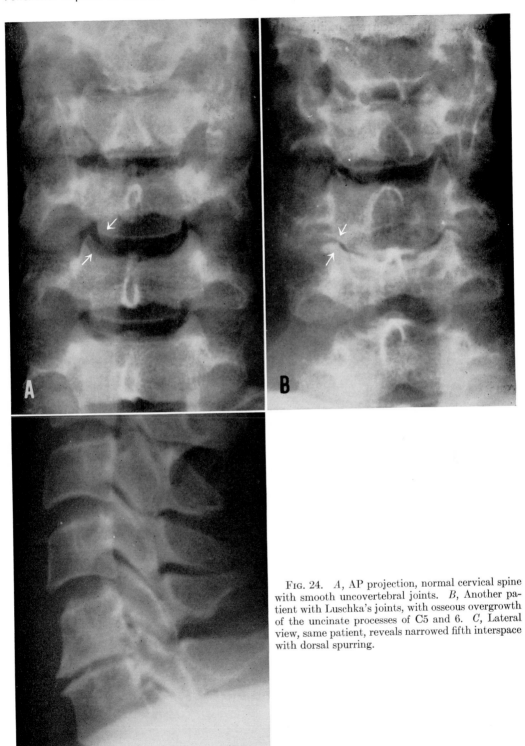

Fig. 24. *A*, AP projection, normal cervical spine with smooth uncovertebral joints. *B*, Another patient with Luschka's joints, with osseous overgrowth of the uncinate processes of C5 and 6. *C*, Lateral view, same patient, reveals narrowed fifth interspace with dorsal spurring.

of the traction type corresponding to the attachments of the longitudinal and intervertebral ligaments of the spine. Calcification occurs in these rings separately, and they fuse with the vertebral bodies at about the age of 18 years. Beginning at about 8 years, they are often present in the thoracic and lumbar regions as irregularly calcified thin, broken circular bands. Less often, ring apophyses are seen in the cervical vertebrae. Later the calcification becomes heavier until final fusion occurs.

Vascular channels are found in the cartilaginous intervertebral plates only during the first three decades of life. Later the discs are almost avascular except for some questionable channels in their peripheries.

In adolescent spines the intervertebral discs may be slightly expanded in the regions of the nucleus pulposus, but this recedes with life's progression of wear and tear. It has been estimated that in the average healthy young adult the gelatinous nucleus pulposus is under a pressure of 30 pounds to the square inch. When cut the turgid nucleus pulposus bulges prominently (Fig. 21). The cartilage plates of the intervertebral discs not infrequently present small irregular breaks in their surfaces, and in some children up to about the age of 10 the cartilage plates dip into the underlying cancellous bone in small grooves.

The annulus fibrosus is composed of a mixture of fibrous cartilage and collagenous fibrous tissue arranged in concentric lamellae passing obliquely across the intervertebral space in alternate directions. The fibers, which arise as continuations of the fibrous cartilages of the apophyseal rings, sweep around in an outward arch to be inserted in the opposite cartilaginous plate and bony ring. Some blend with the fibers of the longitudinal spinal ligaments and others turn over to become embedded in the outer cortex of the vertebral body on the side of the disc from which they originate.

The nucleus pulposus is composed of a chondroid basophilic matrix traversed by a few delicate collagenous fibrils, sometimes

containing stellate cells and large vesiculated balloon cells supposed to represent vestigial notochord. Notochordal remnants also have been identified in the vicinity of the first and second cervical vertebrae and the clivus Blumenbachii.

The spinal column is composed of two series of joints. The amphiarthroses or half joints are formed by the intervertebral discs. The diarthrodeses, or true joints, are formed by the inferior pair of articular processes, hooking down behind the superior segments below. They are encapsulated, and contain synovial lining and articular cartilages. These are designated as apophyseal, or posterior joints. Small joints are present at the posterolateral aspects of the lower five cervical vertebrae in the vicinity of the uncinate processes. Originally described by Luschka in 1858 as true synovial joints, they are important because their relationship to the intervertebral foramina is such that overgrowth may impinge into the foramen and compress the contained nerve trunk. They are today regarded as degenerative alterations, rather than true joints (Fig. 24). Luschka's joints also are referred to as uncovertebral or covertebral joints.

Anteroposterior motion of each vertebra takes place about a transverse axis near the posterior border of its body. Flexion is checked by the supraspinous, interspinous and interlaminal ligaments which bind the adjacent vertebrae together posteriorly. This is aided to some extent by the ligamenta flava, which differ from the other ligaments in that they contain elastic fibers. These ligamentous bindings are so firm that except in the cervical area acute flexion trauma may result in compression of a vertebral body rather than rupture of the posterior check ligaments or dislocation of articular processes. Extension of the back is limited by the anterior vertebral ligaments and the intervertebral discs, which may remain intact in extension injuries, the pedicles and laminae suffering fractures as a result of severe hyperextension.

At the cephalic end of the vertebral

column, the intervertebral ligaments are represented by the heavy craniovertebral group. In the thoracic region the intervertebral ligaments are reinforced by the costovertebral ligaments, and at the lumbosacral region the strong lumbosacral, sacro-iliac and lumbo-iliac structures help stabilize the vertebral column on the pelvis. These groups of ligaments, together with the intertransverse group, determine the degree of normal lateral motion and rotation of the spinal column.

The anterior longitudinal ligament is a heavy, broad band extending from the axis to the sacrum along the ventral aspect of the vertebrae (Fig. 23). It is heaviest in its proximal portion, and is thicker where in apposition to the vertebral bodies. Its dense longitudinal fibers are fixed more firmly to the intervertebral fibrocartilages and the rims of the vertebrae than to their concavities. The ligaments at the sides of the vertebrae extend from these, and are considerably shorter and less dense. The posterior spinal ligament is situated within the spinal canal, extending from the body of the axis to the sacrum. It is heaviest in the thoracic region. This ligament is in intimate approximation to the intervertebral discs, particularly in their midportions. On either posterolateral side the ligament thins out, especially in the vicinity of the intervertebral foramina, where the discs bulge dorsally to occupy a variable portion of the lower half of the foramen. In the thoracic and lumbar regions the ligament follows the concavities of the respective vertebral bodies, but is thickened over the median line where it is separated from the bone by the basivertebral veins.

The ligamentum flavum, composed predominantly of yellow elastic tissue, joins the laminae and articular processes as a continuous structure formed by a medial thicker half uniting the laminae and a lateral thinner portion surrounding the articular joints and blending with their capsules (Fig. 23). The interlaminar fibers are vertically disposed, and are attached inferiorly to the groove on the upper border of the inferior lamina and superiorly to the lower half of the superior lamina. Sharp thin spicules and plaques of bone extend into the ligament from its inferior attachment. These are continuous ligaments, the inner thicker fibers being vertically arranged and the outer thinner ligaments directed obliquely downward and outward. The ligament is so arranged that the inferior half of the lamina is excluded from the vertebral canal. Medially it blends with the opposite side at the bases of the spinous processes. The ligamenta flava are broad and long in the cervical region, and increase in thickness caudally.

The muscles of the back are arranged symmetrically in opposing groups which support the skeleton and control the motion of the back within the limitations set by the ligaments. Posteriorly the short and long intervertebral muscles are attached to the posterior and lateral processes. The vertebral-costal, vertebral-iliac and vertebral-sacral groups produce extension of the back, and with other coordinated groups, rotation and lateral bending. At the cephalic end homologous muscles control the motion of the head and neck. Altogether, the muscles form a heavy coordinated integrated mass making up the posterior wall of the torso. Flexion of the back is produced by contraction of the psoas muscles when the thighs are fixed, by the anterior and lateral abdominal muscles acting through the levers of the thoracic cage and pelvis, and by the anterior neck muscles. Rotation and lateral bending are accomplished by coordinated action of all groups.

At about the 3rd month of gestation, the fetal spine assumes a single, dorsally convex, somewhat coiled posterior curve. Uncoiling begins between the 3rd and 6th months, when the movable portions of the vertebral column straighten out and acquire a second ventral curve. At birth, a posterior thoracolumbar convexity and a sacral curve are present. The head, hips and knees are flexed, and when the face is tipped upwards the anteriorly convex cervical curve develops. When the infant's hips are extended, the lumbar vertebrae are pulled forward by the psoas muscles and hip ligaments forming a typical lumbar curve. This does not become firmly fixed until the child has been walking for several years. In the adult, the cervical spine in the resting position presents a normal anterior curve. The dorsal spine then has a slight dorsal curve and sometimes a curve convex towards the patient's right side. The usual lumbar lordotic curve is demonstrable in the lateral position. This increases somewhat when the patient is in the erect posture.

Two types of curves, a primary or accommodation curve, and a secondary or compensation curve are encountered in the spine. Four of these exist in the sagittal plane, convex forward in the cervical and lumbar regions and concave forward in the dorsal and sacral areas respectively. The dorsal and sacral curves are primary, persisting from the embryonic state. These help accommodate the thoracic and pelvic viscera. The cervical and lumbar curves are convex ventrally and represent secondary curves that appear when the upright posture is attained, and develop by changes in the intervertebral discs. The cervical curve appears in infancy when ventral flexion of the head on the chest begins at about the 3rd month, and with ability to sit at about the 6th month. This cervical curve is not fixed, and is present in the upright but obliterated in the horizontal posture. The lumbar curve between the twelfth thoracic vertebra and the sacral promontory appears between the ages of 9 and 12 months, when the child begins to stand and to walk. This curve becomes relatively fixed in adult life. The anterior prominence of the cervical curve is situated at the body of the fourth cervical vertebra, and the curve ends at about the second dorsal vertebra. The most prominent portion of the dorsal curve is at the seventh or eighth dorsal vertebra, and its termination is at the twelfth thoracic or first lumbar vertebra. The fifth curve occurs in the dorsal spine as a lateral secondary or compensation curve. In most cases it is directed toward the right, and is probably associated with the position of the heart and the greater use of the right hand. This is referred to as physiologic right lateral scoliosis. The lateral curves of accommodation have associated minor morphologic changes in the bodies of the dorsal and sacral regions, while the secondary or compensation curves have associated changes at the intervertebral discs. The alternating curves of the vertebral column are largely responsible for the strength of the spine, which is estimated as sixteen times that of a straight alignment.

A slight, variable flattening of the left side of the dorsal vertebrae from the fourth to tenth dorsal segments inclusive may exist, forming the so-called aortic compression.

The intervertebral foramina are oval in shape, and increase in size from the cephalic to caudal regions. They are bounded anteriorly by the vertebral bodies and intervertebral discs. Above and below are the pedicles. The posterior margins are formed by the superior and inferior articular facets and the ligamentum flavum. By virtue of the movement of the vertebrae the foramina accommodate themselves to the various motions of the spine. When the neck is flexed, the intervertebral spaces are oval and fairly large, but in extension the foramina decrease in size as the gliding surfaces of the articular facets pass one over the other as inclined planes. In the thoracic spine, the intervertebral foramina are relatively small and contain little adipose tissue, since little cushioning of the nerve roots is required because of the restricted motion of the respective dorsal segments. In the lumbar region, posterior extension of the spine causes relative constriction of the intervertebral foramina, while anterior flexion increases the diameter of these openings. It has been estimated that the spinal nerves occupy about one-sixth to one-quarter of the available space of the respective foramina, the rest being utilized by fatty and areolar tissue, vessels, lymphatics and sympathetic nerve fibers.

References

Bailey, D. K.: The Normal Cervical Spine in Infants and Children. Radiology, *59*, 712, 1952.

Beadle, O. A.: The Intervertebral Disks. Medical Research Council, London, 1931. His Majesty's Stationery Office.

Bick, E.: Ring Apophysis of the Human Vertebra. J. Bone & Joint Surg., *33-A*, 783, 1951.

Bick, E. M. and Copel, J. W.: Longitudinal Growth of the Human Vertebra. J. Bone & Joint Surg., *32-A*, 803, 1950.

Boreadis, A. G. and Gershon-Cohen, J.: Luschka's Joints of the Cervical Spine. Radiology, *66*, 181, 1956.

Cattell, H. S. and Filtzer, D. L.: Pseudoluxation and Other Normal Variations in the Cervical Spine in Children. J. Bone & Joint Surg., *47-A*, 1295, 1965.

Compere, E. L. and Keyes, D. C.: Roentgenological Studies of the Intervertebral Discs. Am. J. Roentgenol., *29*, 774, 1933.

Coventry, M. B., Ghormley, R. K. and Kernohan, J. W.: The Intervertebral Disc. J. Bone & Joint Surg., *27*, 105, 233, 460, 1945 (Parts I, II and III).

Davis, P. R.: *Observations on Vertebrae in Different Races.* Actes du VIe Congrès International des Sciences Anthropologiques et Ethnologiques. Paris, 1960; Vol. 1, 443–453.

Eckert, C. and Decker, A.: Pathological Studies of the Intervertebral Discs. J. Bone & Joint Surg., *29*, 447, 1947.

Farkas, A.: The Pathogenesis of Idiopathic Scoliosis. J. Bone & Joint Surg., *36-A*, 617, 1954.

Fineman, S., Borrelli, F. J., Rubinstein, B. M., Epstein, H. and Jacobson, H. G.: The Cervical Spine: Transformation of the Normal Lordotic Pattern into a Linear Pattern in the Neutral Position, J. Bone & Joint Surg., *45-A*, 1179, 1963.

Gaizler, G.: Die Beurteilung der Ruhehaltung der Halzwirbelsaule—eine erledigte Frage. Fortsch. Röntgenstr., *103*, 566, 1965.

Gooding, C. A. and Neuhauser, E. B. D.: Growth and Development of the Vertebral Bodies in the Presence and Absence of Normal Stress. Am. J. Roentgenol., *93*, 388, 1965.

Hadley, L. A.: The Covertebral Articulations and Cervical Foramen Encroachment. J. Bone & Joint Surg., *39-A*, 910, 1957.

————: Anatomico-Roentgenographic Studies of the Posterior Spinal Articulations. Am. J. Roentgenol., *86*, 270, 1961.

Harris, R. I. and Macnab, I.: Structural Changes in the Lumbar Intervertebral Discs. J. Bone & Joint Surg., *36-A*, 304, 1954.

Hirsch, C., Ingelmark, B-E. and Miller, M.: The Anatomical Basis for Low Back Pain. Studies on the Presence of Sensory Nerve Endings in Ligamentous, Capsular and Intervertebral Disc Structures in the Human Lumbar Spine. Acta orthop. scandinav., *33*, 1, 1963.

Inman, V. T. and Saunders, J. B. de C. M.: The Clinico-Anatomical Aspects of the Lumbo-Sacral Region. Radiology, *38*, 669, 1942.

Joplin, R. J.: The Intervertebral Disc. Surg., Gynec. & Obst., *61*, 591, 1935.

Juhl, J. H., Miller, S. M. and Roberts, G. W.: Roentgenographic Variations in the Normal Cervical Spine. Radiology, *78*, 591, 1962.

Keegan, J. J.: Alterations of the Lumbar Curve Related to Posture and Seating. J. Bone & Joint Surg., *35-A*, 640, 1953.

Keyes, D. C. and Compere, E. L.: The Normal and Pathologic Physiology of the Nucleus Pulposus of the Intervertebral Disc. J. Bone & Joint Surg., *14*, 897, 1932.

Knuttson, F.: Growth and Differentiation of the Postnatal Vertebra. Acta radiol., *55*, 401, 1961.

Nachemson, A. and Morris, J. M.: *In vivo* Measurements of Intradiscal Pressure. J. Bone & Joint Surg., *46-A*, 1077, 1964.

Orofino, C., Sherman, M. S. and Schechter, D.: Luschka's Joint—A Degenerative Phenomenon. J. Bone & Joint Surg., *42-A*, 853, 1960.

Penning, L.: Nonpathologic and Pathologic Relationships Between the Lower Cervical Vertebrae. Am. J. Roentgenol., *91*, 1037, 1964.

The Spinal Cord

The spinal cord is derived from the neural groove, a structure of ectodermal origin from which the nervous and neuroglial elements appear. The central canal persists as the rudiment of the embryologic neural canal, communicating with the cerebral ventricles in the same manner that the cord is a direct extension of the brain.

The coverings of the spinal cord are the dura mater, the arachnoid and the pia mater. These originate from the primitive mesenchymal tissue surrounding the nervous system, and are derived from the same tissues which form bone and periosteum. In the embryo the dura mater is separated from the nervous system by loose mesenchymal tissue containing albuminous tissue fluid. The pia mater is formed by mesenchymal cells on the surface of the neural tube. At the onset of secretion of the cerebrospinal fluid, excess fluid passes into the tissue spaces separating the two leaves of the arachnoid into the subarachnoid spaces. Arachnoid trabeculae extend from the pia to the dura. The dura and arachnoid are separated by the thin subdural space containing a small amount of colorless fluid.

The spinal cord originates as an open groove which later closes to form a tube.

The distal portion of the spinal cord, however, develops differently in that it starts as a solid cord of cells rather than a closing or closed neural tube. The central canal in this area is present as a secondary structure rather than as a result of the closing of the original neural groove. Up to the 3rd month of fetal life the spinal cord is about the same length as the spinal canal. During the subsequent growth of the fetus, there is a discrepancy in the rate of growth of the spinal canal as compared with that of the spinal cord. The filum terminale then appears and inserts into the sacrococcygeal region. In the adult the filum terminale consists of an intradural portion about 15 cm long and an external portion about 6 cm long extending below the caudal sac and inserted into the first coccygeal segment. The external portion is invested by dura mater. At birth the lower end of the spinal cord is located at approximately the level of the third lumbar vertebra, while in the adult it usually reaches the superior margin of the second lumbar vertebra.

During the early stages of development, the dura mater is in close proximity to the spinal canal. Later these structures separate and the epidural space is formed. This space becomes filled with areolar tissue and vessels, predominantly large veins. The dura is attached to the intervertebral discs in the lumbar region. In the sacral area the dura is separated from the anterior wall of the spinal canal, merges with the filum terminale and fastens with this structure to the anterior part of the sacral canal. Considerable variation is seen in the configuration of the distal end of the caudal sac. Some differences are noted in its point of termination, which usually is at or below the level of the fifth lumbar intervertebral disc.

The spinal dura mater is fixed to the circumference of the foramen magnum and the second and third cervical vertebrae. It represents only the inner or meningeal layer of the cranial dura mater. The outer or endosteal layer of cranial dura mater terminates at the foramen magnum and is replaced by the periosteum lining the vertebral canal. The dura is connected to the posterior longitudinal ligament, especially at the distal portion of the vertebral canal by fibrous tissue. The dura is quite loose and permits ample space, particularly in the cervical and in the lumbar regions. In the thoracic region, however, the dura is more closely affixed to the spinal canal and the intradural space is considerably less than in other areas. On either side of the dura are the extensions which invest the corresponding spinal nerves. These are short and relatively horizontal in the cervical and upper thoracic regions. Lower in the cord, they become gradually longer and are directly obliquely downward. The dura is poorly supplied with blood vessels and contains a relatively scant nerve supply.

The arachnoid coat of the spinal cord is composed of delicate membranous tissue continuous with the cranial arachnoid. In its distal portion it envelops the nerve roots of the cauda equina. The arachnoid covers the spinal nerves in loose sheaths, and extends with them as they emerge from the canal, forming arachnoidal pouches (Fig. 25). The cerebrospinal fluid circulates in the subarachnoid space, within which are delicate connective tissue septa. The spinal and cranial subarachnoid spaces are in direct communication.

The pia mater is a thin, delicate vascular membrane of areolar tissue, and in the spinal canal consists of two layers. The outer one is composed of bundles of connective tissue fibers arranged in a longitudinal fashion, while the inner is approximated to the cord in a more circular manner. Between these two closely approximated layers of the spinal pia mater is a space which is in continuity with the subarachnoid cavity. This contains a vascular network which supplies the underlying nervous tissue. The pia closely envelops the spinal cord and extends outward along the nerve roots. Along the midline of the anterior aspect of the cord a longitudinal fibrous band termed the linea

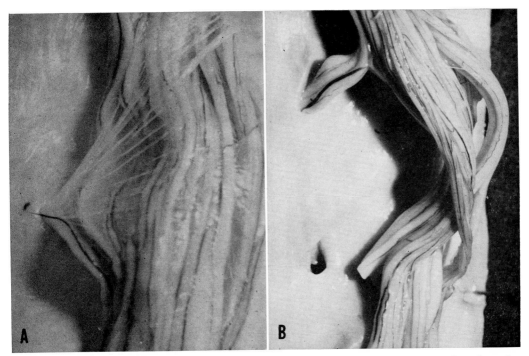

Fig. 25. On opening the dura and leaving the arachnoid intact, the conus and the proximal cauda equina is visible. The arachnoid is stretched to demonstrate the formation of the axillary pouch. *A,* After dissecting away the arachnoid and retracting the cauda equina, the nerve root passing to the dura is seen above, and one segment lower the nerve root has been cut to demonstrate the dural perforation, *B.*

splendens can be demonstrated. This is similar to the dentate ligaments on the lateral aspects of the cord.

The pia mater terminates below the conus medullaris as the filum terminale, which extends downward to form the center of the cauda equina. The filum terminale blends with the dura mater about the level of the second sacral vertebra and then proceeds downward to the coccyx, where it fuses with the periosteum.

The dentate ligaments extend from the midline of both sides of the spinal cord as thin longitudinal septa which originate from a barely perceptible thickening of the pia mater. They extend laterally in a series of triangular folds which insert by apical tips into the dura mater. The first one is located opposite the margin of the foramen magnum between the vertebral artery and the hypoglossal nerve (Fig. 26*A*). The last one is a broader strand of fibrous tissue which unites in a fork-shaped extension merging with the

pia arachnoid around the filum terminale (Fig. 26*B*).

The dentate ligaments can be seen through the translucent intact arachnoid after the dura mater is reflected away. The points of insertion of each triangular fold is extra-arachnoid in position. At the apex of each fold is a small, prong-like continuation of fibrous tissue which joins the dura mater by way of two or three tips about 1 mm in length. These prongs are longer in the cervical than in the thoracic regions, where they may be represented by a single rather heavy fold. The insertional tips are best observed after the dura mater is folded back on itself and extended after it has been incised dorsally and ventrally in the midline (Fig. 27).

When the arachnoid is stripped away, the dentate ligaments can be identified as thin sheets composed of interlacing folds of fibrous tissue, with occasional defects in the triangular leaves. These folds are smaller in

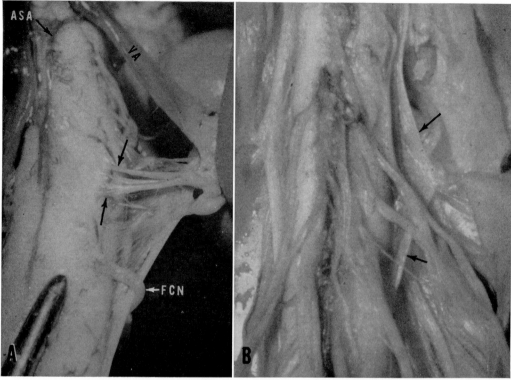

FIG. 26.   A, Dissection of the first dentate fold. The anterior roots of the hypoglossal nerve is stretched (arrows). The vertebral artery (VA) and the anterior spinal artery (ASA) are pulled away. The first cervical nerve passes above the extended dentate ligament (FCN). B, The last dentate ligament is large, broad and merges with the arachnoid covering of the conus (*arrows*). (From Epstein, B. S.: An Anatomic, Myelographic and Cinemyelographic Study of the Dentate Ligaments, Am. J. Roentgenol., *98*, 704, 1966, courtesy of Charles C Thomas, Publisher.)

the cervical region, and increase in size caudally. The ligaments are located between the anterior and posterior nerve roots, dividing the canal into anterior and posterior compartments. The motor pathways are dorsal and the sensory tracts lie ventral to the dentate ligaments. Cerebrospinal fluid circulates around the cord, flowing between the compartments through the spaces between the free edges of the dentate ligaments (Fig. 27).

In the cervical spinal canal the dentate insertions are situated about midway between the successive emerging nerve trunks. They are relatively closely approximated because of the short intervals between the dural sleeves. At rest, the tips are about 2 cm apart. In the upper thoracic region the dural tips are further apart, and are most widely spaced in the lower thoracic region. The thoracic dural tip insertions are heavier and blunter than those in the cervical canal, and are located more caudad in relationship to the emerging nerve roots than those in the cervical region. In the lower thoracic region the points of insertion are close to the caudally placed nerve root exits. The fusion of the tips and the dura is heavy, and a fold directed cephalad is seen when the dura is stretched. The last dentate insertion varies in that it is situated some distance from the adjacent nerve trunks (Figs. 26 and 27).

The free edge of each dentate fold is made up of a rounded cord-like structure. This is a heavy, continuous somewhat elastic strand of fibrous tissue, considerably heavier than the triangular sheets. The prong-like inser-

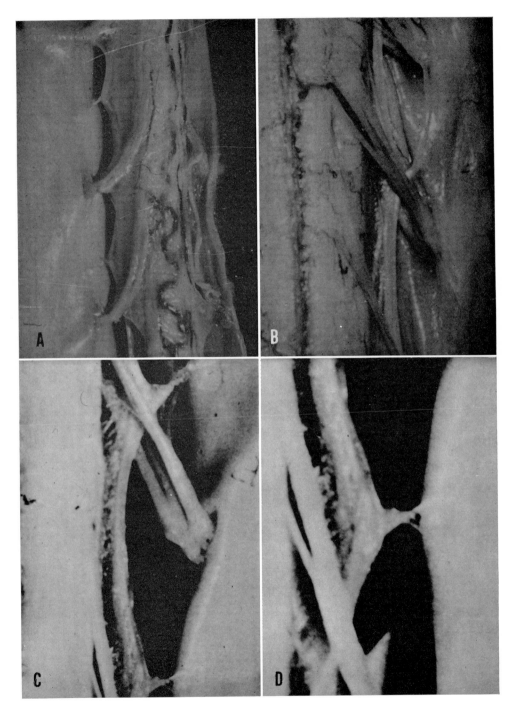

FIG. 27. *A*, The dura has been reflected and the arachnoid stripped away. The dentate tips in the cervicothoracic region are inserted midway between the nerve roots. *B*, In the lower thoracic region the dentate ligaments are broader, and the tips heavier and inserted just above the emerging root. *C*, Magnified photograph of the dentate ligament. Note the rope-like margin and insertion of tip. *D*, The dentate tip inserts into the dura by a prong-like fibrous process which acts as a universal joint permitting rotary movement. (From Epstein, B. S., An Anatomic, Myelographic and Cinemyelographic Study of the Dentate Ligaments, Am. J. Roentgenol., *98*, 704, 1966, courtesy of Charles C Thomas, Publisher.)

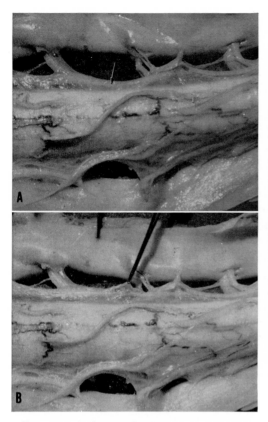

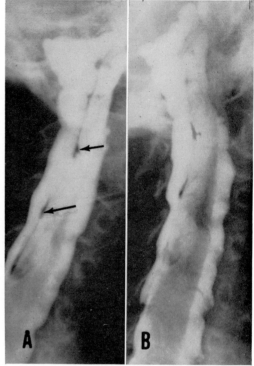

Fig. 29. *A*, Oblique cervical myelogram with the head in slight flexion. The first to the fifth dentate ligament is visible as a linear radiolucency. The tips are represented by the separated broadened markings (*arrows*). *B*, With the head in extension the dentate ligament shortens and rotation occurs at their tips. This is better demonstrated on cinemyelography.

Fig. 28. *A*, One of the dentate tips has been severed and the ligament is retracted against the cord (arrow). *B*, The cut dentate is picked up so that the rounded peripheral ligament is visible. (From Epstein, B. S., An Anatomic, Myelographic and Cinemyelographic Study of the Dentate Ligaments. Am. J. Roentgenol., *98*, 704, 1966. Courtesy of Charles C Thomas, Publishers.)

tions into the dura mater are extensions of these peripheral ligamentous borders. If the dural insertion of a dentate tip is cut, the ligament retracts and the cord-like lateral margins flatten into a straight line against the cord. When the tip is elevated, the rounded margin returns as the triangular fold is extended (Figs. 27 and 28).

On the basis of myelographic and cine-myelographic observations it appears that the dentate tips act as universal joints which permit the dentate ligaments to swivel during rotary motion. During extension of the neck the dentate points approximate each other, while in flexion they come closer together (Fig. 29). It is quite likely

that this indicates shortening and extension of the cord itself during these movements. Breig (1960), on the basis of anatomic investigations, noted that elongation of the spinal canal increased the distances between the dentate attachments, while shortening of the canal brought them closer together. When the column was flexed laterally, the dentate ligaments separated on the convex side and moved closer together on the concave side, so that they converged radially on the axis of curvature. When the canal was elongated in ventroflexion, the dura was drawn out smooth and the dentate ligaments followed this motion, so that the distances between the successive pairs increased in the craniocaudad directions. Stoltmann and Blackwood (1966) observed that the dentate ligaments did not limit anteroposterior movement of the cord, but rather limited cephalocaudad excursions. Jirout (1963) reported that the cervical cord moved backwards and forwards in the supine and prone position for about 2.5 to 4 mm, and occasionally as much as 8 mm. The thoracic cord moves slightly more than 2 mm, but may exceed 4.5 mm. These are physiological movements which occur during motion. His studies were based on air myelograms.

For some time the dentate ligaments were believed to be important in restraining movement of the cord in an anteroposterior direction. Section of the cervical dentate ligaments was, for a while, regarded as helpful in the management of cervical spondylosis (Kahn, 1947), but this practice has been abandoned (Mayfield, 1955; Scoville, 1961; Epstein, Epstein and Lavine, 1963). The tethering effect attributed to the dentate ligaments probably is far less important than that exerted by the emerging nerve roots.

There are 31 pairs of spinal nerves arising from the spinal cord. Each possesses anterior (ventral) and posterior (dorsal)) roots, the latter being identified by the presence of spinal ganglions. There are pairs of 8 cervical nerves, 12 thoracic nerves, 5 lumbar nerves, 5 sacral nerves and 1 coccygeal nerve. The first cervical nerve passes between the occiput and the first cervical vertebra, and the eighth emerges from between the seventh cervical and the first thoracic vertebrae. The first thoracic nerves go through the foramina between the first and second thoracic vertebrae, and so on downwards. Thus, the nerves below the cervicothoracic junction have the numerical designation of the vertebra immediately cephalad, as, for instance, the fifth lumbar nerve coming out from between the fifth lumbar and first sacral vertebrae. Even though there is no anatomic evidence to point towards specific segments in the spinal canal, it has become customary to divide the cord into spinal segments or neuromeres, each of which possesses length equal to the

extent of the attachment of the corresponding pair of spinal nerves. These vary in various portions of the spinal canal. In the cervical region the neuromeres average about 13 mm in length, in the midthoracic region about 26 mm in length, while in the lumbosacral regions they diminish rapidly from 15 mm at the level of the first lumbar nerves to about 4 mm opposite the attachment of the lower sacral nerves.

The spinal cord itself is rather oval, flattened dorsoventrally, and is larger in the cervical and lumbar regions than in the thoracic region. The cervical enlargement, which is the more prominent, extends from approximately the level of the third cervical vertebra to the second thoracic vertebra, reaching its widest diameter at the sixth cervical segment. The lumbar bulge begins at approximately the level of the ninth thoracic vertebra and terminates opposite the twelfth thoracic vertebra. Below this the cord tapers abruptly, forming the conus medullaris and the filum terminale (Fig. 30).

The rootlets of the upper four cervical nerves are smaller than those of the lower four, while the dorsal motor roots are about three times the size of the ventral sensory roots. An exception is the dorsal root of the first cervical nerve, which is smaller than its ventral root. The rootlets emerge from a thin sulcus along the anteromedial and posteromedial aspects of the spinal cord. Those of the cervical region are made up of numerous rootlets which merge and pass horizontally, the dorsal and ventral roots uniting immediately beyond the spinal ganglion to form the nerve trunk, which then passes through the intervertebral foramen. Both nerve roots are covered by pia mater and arachnoid. The arachnoid extends as far as the point where each root penetrates the dura mater. The dura becomes continuous with the epineurium after the roots unite to form the spinal nerve.

The upper cervical nerve roots are more horizontal in their location than those lower down. Here the nerves begin to incline caudad, increasingly so in the thoracic and lumbar regions. The thoracic nerve roots are fairly small, while the lumbar and sacral roots are large. The coccygeal roots are the smallest ones. In the lumbar portion of the spinal canal the nerves assume the configuration which has given rise to the descriptive term cauda equina.

Blood is supplied to the spinal cord by way of the anterior and posterior spinal arteries. In the upper cervical spinal canal the anterior spinal artery is formed by the union of two small vessels originating from the medial aspects of the vertebral arteries above the level of the posterior inferior cerebellar arteries. The originating vessels may be asymmetric, corresponding in size relative to the caliber of the vessels from which they originate. These two rootlets unite in the midline at the level of the medulla oblongata and pass caudally as the anterior spinal artery in the anterior spinal sulcus (Fig. 31). Variations occur in the pattern of fusion of the rootlets of the anterior spinal artery. In some the classic V-shaped configuration is

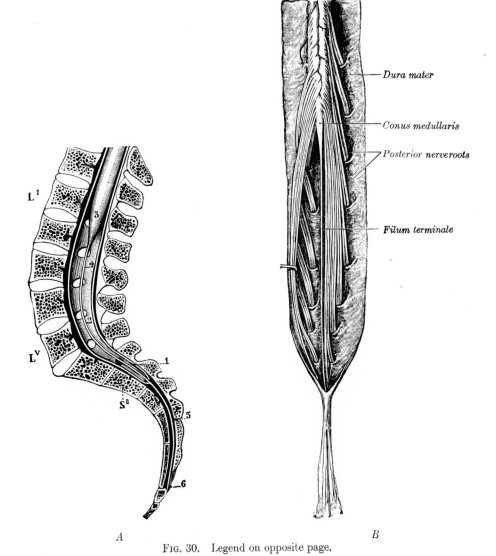

Dura mater

Conus medullaris

Posterior nerve roots

Filum terminale

A   *B*

Fig. 30. Legend on opposite page.

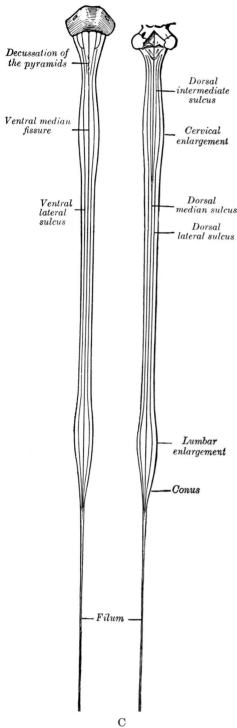

Decussation of
the pyramids

Ventral median
fissure

Ventral
lateral
sulcus

Dorsal
intermediate
sulcus

Cervical
enlargement

Dorsal
median sulcus

Dorsal
lateral sulcus

Lumbar
enlargement

Conus

Filum

C

FIG. 30. *A*, Vertebral canal showing lower end of medulla spinalis and the filum terminale. *B*, Cauda equina and filum terminale, see from behind. *C*, Diagrams of the spinal cord indicating positions of cervical and lumbar enlargement. (*Gray's Anatomy*, Lea & Febiger.)

replaced by multiple rootlets which then unite in the midline, replacing the clean-cut V-shaped origin of the midline trunk.

The anterior spinal artery passes down the midline in the anterior spinal sulcus enveloped in the pial fold of the linea splendens, and terminates along the filum terminale. The respective inferior halves of the spinal cord derive their arterial supply from the sulcal arteries which pass dorsally into the cleft from the anterior spinal trunk. Below the upper cervical level the anterior spinal artery is derived from and receives blood from the ascending branch of the anterior radicular arteries when these vessels reach the midline. The cervical radicular arteries originate from the vertebral and anterior cervical arteries, the latter being branches of the ascending cervical branches of the inferior thyroid artery. The radicular branches to the thoracic portion of the anterior spinal artery are derived from ascending and descending branches of the intercostal arteries. The lumbar radicular arteries arise from the iliolumbar and lateral sacral arteries in the pelvis. Of particular importance is the arteria radicularis magna, known as the artery of Adamkiewicz, which supplies the caudal spinal cord. This vessel usually originates from an intercostal or lumbar artery between the tenth thoracic and second lumbar segments, and passes on a lumbar ventral nerve root to the cord. It is usually located on the left side. It has a somewhat characteristic course, first directed cephalad, then making a sharp turn into a median descending segment which at first is straight and then terminates in a sinuous fashion.

There are usually from 6 to 8 large anterior radicular arteries, the largest of which is the arteria radicularis magna. Next in size are those in the cervical and the lower thoracic region. The cervical radicular arteries appear at the third, fourth, fifth or sixth segments, and are quite variable in size and distribution. As a rule, one is present in the upper cervical region, and two or three in the lower cervical region. In the thoracic

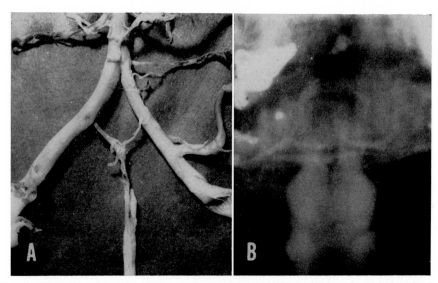

FIG. 31. *A*, Dissection of rootlets of the anterior spinal artery derived from the two vertebral arteries. *B*, Myelographic demonstration of junction of rootlets to form the anterior spinal artery (from Epstein, B. S., The Myelographic Demonstration of the Anterior Spinal and Radicular Arteries, Am. J. Roentgenol., *91*, 247, 1964, courtesy of Charles C Thomas, Publisher).

spinal canal one or two are usually seen in the upper and lower thoracic regions respectively.

The anterior spinal artery thus is formed by anastomosing vessels which originate from the ascending and descending branches of the various radicular arteries. The areas of the cord best supplied with blood are those in proximity to the radicular arteries and their origins. The caudad and cephalad ends of the respective vessels usually provide less blood to their spinal segments. In general this occurs mainly at about the fourth or fifth thoracic level, and to a lesser degree at the thoracolumbar junction. The anterior spinal artery supplies the anterior two-thirds of the transverse area of the spinal cord. The posterior aspect of the cord is supplied from the two posterior spinal arteries, one on either side of the midline. These anastomose freely, and send vessels to communicate with those of the anterior spinal artery. Variations in the main supplying arteries are not at all uncommon (Fig. 32). Aortography, both midstream and selective injections, have been found helpful in identifying and visualizing the arteries of the cord.

The anterior venous trunk is derived from the radicular veins, which do not correspond in location to the arteries, but are of approximately the same size. The truncus venosus anterior lies slightly to the side of the anterior spinal artery and just dorsal to it. It is also invested by the linea splendens.

INTRASPINAL DIMENSIONS

The width of the spinal cord at the level of the first cervical vertebra is approximately 10 mm, and it is but slightly narrower in the lower cervical region. For practical purposes its width is about 10 mm in the sagittal plane and about 15 mm in the coronal plane, and it is shaped like a flattened ovoid. Two enlargements are present, one in the lower cervical and the other in the lower thoracic region, where the nerves for the extremities originate (Fig. 30). The shape of the cord varies somewhat with movement. Such changes can be made out fairly well in the frontal plane on positive contrast myelograms. In the sagittal plane the configuration of the cord is better identified on air contrast myelograms with laminagraphy

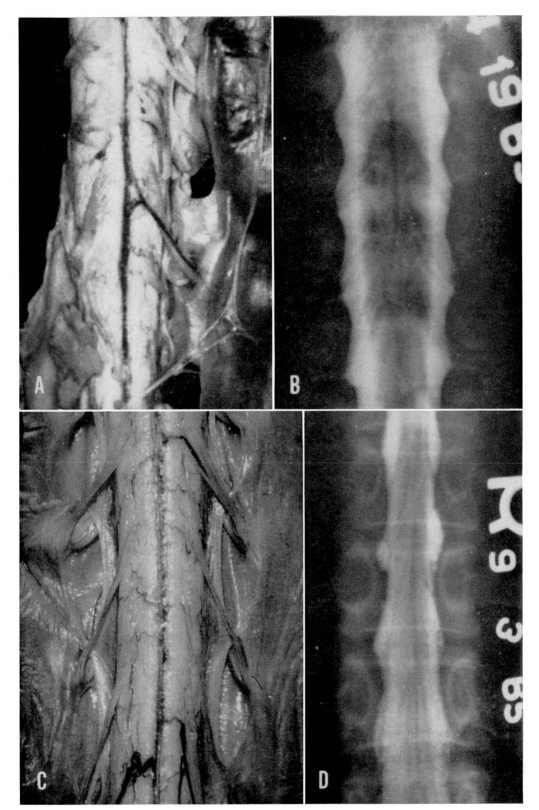

Fig. 32. *A*, Dissection showing anterior spinal artery and a supplying vessel passing along nerve root. *B*, Myelographic representation of the midline anterior spinal artery. *C*, Anterior spinal artery in the mid-thoracic region. *D*, Myelographic representation of the anterior spinal artery in the same region. Some of the nerve roots are visible directly obliquely laterally and downwards.

The coverings of the spinal cord permit it to move about within the limitations imposed by the tethering action of the nerve roots, the cranial and caudad attachments and the dentate ligaments. The dural sac itself often changes configuration markedly during strain and exertion. This can be demonstrated myelographically by having the patient strain, producing a narrowed, tapered configuration of the thecal sac and an upward movement of the pantopaque column which may exceed two or three vertebral segments. This is attributed to venous engorgement in the epidural space, causing a corresponding diminution in the thecal sac. It is reasonable to assume that this kind of pumping action may play an important part in the circulation of the cerebrospinal fluid (Fig. 33).

Changes occur in the position of the cord when the patient is supine or prone (Fig. 34), or on moving from side to side. With postural alterations the cord follows the contours of the canal, descending to the roof or the floor in accordance with body position. A lesser degree of displacement takes place from side to side when the lateral recumbent position is assumed. Flexion of the head and neck stretch the cord, and similar changes take place to a lesser degree lower down on forward bending. Extension of the head and neck shortens the cord, and to a lesser extent backward bending produces the same effect in the thoracolumbar region.

The subarachnoid space varies according to its situation in the spinal canal. In the middle and lower cervical areas the dural sac follows the cord contours rather closely, being flattened dorsoventrally. In the thoracic spinal canal the dura assumes an almost circular configuration, and as it invests the cord it is smaller than in either the cervical or the lumbar area. In the lumbar spinal canal the dural sac is triangular in the cephalad segments and almost pentagonal in the last two caudad vertebrae, with rounded angles following the general configuration of the region. The sacral dural envelope again becomes almost circular, but considerable variation in size and contour occurs here as well as in the lumbar vertebrae.

Considerable importance is attached to accurate determination of the sagittal measurement of the spinal canal. The available space varies in proportion to the anteroposterior as well as the side-to-side dimensions. Inasmuch as the spinal cord maintains a relatively constant size, while the dimensions of the bony confines varies considerably, it can be readily understood why a small lesion intruding into a small spinal canal and intervertebral foramen may produce changes which in a large space would not cause significant encroachment on the cord or the emerging nerve trunks.

Measurement of the cervical spinal canal can be made readily on true lateral roentgenograms, best made at a 72-inch target-film distance. On examinations made at a 40-inch distance a magnification error of about 2 to 3 mm is encountered. Another factor which may cause some error is that incident to the distance of the subject's neck from the film, varying according to the breadth of his shoulders. The bony landmarks used for determining the sagittal diameter of the cervical spinal canal are taken from the middle of the posterior aspect of the respective vertebral bodies to the thickened cortical line where the spinous process and lamina of the corresponding vertebra meet. If the measurement is made from the upper or lower aspect of a vertebral body to the junctional point of the spinous process and lamina, the measurement may be diminished if osteophytes are present. Both measurements are useful.

The measurements of the cervical spinal canal at the level of the first cervical vertebra vary from 16 to 27 mm in adults. At the second cervical segment the sagittal diameter is between 15 and 25 mm. Below this the lower limit of normal is about 12 mm, while the upper limit varies between 21 and 23 mm. Measurements of the sagittal diameter of the cervical spinal canal in children by Hinck, Hopkins and Savara (1962) indicate that these are but slightly

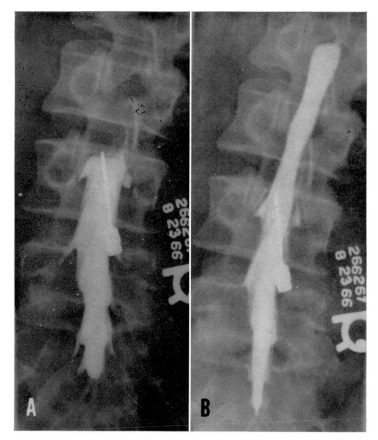

FIG. 33. *A*, Erect myelogram with patient breathing normally. A herniated disc is seen on the left side of the fifth lumbar interspace. *B*, With strain the pantopaque column moves upward, narrowing the thecal sac and practically obliterating the discal defect.

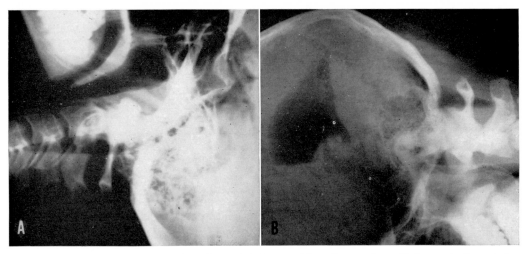

FIG. 34. *A*, Transcervical view of cervico-occipital area with patient supine. Air is seen in the anterior cervical spinal canal up to the medullary and pontine cisterns. *B*, Transcervical view, prone position. Air moves above the cord in the upper cervical canal and the cisterna magna.

less than in adults, despite the differences in the length of the vertebral column.

An important measurement in the cervical spine is that between the atlas and the dens. In children this varies between 3 and 5 mm, and in adults this distance is approximately 2 to 4 mm. A decrease in this space becomes apparent with advancing age. This line usually is drawn between the midportion of the posterior aspect of the dens to the convexity of the midportion of the anterior arch of the atlas. Changes produced during flexion and extension may be important.

The thoracic spinal canal varies between 17 and 22 mm in diameter. It is of interest that developmental narrowing in this region apparently does not take place with the same symptomatic impact as occurs when the sagittal diameter of the cervical or lumbar canal is affected.

The lumbar spinal canal varies in its sagittal diameter from 15 to 23 mm in the upper three lumbar segments, and from about 13 to 20 mm below this. Measurements are a little more difficult to obtain here than in the cervical region. However, a fairly good approximation can be had by measuring the height of the respective intervertebral foramina. In measuring the

sagittal diameter of the spinal canal in dried specimens a slight but definite difference is observed in the elevation of the cephalad and caudad aspects of the neural arches. The latter is tilted upwards and is approximately 3 to 5 mm higher than the cephalad margin, a situation which permits overlapping of the vertebral arches during movement. This results in some discrepancy in the measurements of specimens as contrasted with those made in patients. In addition, a 2- to 4-mm discrepancy occurs if measurements are made from the midportion of the hollow of the dorsal aspect of the vertebral bodies rather than from the upper or lower margins. A correlation exists between the configuration of the pedicles, the neural arches and the configuration of the lateral recesses of the spinal foramina. With narrowing of the sagittal diameter the pedicles tend to be heavier and the laminae converge towards the midline rather than splay apart. These are useful hints as to the available space in the canal (Fig. 36). It is important to realize that narrowing of the spinal canal, particularly in the lumbar region, may be quite marked in the lowermost two or three segments while above the canal has a normal configuration. Occasionally the midlumbar canal alone is narrowed.

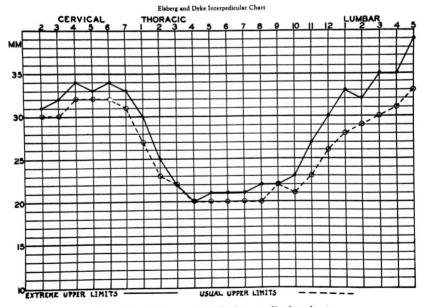

Fig. 35.   Elsberg and Dyke interpedicular chart.

TABLE 1. MEASUREMENT OF THE NORMAL INTERPEDICULAR SPACE IN THE CHILD
(From Landmesser, and Heublein, courtesy of Connecticut State Med. J.)

Age	Vertebra																
	Dorsal												Lumbar				
	1	2	3	4	5	6	7	8	9	10	11	12	1	2	3	4	5
1	16–20	14–19	13–17	13–17	13–17	13–17	13–17	14–17	14–17	14–17	14–17	15–19	15–20	17–20	17–20	18–22	19–23
2	17–21	14–19	14–17	14–16	14–16	14–16	13–17	13–17	14–19	14–19	15–19	15–20	17–21	18–21	18–22	19–22	21–26
3	17–22	16–19	14–18	14–17	14–17	15–17	15–17	15–18	15–18	16–19	16–20	18–22	19–22	19–23	19–23	20–25	20–27
4	19–23	16–21	15–19	15–19	15–19	14–19	14–19	15–19	15–19	15–19	16–21	19–23	20–23	19–23	19–23	19–25	23–28
5	20–24	17–21	15–20	15–19	15–19	15–19	15–19	15–19	15–19	15–19	18–20	18–24	18–24	19–25	19–25	23–26	24–29
6	20–24	16–21	16–19	15–19	15–19	15–19	15–19	15–20	15–20	15–20	17–21	19–24	20–24	20–26	21–26	21–28	22–29
7	20–26	17–23	15–21	15–20	15–19	15–19	15–19	15–20	15–20	16–20	17–21	19–24	21–25	21–26	22–27	23–29	25–32
8	19–26	16–22	15–20	15–19	15–19	15–19	15–20	15–21	15–21	16–21	17–22	19–24	20–25	21–25	22–27	23–27	26–32
9	20–26	17–21	16–20	16–20	16–19	15–19	15–19	15–20	15–20	16–21	17–21	20–24	21–25	22–26	23–27	23–27	25–31
10	23–26	18–22	17–21	16–20	15–19	15–19	15–20	15–21	15–21	17–21	18–21	19–25	21–26	23–26	23–27	24–29	26–32
11	21–25	18–22	16–21	16–21	16–20	16–19	16–20	16–21	16–21	17–21	18–22	21–25	22–26	22–26	23–27	24–28	24–32
12	19–26	17–23	15–21	15–20	15–20	15–19	15–19	16–20	16–21	17–21	17–22	21–25	21–26	22–26	23–27	24–29	24–32
13	21–26	18–23	16–21	15–21	15–20	15–20	16–20	15–21	15–21	15–21	16–22	18–25	20–27	21–27	22–29	23–30	25–32
14	22–27	18–23	17–21	16–21	16–20	16–20	16–20	16–20	16–21	17–21	17–23	20–25	22–26	22–27	22–28	23–29	28–35
15	22–27	18–23	17–21	16–20	16–20	15–20	15–20	15–21	15–21	16–22	18–24	21–26	23–27	23–27	24–28	24–30	26–34

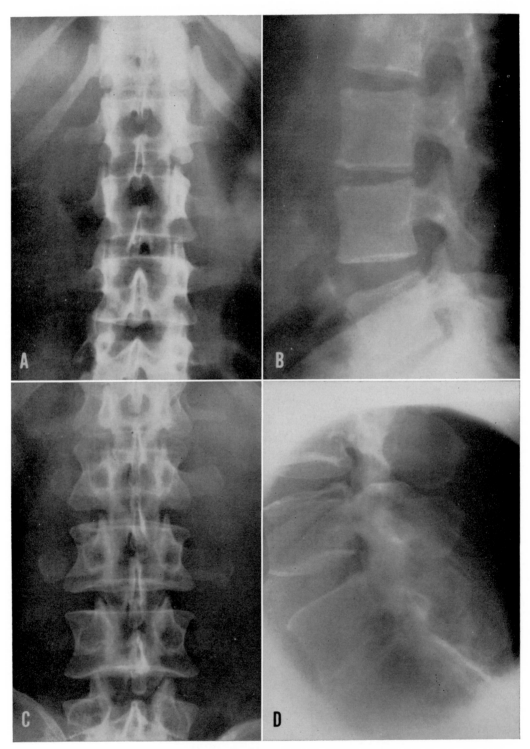

FIG. 36.   *See legend on facing page.*

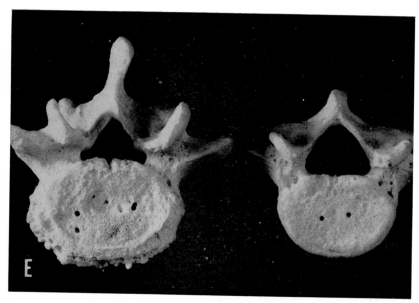

FIG. 36. *A,* AP view, normal lumbar spine with wide canal. The laminae are divergent and the pedicles are average. *B,* Lateral view shows the intervertebral foramina to be wide. *C,* AP view of lumbar spine with narrow canal. The pedicles are heavy and relatively closely spaced. The laminae are heavy and converge. *D,* Lateral view. The pedicles are short and the intervertebral foramina elongated and flattened. *E,* The spinal foramina of a narrow spinal canal is compared with a normal canal.

The normal range of measurements between the pedicles of the cervical, thoracic and lumbar vertebrae in adults was established by Elsberg and Dyke (1934) (Fig. 30). Upper and lower limits of normal were defined, and the usefulness of these determinations in evaluating localized widening of the spinal canal due to tumors is well known. Similar values were determined for infants and children by French and Peyton (1942), who published two sets of curves for infants from birth to 5 years of age and from 5 to 10 years. A more detailed survey was made by Simril and Thurston (1955). Landmesser and Heublein (1953) published a table of measurements in children from 1 to 15 years old (Table 1). Hinck, Clark and Hopkins (1966) reinvestigated this subject quite intensively, and reported on the normal interpedicular distances in children and adults. In general, the lower margin of their values is from about 2 to 4 mm below that shown by Elsberg and Dyke. These authors commented that their investigations indicated that congenital stenosis of the spinal canal in the sagittal diameter may or may not be associated with diminished interpedicular distances. In view of the importance of establishing an idea as to the available space in the spinal canal, it is apparent that diminished as well as increased interpedicular measurements are of considerable interest. On the other hand, localized enlargement of the spinal canal beyond the upper range on the Elsberg-Dyke chart is occasionally observed in the absence of any pathological change (Jefferson, 1955).

References

Arnell, S.: Myelography with Water Soluble Contrast. Acta radiol, Supp., *75,* 1948, Stockholm.

Boijsen, E.: The Cervical Spinal Canal in Intraspinal Expansive Processes. Acta radiol., *42,* 101, 1954.

Breig, A.: *Biomechanics of the Central Nervous System.* The Year Book Publishers, Chicago, 1960.

Breig, A. and Marions, O.: Biomechanics of the Lumbosacral Nerve Roots. Acta radiol., *1,* 1141–1160, 1963.

Burrows, E. H.: The Sagittal Diameter of the Spinal Canal in Cervical Spondylosis, Clinical Radiol., *14,* 77–86, 1963.

Djindjian, R., Fauré, C. and Hueth, M.: *Explora-tions Artériographiques des Anéurysmes Artério-veineux della Moelle Épinière.* Les Monographies des Annales de Radiologie. Expansion Scientifique Française, Paris, 1966.

Elsberg, C. A. and Dyke, C. G.: Diagnosis and Localization of Tumors of Spinal Cord by Means of Measurements Made on X-ray Films of Verte-brae, and the Correlation of Clinical and X-ray Findings. Bull. Neurol. Inst. New York, *3*, 359, 1934.

Epstein, B. S.: Effect of Increased Pressure on the Movement of Iodized Oil within the Spinal Canal. Am. J. Roentgenol., *52*, 196, 1944.

————: The Myelographic Demonstration of the Anterior Spinal and Radicular Arteries. Am. J. Roentgenol., *91*, 427–430, 1964.

————: An Anatomic, Myelographic and Cine-myelographic Study of the Dentate Ligaments, Am. J. Roentgenol., *98*, 704, 1966.

Epstein, B. S., Epstein, J. A. and Lavine, L.: The Effect of Anatomic Variations in the Lumbar Vertebrae and Spinal Canal on Cauda Equina and Nerve Root Syndromes. Am. J. Roentgenol., *91*, 1055–1063, 1964.

Epstein, J. A., Epstein, B. S. and Lavine, L.: Cervical Spondylotic Myelopathy. Arch. Neurol., *8*, 307, 1963.

Hinck, V. C., Clark, W. M. and Hopkins, C. E.: Normal Interpedicular Distances (Minimum and Maximum) in Children and Adults. Am. J. Roentgenol., *97*, 141–153, 1966.

Hinck, V. C., Hopkins, C. E. and Clark, W. M.: Sagittal Diameter of the Lumbar Spinal Canal in Children and Adults. Radiology, *85*, 929–937, 1965.

Hinck, V. C., Hopkins, C. E. and Savara, B. S.: Sagittal Diameter of the Cervical Spinal Canal in Children. Radiology, *79*, 97–108, 1962.

Jefferson, A.: Localized Enlargement of the Spinal Canal in the Absence of Tumor: A Congenital Abnormality. J. Neurol., Neurosurg. & Psychiat., *18*, 305–309, 1955.

Jirout, J.: Mobility of the Thoracic Spinal Cord Under Normal Conditions. Acta radiol., *1*, 729–735, 1963.

Kahn, E. A.: Role of Dentate Ligaments in Spinal Cord Compression and the Syndrome of Lateral Sclerosis. J. Neurosurg., *4*, 191, 1947.

Landmesser, W. E. and Heublein, G. W.: Measure-ment of the Normal Interpedicular Space in the Child, Connecticut M. J., *17*, 310, 1953.

Locke, G. R., Gardner, J. I. and Van Epps, E. F.: Atlas-dens Interval (ADI) in Children. A Survey Based on 200 Normal Cervical Spines. Am. J. Roentgenol., *97*, 135–140, 1966.

Mayfield, F.: Symposium on Cervical Trauma: Neurosurgical Aspects. Clin. Neurosurg., *2*, 83, 1955.

Porter, E. C.: Measurement of the Cervical Spinal Cord in Pantopaque Myelography. Am. J. Roentgenol., *76*, 270–272, 1956.

Retan, H.: Movements of Fluid Inside Cerebro-spinal Space. Acta radiol., *22*, 762, 1941.

Scoville, W. B.: Cervical Spondylosis Treated by Bilateral Facetectomy and Laminectomy. J. Neu-rosurg., *18*, 423, 1961.

Simril, W. A. and Thurston, D.: The Normal Interpediculate Space in the Spines of Infants and Children. Radiology, *64*, 340, 1955.

Stoltmann, H. F. and Blackwood, W.: An Anatom-ical Study of the Role of the Dentate Ligaments in the Cervical Spinal Canal. J. Neurosurg., *24*, 43–46, 1966.

Teng, P.: Myelographic Identification of the Den-tate Ligament. Radiology, *74*, 944–946, 1960.

————: Ligamentum Denticulatum. (An ana-tomical review and its role in various neurosurgical problems of the spinal cord.) J. Mt. Sinai Hosp., *32*, 567–577, 1965.

Turnbull, I. M., Breig, A. and Hassler, O.: Blood Supply of Cervical Spinal Cord in Man. A micro-angiographic Cadaver Study. J. Neurosurg., *24*, 951–965, 1966.

Wolf, B. S., Khilnani, M. and Malis, L. I.: Sagittal Diameter of the Bony Cervical Spinal Canal and its Significance in Cervical Spondylosis. J. Mt. Sinai Hosp., *23*, 283, 1956.

Radiologic Examination of the Normal Spine

THE CERVICAL SPINE

The technic involved in achieving a sharp, detailed study of the cervical spine in an infant or child is more difficult than in the older child or adult. The cervical spine in infants is examined by means of recumbent anteroposterior and lateral views. In the lateral projection it has been found helpful to extend the child's neck manually, and simultaneously to bring the arms as far dorsally as possible with the shoulders drawn down. In this position, the entire cervical spine and sometimes the upper thoracic vertebrae are brought into view. The study is made with an extension cylin-der cone at $\frac{1}{60}$ of a second, without the Bucky diaphragm, using screens of the finest definition. Unless specifically needed for some unusual possibility, oblique and flexion and extension studies are not re-quired (Fig. 37).

In young children, adolescents and adults, the technic of examination of the cervical spine is varied according to the information desired. Study is directed towards visual-ization of the vertebral bodies, the inter-vertebral discs and foramina, the apophyseal

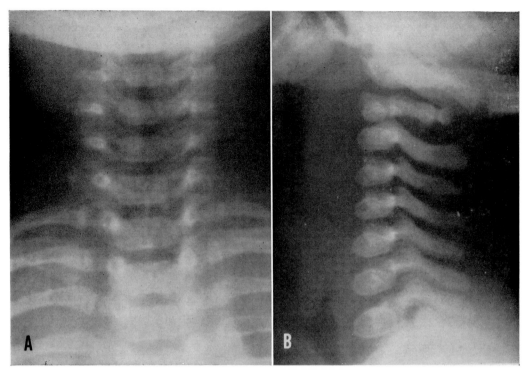

FIG. 37. *A,* Normal infant cervical spine. The pedicles are widely spaced, normal in this age group. *B,* Lateral neck. The vertebral bodies are rounded and the canal is wide. The dens is attached to the body of C2 by a cartilaginous band.

joints, the transverse and spinous processes and the paravertebral soft tissues, utilizing anteroposterior views, special studies for the atlantoaxial articulation, right and left oblique views and lateral views in the neutral position and laminagrams in flexion and in extension as required (Figs. 15, 38, 39, 40). Clinical judgment should be exercised in the selection of those projections required to answer a specific question.

Inasmuch as the present volume does not undertake to present radiologic technic in detail, no attempt is made to provide such information. Suffice it to say that the interpretation of roentgenograms of the spine rests upon a foundation of proper technic, and films that are poorly exposed, made with the patient in motion or in improper position may lead to diagnostic error. The importance of stereoroentgenographic views often is insufficiently recognized. These studies provide a three-dimensional index for the separation of bony shadows. The disadvantages of additional time and expense is well compensated for by the additional information available. Laminagraphic examinations of the cervical spine are helpful, especially in visualization of the atlantoaxial articulation and the first and second cervical segments, particularly the odontoid process. Better visualization of the atlas and axis can be obtained by keeping the mandible in motion during the roentgenographic exposure (Fig. 39) (Ottonello, 1930), the principle being that continued motion of the mandible during a rather long exposure eliminates its shadow, leaving the upper cervical spine in sharper relief. A similar benefit can be obtained on thoracic roentgenograms taken while the patient is breathing quietly, so that rib shadows are blurred out.

In newborn infants, the odontoid process is cartilaginous and hence not visible. Its

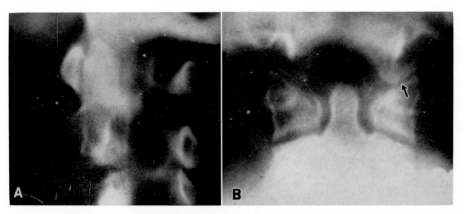

Fig. 38. Lateral (*A*) and anteroposterior (*B*) body section roentgenograms of first and second cervical vertebrae. Note articulation of atlas with cranial occipital condyles (*arrow*).

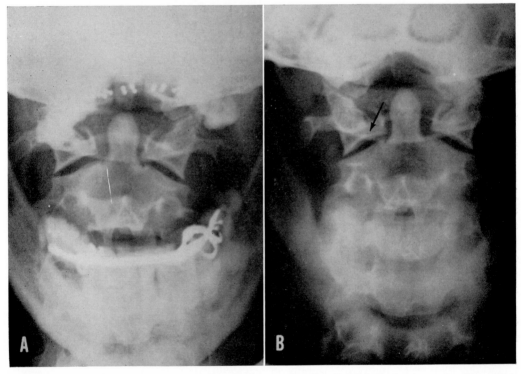

Fig. 39. *A*, AP study of atlas and axis through the open mouth. *B*, With the jaw in motion (Ottonello's technic) the upper cervical vertebrae are better seen. A pseudonotch is visible in the supramedial aspect of the lateral masses of C1 (arrow).

absence should cause no doubt. In later infancy and early childhood, as the odontoid begins to calcify, its structural characteristics become manifest. These are seen as a ventral, split bar in the 2nd and 3rd year of life delineated from the anterosuperior aspect of the body of the second cervical vertebra by a thin line of cartilage. The tip of the odontoid is cleft by a small V-shaped defect (Figs. 40, 41), which later is occupied by a calcified epiphysis which ultimately fuses with the mass of the dens. Considerable variability exists in the size and shape of the apical odontoid epiphysis. The

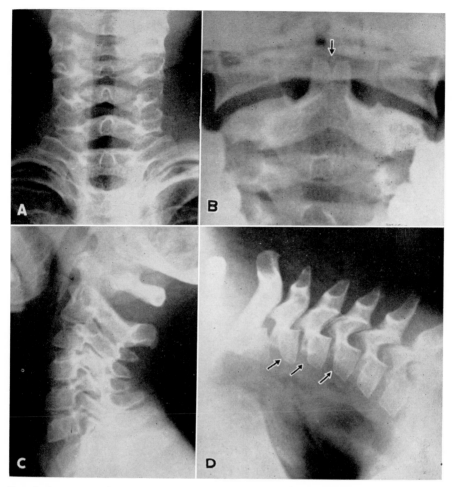

Fig. 40. *A,* Anteroposterior view of cervical spine of normal 5-year-old child. *B,* Atlas and axis. Note cleft in dens, with small center of ossification in midline (*arrow*). *C,* Lateral view. *D,* Lateral view in flexion. Note range of motion of vertebral bodies and their spinous processes. The anterosuperior aspects of the bodies are rounded (*arrows*).

vertical cleft between the two lateral masses of the odontoid occasionally persists into adolescence (Figs. 41, 42), while the cartilage between the base of the dens and the subjacent body of the second cervical vertebra may be visible up to about the age of 10 years. This sometimes is mistaken for a fracture, particularly when observed in the anteroposterior or lateral views as a thin radiolucent line. However, when this line is sclerotic no difficulty is encountered.

The articulations between the occipital condyles and the first cervical vertebra can best be demonstrated in the anteroposterior position by means of laminagrams. These cup-like articulations also are visible on films made with the patient's mouth open. The superior facets of the body of the first cervical vertebra can be observed on lateral neck roentgenograms. Under ordinary circumstances these may vary in the angle of inclination from about 30 to 60 degrees (Fig. 38). Delineation of this region is important in the demonstration of congenital malformations of the craniovertebral junction.

The relationship between the articular surfaces of the first and second cervical

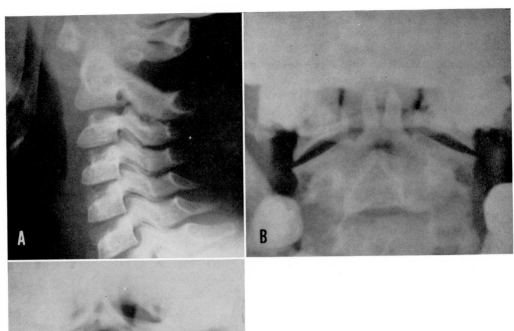

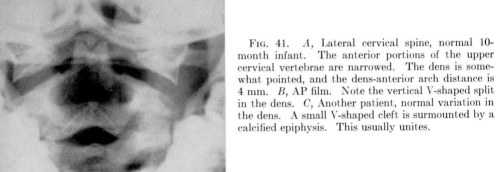

Fig. 41. A, Lateral cervical spine, normal 10-month infant. The anterior portions of the upper cervical vertebrae are narrowed. The dens is somewhat pointed, and the dens-anterior arch distance is 4 mm. B, AP film. Note the vertical V-shaped split in the dens. C, Another patient, normal variation in the dens. A small V-shaped cleft is surmounted by a calcified epiphysis. This usually unites.

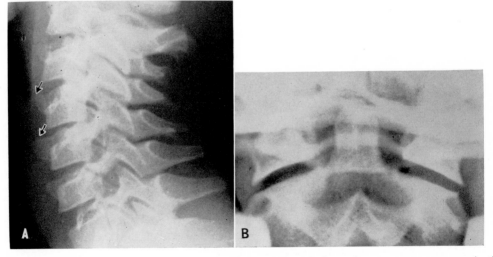

Fig. 42. A, Normal cervical spine in 12-year-old child. Note shadows of transverse processes projecting in front of vertebral bodies (arrows). B, Same patient, anteroposterior view of atlas and axis. Thin white streak in midportion of dens represents line of ossification.

vertebrae is of interest. In the normal individual these edges are in correct anatomic position when they are in the same line. However, if the head is turned forcibly to the right or left side, or if there is a pronounced spasm of the occipito-cervical muscular groups, it is not uncommon for the edge of one articular surface of the first cervical vertebra to be shifted laterally for 2 to 3 mm, while the opposite one overlies the articular surface beneath by about the same distance. Caution should be exercised in interpreting such variations from the normal as dislocations (Fig. 15). As seen in the lateral projection, the tip of the odontoid process may rest at the level of the superior portion of the anterior arch of the first vertebral body, or may be slightly above or beneath it, and space between the articular surfaces varies from 2 to 4 mm and is somewhat increased during flexion. In children, films made in extension sometimes show an apparent overriding of the anterior arch of the atlas on the dens. This probably is caused by a lack of calcification of the

distal tip of the dens, rendering this structure invisible on the roentgenogram. The relationship between the tip of the odontoid process and the base of the skull is useful in the diagnosis of basilar impression. A line drawn between the dorsal aspect of the hard palate and the posterior rim of the foramen magnum (Chamberlain's line) passes above the odonotid tip under normal conditions. If the odontoid extends above this line some degree of basilar invagination presumably is present.

Occasionally a variable radiolucent notch-like shadow appears in the medial portion of the articular mass of the atlas. This "pseudonotch" is formed medially (Fig. 39) by the margin of the medial tubercle of the lateral mass which is continuous inferiorly with the articular surface of the inferior articular facet, and laterally by the concavity of the superior facet. This formation is attributed in part to the nutrient artery entering the atlas just posterior to the medial tubercle (Meghrouni and Jacobson, 1959). Another variable structure of anatomic interest is the

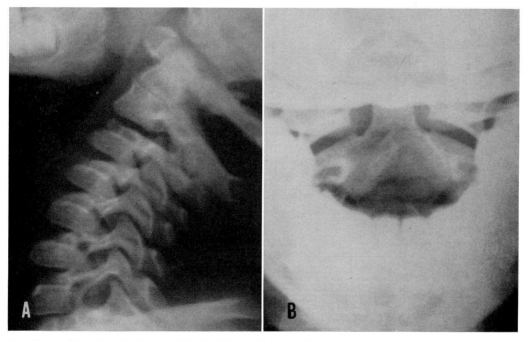

Fig. 43. *A*, Lateral neck, 11-year-old girl with a radiolucent linear zone at the base of the dens. *B*, Open mouth view again shows the radiolucent line.

presence of an anomalous ossification center in the oblique atlantooccipital ligaments. When this calcifies, a bony arch is formed which encloses the sulcus for the vertebral artery, and through which the vertebral artery and the suboccipital nerve pass (Fig. 44). Pyo and Lowman (1959) found this to be present in 12.6 per cent of normal skulls. In 4 per cent of 300 skull roentgenograms this structure was unilateral. In some instances complete arching was present while in others the fusion was incomplete. A wide range of anatomic variation in the "ponticulus posticus" is found.

In the lateral projection, the anteroinferior aspect of the second cervical vertebra frequently overlaps the corresponding superior surface of the body of the third cervical vertebra. Similar change of lesser degree may be observed between the third and fourth, fourth and fifth and sometimes between the fifth and the sixth cervical segments. The tips of the transverse processes of the cervical segments overlap the anterior aspects of the bodies of the cervical vertebrae and the respective intervertebral discs (Fig. 40). These overlapping shadows are apparent on oblique as well as lateral roentgen-

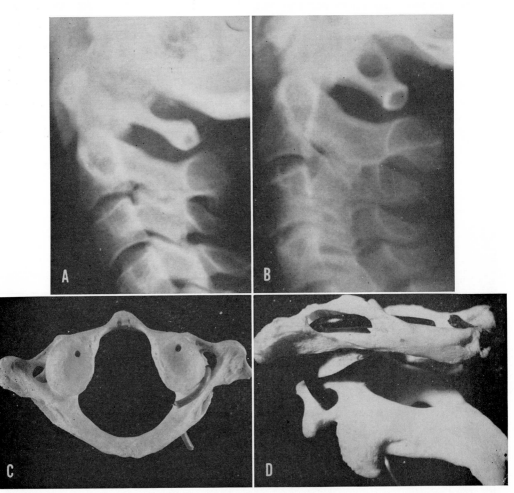

FIG. 44. *A*, A small calcareous linear deposit is seen in the oblique antlantooccipital ligament just above the lamina of C1. *B*, Complete calcification in this ligament, forming a foramen through which the vertebral artery and suboccipital nerve pass (ponticulus posticus). *C*, Cranial view of 1st cervical vertebra. A wire is threaded along the groove for the vertebral artery. *D*, Another specimen with a complete ponticulus posticus. A wire is threaded through the foramina transversaria and the ponticulus.

ograms of the cervical spine. The foramen transversarium of the second cervical vertebral transverse process overlying the anterior aspect of the inferior margin of the second cervical vertebrae is often visible (Fig. 45), but the corresponding foramina of the transverse processes of the third, fourth, fifth and sixth cervical vertebrae cannot be seen on lateral or oblique views. The size of the foramina transversaria of the first cervical vertebra can be demonstrated on roentgenograms taken for the base of the skull. This, and the second foramen transversarium are useful in attempting to estimate its condition when associated with dilatation of the vertebral arteries, as, for example, arteriovenous malformations in the posterior cranial fossa which derive a large blood supply from the vertebral arteries. The intervertebral foramina are best observed on oblique roentgenograms, preferably right and left anterior oblique stereoroentgenographic studies. On these the foramina on the same side near the film are visualized. An additional unfused ossification center and epiphysis occasionally is identified on the inferior lamina of a cervical

vertebrae or a spinal process. A small accessory bone occasionally appears beneath the anterior arch of the atlas as well, best seen on lateral films. These should not be misinterpreted as fractures.

The relative positions of the cervical vertebral bodies in flexion and extension vary considerably, depending largely upon the body habitus and muscular propensities of the individual. Thus, a patient with a long slender neck may show a much greater degree of movement in flexion and extension than a stocky individual with a short neck. During flexion and extension the articular facets of the cervical vertebrae glide forwards and backwards, resulting in relatively smooth spinal curves. The range of sliding of the cervical facets is progressively more pronounced in the articulations between the second and third, the third and fourth, the fourth and fifth and sometimes in the fifth and sixth neural arches (Fig. 46). The variations which take place under certain conditions are striking. In patients who have had muscular injuries the usual cervical lordotic curve may be straightened, and the range of motion considerably lim-

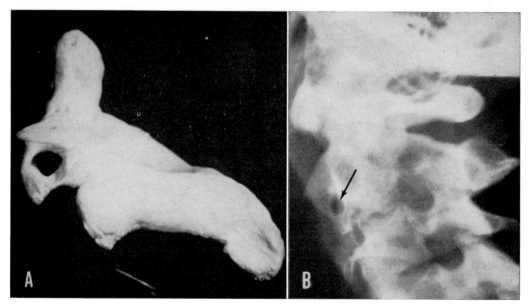

FIG. 45. *A*, Specimen of normal second cervical vertebra in oblique position to demonstrate the foramen transversarium. *B*, Oblique upper cervical spine film with the foramen transversarium brought into view (arrow).

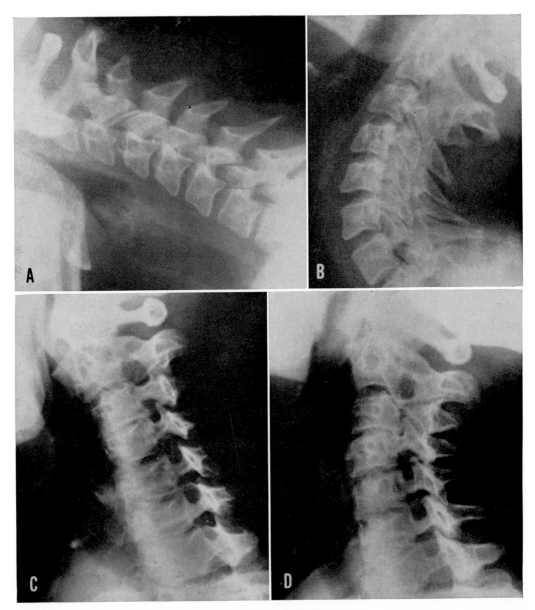

Fig. 46. *A*, Cervical spine, extreme flexion with mild restriction of movement of midcervical segments. *B*, the range of extension is normal. *C*, Oblique film with head slightly flexed. The intervertebral foramen between C3 and 4 is impinged upon by a spur. *D*, With the head in extension and rotated the intervertebral foramina between C2, 3 and 4 are markedly altered. There were no symptoms associated with this change in position.

ited. Forward placement of one of the upper cervical vertebrae on the subjacent vertebra occasionally is so striking that a diagnosis of subluxation is made erroneously. The effect of muscle spasm on the alignment of the cervical vertebrae is such that pronounced changes in movement and alignment at rest may simulate gross changes in anatomic position. Absence of the normal lordotic curve, apparent changes in alignment of the upper cervical vertebrae, apparent changes in the range of motion of the neck as seen on lateral roentgenograms all may be encountered in normal individuals (Figs. 18 and 19).

The shapes of the cervical vertebral bodies differ in infancy, adolescence and adult life. In infants the anterior margins tend to be rounded, so that the vertebral bodies present a somewhat ovoid appearance (Fig. 37). This is less apparent in childhood, but some flattening and rounding of the antero-superior aspects of the cervical vertebrae, particularly in the midcervical region, may be quite prominent (Fig. 43). Later in life the vertebral bodies are rather square in appearance, but downward inclination of the anterosuperior surfaces persists (Fig. 46).

The sagittal diameter of the infant spinal canal is large in relationship to the size of the vertebral bodies. Measured from the neuro-central synchondrosis to the apex of the neural arch at the base of the spinous processes, the average depth in the newborn infant to about 3 months of age is approximately 1.0 cm. The transverse measurement exceeds this, and at times the apparent widening of the interpedicular spaces in infancy is deceptive, so much so that occasionally one is tempted to consider the possibility of a congenital malformation such as a meningocele. The neural arches usually are united early in infancy. With growth of the child the dimensions of the spinal canal increase slowly in comparison to the growth of the vertebra itself.

In infants and children, and sometimes in adults as well, the transverse processes are directed anteriorly, and project over the intervertebral discs (Figs. 41 and 43), simulating discal calcifications.

In the lateral projection, the position of the spinous processes sometimes help indicate restriction or unusual degrees of mobility of the cervical spine. Normally with the head in extension, the tips of the spinous processes of the middle cervical vertebrae are practically in opposition to each other. In flexion, separation of the spinous processes occurs. Their tips present characteristic configurations, that of the second being bul-

bous and prominent, the third, fourth and fifth being shorter and smaller, the sixth larger in size, while the seventh is the most prominent of the group. The tips of the spinous processes not infrequently are bifid and irregular. On routine roentgenograms of the cervical spine, these structures may be obliterated by overpenetration because of their relative thinness. However, this can be overcome by viewing the films through a bright light. If structural changes are suspected, underexposed roentgenograms prove helpful. The spinous processes may be identified on anteroposterior films as tear-shaped shadows with calcific rims lying in the midline at a point beneath the inferior margin of the vertebra of origin (Fig. 24).

The cervical nerves occupy about 20 to 25 per cent of the available area of their respective intervertebral foramina. The remainder of the space is filled by fatty tissue, lymphatics and blood vessels. With the neck in the neutral or flexed position, the intervertebral foramina are fairly large, but in extension they decrease in size as the gliding surfaces of the articular facets pass over each other as inclined planes. This is most pronounced in the midcervical region, where the range of motion is greatest.

THE THORACIC SPINE

The thoracic spine in infants is usually seen adequately on lateral roentgenograms of the chest, and should be scrutinized as part of such examinations. Incomplete fusion of the spinous processes of the upper dorsal segments is seen until about 6 months of age and is of no pathologic importance. At birth the thoracic and lumbar vertebrae are rather rounded. The superior and inferior aspects of the vertebral bodies are more densely calcified than the intermediate area in most instances (Fig. 47), but occasionally the periphery is fairly densely calcified and contains a small, central core which represents the ossification center (Fig. 48B). The anterior aspect of the vertebral bodies is indented in its midportion by the opening

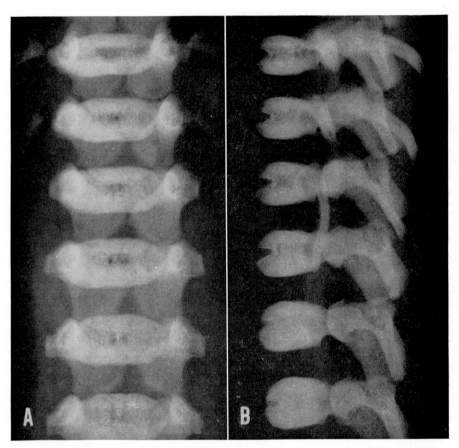

Fig. 47. *A*, AP view, normal thoracolumbar spine of a newborn infant. The neural arches are ununited and the pedicles are widely spaced. The vertebral bodies are ovoid in configuration. The radiolucent focus in the center of each body represents vascular channels in the cancellous bone. *B*, The grooves for the anterior spinal veins are prominent. Increased density at the upper and lower aspects of the vertebral bodies is normal. The spinal canal is wide, exceeding the AP diameter of the adjacent vertebral bodies.

for the vertebral vein. Similar openings are present on the dorsal surfaces, either as a single or more often as a double opening (Fig. 48). The dorsal vascular channels persist into adult life, and often can be identified on body section roentgenograms as somewhat funnel-shaped structures opening into the dorsal aspect of the vertebral bodies (Fig. 49). The neurocentral synchondroses are prominent at birth, and unite with the centrums at about 3 or 4 years of age.

Examination of the thoracic spine is usually accomplished by anteroposterior and lateral roentgenograms. Stereoscopic views are advised when detail of the pedicles or the neural arches is desired. In addition, it is

sometimes advantageous to obtain oblique roentgenograms when information concerning the costovertebral articulations or the articular facets is required. In obtaining the anteroposterior views of the thoracic spine, the influence of the difference in the anteroposterior diameter of the lower half of the chest compared with the upper half must be taken into account. It is sometimes advisable to use wedge filters, or to obtain studies of the upper and lower halves of the thoracic spine on separate films. Cone-down roentgenograms for the sharpest possible detail are desirable. Lateral roentgenograms of the thoracic spine usually visualizes the third to the tenth dorsal ver-

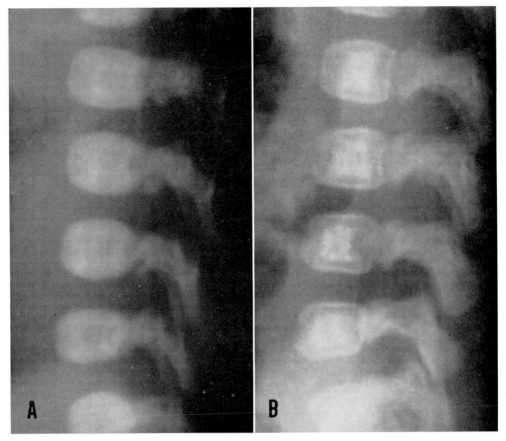

FIG. 48. *A*, Lateral newborn spine. Calcification is proceeding beneath the cartilaginous plates. The openings for the anterior and posterior vascular channels are indistinct. *B*, Another newborn spine with a calcific center of ossification in the middle of each vertebral body.

tebrae adequately. Special technics are required for proper demonstration of the first, second and third thoracic vertebrae. In such studies a modified oblique projection is utilized, the lower cervical and upper dorsal segments being seen through the thoracic inlet. Lateral laminagrams of the upper thoracic vertebrae sometimes portray these structures to better advantage. In the evaluation of the lower thoracic segments, one must consider the relative position of the diaphragm and the abdominal viscera. If these overlap the lower dorsal vertebrae, a technic which shows the middle thoracic vertebrae will be too light, and additional views coning down over the thoracolumbar segments are required.

The intervertebral foramina of the dorsal spine are relatively smaller and are rounder than those in the cervical or lumbar regions. Relatively little adipose tissue is present in these intervertebral foramina, inasmuch as the nerve roots in this area are less mobile.

Beginning at approximately the 6th year of life a ring apophysis appears on the superior and inferior surfaces of the middle and lower thoracic vertebrae and the upper three or four lumbar vertebrae. Less frequently such apophyses also appear in the cervical and upper thoracic regions. These occur as incomplete thin rims of bone slightly apart from the vertebrae, visible both in the lateral and the anteroposterior views. Ossification of these structures is most pronounced at about the age of 13 years, and fusion with the vertebral

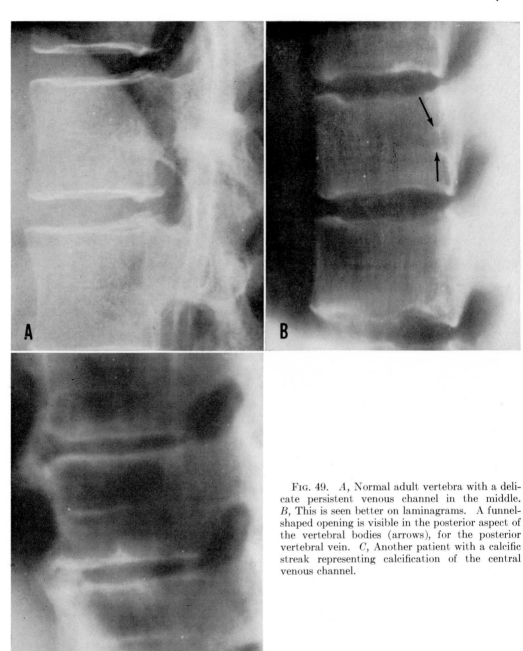

Fig. 49. *A*, Normal adult vertebra with a delicate persistent venous channel in the middle. *B*, This is seen better on laminagrams. A funnel-shaped opening is visible in the posterior aspect of the vertebral bodies (arrows), for the posterior vertebral vein. *C*, Another patient with a calcific streak representing calcification of the central venous channel.

bodies occurs by the time the patient reaches the age of 18. These structures lie outside the true vertebral epiphyseal plates and are unassociated with the growth of the vertebral body itself (Fig. 22).

Inspection of the paravertebral regions on anteroposterior roentgenograms of the thoracic spine is important. To the left one can frequently observe a line of increased density which extends from the fourth to approximately the level of the tenth or eleventh thoracic vertebra. This line represents the reflection of the medial pleura of the left lung (Fig. 50). It should be differentiated from the lateral margin of the descending thoracic aorta which usually follows a more oblique course, situated laterally in the upper and medially in the lower aspect as it approaches the aortic hiatus of the diaphragm. This line sometimes indicates, by change in its position, disease of the adjacent spine such as osteomyelitis, tumor, hematoma, or occasionally, pleural effusion. In the lower right hemithorax, because of the shelving characteristics of the posteromedial aspect of the lung due to the azygos vein, the right posteromedial pleural line is usually not as apparent, and may be continuous with the psoas shadow below the right crus of the diaphragm.

THE LUMBOSACRAL SPINE AND COCCYX

During the newborn period, the bodies of the lumbar vertebrae present a somewhat biconvex appearance with slightly lower or straight anterior and posterior walls (Fig. 47). In some, the remnants of a center of ossification is seen in the middle of the spongiosa of the centrum while the peripheries are thin and sharply defined. In others, superior and inferior plates of dense bone are separated by less densely calcified spongiosum (Fig. 48). Fissures at the middle of the anterior and posterior aspects of the middle and lower thoracic vertebrae and the upper lumbar vertebral bodies correspond to sinusoidal venous reservoirs (Fig. 49). The neurocentral arches are incompletely fused, the pedicles are relatively heavy and the laminae are well formed but are poorly seen because they are still largely cartilaginous. The spinous processes, being unossified, cannot be demonstrated.

On lateral views there is usually a slight lumbar curve convex anteriorly at the lumbosacral junction. The intervertebral discs are relatively large and are wider at their anterior and posterior aspects. The intervertebral foramina likewise are quite large. The intervertebral discs increase in width slightly from the upper to the lower lumbar areas. I have not seen narrowing of the lumbosacral interspace in the normal newborn. The sagittal diameter of the spinal canal is wider than that of the vertebral bodies. Average measurements are 1 cm for the vertebral bodies and 1.0 to 1.3 cm for the canal at the midlumbar level (Fig. 48).

The bodies of the sacral vertebrae are separated from each other by intervertebral discs which are better identified on lateral than on frontal roentgenograms. In the newborn period the transverse processes may

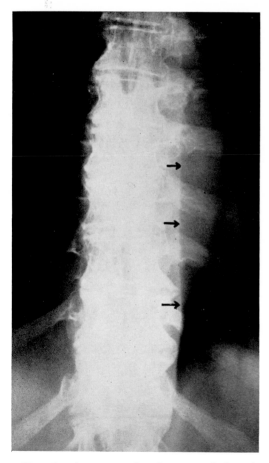

FIG. 50. Anteroposterior view, normal thoracic spine. Left paravertebral pleural reflection line (arrows) lies medial to arcuate shadow of descending thoracic aorta.

be unfused with the vertebral bodies. The first segment of the coccyx is ossified at birth, but the remaining components usually are not visible. The dorsal plate of the sacrum, corresponding to the neural arches, can be identified on lateral films, and likewise are separated by radiolucent cartilaginous bands.

During childhood lumbar vertebrae ossify slowly. By approximately the 3rd to 4th year of life, the neurocentral synchondroses fuse with the vertebral bodies. Ossification of the neural arch proceeds so that articular facets and laminae become increasingly visible because of the increased calcium content. The spinous processes likewise begin to appear radiologically, and are visible by the time the 5th or 6th year has been reached. The anterior sinusoidal venous channels gradually vanish, while their posterior counterparts may remain visible well into adult life (Fig. 49).

Radiologic examination of the lumbar spine from childhood to old age is accom-

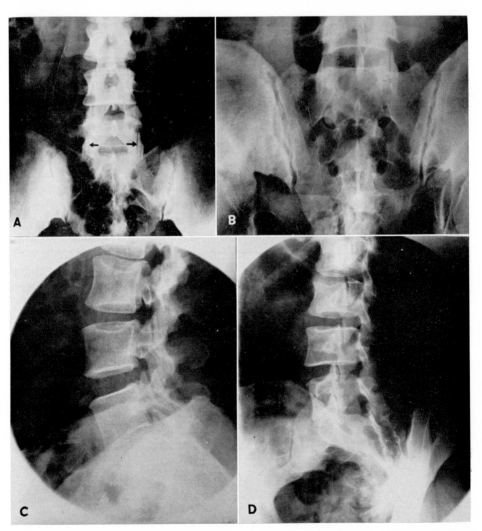

Fig. 51. *A*, Anteroposterior view, lumbosacral articulation, normal adult spine. Note vertical position of articular facets (arrows). *B*, 45 degree tilt-up view. *C*, Lateral conedown view of lumbosacral articulation. *D*, Posterior oblique view showing articular facets. The right posterior projection brings out the right articular facets.

plished in a variety of ways, each designed to provide information concerning some specific point. A routine roentgenographic examination should consist of anteroposterior and lateral views, and when indicated, oblique views for demonstration of the articular facets and the neural arches (Fig. 51). If information concerning the mobility of the spine is required, studies may be made in the erect frontal views with the patient bending sharply towards the right and left side for demonstration of change in the interspaces between the various lumbar vertebrae. Additional lateral studies should be made in flexion and extension. A variety of views have been proposed for examination of the lumbosacral articulation, sacrum and sacro-iliac joints. This is best accomplished by means of cone-down roentgenograms in the lateral and oblique projections, centering on the lumbosacral articulation or mid-sacrum as required and with "tilt up" views

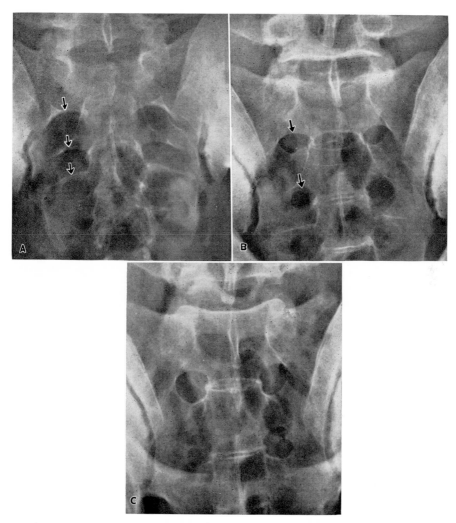

Fig. 52. A, Direct anteroposterior view of normal adult lumbosacral junction. The sacral foramina are foreshortened, and their superior rims are presented as rather dense lines (arrows). B, Tilt-up view with beam directed 30 degrees towards patient's head. The lumbosacral joint is better visualized, and the sacral foramina are projected as oval structures (arrows). C, 45-degree tilt-up view. The upper two sacral foramina are practically circular. Note the difference in the appearance of the sacro-iliac joints on the three projections.

of the sacrum and lumbosacral joints in the anteroposterior position. The latter have to be made with consideration of the configuration of the sacrum in the particular individual (Fig. 52). Usually, it is possible to obtain a study of the sacrum in which the intervertebral foramina are rendered as circular or almost circular shadows if the tube is tilted 15 to 25 degrees towards the patient's head with the central ray passing through the body of the first sacral vertebra. Stereoscopic views of the lumbosacral spine and the sacrum are helpful in identifying areas of altered bony density. Laminagraphic studies are also useful, particularly in demonstrating the neural arches (Fig. 53) and small areas of bone destruction. Laminagrams of the lumbosacral joint and sacrum in the lateral view portray the dorsal and ventral walls of the sacral canal to better advantage than can be observed on straight films. Anteroposterior laminagrams of the sacrum and of the sacro-iliac joints may prove informative.

The configuration of the spinal foramina of lumbar vertebrae has clinical importance. The first and second lumbar vertebral canals are rather triangular, with the lateral aspects well rounded. The last three lumbar vertebral foramina tend more to a pentagonal configuration, but their heights are less than the upper two. Measurements made on lateral roentgenograms indicate that the average height of the first two lumbar spinal foramina is approximately 14 to 22 mm, while the lower three is between 13 and 20 mm. From the clinical viewpoint the dimensions of the lateral recesses of the spinal canal are significant because it is here that diminished space increases the possibility of nerve root compression. Unfortunately, these areas cannot be measured, but some inference as to the available space can be made by determining the sagittal measurement of the lumbar canal. If significantly narrowed, particularly in the lowermost two lumbar segments, where a measurement of less than 13 mm is significant, the effects of

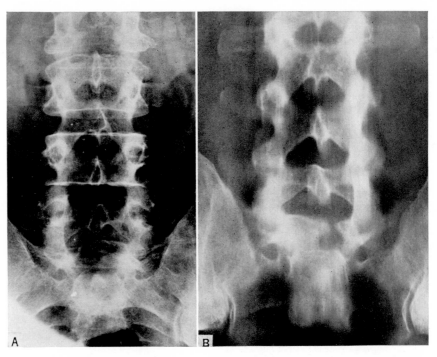

Fig. 53. *A*, Anteroposterior roentgenogram of lumbar spine. Incomplete fusion of spinous process of L5. *B*, Body section roentgenogram. The neural arches are sharply in focus, and the malformation of the spinous process of L5 is better seen.

spondylotic ridges or discal herniations may be augmented (Fig. 17).

Examination of the neural arches is helpful in evaluating the configuration of the spinal foramina. In the presence of congenital narrowing in the sagittal plane there is a definite tendency for the laminae to be heavy and for the posterior aspects of the neural arches to be directed medially. The distal portions of the posterior articular facets are bulbous and rounded, so that they come quite close to the spinous processes. The pedicles are heavy, rounded, and the interpedicular spaces are somewhat narrowed so that the measurements are at the lower range or slightly less than average. This tendency is increased later in life when superimposed spondylotic changes produce thickening of the neural arches. As a consequence of the structural variations the lateral recesses of the spinal foramina are constricted so that the available space for passage of the respective nerve roots is diminished (Fig. 54) here and in the intervertebral foramina.

A study of the lumbosacral articulation alone could well be the subject of a monograph. The numerous variations discovered as incidental findings during roentgenographic examinations made for purposes other than investigation of the lumbosacral spine indicate that many anatomic variations exist in this area without clinical evidence of impairment of spine function. However some observers have come to other conclusions as to the significance of minor lumbosacral articulation malformations. Howard (1942) mentioned that symmetrical articulations of the lumbosacral apophyseal joints may predispose to back pain. Ferguson (1934) stated that sagittal positions of the articular facets of the fourth and fifth lumbar vertebrae and fifth lumbar and first sacral vertebrae were advantageous from a mechanical point of view, while an anteroposterior position (coronal articular facets) was a predisposing factor to weakness of the structural function of the lower lumbar spine and might be a causative factor in the production of pain. He was of the opinion that

mixed or asymmetrical articular facets in the lumbosacral spine predisposes many people to pain because of structural weakness. The incidence of pain was found to be more frequent in those with narrow lumbosacral interspaces in a ratio of 4.5 to 1 by Hodges and Peck (1937). In individuals with low back pain developmental anomalies in the lumbosacral region occurred with an increased frequency of 2 to 1. On the other hand, Mitchell (1934) mentioned that asymmetry of articular facets of the lumbosacral spine was favorable in that it permitted a certain degree of rotation, whereas purely sagittal or coronal arrangements prevented such movement. It was his opinion that arrangement of articular facets in a coronal plane caused these to impinge upon one another so that any tendency towards forward slip was inhibited. Pheasant and Swenson (1942) concluded that the lumbosacral articulations in normal individuals were arranged most frequently in an oblique or coronal plane. Purely oblique or sagittal planes of articulation were not encountered. Roentgenologically the facets may appear to be situated coronally or sagittally (Fig. 55) depending on which component predominates. They concluded that asymmetry of the lumbosacral region occurs in approximately one quarter of all human spines, varying in degree, and accompanied by alterations in force transmission of varying significance.

Narrowing of the lumbosacral interspace in itself is not necessarily significant. It has also been my experience that location of the lumbosacral articular facets in an oblique or sagittal plane does not indicate the cause of a patient's complaints. A review of a long series of spine studies in patients admitted for conditions other than back pain, showed that many normal individuals have minor congenital variations at the lumbosacral articulation. I do not, therefore, regard the demonstration of a narrowed lumbosacral interspace or to variation in articular facets between the fourth and fifth lumbar and fifth lumbar and first sacral segments as a

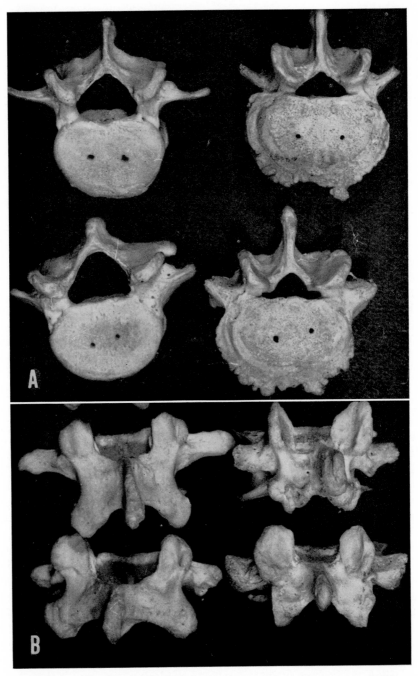

Fig 54. *A*, Fourth and fifth lumbar vertebrae with a normal and a narrow canal. *B*, The neural arches of the normal vertebrae have divergent laminae, those of the specimen with a narrow canal have heavier, convergent laminae.

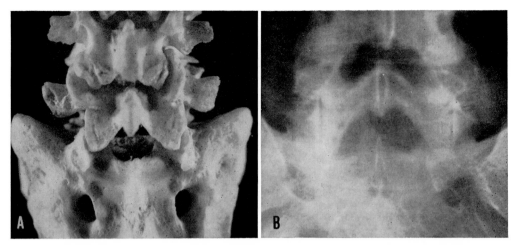

FIG. 55. *A*, Specimen of lumbosacral spine, dorsal view. The articular facets between L5 and S1 are sagittally placed. *B*, Roentgenogram of a normal lumbosacral articulation with sagittally placed facets.

definite cause for pain. This must be sought for in disturbances which may not be visible on plain roentgenograms, such as torsional and stress disturbances of the soft tissues of the back. The possibility of discal herniation must be considered with recurrent pain, especially if radicular symptoms are present.

Congenital malformations of the neural arches of the first, second or third lumbar vertebrae are infrequent. Occasionally small fissures are present across various portions of the arch or the articular facets, usually across the distal portion of the inferior articular facet (Figs. 56, 57). In 1939, Hipps examined such an anomaly. Microscopic and gross studies showed that the zone of rarefaction was not a fracture, but a developmental abnormality in the nature of an apophyseal line. This fissure line was found to be composed of hyaline cartilage, and the microscopic picture ruled out the possibility of an ununited fracture. These fissures represent failures of fusion of an ossification center at the tip of an articular facet. The lesion is usually unilateral, but occasionally is bilateral and mostly occurs in the second and third lumbar neural arches. The superior articular facet is rarely involved.

The angle of inclination of the lumbosacral articulation is of interest. It was pointed out by Ferguson (1949) that the normal angle formed in the horizontal plane with the articular surface of the first sacral segment is 34 degrees. If this angle is significantly exceeded, Ferguson felt that instability of the lumbosacral junction exists.

Anomalies of articulation of the fifth lumbar vertebra in relationship to the first sacral segment are frequent (Figs. 20, 58). A transitional fifth lumbar vertebra in which one or both transverse processes as well as the inferior aspect of the body partially fuses with the sacrum, is regarded as a "sacralized fifth lumbar vertebra." The opposite process in which a first sacral segment is significantly separated from the remainder of the sacrum is referred to as a "lumbarized first sacral segment." It is not at all infrequent to observe 6 lumbar vertebrae. In such instances it is preferable to designate the distal lumbar segment as the first presacral vertebra. To definitely establish whether or not such a transitional form exists, a count of the entire spine from the first cervical segment down is necessary.

The structure of the transverse processes of the fifth lumbar and first sacral segments often is of interest, particularly if articulations are formed between the tips of the transverse processes of the fifth lumbar vertebrae and the adjacent sacrum and iliac bones (Figs. 58, 59). It is believed that if

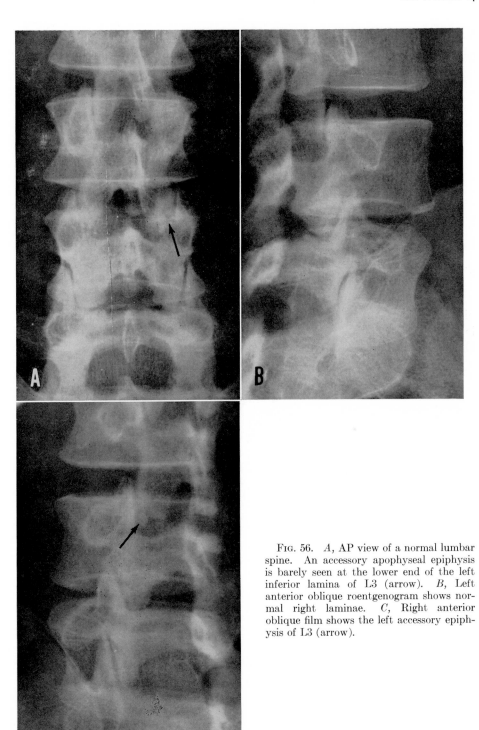

Fig. 56. *A*, AP view of a normal lumbar spine. An accessory apophyseal epiphysis is barely seen at the lower end of the left inferior lamina of L3 (arrow). *B*, Left anterior oblique roentgenogram shows normal right laminae. *C*, Right anterior oblique film shows the left accessory epiphysis of L3 (arrow).

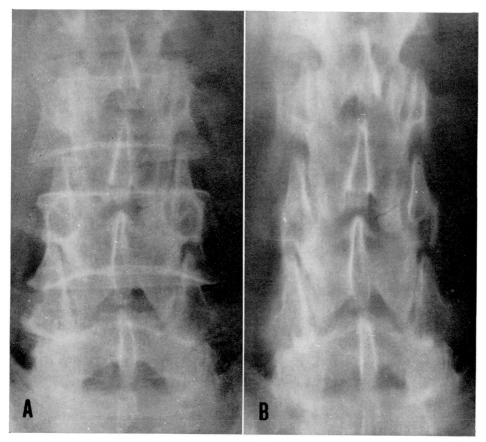

FIG. 57. *A*, AP view of a normal lumbar spine with a large accessory left laminar epiphysis of the inferior lamina of L3. *B*, This is better seen on a laminagram.

this change is bilateral, no weakening of the lumbosacral articulation exists. However, if it is unilateral, changes in stress can result in painful syndromes and arthritic manifestations may appear. Such changes have often been observed in patients who had no symptoms, and unless examination fails to disclose any other reason for pain in the lumbosacral region, I would hesitate before deciding such an anatomic variation is the cause of complaints. Calcification of the ileo-lumbar ligaments occasionally appear, and are of no specific importance (Fig. 60).

There has been much discussion about the demonstration and importance of abnormal mobility of the lower lumbar spine as a cause of persistent low midback pain. Various patterns of minor shifts of the lower lumbar vertebrae have been reported, based on ex-

aminations made with the patient in strained flexed and extended positions. While of interest in demonstrating the range of motion, it is noteworthy that many patients have long intervals of freedom from pain with no anatomic changes which can be demonstrated radiologically. At present no definite correlation between such symptoms, often indefinite and of variable intensity, and the bony configuration of the lower vertebral column can be regarded as established with certainty. Discussion of deformities such as spondylolysis and spondylolisthesis is assigned to a later chapter.

Variations in the structure of the sacrum sometimes are observed on plain films. Among these are changes in the diameter of the sacral canal pointing to the presence of an occult meningocele, obliteration of the

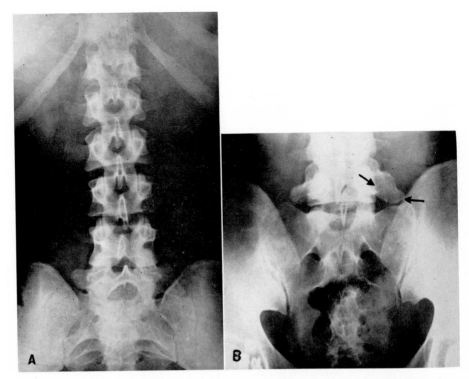

Fig. 58. *A*, Anteroposterior view normal adult lumbosacral spine. The presacral vertebra is not united to the sacrum, and represents a sixth lumbar vertebra. *B*, Tilt-up view. Note the prolonged transverse process of the presacral vertebra (arrows), and the spina bifida occulta of the uppermost sacral vertebra.

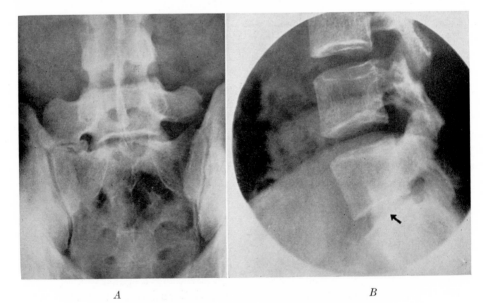

A   *B*

Fig. 59. *A*, The right transverse process of the fifth lumbar vertebra articulates with the iliac bone and the sacrum. *B*, Lateral cone-down view. The enlarged right transverse process is projected across the lumbosacral articulation (arrow).

lumen of the sacral canal, shortening or other bony deficiencies of the sacrum, and coccygeal abnormalities. Some are of practical interest when caudal anesthesia is contemplated. Another interesting change occurs in the inferolateral aspects of the sacroiliac region on the iliac side. This is the

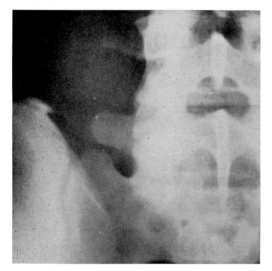

FIG. 60. The right iliolumbar ligament is calcified at its point of origin from the iliac crest.

"paraglenoid foramen" an anomalous notch for the iliac artery (Fig. 61).

The importance attributed to roentgenographic examination of the spine in industry is attested by reports of pre-employment surveys. O'Connor (1946) found that pre-employment spine roentgenograms helped to reduce the incidence of back strains by enabling each person to enter a job suited for his own physical capacities. Barton and Biram (1946) reported on routine anteroposterior and lateral roentgenograms of the lumbosacral regions in 1,000 consecutive preplacement examinations. They found 856 defects in 498 patients, and concluded that spondylolisthesis, arthritis and in some cases transitional lumbosacral vertebrae were significant factors in back strain in workers over 45 years of age. A report on a series of 3,000 preplacement examinations of the lumbosacral spine over a 2-year period was made by Allan and Lindem (1950) who encountered a large number of asymptomatic conditions, including degenerative processes and congenital or developmental anomalies. These authors were of

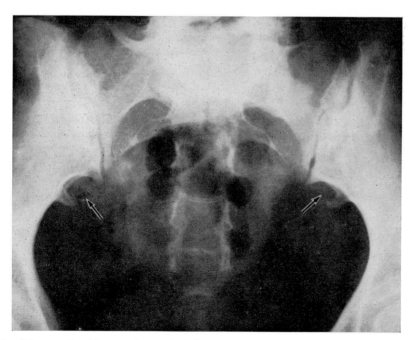

FIG. 61. The paraglenoid fossae (arrows) of the inferior aspect of the iliac bones adjacent to the sacro-iliac joints.

the opinion that in industries requiring physical exertion, preplacement examinations of the spine may well be compared with survey roentgenograms of the chest. It would appear reasonable to check any individual who is required to exert himself or who might be subjected to strains of the back before employment. In this way, incidence of chronic low back pain might be minimized by the avoidance of undue strain in individuals who appear to be susceptible to such disturbances by reason of an anatomic variation in their spines. This statement might appear contradictory in view of what has been said before in the present chapter. In mitigation of this apparent discrepancy, I remind the reader that the result of a survey of over 1,000 patients is applicable to industry on a broad scale, while an individual's variation has to be evaluated in the light of his existing symptoms.

A few comments may be made here as to the relative importance of the various components of a vertebra in casting a roentgenographic shadow. One must keep in mind that we are dealing with a composite picture, the cortex being relatively radioopaque, while the spongiosa is considerably more radiotransparent. The spongiosa is made up of interlacing trabeculae which in general assumes a vertical and horizontal distribution. Snure and Mainer (1937) came to the conclusion that most of the detail of the osseous structures portrayed on roentgenograms is caused by the cortical bone, while the spongiosa accounts for the general density of the vertebral body. They noted that when areas of cortical bone 1 cm square were removed from the lateral surfaces of a vertebral body and the excavated area was filled with paraffin, their locations could be demonstrated on roentgenograms. Three fine holes extending almost across the vertebral body through the spongiosa, however, when filled with paraffin were practically invisible. On the other hand, Wagoner, Hunt and Pendergrass (1945) came to the conclusion that the spongiosa was the more important component in the production of the roentgenographic shadow pattern of a normal vertebral body. I have made roentgenograms of lumbar and thoracic vertebrae in which relatively large holes were present in the spongiosa. Unless these were quite large, exceeding 1.0 cm in diameter, the shadows were obscured by the overlying cortex. On the other hand if a small bit of cortex was removed, the density of the remainder of the cortex as well as the relatively intact spongiosa did not necessarily prevent identification of the injured area if the injured site was tangentially placed so that the defect could be seen. This required multiple, detailed views.

It is difficult to transpose such evidence into clinical terms and to state that fairly extensive destruction of either cortex or medulla is required to identify the change roentgenologically in the living. The results of experiments on dead tissue can hardly be transposed because the effect of overlying tissues, water content, motion and strain is eliminated. Thus it is possible for a vertebra to appear quite normal roentgenologically on one examination, and only a few days later to observe a change in its contour secondary to compression. This may be the first radiologic indication of disease of the bone. A considerable amount of destruction of either the cortex or the spongiosa must exist before the lesion can be identified *in vivo*. Roentgenograms of the spine often are deficient in demonstrating small diseased areas. The help of multiple views, stereoroentgenograms and body section radiography in the identification of minimal destruction areas should not be forgotten. In addition, radioactive strontium scans can provide useful information.

References

Allen, M. L. and Linden, M. C.: Significant Roentgen Findings in Routine Pre-Employment Examination of the Lumbosacral Spine, Am. J. Roentgenol., *80*, 762, 1950.

Barton, P. N. and Biram, J. H.: Replacement Examination of Lower Back, Industrial Med., *15*, 319, 1946.

Chamberlain, W. E.: Basilar Impression (Platybasia). Yale J. Biol. & Med., *11*, 487, 1939.

Cimmino, C. V.: Further Notes on the Esophageal-Pleural Stripe. Radiology, *77*, 974, 1961.

Farmer, H. L.: Accessory Articular Processes in Lumbar Spine, Am. J. Roentgenol., *36*, 763, 1936.

Ferguson, A. B.: Clinical and Radiographic Interpretation of Lumbosacral Anomalies, Radiology, *22*, 548, 1934.

Ferguson, G. H.: Roentgen Diagnosis of the Extremities and Spine, Annals of Roentgenology, 2nd ed., New York, Paul B. Hoeber, Inc., 1949.

Gianturco, C.: Motion of Lower Lumbar Vertebrae in Normal Individuals and in Patients with Low Back Pain, Am. J. Roentgenol., *52*, 261, 1944.

Hadley, L. A.: Secondary Ossification Centers and the Intra-Articular Ossicle, Am. J. Roentgenol., *76*, 1095, 1956.

————: *Anatomico-Roentgenographic Studies of the Spine.* Springfield, Charles C Thomas, 1964.

Harris, R. I. and Macnab, I.: Structural Changes in the Lumbar Intervertebral Discs, J. Bone & Joint Surg., *36-B*, 304, 1954.

Hasner, E., Schalimtzek, M. and Snorrason, E.: Roentgenological Examination of the Function of the Lumbar Spine, Acta radiol., *17*, 141, 1952.

Hipps, H. E.: Fissure Formation in Articular Facets of Lumbar Spine, J. Bone & Joint Surg., *21*, 289, 1939.

Hodges, F. J. and Peck, W. W.: Low Back Pain with Sciatic Radiation, Am. J. Roentgenol., *37*, 461, 1937.

Howard, L. G.: Low Back Pain and Lumbosacral Joint, M. Clin. North America, *26*, 1551, 1942.

Knuttson, F.: Instability Associated with Disk Degeneration in Lumbar Spine, Acta radiol., *25*, 593, 1944.

Lachman, E.: Comparison of Posterior Boundaries of Lungs and Pleura as Demonstrated on Cadaver and on Roentgenograms of Living, Anat. Rec., *83*, 521, 1942.

Leikkonen, O.: Low Back Pain and Sciatica, Acta orthop. Scandinav., Suppl. 40, Copenhagen, 1959.

Letterman, G. S. and Trotter, M.: Variations of Male Sacrum, Surg., Gynec. & Obst., *78*, 551, 1944.

Meghrouni, V. and Jacobson, G.: The Pseudonotch of the Atlas, Radiology, *72*, 260, 1959.

Millard, D. G.: Displacement of the Linear Thoracic Paraspinal Shadow of Brailsford. An Early Sign in Osteomyelitis of the Thoracic Spine. Am. J. Roentgenol., *90*, 1231, 1963.

Mitchell, G. A. B.: The Lumbosacral Junction, J. Bone & Joint Surg., *16*, 233, 1934.

Norman, A.: Segmental Bulge of the Linear Thoracic Paraspinal Shadow (Paravertebral Line). An Early Sign of Disease of the Thoracic Spine. J. Bone & Joint Surg., *44-A*, 352, 1962.

O'Connor, R. B.: Physical Capacities Appraisal of Industrial Back, Industrial Med., *15*, 639, 1946.

Oppenheimer, A.: Longitudinal Fissures in Vertebral Articular Processes, J. Bone & Joint Surg., *23*, 280, 1941.

————: Supernumerary Ossicle at Isthmus of Neural Arch, Radiology, *39*, 98, 1942.

————: Disease of Vertebral Column, Am. J. Roentgenol., *53*, 348, 1945.

Ottonello, P.: Nuovo Metodo per la Radiografia della Colonna Cervicale Completa in Proiezione Sagitalle Ventro-Dorsale, Riv. di. Radiol. e. Fis. Med., *2*, 291, 1930.

Pheasant, H. C. and Swenson, P. C.: Lumbosacral Region, J. Bone & Joint Surg., *24*, 299, 1942.

Pyo, J. and Lowman, R. M.: The "Ponticulus Posticus" of the First Cervical Vertebra, Radiology, *72*, 850, 1959.

Reid, J. D.: Effects of Flexion-Extension Movements of the Head and Spine Upon the Spinal Cord and Nerve Roots, J. Neurol., Neurosurg. & Psychiat., *23*, 214, 1960.

Romanus, T. and Tovi, A. A.: Variation of the Atlas. Roentgenographic Incidence of a Bridge over the Groove on the Atlas for the Vertebral Artery. Acta radiol., *2*, 289, 1964.

Snure, H. D. and Maner, G. D.: Metastatic Malignancy in Bone, Radiology, *28*, 172, 1937.

Trackler, R. T. and Brinker, R. A.: Widening of the Left Paravertebral Pleural Line on Supine Chest Roentgenograms in Free Pleural Effusions. Am. J. Roentgenol., *96*, 1027, 1966.

Trotter, M. and Letterman, G. S.: Variations of the Female Sacrum, Surg., Gynec. & Obst., *78*, 419, 1944.

Wagoner, G. and Pendergrass, E. P.: The Anterior and Posterior "Notch" Shadows seen in Lateral Roentgenograms of the Vertebrae of Infants, Am. J. Roentgenol., *42*, 663, 1939.

Wagoner, G. W., Hunt, A. D., Jr. and Pendergrass, E. P.: Relative Importance of Cortex and Spongiosa in Production of Roentgenogram of Normal Vertebral Body, Am. J. Roentgenol., *53*, 40, 1945.

Myelography

Contrast examination of the spinal canal is accomplished by the introduction of either a positive or negative contrast agent into the subarachnoid space. Gas myelography with either air or oxygen renders the subarachnoid space more transparent than the adjacent tissues, thereby bringing the spinal cord into relief as a shadow of increased density. The cauda equina is not shown as advantageously. Positive contrast agents instilled into the subarachnoid space are either of the absorbable or non-absorbable varieties. The water-soluble absorbable material, Abrodil (sodium mono-iodomethyl sulphonyl), is limited in its application to the lumbar region, and does not have to be removed from the spinal canal. The positive contrast agent first used for myelography was Lipiodol, now replaced by Pantopaque (ethyl iodophenylundecylate). This substance can be used to opacify the entire spinal canal and the posterior cranial fossa, and for demonstrating the fourth ventricle, the aqueduct of sylvius and the posterior portion of the third ventricle. Pantopaque is relatively unabsorbable, and should be removed as completely as possible after myelography.

In 1919 Dandy recognized the diagnostic possibilities of air contrast in the investigation of the spinal canal for tumors. This was also noted by Jacobaeus in 1921. Because of the technical difficulties encountered at the time in obtaining adequate roentgenograms, relatively little was accomplished. However, interest in the radiologic investigation of the spinal canal was stimulated by the pioneer work of Sicard and Forestier (1922), who established Lipiodol myelography as one of the significant advances in neuroradiology. Lipiodol was first conceived of as a therapeutic agent for sciatic and other neuralgic pains. Sicard and Forestier injected Lipiodol into the epidural space in an effort to alleviate this kind of pain. Quite by accident they discovered that when Lipiodol entered the subarachnoid space, it flowed freely and produced no perceptible ill effects. They immediately recognized the importance of this observation in the diagnosis of spinal cord tumors. By 1923, Sicard, Paraf and Laplane reported on the examination of the spinal meningeal spaces in about 150 patients. They first utilized the cisternal approach, as suggested by Ayer (1920), with the aim of assuring descent in the spinal canal in order to identify various obstructive lesions. However, they also carefully considered the advantages of lumbar instillation.

One of the first to use Lipiodol in the United States was Mixter, who later contributed so much to the diagnosis and treatment of herniated intervertebral discs. He reported on the application of Lipiodol to the diagnosis of spinal canal tumors in 1925. In 1924 Ayer and Mixter had described marked cellular reactions in the cerebrospinal fluid of cats following introduction of Lipiodol. They had some hesitation in using Lipiodol in patients, recommending that its use be limited to those patients with evidence of intraspinal block Credit for the radiological aspects of this work was given to J. D. Camp, who continued to advance our knowledge of myelography for many years. It was he who helped establish fluoroscopy as an essential part of the examination by his development of the tip-table. In a personal communication, Camp wrote "Dr. Mixter, through friendship with Sicard in France, received from him some of the first Lipiodol that was sent to this country. Those were days before mechanized tables. The procedure at that time was for Dr. Mixter to perform a cisternal puncture with the patient in the erect position behind the screen of a vertical fluoroscope. Five-tenths cc of Lipiodol was injected and the flow of the media to the sacral cul-de-sac was observed fluoroscopically. Naturally, because of the small amount of oil used, only obstructing lesions were identified. Realizing that a better control of the oil could be obtained in the horizontal position with some means of varying the angle of the table, we improvised some rather crude methods of elevating the head or foot of the horizontal table by means of wooden blocks to expedite the movement of the oil in one direction or the other. I am not certain how many tumors we were able to localize with this procedure, but the results were good enough to stimulate us to use a greater amount of oil, not over 2 cc, in an attempt to get greater information and perhaps localize some smaller lesions."

The term "myelography" was first used by Berberich in 1923 at a meeting of the Medical Society of Frankfurt. Sicard and Forestier preferred the appellation "epréuve du Lipiodol sous arachnoidien" [the subarachnoid Lipiodol test] because they considered the word "myelography" a misnomer, inasmuch as the medulla itself was not outlined. The superior accuracy of myelography for localizing spinal cord tumors over clinical methods was recognized, and surgeons availed themselves of this information for more precise planning of their operations.

On September 30, 1933 Mixter and Barr addressed the New England Surgical Society on the clinical significance of rupture of the intervertebral discs with involvement of the spinal canal. They reported on 19 cases. Of these, 4 had involvement of the cervical spinal canal. Lipiodol block was encountered in 3, and in 1 patient Lipiodol examination was not done. There were 4 patients with thoracic herniated discs. Of these one had a block at D6-7, and in the others Lipiodol examination was not done. Of 11 patients with herniated lumbar discs 6 had evidence of block, and in 3 Lipiodol examinations were reported as negative. No Lipiodol examination was done in the remaining 2 patients.

In a paper published August 29, 1935, Mixter and Ayer clearly recognized the great importance of myelography, and commented that "in our earlier use of Lipiodol, the lesion was not clearly disclosed; with our present technique, elaborated particularly by Dr. A. O. Hampton of the x-ray department, we were frequently able to obtain results which were almost pathognomonic for herniation of the disc."

"The technique is simple enough if two things are constantly kept in mind, i.e., that we are trying to show a small mass which seldom causes compression of the whole cauda equina, and that the lesion always lies anterior to the dura. It is not our aim to show subarachnoid block, but to show a defect in the Lipiodol shadow at the site of a protruded intervertebral disc. For this purpose the usual 1.5 or 2 cc. of Lipiodol, sufficient to demonstrate block, is not enough, and we now use 5 cc. in order nearly to fill the lumbosacral canal. The injection is best made by puncture a little above the suspected lesion to prevent a breaking up of the oil into globules.

"The patient in the prone position is then examined fluoroscopically on the tip-table, films being taken when an excavation in the Lipiodol shadow at the level of a disc be-

comes apparent. . . ." The great importance of recognizing the close resemblance to back strain, lumbosacral or sacro-iliac strain, and providing adequate surgical relief was stressed. The discussion continued with a recounting of their experiences with cervical and thoracic herniated discs. They used cisternal instillation for these patients, and concluded that the diagnosis of herniation of the intervertebral disc in the cervical region could be only tentative, and that true neoplasm is always a possibility in these cases. Three patients had thoracic discal herniations, which were not discussed except to note that the diagnosis of ruptured disc was not made before operation.

The question of untoward reactions to the subarachnoid instillation of Lipiodol was investigated soon after it came into use. In a discussion of a paper by Globus and Strauss on intraspinal "iodolography" in 1929, Elsberg remarked that he had seen fresh adhesions and marked congestion of the meninges and nerve roots "which are not ordinarily observed when the spinal cord is exposed during the course of a laminectomy, and have always explained this as a result of the irritating qualities of this foreign substance." In 1941 Marcovich, Walker and Jessico reported in detail on the irritant properties of intrathecal Lipiodol.

Lipiodol myelography lost some of its disadvantages when Kubik and Hampton (1941) described a method for removal of Lipiodol from the spinal canal. They advocated leaving the needle in situ during myelography, and using it for aspiration of the radioopaque after the examination had been completed. However, even with gentle suction, using a 2-cc. syringe, pain was a frequent and feared concomitant of both Lipiodol, and later, of Pantopaque myelography. In 1964 I described a method of syphoning Pantopaque from the spinal canal which permits evacuation of the contrast medium with little or no pain.

Because of the irritant qualities of Lipiodol, and the increasing importance of myelography, investigations into the use of air myelography were again undertaken after 1935. Considerable progress was made, but the superior diagnostic capacities of Lipiodol soon established this as the contrast agent of choice.

Epidurography (Sanford and Doub, 1941) as a diagnostic method also was suggested, but never came into common use. In the 1930's Thorotrast was occasionally advocated as a contrast agent because of its

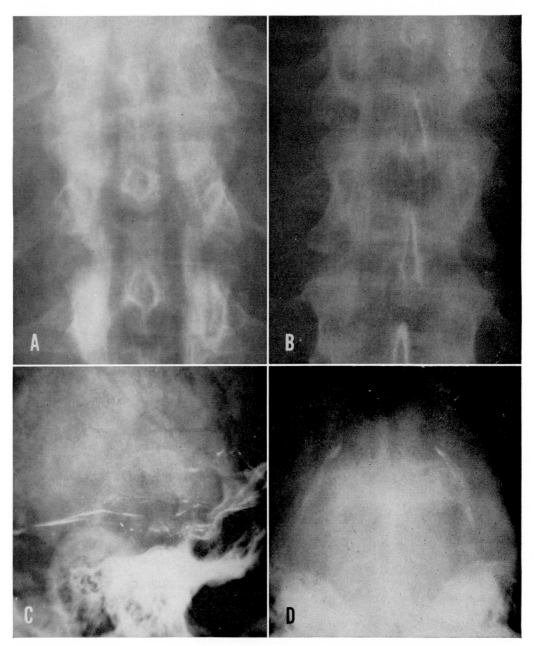

FIG. 62. A, The lower thoracic spinal cord is outlined by Thorotrast from a myelogram done about 15 years before. B, The fila of the cauda equina also are visible due to impregnation with Thorotrast. C, Thorotrast also is deposited in the ependymal lining of the cerebral ventricles seen on lateral and, D, Towne's projections.

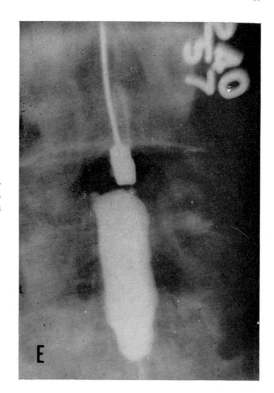

Fig. 62 (*Continued*). *E*, On myelographic examination with Pantopaque a normal flow was present and the contrast medium was readily aspirated from the spinal canal.

superior opacity, fluidity and ability to outline the spinal canal and the cauda equina with apparent lack of toxicity. Forced drainage of the spinal canal was utilized to evacuate the Thorotrast (Nosik, 1943). This method never gained acceptance. Years later delayed effects of Thorotrast resulting in severe cauda equina irritation were reported by Maltby (1964) and by Tucker, Sibley and Laphan (1964). In the second edition of this book a case was cited in the section on arachnoiditis which is worth some elaboration here. The patient, a 43-year-old man, had a Thorotrast myelogram 18 years before he was seen by us. He came because of fluctuating pain in both legs, some difficulty in starting the urinary stream, low back pain and diminished potency. A review of his history disclosed that these complaints were quite similar to those he had prior to the Thorotrast myelogram.

On plain film roentgenograms of his spine thin linear opacities corresponding to the roots of the cauda equina were noted in the spinal canal. Opacification of the ependymal lining of both lateral ventricles and choroid plexuses were noted on skull films. The distal portion of his cord could be clearly seen in the lower thoracic spinal canal. It was assumed that Thorotrast had impregnated the pial covering of his cauda equina, spinal cord and cerebral ventricles. No free contrast agent was visible, so it was assumed that the Thorotrast probably had been removed by drainage (Fig. 62).

Because it was felt that he might have a Thorotrast arachnoiditis, and after much discussion, Pantopaque myelography was done. A normal flow was present from the caudal sac to the cervical level, and the Pantopaque was readily removed from his spinal canal. The relationship between his complaints and the impregnation of his pial membranes with Thorotrast remained in question.

Maltby (1964) followed 3 patients who had undergone Thorotrast myelography in the early 1940's and found that years later severe pain and neurogenic bladder symptoms appeared. Two patients died, and he attributed this to complications directly due to damage to the nervous system as a result of biologic changes produced by the Thorotrast. It was of interest that in his patients there was no apparent ill effect from the retained contrast material for about 8 years. Then insidious indications of a progressive cauda equina lesion appeared, first with motor symptoms and then with weakness and progressive paralysis.

Tucker, Sibley and Lapham (1964) commented that all 4 of their patients had normal Pantopaque myelograms after cauda equina damage appeared following Thorotrast myelography. The interval between myelography and the onset of neurologic disturbances varied from 5 to 18 years. They observed that the length of the latent period was inversely proportional to the estimated amount of retained Thorotrast in the spinal canal, and attributed the neurologic picture to injury of the cauda equina rather than to the lower lumbar and sacral spinal cord. In one of their cases, exploration showed the arachnoid to be excessively thickened, adherent to the nerve roots, and to be composed of dense hyalinized connective tissue.

The use of absorbable radioopaque contrast agents is advocated by Scandinavian workers. In 1931 Arnell and Lidström reported on myelography with Abrodil (sodium mono-iodomethyl sulphonyl). For a while this was neglected, but by about 1944 Arnell and others revived interest in this technic, and presently it is the method of choice in Scandinavian clinics. However, it never gained general acceptance in the United States and England because of certain handicaps. Among these are limitation of the examination to the lumbar region, the need for spinal anesthesia as a preliminary step, and the possibility of adverse reactions, which, from the reports in the literature, are slight. However, some instances of shock and other postmyelographic reactions have been mentioned. Its main advantage is

superior portrayal of the nerve roots. The examination is made by film only, and must be completed in about 15 minutes because the contrast agent is absorbed rapidly.

In 1942 Strain, Plati and Warren reported on a new contrast material for myelography. This preparation, ethyl iodophenylundecylate (Pantopaque) was less viscous than Lipiodol, flowed smoothly, and provided excellent contrast. Some object to the density of Pantopaque, and efforts to achieve a similar opaque agent with a lesser density are still in progress. At first it was thought that Pantopaque was absorbable, but over the years it has been established that it is absorbed slowly, if, indeed, at all, in many instances. Recently I had the opportunity of reexamining 2 patients with Pantopaque in their cranial cavities after cervical myelography 8 and 10 years before. Over this time the droplets had disappeared completely in one, and had diminished markedly in the other (Fig. 63). I had another instance of an infant who had Pantopaque instilled inadvertently into a lumbar intervertebral disc during myelography for demonstration of spinal canal invasion by a mediastinal neuroblastoma. The child survived operation and x-ray therapy. Reexamination a year later showed that the Pantopaque had disappeared, the intervertebral disc retaining its normal appearance (Fig. 64). In many other patients persistence of small quantities of Pantopaque in the lumbar sac has been noted for several years after myelography. Gradual disappearance of epidural Pantopaque had also been observed (Fig. 65).

There has been much argument as to whether or not Pantopaque should be removed routinely. In England it has been the practice of neuroradiologists to use about 6 ml of Pantopaque, and to leave it in the spinal canal. They found that Pantopaque in these quantities was well tolerated, and that no significant reaction to its presence had been observed over the years. The amount used was enough to permit adequate visualization of the spinal canal if the exam-

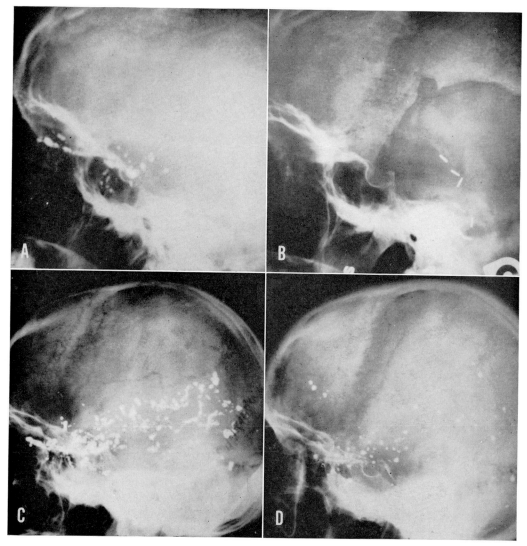

Fig. 63. *A*, Pantopaque has entered the middle and anterior cranial fossa during a cervical myelogram. Ten years later, *B*, the Pantopaque has disappeared. The bone defect is incident to operation for a temporal lobe meningioma. *C*, Another patient with a large quantity of Pantopaque in the cranium after cervical myelography. *D*, Ten years later considerable diminution has taken place in the quantity of contrast material visible.

ination was performed in both the supine and prone positions. Their main objection to removing the Pantopaque was the pain associated with aspiration. Because of the ease of syphonage removal, the use of larger quantities of Pantopaque has become routine in my work. Under certain conditions this makes for a more efficient study, especially of the thoracic and cervical regions.

At the present time very few people doubt the importance of myelography before exploration of the spinal canal, or indeed in the investigation of lesions which might even remotely resemble spinal cord tumors. Patients suspected of demyelinating diseases undergo myelographic examination in the hope that every now and then one is encountered with an unsuspected spinal cord

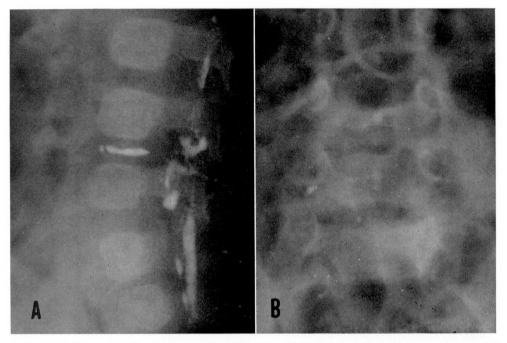

Fig. 64. *A*, Pantopaque has inadvertently entered the epidural space and the nucleus pulposus of the fourth lumbar disc in this infant with epidural invasion of the thoracic canal by a mediastinal neuroblastoma. *B*, One year later the Pantopaque has practically disappeared.

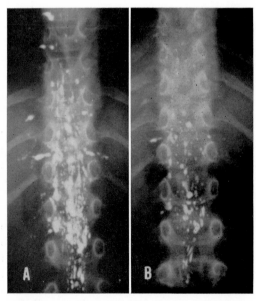

Fig. 65. *A*, Epidural Pantopaque with extension along the nerve roots. *B*, One year later there has been a diminution in the quantity of Pantopaque seen in this region.

tumor which is amenable to treatment, and which does not display a characteristic clinical picture.

Myelography, like other diagnostic procedures, is subject to individual variations in the elegance of performance and interpretation of observations. Considerable disparity in the diagnostic accuracy of myelography has been reported. In my own experience of over 3500 myelograms, this has been about 90 per cent. Published figuers vary from about 65 per cent to a high of 96 per cent. The accuracy is greater when the examinations are conducted by one individual, when the patients are carefully selected, and when the clinical problem is clearly understood before proceeding with the study.

It is apparent from the earlier literature that not all were in enthusiastic accord with the opinion that myelography should precede exploration of the spinal canal. In 1941, Dandy published a paper entitled "Concealed Ruptured Intervertebral Discs." and included in the heading the statement

"A plea for elimination of contrast examinations in diagnosis." Deery (1943) believed that physical examination was sufficient to indicate the level of the lesion and that contrast examinations were unnecessary, an opinion echoed by O'Connell in 1951, and others. Other authors such as Key (1952) advocated that myelography be used only in those instances when the clinical picture was confusing. Svien, Dodge and Camp (1951) pointed out the danger of overlooking spinal lesions because of reluctance to use myelography. These authors reported an analysis of 1245 surgical cases of herniated lumbar discs and 51 patients with spinal cord tumors at or below the 10th dorsal vertebra. They found that in 20 cases of spinal cord tumor the preoperative diagnosis had been herniated disc. In 7 others the possibility of a herniated disc or spinal cord tumor had been considered. The signs and symptoms of all 27 cases strongly suggest the discal lesions of the lower two lumbar interspaces, but in only 5 were the tumors located there. In the other 22 the lesions were cephalad to the fourth lumbar level. I have had similar experiences, so much so that no myelographic examination is considered complete unless the patient is investigated from the caudal sac to the upper cervical area, and when indicated, the posterior fossa. This is done even in the presence of a clearly defined lower lumbar discal lesion. It is so easy to explore the entire intrathecal area, particularly with image intensification fluoroscopy, and it is possible to record the examination so thoroughly on cineradiographic and spot film examinations, that this is done as a routine.

Positive Contrast Myelography (Pantopaque)

Myelography is a radiologic examination which should be performed by well-trained radiologists as a preliminary step in determining the patient's requirements for surgical intervention, and not out of a desire to satisfy diagnostic curiosity. It is an essential investigation in so-called degenerative diseases of the spinal cord because often enough a tumor which produces similar symptoms is uncovered. Pantopaque myelography has definite advantages in the identification of mass lesions, be they tumors or discal herniations, and with care, is helpful in the diagnosis of meningeal inflammatory disorders such as arachnoiditis. It can identify intramedullary masses, intradural extramedullary tumors, extradural tumors, and impingement into the spinal canal produced by lesions in the bone and the adjacent soft tissues. Exploration of the subarachnoid space from the caudal sac to and including the posterior cranial fossa can be undertaken, and the fourth ventricle, the aqueduct of sylvius and the posterior portion of the third ventricle also can be investigated if necessary. The great advantage of Pantopaque myelography is that it permits a complete investigation of the spinal subarachnoid space and the posterior cranial fossa.

Even now there are some misgivings about myelographic examinations. Occasionally one hears remarks not only from patients, but from physicians as well, to the effect that myelography is so fearsome that laminectomy is preferable. Fortunately, this unrealistic and unwarranted attitude is diminishing. Properly performed, myelography can be accomplished with little or no discomfort except for the unpredictable postmyelographic sequelae such as headaches. With the aid of syphonage all or almost all of the contrast agent can be removed quite painlessly in most patients.

Image intensification fluoroscopy and cineradiography have added greatly to the ease and accuracy of myelography. Cinemyelography is especially helpful as a "frozen memory," permitting review of the fluoroscopic changes. It is of the utmost importance in refreshing one's memory about small or transient defects, in establishing changes incident to motion, in studying pulsatile changes in the subarachnoid space, and in establishing a common basis for reviewing an examination in consultation with the referring physician or other interested colleagues.

The procedure is instituted by instillation of Pantopaque into the lumbar subarachanoid space. An accurate, proper lumbar puncture is important. I prefer to use a 17 or 18-gauge needle with a short bevel, and as a rule perform the tap with the patient sitting. Because strain may narrow the intrathecal space perceptibly, it is important that the patient be relaxed. The needle is inserted with its bevel directed parallel to the long axis of the spine, so that its point passes through rather than cuts the longitudinal fibers. If there is any difficulty in performing the tap, or if the patient is restless and apprehensive, the needle is introduced with the patient face down on the table under image intensification fluoroscopic control. It is preferable to get a midline position of the needle tip, but quite often the tip is laterally placed. If a free flow of cerebrospinal fluid is obtained, the procedure can be continued. However, if there is an intermittent flow and the needle tip is far lateral in position, it is better to repeat the tap at an interspace above or below the original placement.

If the patient complains of pain when the needle is inserted, it is an indication that the needle tip is laterally placed towards the affected side. This can be used as a guide for a second attempt. Should pain again occur, it is better to continue the procedure under fluoroscopic guidance with the patient prone. At times one can almost tell from the way the spinal fluid flows from the lumbar puncture needle whether or not the canal is of normal width. Usually a ready flow follows a painless tap. Should there be, however, an intermittent flow, with the needle tip well placed, it is probable that a narrow canal is present. Gentle instillation of a small quantity of Pantopaque with the patient semierect under fluoroscopic control helps identify the placement of the contrast agent in the subarachnoid space by caudad flow. Epidural injection is noted by the spreading of the Pantopaque paraspinally and along emerging nerve roots. Subdural Pantopaque flows slowly and produces bizarre defects. These changes will be described later (p. 128).

Samples of cerebrospinal fluid are collected after manometric determinations are made. Often manometric readings are not done because the entire canal is investigated during myelography. If a spinal fluid block is suspected, the examination is conducted with about 1.5 ml of Pantopaque. Additional quantities are added as desired if a free flow through the spinal canal is present.

With the patient comfortably placed in a face-down position, the stylet is replaced with a right angle connector joined to a 50-cm sterile plastic tube and a 20-ml syringe, both previously filled with from 12 to 18 ml of Pantopaque. A one-way valve at the syringe end, or a small clamp on the tube, permits control of the flow (Fig. 66). About 8 ml of air, sterile saline solution or cerebrospinal fluid is floated above the Pantopaque in the syringe, so that the contrast material in the tube can be injected into the spinal canal should this be required. The patient is then brought into a semierect position and the Pantopaque is introduced into the subarachnoid space under image intensification fluoroscopy. Cineradiographic recording usually is made of the flow of the initial 3 or 4 ml. Prior to this, the patency of the system is checked by observing the ease of flow of cerebrospinal fluid back and forth in the plastic tube as thumb pressure is taken off and reapplied to the plunger of the syringe.

The quantity of Pantopaque used varies with the requirements of the examination. In patients suspected of spinal canal obstructions about 1.5 ml is first used. Generally, the amount used should be that sufficient to fill the lumbar canal up to the level of the midportion of the body of the third lumbar vertebra with the patient erect or semierect. In a canal of average dimensions about 10 to 12 ml is required. Narrow canals fill up to this level with as little as

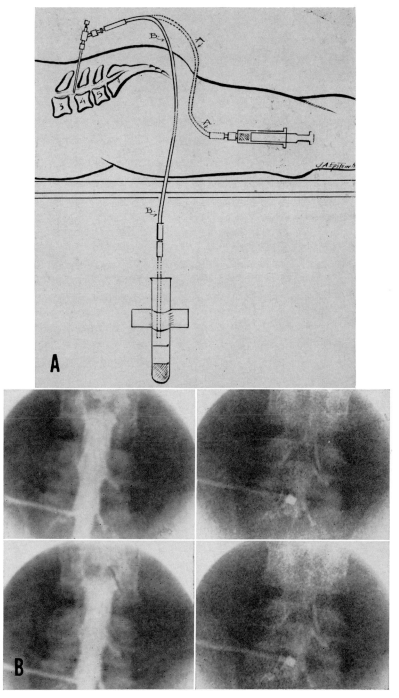

FIG. 66. *A*, Diagram demonstrating placement of the spinal needle, syringe for injection and later use of the sterile polyethylene tube for drainage by means of syphonage. *B*, Frames from a cinemyelographic examination during syphonage (*A*, from Epstein, B. S. and Epstein, J. A., Myelography, Medical Radiography and Photography, *42*, 9, 1966); (*B*, from Epstein, B. S., Evacuation of Pantopaque from the Lumbar Spinal Canal by Syphon Action, Radiology, *93*, 472, 1964.)

4 to 5 ml, while wide canals accept up to 25 or 30 ml (Fig. 67). A larger quantity, about 15 to 18 ml usually is preferable for thoracic and cervical problems. If doubt exists as to filling defects in the lower thoracic or upper lumbar regions, I do not hesitate to fill the canal to the required level, even if over 30 ml of Pantopaque is required.

Having filled the canal to the desired level, the tube-syringe assembly may be removed and replaced with the stylet. If the entire quantity of Pantopaque has been injected so that the tube is radiotransparent, except for a few droplets which adhere to the tube walls, and if the examination is basically for the thoracic or cervical regions, the stopcock is closed and the assembly is taped to the patient's buttock. This minimizes manipulation of the stylet in and out of the shaft of the needle, reducing the possibility of infection. It also facilitates later syphon removal of the contrast material.

Inasmuch as little sedation is required, the patient usually is cooperative enough to perform the desired maneuvers promptly. One must take the time before the examination to review carefully the purposes and technic of the study and the part played by the patient. A "dry run" before instillation of Pantopaque often is helpful.

With the Pantopaque at the desired level, the erect patient is turned under fluoroscopic control into the oblique and the lateral positions. Cineradiographic runs and spot film roentgenograms are made as desired. The effects of strain, motion, bending or twisting can be recorded especially well with cineradiography. Under fluoroscopic inspection the table then is tilted downwards. The flow of Pantopaque is observed and records made as desired as the patient is turned into various positions. Cross-table lateral roentgenograms are also obtained as required.

Passage of Pantopaque through the thoracic canal is facilitated by placing the patient into either the right or left oblique or lateral positions. In those with dorsal kyphoses this maneuver can be most helpful. As a rule it is not necessary to use restraining devices other than shoulder rests because the flow of Pantopaque can be controlled quite readily. Passage into the cranium is prevented by keeping the head extended. It usually is not necessary to tilt the table more than about 45 degrees in the head-down position to get good passage through the thoracic spinal canal and to obtain practically a full column filling of the cervical spinal canal

Examination of the thoracic canal usually is made in both oblique, the lateral and the frontal positions. Decubitus, recumbent and cross-table films are obtained as required. Here the use of 15 ml or a larger volume of Pantopaque is helpful in getting adequate filling of the thoracic spinal canal. Cineradiographic recording of the passage of Pantopaque is essential because it permits repeated reexamination of the area. Usually it is not necessary to turn the patient on his back to fill the dorsal aspect of the canal because the larger volumes used permit adequate filling of the canal. Should this, however, be deemed essential, the needle can be removed and reinserted later for removal of the Pantopaque. It is of interest that when this is done no extravasation takes place, causing one to wonder why the belief exists that a second puncture should not be made for myelography for 10 days after a preceding tap. This is a rule that might be reconsidered. I do not usually adhere to it.

For examination of the cervical spinal canal, the region of the foramen magnum and the posterior cranial fossa, the patient is kept in an oblique position with his head extended until all the Pantopaque has entered the cervical spinal canal. The table is then brought back to an almost horizontal position, and the investigation continued in the frontal and oblique projections with the neck in the flexed, neutral and extended positions. Spot roentgenograms and cineradiographic runs are made as indicated. For filling the posterior cranial fossa, the table is tilted slightly downwards while the patient is held in an oblique position with

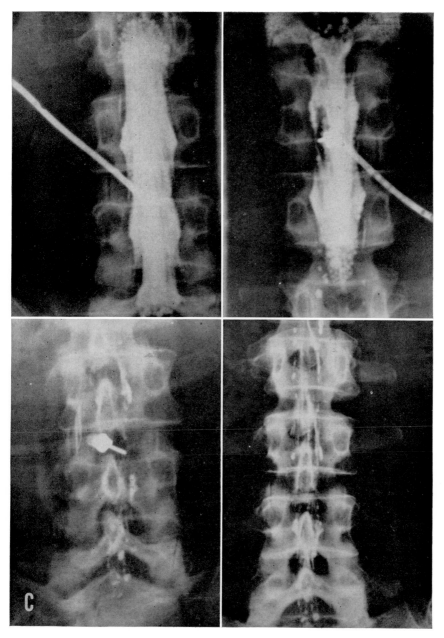

FIG. 66 (*Continued*). *C*, Spot films made during removal of Pantopaque by syphonage. Droplets are scattered along the lateral aspects of the canal. No pain during syphonage, but pronounced, sharply localized pain on aspiration gently with 2-ml syringe.

the head extended. The Pantopaque is introduced under image intensification fluoroscopy, filling the anterior aspect of the posterior cranial fossa with the head slightly flexed and the posterior aspect with the head extended. The exact positioning is controlled by the myelographer at all times. After checking one side, the Pantopaque is returned to the cervical spinal canal by extending the head and bringing the table to a horizontal position. The patient then is turned into the opposite oblique and the

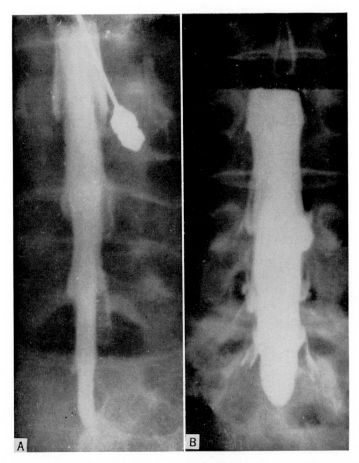

FIG. 67. *A*, Narrow caudal sac. Six ml of Pantopaque have filled the sac up to the level of the third lumbar vertebra. Erect examination. *B*, A wide spinal canal, erect examination using 24 ml of Pantopaque.

procedure repeated. If it is desired to bring the Pantopaque over the clivus, cross-table laterals are obtained with the head extended and straightened. Control of the column can be maintained by cross-table Polaroid exposures, or if available, bi-plane fluoroscopic inspection.

Care should be taken to prevent passage of Pantopaque into the middle and anterior cranial fossae. While this usually has no ill effect, it is nevertheless important to avoid such an occurrence for medicolegal reasons, if for nothing else. Pantopaque is held up in the interpeduncular cistern by a transverse arachnoidal membrane suspended between the oculomotor nerves. This membrane can be demonstrated anatomically

after removal of the broad covering membrane over the pons and the interpeduncular cistern. On either side in the broad basement membrane are openings through which the oculomotor nerves and adjacent structures pass, and through which Pantopaque flows if the head is tilted downwards or to one side or the other (Fig. 68). It is possible to evacuate Pantopaque completely from the posterior cranial fossa in most patients, but I still have to accomplish this from the middle or anterior fossae. Introduction of air into the subarachnoid intracranial cisterns and ventricles has not in my experience resulted in the return of Pantopaque into the spinal canal from the supratentorial spaces.

The fourth ventricle, the sylvian aqueduct and the posterior aspect of the third ventricle can be opacified by placing the patient on his back after removing the spinal needle, and tilting the table downwards so that the Pantopaque enters the fourth ventricle. The head is flexed anteriorly during this maneuver, and films are made in the antero-posterior and cross-table lateral projections (Mones and Weman, 1959) (Fig. 69). It is of historic interest that this possibility was recognized by early workers, notably Sicard and Forestier and by Peiper and Klose (1925).

The Normal Lumbar Myelogram

When adequately filled and with the patient in the erect position, the caudal sac appears as a tapered structure which terminates in a rounded or pointed fashion at the level of about the second sacral segment. A wide variability exists in the appearance of the caudal sac and its location in relationship to the lumbosacral vertebrae. It is not possible, as a rule, to anticipate either the terminal point or the configuration of the caudal sac from plain film roentgenograms of the spine. It is possible, however, to estimate the sagittal diameter of the lumbar

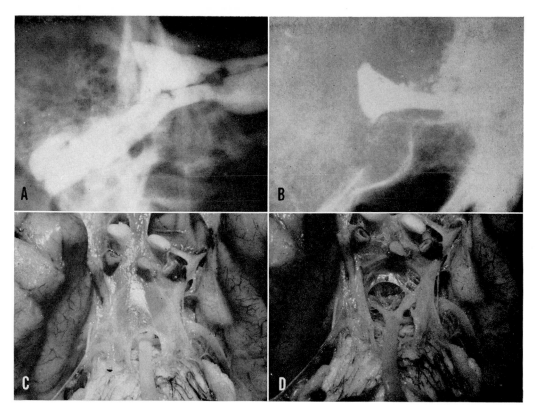

Fig. 68. *A*, Oblique myelogram cervico-occipital region. Pantopaque in the posterior fossa outlines the cerebellar tonsil. Immediately beneath are the dentate ligament and the hypoglossal nerve. Pantopaque enters the medullary, pontine and interpeduncular cisterns. *B*, Transcervical myelogram shows Pantopaque held back by the transverse membrane across the interpeduncular cistern. *C*, Base of the brain with intact basilar membrane over the interpeduncular cistern. Note the foramen for the basilar artery. The oculo-motor nerves traverse the lateral aspects of this membrane. *D*, After the basilar membrane is dissected away, a transverse membrane is seen across the interpeduncular cistern anterior to the bifurcation of the basilar artery. It is this membrane which holds the Pantopaque back, as seen in *B*. (From Epstein, B. S.: The Role of a Transverse Arachnoidal Membrane within the Interpeduncular Cistern in the Passage of Pantopaque into the Cranial Cavity, Radiology, *85*, 914, 1965.)

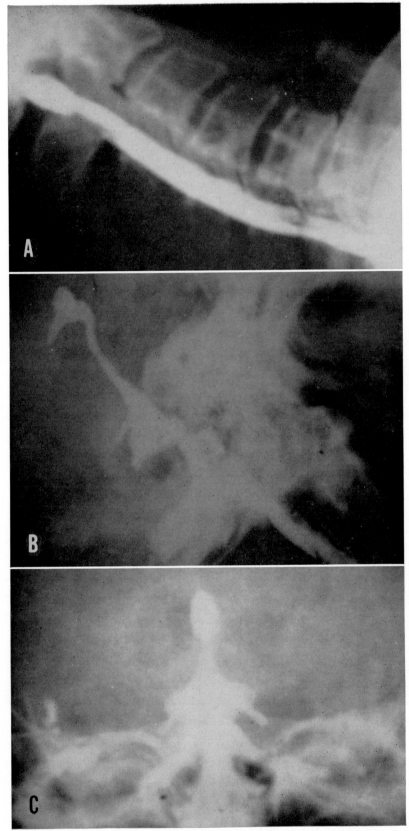

FIG. 69. *A*, With the patient supine Pantopaque is passed into the cervical spinal canal. *B*, After filling the cisterna magna and the vallecula, Pantopaque enters the fourth ventricle, the sylvian aqueduct and the posterior portion of the third ventricle. The internal auditory canal on the right side also is filled (*C*).

spinal canal by determining the height of the intervertebral foramen at the respective interspaces, which usually is a millimeter or two more than this measurement. A sagittal diameter of less than 1.3 cm may be taken as a fair indication that the canal is narrowed. This observation also can be made when the intervertebral foramina assume an elongated appearance in the caudad-cephalad aspect, the pedicles are ovoid and heavy and the inferior laminae seen in the frontal projection converge towards the midline (Figs. 36, 54). A better indication of diminished space within the thecal sac is given by the quantity of Pantopaque necessary to fill it to the level of the middle of the third lumbar vertebra. Normally about 8 to 12 ml are required. If less than 6 ml fills the canal to this level, the column of Pantopaque is slender, usually terminates at about the fifth lumbar interspace, and, as a rule, the axillary pouches of the low lumbar segments are rather inconspicuous (Fig. 67).

The configuration of the caudal sac should be carefully scrutinized, particularly in regard to its point of termination and its width in relation to that of the spinal canal. When the sac ends in a high position, or when it is narrow in relation to the interpedicular space, laterally placed discal herniations may exist without producing visible defects (Fig. 70). However, in these instances even a slight deformity of an axillary pouch becomes significant. The position of the distal aspect of the thecal sac in relation to the posterior surfaces of the vertebral bodies is variable, especially at the fifth lumbar interspace. Here the sac has a tendency to be separated from the floor of the canal (Fig. 71). There are times when one can only note that no definite myelographic defects are present, and that the clinical picture then may be more important than the myelogram.

With normal or wide lumbar canals the lateral margins present downward, obliquely directed axillary pouches of the emerging nerve roots. These nerve sleeves are rather variable in appearance. At times they become more prominent after the patient has been erect for a short time. Arachnoidal diverticula are identified as saccular structures continuous with the subarachnoid space. These occur most frequently in the lower lumbar region, and appear less often in the upper lumbar or cervical areas. A free flow of Pantopaque into and out of some

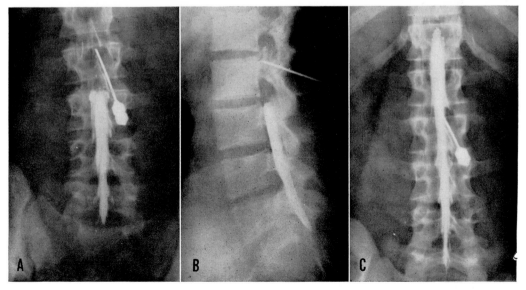

Fig. 70. *A*, Erect myelogram, 16-year-old male patient after instillation of 4 ml of Pantopaque. The canal is narrow. *B*, Lateral view. *C*, When the patient strains, the Pantopaque rises to the level of the 12th thoracic vertebra. The patient had a lateral discal herniation at the L5 interspace on the right side.

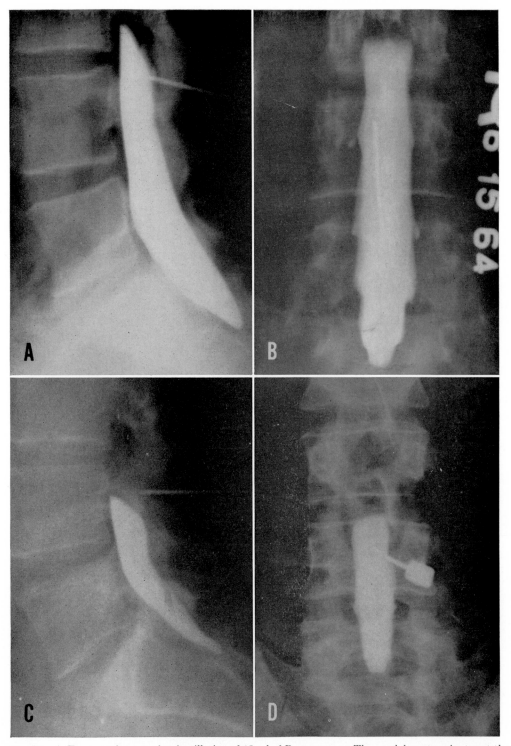

Fig. 71. *A*, Erect myelogram after instillation of 18 ml of Pantopaque. The caudal sac terminates at the second sacral level. The sac is wide, and its anterior aspect is close to the floor of the canal. *B*, AP myelogram, same patient. *C*, Erect lateral of another patient. The caudal sac terminates at the second sacral level, but its anterior aspect is elevated from the floor of the canal. *D*, Same patient, erect AP myelogram.

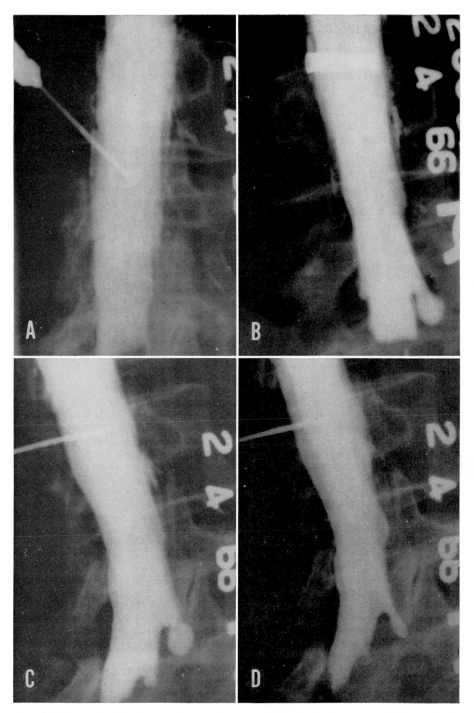

Fig. 72. *A*, Fifteen ml of Pantopaque has been introduced into the lumbar canal with the patient recumbent. *B*, As the patient is brought to the erect position a large diverticulum appears at the right fifth axillary pouch. *C*, Oblique projection shows the diverticulum and the first sacral root beneath. *D*, When the patient strains, the axillary pouches and the diverticulum become less conspicuous.

arachnoidal diverticula is observed (Fig. 72), while in others the diverticula fill slowly and become evident only after several hours have passed. As a rule, these arachnoidal sleeves, or diverticula, are not of any great significance. Exceptions to this rule occur when such sacs become large, distend with cerebrospinal fluid and sometimes produce sufficient pressure against the adjacent nerve root to warrant surgical intervention for relief. Observation of the Pantopaque column in the oblique projections render the axillary pouches and arachnoidal diverticula more prominent, so that when the patient is turned into the right anterior oblique position, for example, the left axillary pouches become conspicuous and the right are obscured.

If relatively small quantities of Pantopaque are used in wide canals with the patient prone, the contrast agent pools into the hollows of the dorsal aspect of the respective lumbar vertebrae. This produces a broken or "hour-glass" configuration of the column, which can be eliminated by adding an adequate amount of Pantopaque (Fig. 73). Fluoroscopic inspection of the advancing head of the column both in the cuadad or cephalad flow is most important in identifying small defects and central veil-like lesions. This must be done in the oblique as well as the frontal positions if one is to derive the greatest diagnostic benefit from the examination. It should not be left to the technician to take films of his choice, but rather it is the radiologist's duty to make a full fluoroscopic inspection, rotating the patient from the prone to the lateral positions on the right and left sides. Transabdominal and lateral views are required to identify indentations into the ventral and dorsal aspects of the opaque column.

The effect of coughing or straining on the configuration of the Pantopaque has been mentioned before (Figs. 33, 70, 72). The constriction and elevation of the column sometimes is considerable, but more often this change is moderate. Such movement takes place in the recumbent as well as the erect position, and is more vigorous in narrow than in wide thecal sacs. It is not infrequent for the contrast agent to rise two or more interspaces during vigorous strain. In those patients the caudal sac may be reduced to a narrow thread-like appearance. The fila of the cauda equina sometimes are more visible in the semi-erect prone position during strain.

The roots of the cauda equina often can be delineated with the patient erect or semierect if adequate penetration is used in making the roentgenograms. These nerve trunks appear as parallel or slightly divergent radiolucent linear markings. It is quite difficult to determine whether the shadows represent normal or abnormal fila unless they are unusually heavy. Displacement of cauda equina roots by the lumbar puncture needle is seen frequently, and is not associated with pain unless aspiration is attempted. Here the patient will complain of sharply localized pain as soon as the nerve is brought into the needle tip, even with very gentle suction (Fig. 74).

After the lower lumbar canal is investigated, the patient is tilted slowly, head downward, and the flow of Pantopaque into the upper lumbar and the lower thoracic canal is studied. It is often possible to identify the conus of the spinal cord as a tapered radiolucency in the lowermost thoracic and upper lumbar levels. Occasionally the proximal aspects of the roots of the cauda equina are seen in the frontal projection. The conus and some nerve roots also appear on lateral cross-table roentgenograms in the upper aspect of the spinal canal. The nerve roots pass caudally as straight lines directed slightly dorsad. The filum terminale is visible on frontal views as a thin straight line in the middle of the canal. If information about the conus and the filum terminale is desired, it is helpful to withdraw the lumbar puncture needle and place the patient on his back. Careful tilting of the patient pools the contrast material about the conus and the filum terminale, a useful procedure in instances when shortening of the filum

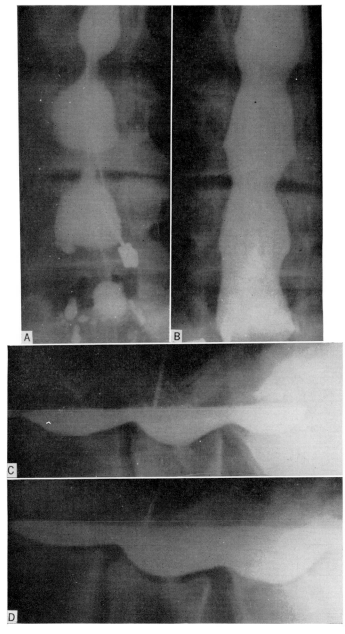

Fig. 73. *A*, Anteroposterior myelogram, 6 ml of Pantopaque. Note the multiple hourglass defects. The one at the narrowed third lumbar interspace is of particular interest.

B, Same patient, 18 ml of Pantopaque. Note that the defect at the third lumbar interspace is eliminated, as are those above and beneath.

C, Same patient, 6 ml transabdominal examination. The Pantopaque fills the concavities in the dorsal aspect of the vertebral bodies. Indentations at the level of the intervertebral discs are responsible for the hourglass deformities of the column, attributed to the large capacity of the spinal canal.

D, Same patient, 18 ml transabdominal examination. After adding an adequate quantity of Pantopaque, the defects at the intervertebral discal levels are no longer present. This was a capacious canal and proper examination required larger amounts of Pantopaque.

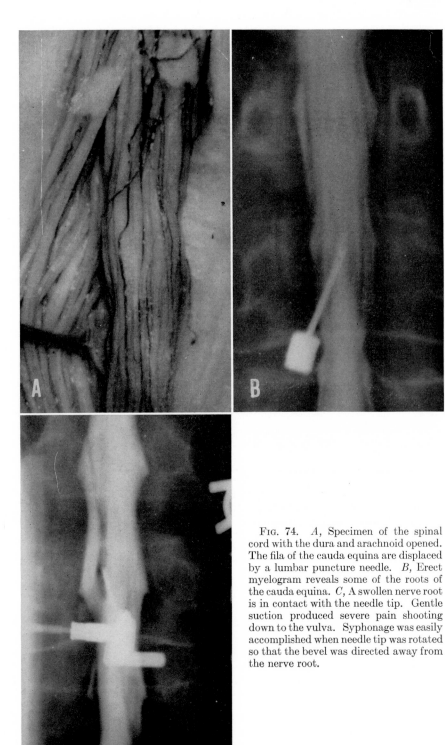

Fig. 74. *A*, Specimen of the spinal
cord with the dura and arachnoid opened.
The fila of the cauda equina are displaced
by a lumbar puncture needle. *B*, Erect
myelogram reveals some of the roots of
the cauda equina. *C*, A swollen nerve root
is in contact with the needle tip. Gentle
suction produced severe pain shooting
down to the vulva. Syphonage was easily
accomplished when needle tip was rotated
so that the bevel was directed away from
the nerve root.

terminale and a consequent lower position of the conus is suspected. Demonstration of the anterior spinal artery below the first lumbar vertebra either in the prone or supine position helps identify a low-lying conus (Figs. 75A, B and C).

Myelographic identification of the filum terminale within the sacral canal is rare. I have observed one such instance (Fig. 75D and E) in a 24-year-old patient who had a normal myelogram. Six days later an intravenous urogram was done. On this a thin line of Pantopaque could be seen in the midline in the sacral canal in the anteroposterior projection. On the lateral study the insertion of the filum terminale into the anterior aspect of the canal at the level of the fourth sacral segment could be clearly seen. Inasmuch as none of the Pantopaque had entered the subdural space or the central canal, it must be presumed that the caudal sac ended in a thin linear cavity continuous with the subarachnoid space.

Thoracic Myelogram

As the patient is tilted head downward in the prone position, Pantopaque passes along the anterior and lateral aspects of the canal, outlining the spinal cord as a central radiolucent shadow. The axillary pouches in the thoracic region are less prominent than those caudad, and project only slightly laterally. The anterior spinal artery is identified as a relatively straight line in the middle of the cord. Passing obliquely downward occasionally are radicular arteries directed towards the axillary pouches. Lateral to the spinal cord obliquely placed radiolucent linear shadow representing some of the thoracic nerves can be seen (Figs. 32 and 75). With the patient turned into an oblique position, the dentate ligament occasionally can be demonstrated as a thin line on fluoroscopic, cineradiographic and spot film examinations. It is possible to see Pantopaque flow more rapidly below the lower dentate ligament, while that above it moves somewhat slower. However, the columns unite quickly as the

Pantopaque flows into the supraligamentous from the infraligamentous aspects of the canal through the spaces between the dentate insertions into the dura mater. This observation is best made with cineroentgenographic studies. On lateral films and cineradiograms the dentate ligament is about midline in position, while on oblique studies the line moves from the anterior towards the posterior aspect of the canal (Fig. 76). The pulsatile activity in the lower and midthoracic region is moderate, and is more prominent in the upper thoracic area.

Inspection of the caudad flow of Pantopaque is an essential part of thoracic myelography. This is accomplished as the patient is returned to the erect position after the cervical canal has been studied. It is at this time that arachnoidal diverticula can be demonstrated. These vary in size from a millimeter or two to over a centimeter in diameter, and are observed quite frequently. As the patient is brought to the erect position, the Pantopaque descends in globules below the level of the upper third of the thoracic spinal column. Above this, it is usually possible to keep the column together, permitting an excellent opportunity to check on the cord and axillary pouches at the cervicothoracic junction in the frontal position. By use of the recumbent "swimmer's position," made with one arm brought along the head and the other along the back, oblique to lateral examinations of the cervicothoracic area are possible (Fig. 77).

Arachnoidal diverticula occur singly, or two or three may be present. They appear more often in the midthoracic region, but are seen above or beneath this level fairly frequently. Usually they are situated in the midline over the dorsal aspect of the cord (Fig. 78). They retain Pantopaque, and sometimes it is necessary to reinvert the patient to empty the sac. Evacuation can be facilitated by having the patient cough vigorously, forcing the Pantopaque out of the sac back into the mainstream of the

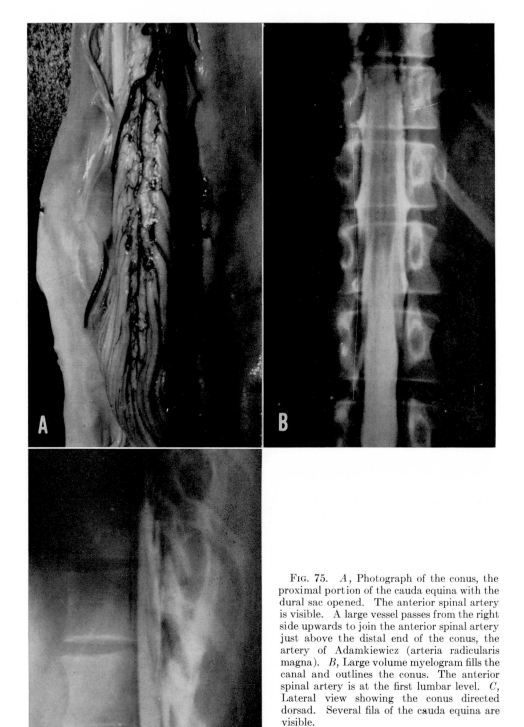

Fig. 75. *A*, Photograph of the conus, the proximal portion of the cauda equina with the dural sac opened. The anterior spinal artery is visible. A large vessel passes from the right side upwards to join the anterior spinal artery just above the distal end of the conus, the artery of Adamkiewicz (arteria radicularis magna). *B*, Large volume myelogram fills the canal and outlines the conus. The anterior spinal artery is at the first lumbar level. *C*, Lateral view showing the conus directed dorsad. Several fila of the cauda equina are visible.

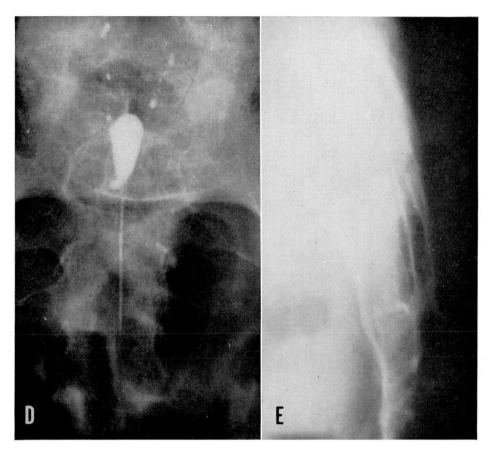

Fig. 75 (*Continued*). *D,* Another patient, a 24-year-old man with complaints referable to both lower extremities. The spinal canal is abnormally wide, but no gross defects are seen. This film 6 days later shows the terminal filum terminale down to its insertion in the lower sacrum. *E,* Lateral view. The filum terminale passes through the sacral canal and inserts in the fourth segment.

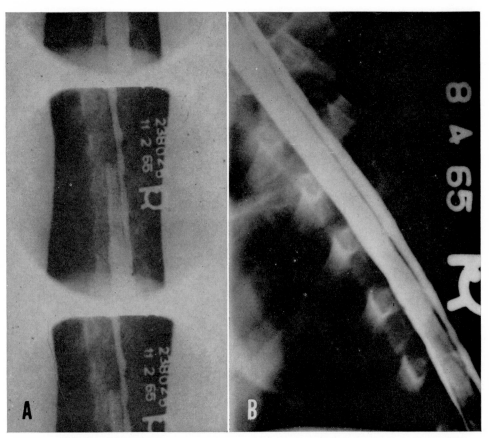

Fig. 76. *A*, Frames from a cinemyelographic examination of the thoracic spinal canal. In the lowermost frame the advancing Pantopaque column is separated by the dentate ligament. The lower stream is ahead of the upper one. *B*, Oblique roentgenogram of the thoracic dentate ligaments in a filled canal.

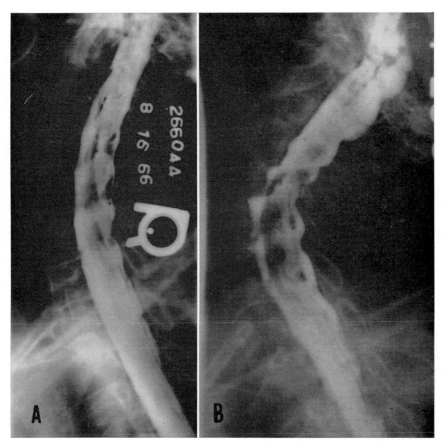

Fig. 77. *A*, "Swimmer's position" outlines the cervical and upper thoracic spinal canal. *B*, With the head extended wrinkles appear in the dorsal aspect of the column incident to infolding of the yellow ligaments.

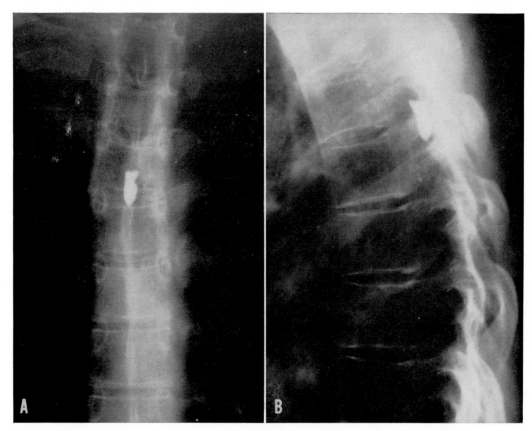

Fig. 78. *A*, Pantopaque is retained in a small arachnoidal diverticulum in the upper thoracic canal. The patient is erect. *B*, Lateral projection, the diverticulum is situated in the dorsal aspect of the canal. On coughing, the diverticulum emptied partially and the Pantopaque descended in the spinal canal. A small amount could not be evacuated.

subarachnoid space, so that the globules descend to the caudal sac. This maneuver is not always successful, especially if the sac is fairly large. Not infrequently Pantopaque also collects in the lateral recesses of the thoracic spinal canal. Coughing and straining is required to mobilize these droplets so that they can fall caudally. The range of movement in the spinal canal during coughing and straining is best studied by cineradiographic recordings. It is of considerable interest that globules caught in the midthoracic region may be pushed up into the lower cervical space during a cough. Probably this movement, imparted to the fluid column, also plays a part in the circulation of the cerebrospinal fluid.

Thoracic arachnoidal diverticula usually are innocuous. However, they assume clinical importance when they become large enough to cause spinal cord compression. When they close off and become noncommunicating cysts, they act like extramedullary lesions, and may produce osseous changes in the adjacent vertebrae.

Cervical Myelograms

I prefer to fill the cervical subarachnoid space with the patient in an oblique position, keeping his head extended. A cineradiographic record is made as the Pantopaque enters the cervical subarachnoid space. A hesitation and transitory "U"-shaped configuration of the Pantopaque column at the cervicothoracic junction should not be mis-

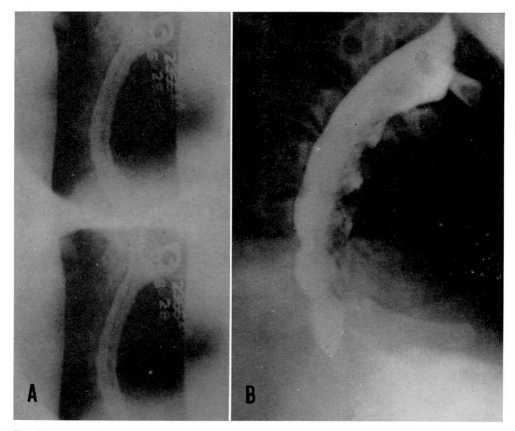

Fig. 79. Frames from a cinemyelographic examination of the cervical canal with the patient in the right lateral position. A full column is attained by using 18 ml of Pantopaque, so that the entire canal is opacified. The dentate ligaments are visible. B, Same patient, cross-table lateral with the head in extension.

interpreted as a discal or spondylotic lesion. Adequate filling of the cervical subarachnoid space gives the advantages of a full column. Good lateral myelograms can be obtained with the patient turned into a lateral horizontal position with the head tilted upwards (Fig. 79). When the Pantopaque has filled this area, and it is preferable to utilize the entire amount instilled, the table is brought back to a horizontal position. Spot roentgenograms are made first in the oblique position, recording various angles as indicated by the fluoroscopic examination. The effects of flexion and extension are investigated. Pantopaque is brought up to the foramen magnum, and into the cisterna magna if necessary (Fig. 80).

Following the first oblique inspection the head is extended and the patient turned face down. The study is then continued, again recording observations on spot films and cineradiographically. The procedure is repeated in the opposite oblique and the lateral positions. Cross-table laterals are then made with the head extended and flexed, using Polaroid 10-second developing technics followed by conventional roentgenograms made as soon as the Polaroid film is inspected. This time can be shortened if cross-table image intensification apparatus is available.

In the frontal prone position the spinal cord usually is demonstrable in the middle of the subarachnoid space. Pantopaque covers the floor of the canal in a thin layer, and continues as lateral rivulets which outline the outer margins. The axillary pouches are directed laterally, almost perpendicular

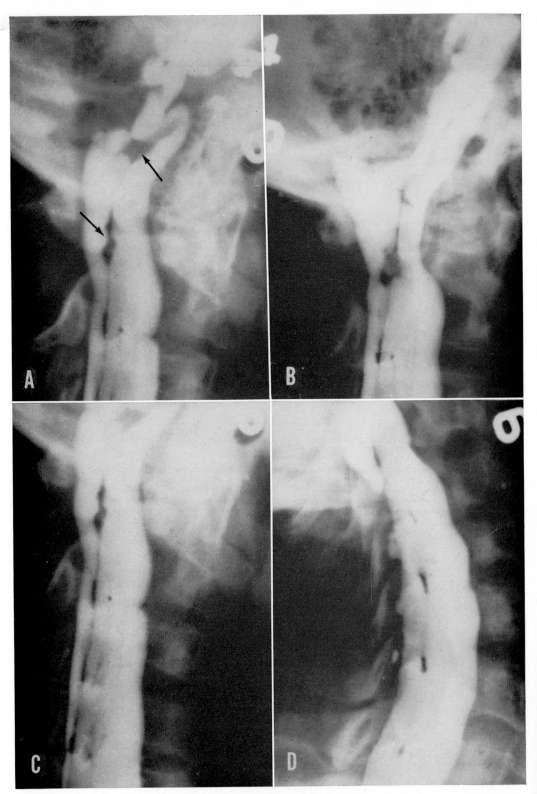

Fig. 80. *A*, Pantopaque in the upper cervical canal and the posterior fossa. The upper dentate ligament and the hypoglossal nerve are visible, and above is the vertebral artery (arrows). *B*, When the head is flexed, the medullary, pontine and part of the interpeduncular cisterns fill. The ipsilateral cerebellar tonsil is visible. *C*, The dentate ligament is seen as a strip interrupted by slightly widened areas corresponding to the dentate tips. *D*, With the head extended the configuration of the dentate ligament changes. A swiveling motion is attained at the tips, better seen on the cinemyelographic examination.

to the main column. These present a central radiolucency which indicates the respective emerging cervical nerves. Usually the lower pouches are more prominent than those above the fourth cervical interspace, but they vary somewhat in size (Fig. 32). Cervical axillary diverticula are infrequent, and are less prominent than those in the thoracic or lumbar regions. They present as small, round blobs of Pantopaque somewhat distal to the nerve root. If of some size, they may empty, but, as in the lumbar and thoracic areas, also can retain Pantopaque for quite a while (Fig. 81). As a rule no clinical significance is attributed to cervical arachnoidal diverticula. I am not aware of any associated with changes such as occur with large diverticula in the thoracolumbar meninges. These should not be confused with the prominent arachnoidal sacs seen in some patients with neurofibromatosis.

The anterior spinal artery appears as a centrally located relatively straight line. Often it is discontinuous where the cord crosses the intervertebral discs, especially if the canal is wide and incompletely filled. Passing obliquely downwards from the anterior spinal artery are radicular branches which extend with the nerve root to the axillary pouch from which it enters. These vessels are variable in size and position, and are visible more often in the lower aspect of the cervical cord (Fig. 32).

Individual bundles of nerve rootlets, usually of the anterior roots, can also be identified passing obliquely and laterally to the respective axillary pouches. In the oblique position, the laterally directed nerve roots and the dentate ligaments become visible (Fig. 82). The latter can be clearly seen with image intensification fluoroscopy, and its movement during neck movement recorded on cineroentgenograms. As Panto-

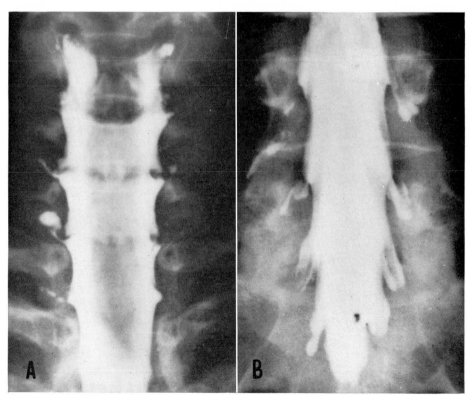

FIG. 81. *A*, Cervical arachnoidal diverticula in a 47-year-old man. *B*, Same patient, lumbar diverticula. These were asymptomatic.

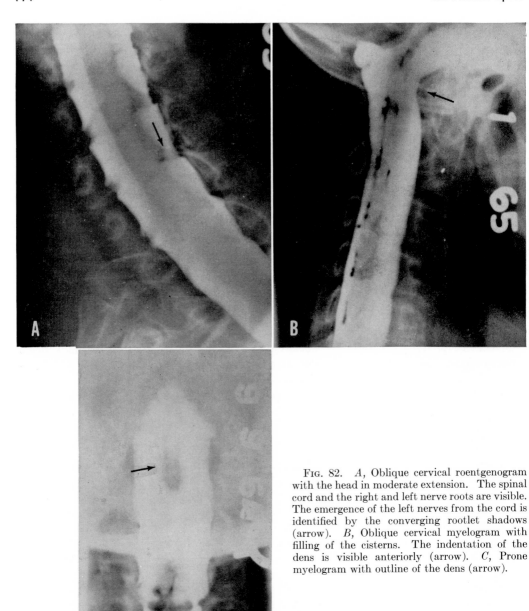

FIG. 82. *A*, Oblique cervical roentgenogram with the head in moderate extension. The spinal cord and the right and left nerve roots are visible. The emergence of the left nerves from the cord is identified by the converging rootlet shadows (arrow). *B*, Oblique cervical myelogram with filling of the cisterns. The indentation of the dens is visible anteriorly (arrow). *C*, Prone myelogram with outline of the dens (arrow).

paque flows into the dependent portion of the cervical spinal canal, the stream often is split, some flowing beneath and some above the lowermost dentate ligament. The dural insertions of the dentate tips are identifiable as rounded shadows when the head is extended. These become elongated as the head is brought to the neutral position, and with the head flexed the dentate tips become inconspicuous. The linear configuration of the dentate ligament is brought out best in flexion. Its shadow is broken at the levels of the dentate tips in extension. The range of motion of the spinal cord can be estimated from the change in the position of the dentate tips, which approximate each other as the head is extended and separate as the head is flexed. The range of motion is from 0.5 to about 1 cm in the cervical region (Fig. 80).

It is possible to obtain good lateral cine-myelographic and spot film studies of the cervical spine when an adequate quantity of Pantopaque produces a full column for examination. The head is kept tilted upwards to prevent undue flooding of the posterior fossa. In this position the dentate ligament is in the midline. Often a double shadow is seen if the patient is not in a true lateral posture (Fig. 83). The changes resulting from flexion and extension are the same as those noted on oblique studies. Most of the time only the lowermost ligament is outlined. Above and beneath the dentate ligament are the shadows of the dorsal and ventral nerve rootlets. The cord itself often can be identified, but not as well as can be demonstrated on cervical gas myelograms with laminagraphy. Indentations into the dorsal aspect of the cervical spinal canal are produced to a varying extent when the head is extended by infolding of the ligamenta flava and the change in position of the articular surfaces of the laminae (Fig. 83).

The pulsatile activity in the cervical spinal canal is much more vigorous than in the lumbar or thoracic regions. The range of movement with each heart beat varies considerably. In some patients an upward and downward movement of the Pantopaque column and droplets exceeds an interspace with the patient at rest. In others the range of motion is only a few millimeters. Movement of the column is markedly affected by strain and cough in the erect and recumbent posture. Droplets, or a portion of the column, can be pushed up into the cranial fossa from the lower cervical segments in some patients by means of a vigor-

ous cough. The synchronization of the pulsatile movement with the heart beat can be demonstrated by having the patient perform a Valsalva maneuver, which pushes the column up and slows down the pulsatile activity considerably. Pulsatile activity in the axillary pouches occurs, but to a distinctly diminished extent as compared with the main column. Pantopaque also is pushed across the midline by the pulsatile activity in the cervical subarachnoid space as well as by the force of gravity produced by the altered positions of the patient. This probably has a part in the cerebrospinal fluid circulation mechanics.

The displacement of Pantopaque by coughing provides a mechanism whereby droplets caught in the lateral recesses can be brought back to the middle of the canal, so that they can descend to the caudal sac for removal (Fig. 84). In several patients with arachnoidal diverticula no pulsatile activity could be seen in the pouches. Evacuation of these pouches was incomplete as compared with that which occurs in lumbar arachnoidal diverticula.

The pulsatile activity in the cervical subarachnoid space is affected by the width of the canal and the presence of osteophytic changes or other mass lesions. This will be discussed later.

Examination of the region of the foramen magnum and the posterior fossa is required when there is any suspicion of a high cervical lesion. Under image intensification fluoroscopy the contrast agent is brought into the cerebellopontine angles, the cisterna magna and over the clivus (Fig. 86). The internal auditory canal can be demonstrated (Fig. 85), providing a method for the diagnosis of cerebellopontine angle and auditory nerve tumors. The vertebral arteries, the origin of the inferior spinal artery and the hypoglossal nerve (Fig. 80) become visible in the oblique positions, while the basilar artery and its branches are demonstrable in the prone position as Pantopaque flows around the dens over the clivus (Figs. 82 and 86). Control of the Pantopaque column over the

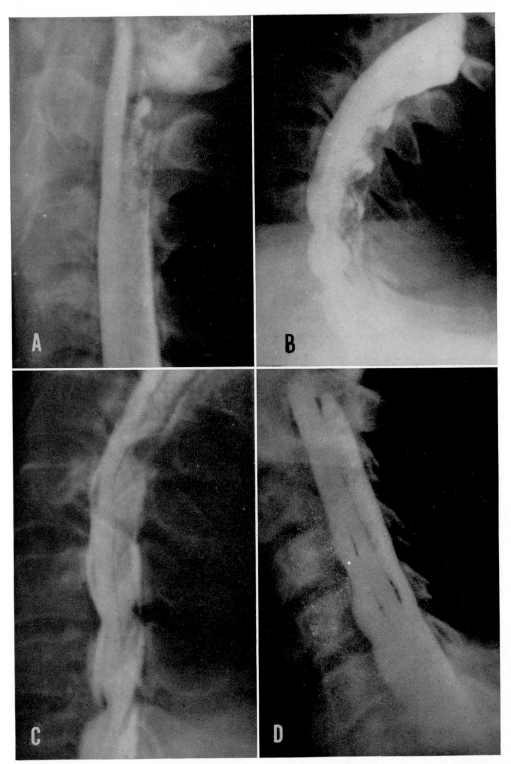

Fig. 83. *A*, Cross-table lateral cervical myelogram. The cord is seen in the upper aspect of the canal, its lower portion below the dentate ligaments being obscured by the Pantopaque. *B*, In extension the yellow ligaments infold and indent the superior aspect of the Pantopaque column. Slight upward bulging of the fourth, fifth and sixth intervertebral discs. *C*, Another lateral cervical myelogram with both dentate ligaments exactly parallel so that they project as one line. The anterior identations are incident to slight spurring. *D*, With the patient's head and neck turned the right and left dentate ligaments are visible as two almost parallel radiolucent streaks.

116

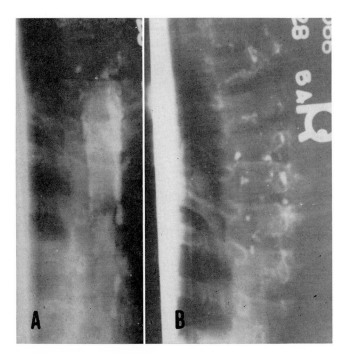

Fig. 84. *A*, Pantopaque is caught in the cervicothoracic spinal canal. *B*, With a vigorous cough the Pantopaque is forced upwards into the middle of the canal, and then drops to the caudal sac. Residual droplets left were also cleared by further coughing.

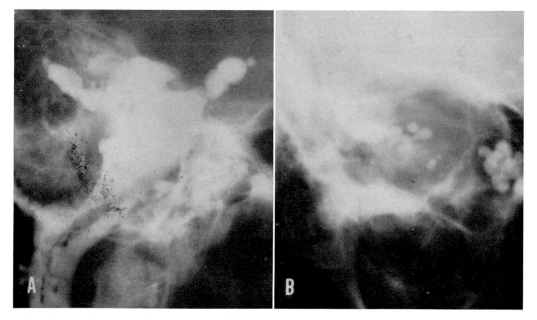

Fig. 85. *A*, Pantopaque has been introduced into the posterior fossa so that the vertebral artery, the cerebellar tonsil and the basal cisterns are opacified. The cerebellopontine angle is filled. *B*, On turning the patient into the prone position, some of the Pantopaque is seen in the left auditory canal.

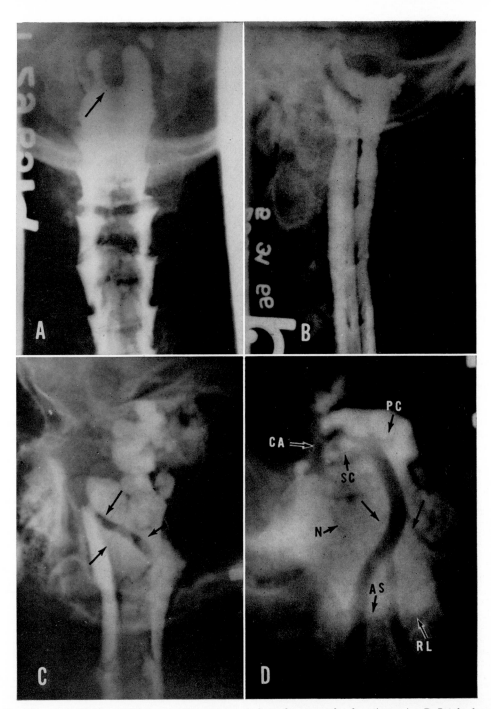

Fig. 86. *A*, With the patient prone, Pantopaque is brought up to the dens (arrow). *B*, In the lateral position the dentate ligaments, the vertebral artery and the cerebellar tonsil are visualized. *C*, As the patient is rotated anteriorly and the head brought slightly upwards, the vertebral artery and the medulla oblongata are seen (arrows). Several delicate vessels emerge from the vertebral artery, branches of the posterior inferior cerebellar artery. *D*, With the patient again prone and the head tilted downwards, the union of the vertebral arteries and the basilar artery are seen. The anterior inferior cerebellar arteries are visible (arrows). The right vertebral artery is smaller than the left. The bifurcation of the basilar artery and the origins of the posterior cerebral (PC) and the superior cerebellar (SC) arteries is visible. The sixth cranial nerve (N) passes along the belly of the pons. The anterior spinal artery (AS) coming from rootlets derived from the vertebral arteries can be made out. The broad lateral shadow (CA) is presumed to be the internal carotid artery. In this projection with the patient prone and the head tilted sharply upwards, some Pantopaque extends to the cerebellopontine angle.

clivus is apt to be rather difficult, but can be managed with image intensification and bi-plane fluoroscopy or Polaroid roentgenograms. Visualization of the posterior fossa by means of positive contrast often is helpful in identification of tumors of the cerebello-pontine angle and of vascular deformities such as vertebral or basilar artery aneurysms. It also has been most helpful in the demonstration of cerebrospinal fluid fistulae associated with disease of the temporal bone. Pribram, Hass and Nishioka (1966) in reporting a fistula from the dural sleeve at the fifth nerve, recommend that for such investigations the Pantopaque be left in place for about 15 minutes, and that laminagrams as well as plain film roentgenograms be taken.

References

Arbuckle, R. K., Shelden, C. H. and Pudenz, R. H., Pantopaque Myelography: Correlation of Roentgenologic and Neurologic Findings, Radiology 45, 356, 1945.

Ayer, J. B.: Puncture of the Cisterna Magna, Arch. Neurol. & Psychiat., 4, 529, 1920.

Ayer, J. B. and Mixter, W. J.: Abstract, Arch. Neurol. & Psychiat., 11, 499, 1924.

Baker, Jr., H. L.: Myelographic Examination of the Posterior Fossa with Positive Contrast Medium, Radiology, 81, 791, 1963.

Barr, J. S. and Mixter, W. J.: Posterior Protrusion of the Lumbar Intervertebral Discs. J. Bone & Joint Surg., 23, 444, 1941.

Batts, M., Jr.: Rupture of the Nucleus Pulposus. An Anatomical Study, J. Bone & Joint Surg., 21, 121, 1939

Beadle, O. A.: The Intervertebral Disks: Observations on their Normal and Morbid Anatomy in Relation to Spinal Deformities, Medical Research Council, Special Report Series No. 161, London, His Majesty's Stationery Office, 1931.

Berberich, J.: Personal communication.

Bream, C. A., Jenkins, R. and Farmer, T.: Cineradiographic Diagnosis of Neurological Diseases, Neurology, 15, 973, 1965.

Breig, A.: Biomechanics of the Central Nervous System, Chicago, The Year Book Medical Publishers, Inc., 1960.

Breig, A. and Marions, O.: Biomechanics of the Lumbosacral Nerve Roots, Acta radiol., 1, 1141, 1963.

Brierre, J. T. and Colclough, J. A.: Total Myelography. Complete Visualization of the Spinal Subarachnoid Space, Radiology, 64, 81, 1955.

Brown, F. M. and Aye, R. C.: Myelographic Demonstration of the Basilar Artery, Am. J. Roentgenol., 73, 32, 1955.

Bucy, P. C.: Chondroma of the Intervertebral Disk, J.A.M.A., 94, 1552, 1930.

Bunts, A. T.: Surgical Aspects of Ruptured Intervertebral Disc: With Particular Reference to Thorotrast Myelography, Radiology, 36, 604, 1941.

Burrows, E. H.: The Sagittal Diameter of the Spinal Canal in Cervical Spondylosis, Clinical Radiol., 14, 77, 1963.

Camp, J. D.: Multiple Tumors within the Spinal Canal: Diagnosis by means of Lipiodol Injected into the Subarachnoid Space, Am. J. Roentgenol., 36, 775, 1936.

———: The Roentgenologic Diagnosis of Intraspinal Protrusion of Intervertebral Disks by means of Radiopaque Oil, J.A.M.A., 113, 2024, 1939.

———: Contrast Myelography, Med. Clin. North America, 25, 1067, 1939.

———: Contrast Myelography, Past and Present, Carman Lecture, Radiology, 54, 477, 1950.

———: Personal communication, 1959.

Camp, J. D. and Addington, E. A.: Intraspinal Lesions Associated with Low Back Pain and Sciatic Pain, and their Localization by means of Lipiodol within the Subarchnoid Space, Radiology, 33, 701, 1939.

Copelman, B.: Roentgenographic Diagnosis of Small Central Protruded Intervertebral Disc, Am. J. Roentgenol., 52, 245, 1944.

Craig, R. L.: Effect of Iodized Poppy-Seed Oil on the Spinal Cord and Meninges, Arch. Neurol & Psychiat., 48, 799, 1942.

Craig, W. M.: Use and Abuse of Iodized Oil in Diagnosis of Lesions of Spinal Cord, Surg., Gynec. & Obst., 49, 17, 1929.

Dandy, W. E.: Ventriculography Following Injection of Air into the Cerebral Ventricles, Ann. Surg., 68, 5, 1918.

———: Roentgenography of the Brain after Injection of Air into the Spinal Canal, Ann. Surg., 70, 397, 1919.

———: Loose Cartilage from Intervertebral Disk Simulating Tumor of the Spinal Cord, Arch. Surg., 19, 660, 1929.

———: Concealed Ruptured Intervertebral Disks: Plea for Elimination of Contrast Mediums in Diagnosis, J.A.M.A., 117, 821, 1941.

———: Recent Advances in the Diagnosis and Treatment of Ruptured Intervertebral Discs, Ann. Surg., 115, 514, 1942.

Deery, E. M.: Herniation of the Nucleus Pulposus as a Complication of Pre-existing Low Back Instability, Surg. Gynec. & Obst., 77, 79, 1943.

Djindjian, R., Fauré, C. and Hurth, M.: Explorations Artériographiques des Anéurysmes Artério-Veineux de la Moelle Epinière, Les Monographies des Annales de Radiologie, Expansion Scientifique Française, 1966.

du Boulay, G. H.: Pulsatile Movements in the Cerebrospinal Fluid Pathways, Brit. J. Radiol., 39, 255, 1966.

du Boulay, G. H. and Monson, E. M.: Telecine Technique Applied to Neuroradiology, Brit. J. Radiol., 37, 814, 1964.

Echlin, F. A., Ivie, J. McK. and Fine, A.: Pantopaque Myelography as an Aid in the Pre-operative Diagnosis of Protruded Intervertebral Discs, Surg., Gynec. & Obst., *80*, 257, 1945.

Elsberg, C. A. and Dyke, C. G.: Diagnosis and Localization of Tumors of the Spinal Cord by Means of Measurements Made on X-ray Films of the Vertebrae, and the Correlation of Clinical and X-ray Findings, Bull. Neurol. Inst., New York, *3*, 359, 1934.

Epstein, B. S.: The Effects of Increased Intraspinal Pressure on Movements of Iodized Oil Within the Spinal Canal, Am. J. Roentgenol., *52*, 196, 1944.

————: The Evacuation of Pantopaque from the Lumbar Spinal Canal by Siphon Action, Radiology, *83*, 472, 1964.

————: The Myelographic Demonstration of the Anterior Spinal and Radicular Arteries, Am. J. Roentgenol., *91*, 427, 1964.

————: *Myelography in Classic Descriptions in Diagnostic Roentgenology*, Springfield, Charles C Thomas, 941, 1964.

————: The Role of a Transverse Arachnoidal Membrane within the Interpeduncular Cistern in the Passage of Pantopaque into the Cranial Cavity, Radiology, *85*, 914, 1965.

Epstein, B. S. and Davidoff, L. M.: The Roentgenologic Diagnosis of Dilatation of the Spinal Cord Veins, Am. J. Roentgenol., *49*, 476, 1943.

Epstein, B. S. and Epstein, J. A.: Syphonage Technic for Removal of Pantopaque, Acta radiol., *5*, 1007, 1966.

Epstein, B. S., Epstein, J. A. and Lavine, L.: The Effect of Anatomic Variations in the Lumbar Vertebrae and Spinal Canal on Cauda Equina and Nerve Root Syndromes, Am. J. Roentgenol., *91*, 1055, 1964.

Frazier, C. H. and Glaser, M. A.: Iodized Rape-Seed Oil (Campiodol) for Cerebrospinal Visualization, J.A.M.A., *91*, 1609, 1928.

Hampton, A. O.: Iodized Oil Myelography: Use in Diagnosis of Rupture of the Intervertebral Disk into the Spinal Canal, Arch. Surg., *40*, 444, 1940.

Hampton, A. O. and Robinson, J. M.: The Roentgenographic Demonstration of Rupture of the Intervertebral Disc into the Spinal Canal after the Injection of Lipiodol. With Special Reference to Unilateral Lumbar Lesions Accompanied by Low Back Pain with "Sciatic Radiation," Am. J. Roentgenol., *36*, 782, 1936.

Hinck, V. C., Clark, W. M. and Hopkins, C. E.: Normal Interpedicular Distances (Minimum and Maximum) in Children and Adults, Am. J. Roentgenol., *97*, 141, 1966.

Hinck, V. C., Hopkins, C. E. and Clark, W. M.: Sagittal Diameter of the Lumbar Spinal Canal in Children and Adults, Radiology, *85*, 929, 1965.

Hinck, V. C., Hopkins, C. E. and Savara, B. S.: Sagittal Diameter of the Cervical Spinal Canal in Children, Radiology, *79*, 97, 1962.

Jacobaeus, H.: On Insufflation of Air into the Spinal Canal for Diagnostic Purposes in Cases of Tumors in the Spinal Cord, Acta m◠l. Scandinav., *55*, 555, 1921.

Jefferson, A.: Localized Enlargement of the Spinal Canal in the Absence of Tumor: A Congenital Abnormality, J. Neurol., Neurosurg., & Psychiat., *18*, 305, 1955.

Jirout, J.: Mobility of the Thoracic Spinal Cord under Normal Conditions, Acta radiol., *1*, 729, 1963.

Jones, M. D.: Cineradiographic Studies of the Collar-Immobilized Cervical Spine, J. Neurosurg., *17*, 633, 1960.

Kahn, E. A.: The Role of the Dentate Ligaments in Spinal Cord Compression and the Syndrome of Lateral Sclerosis, J. Neurosurg., *4*, 191, 1947.

Key, J. A.: Indications for Operation in Disc Lesions in the Lumbosacral Spine, Ann. Surg., *135*, 886, 1952.

Kubik, C. S. and Hampton, A. O.: Removal of Iodized Oil by Lumbar Puncture, New England J. Med., *224*, 455, 1941.

Kvernland, B. N., Grewe, R. V., Woolley, I. M. and Lee, I. R.: Upright Large Volume Dynamic Myelography, Radiology, *72*, 562, 1959.

Left, H. H. and MacLean, Jr., J. A.: Visualization of the Brain and Spinal Cord with Diiodotyrosine-Gelatin Contrast Medium, Including Observations on the Fate of this Material, Arch. Neurol. & Psychiat., *48*, 343, 1942.

Liliequist, B.: The Subarachnoid Cisterns. An Anatomic and Roentgenologic Study, Acta radiol., Supp. 185, 1959.

Lindblom, K. and Rexed, B.: Spinal Nerve Injury in Dorso-Lateral Protrusions of Lumbar Disks, J. Neurosurg., *5*, 413, 1948.

Locke, G. R., Gardner, J. I. and Van Epps, E. F.: Atlas-Dens Interval (ADI) in Children. A Survey Based on 200 Normal Cervical Spines, Am. J. Roentgenol., *97*, 135, 1966.

Love, J. G. and Walsh, M. N.: Intraspinal Protrusion of Intervertebral Disks, Arch. Surg., *40*, 455, 1940.

————: Protruded Intervertebral Disks, Surg., Gynec. & Obst., *77*, 497, 1943.

Malis, L. I.: The Myelographic Examination of the Foramen Magnum, Radiology, *70*, 196, 1958.

Malis, L. I., Newman, C. M. and Wolf, B. S.: Full-Column Technic in Lumbar Disk Myelography Radiology, *60*, 18, 1953.

Maltby, G. L.: Progressive Thorium Dioxide Myelopathy, New England J. Med., *270*, 490, 1964.

Marcovich, A. W., Walker, A. E. and Jessico, C. M.: Immediate and Late Effects of Intrathecal Injection of Iodized Oil, J.A.M.A., *116*, 2247, 1941.

Mayfield, F.: Symposium on Cervical Trauma: Neurosurgical Aspects, Clin. Neurosurg., *2*, 83, 1955.

McRae, F. L.: Asymptomatic Intervertebral Disc-protrusions, Acta radiol., *46*, 9, 1956.

Mixter, W. J.: Use of Lipiodol in Tumor of the Spinal Cord, Arch. Neurol. & Psychiat., *14*, 35, 1925.

————: Rupture of the Intervertebral Disk. A Short History of its Evolution as a Syndrome of Importance to the Surgeon, J.A.M.A., *140*, 278, 1949.

Mixter, W. J. and Ayer, J. G.: Herniation or Rupture of the Intervertebral Disc into the Spinal Canal, New England J. Med., *213*, 385, 1935.

Mixter, W. J. and Barr, J. S.: Rupture of the Intervertebral Disc with Involvement of the Spinal Cord, New England J. Med., *211*, 210, 1934.

Mones, R. and Werman, R.: Pantopaque Myeloencephalography, Radiology, *72*, 803, 1959.

Nichols, B. H. and Nosik, W. A.: Myelography with the Use of Thorium Dioxide Solution (Thorotrast) as a Contrast Medium, Radiology, *35*, 459, 1940.

Nosik, W. A.: Intraspinal Thorotrast, Am. J. Roentgenol., *49*, 214, 1943.

Nosik, W. A. and Mortensen, O. A.: Myelography with Thorotrast and Subsequent Removal by Forced Drainage, Experimental Study, Am. J. Roentgenol., *39*, 727, 1938.

O'Connell, J. E. A.: Protrusion of the Lumbar Intervertebral Discs: A Clinical Review Based on 500 Cases Treated by Excision of the Protrusion, J. Bone & Joint Surg., *33-B*, 8, 1951.

Odin, M. and Runstrom, G.: Iodized Oil as an Aid to the Diagnosis of Lesions of the Spinal Cord and a Contribution to the Knowledge of Adhesive Circumscribed Meningitis, Acta radiol., Supp. 7, Stockholm, 1928.

Peacher, W. G. and Robertson, R. C. L.: Pantopaque Myelography: Results, Comparison of Contrast Media and Spinal Fluid Reaction, J. Neurosurg., *2*, 220, 1945.

Peiper, H. and Klose, H.: Uber die Grundlagen einer Myelographie, Arch. Klin. Chirurg., *134*, 303, 1925.

Porter, E. C.: Measurement of the Cervical Spinal Cord in Pantopaque Myelography, Am. J. Roentgenol., *76*, 270, 1956.

Pribram, H. F. W., Hass, A. C. and Nishioka, H.: Radiographic Localization of a Spontaneous Cerebrospinal Fluid Fistula, J. Neurosurg., *24L*, 1031, 1966.

Ramsey, H. G. S. and Strain, W. H.: Pantopaque; New Contrast Medium for Myelography, Radiolog. & Clin. Photog., *20*, 25, 1944.

Ramsey, G. H., French, J. D. and Strain, W. H.: Iodinated Organic Compounds as Contrast Media for Radiographic Diagnosis. IV. Pantopaque Myelography, Radiology, *43*, 236, 1944.

Reiser, E.: Theoretiches und Kasuistiches zur Myelographie, Fortschr. a.d. Geb.d. Röntgenstrahlen, *34*, 443, 1926.

Richter, Hs. R. and Nidecker, H. J.: Röntgenkinomatographische Untersuchungen mit Positiven und Negativen Kontrasten im Wirbelkanal, Acta radiol., *1*, 751, 1963.

Rockett, F. X., Wittenborg, M. H., Shillito, Jr., J., and Matson, D. D.: Pantopaque Visualization of a Congenital Dural Defect of the Internal Auditory Meatus Causing Rhinorrhea, Am. J. Roentgenol., *91*, 640, 1964.

Sanford, H. and Doub, H. P.: Epidurography: A Method of Roentgenologic Visualization of Protruded Intervertebral Disk, Radiology, *36*, 712, 1941.

Scanlan, R. L.: Positive Contrast Medium (Iophendylate) in Diagnosis of Acoustic Neuroma, Arch. Otolaryngol., *80*, 698, 1964.

Schmorl, G.: *Die Gesunde und Kranke Wirbelsäule im Röntgenbild.*, Fortschr. a. d. Geb.d. Röntgenstraheln, Erganzungsband XLIII, Leipzig, Georg Thieme, 1932.

Shafron, M. and Wiener, S. N.: Pantopaque Examination of the Cerebellopontine Angle, Radiology, *85*, 921, 1965.

Sicard, J. A. and Forestier, J.: Méthode Génerale d'Exploration Radiologique par l'Huile Iodée (Lipiodol), Bull. et Mém. Soc. d. Hôp. de Paris, *46*, 463, 1922.

————: Roentgenologic Exploration of the Central Nervous System with Iodized Oil (Lipiodol), Arch. Neurol. & Psychiat., *16*, 420, 1926.

Sicard, J. A., Haguenau and LaPlane: Transition Lipiodole Rachidien, Technique Sou-Arachnoidienne, Resultats Diagnostiques, Rev. Neurologique, *1*, 1, 1924.

Smith, F. P., Pitts, Jr., F. R. and Rogoff, S. M.: Cinemyelography, J. Neurosurg., *17*, 1112, 1960.

Stoltmann, H. F. and Blackwood, W.: An Anatomical Study of the Role of the Dentate Ligaments in the Cervical Spinal Canal, J. Neurosurg., *24*, 43, 1966.

Stookey, B.: Compression of the Spinal Cord Due to Ventral Extradural Cervical Chondromas: Diagnosis and Surgical Treatment, Arch. Neurol. & Psychiat., *20*, 275, 1928.

Strain, W. H., Plati, J. T. and Warren, S. L.: Iodinated Organic Compounds as Contrast Media for Radiographic Diagnosis. I. Iodinated Aracyl Esters, J. Am. Chem. Soc., *64*, 1436, 1942.

Suh, T. H. and Alexander, L.: Vascular System of the Human Spinal Cord, Arch. Neurol. & Psychiat., *41*, 659, 1939.

Teng, P.: Myelographic Identification of the Dentate Ligament, Radiology, *74*, 944, 1960.

————: Ligamentum Denticulatum. (An Anatomical Review and its Role in Various Neurosurgical Problems of the Spinal Cord.) J. Mt. Sinai Hosp., *32*, 567, 1965.

Tucker, H. J., Sibley, W. A. and Lapham, L. W.: Cauda Equina Damage After Thorium Dioxide Myelography, Acta radiol., *5*, 1147, 1966.

Turnbull, I. M., Breig, A. and Hassler, O.: Blood Supply of Cervical Spinal Cord in Man. A Microangiographic Cadaver Study, J. Neurosurg., *24*, 951, 1966.

Wideroe, S.: On Intraspinal Injections of Air and their Diagnostic Value in Diseases of the Cord, Especially Tumors, Norsk. Mag. f. Laegevidensk, *32*, 491, 1921.

Worth, H. M.: The Use of Lipiodol in the Localization of Spinal Tumors, Brit. J. Radiol., *11*, 211, 1938.

Arachnoidal Diverticula

Arachnoidal diverticula, or cysts, are found proximal to the dorsal root ganglion and are intimately associated with this root'

The ventral nerve root has never been found to be the point of origin of these structures. They are in free communication with the subarachnoid spaces in many instances, and cineradiographic examinations of the emptying and filling of some arachnoid cysts indicate a considerable variation in the passage of fluid in and out. Apparently some have rather widely patent mouths, and others present constricted necks. On microscopic examination the cavities are lined with arachnoid, and proliferative layered accumulations of arachnoid form a significant portion of the cyst wall. Dense collagenous fibers derived from and continuous with the dura mater of the dorsal root sleeves consti-

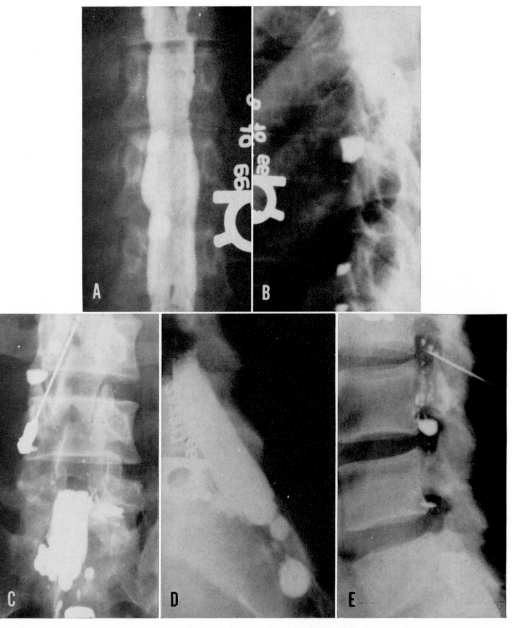

FIG. 87. *A*, Multiple thoracic arachnoidal diverticula, AP view and *B*, lateral view. *C*, *D* and *E*, Multiple lumbar diverticula also are present, as well as several sacral sacs. Same patient.

tute the outermost layer. The nerve root does not lie free within the cavity, but the nerve fibers are compressed by the fluid-filled structures and may be incorporated in its wall. On the other hand, spinal extra-dural cysts do not contain nerve fibers. The cause of these pouch-like diverticula sup-posedly is related to hydrostatic pressures in the subarachnoid space (Smith, 1961). The possibility that they represent a congenital variation is suggested by the wide variability encountered in these structures. In some, the diverticula extend for only a few milli-meters along the nerve root, and are some-what cylindrical in configuration. In others, they are grossly saccular. They occur singly, but more often are multiple (Fig. 87). Considerable extension along the nerve roots also is observed, in some extending for as much as 5 or 10 cm distally. In the latter group the emptying of the Pantopaque from the elongated arachnoidal diverticula, is slow. No untoward symptoms have been observed as a complication of filling of these diverticula, even though Pantopaque is re-tained for a long while. In differential diagnosis arachnoidal cysts have to be dis-tinguished from those associated with von Recklinghausen's disease, with congenital malformations such as meningoceles, symp-tomatic spinal extradural cysts, and intra-dural cysts of the spinal meninges variously described as circumscribed serous spinal meningitis, localized adhesive spinal arach-noiditis, arachnitis adhesive circumscripta, or meningitis serosa circumscripta spinalis. In the latter group are loculated fluid accu-mulations caught in arachnoid scar tissue which binds the dura to the surface of the cord rather than smooth-lined arachnoidal cystic extensions. The lesions result from a variety of infectious, chemical or traumatic processes.

Occasionally arachnoidal cysts become large enough to cause nerve root compression (Fig. 88). These sometimes can be identi-

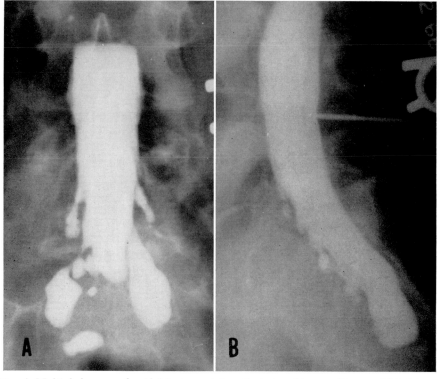

Fig. 88. *A*, Multiple large arachnoidal first sacral diverticula in a 34-year-old man with left buttock and right sciatic pain. Relief followed unroofing of these foramina and the upper sacrum, freeing nerve roots compressed by the sacs. *B*, Lateral lumbosacral myelogram.

fied on plain film roentgenograms because their erosive effects produce a smoothly rounded indentation in the adjacent vertebra or sacrum. They should be differentiated from the perineurial or extradural sacral cysts described by Tarlov (1953) as occurring at the junction of the posterior nerve root with the dorsal root ganglion, in the space between the perineurium and endoneurium as nearly solid masses containing nerve fibers and ganglion cells. The latter do not communicate with the cerebrospinal fluid spaces, so that they do not fill with Pantopaque, nor do they, as a rule, produce bone erosion unless they are quite large.

References

Abbott, K. H., Retter, R. H. and Leimbach, W. H.: The Role of Perineurial Sacral Cysts in the Sciatic and Sacrococcygeal Syndrome, J. Neurosurg., *14*, 5, 1957.

Fahrenkrug, A. and Hojgaard, K.: Multiple Paravertebral Lumbar Meningocele, Brit. J. Radiol., *36*, 574, 1963.

Jacobs, L. G., Smith, J. K. and Van Horn, P. S.: Myelographic Demonstration of Cysts of Spinal Membranes, Radiology, *62*, 215, 1954.

Lombardi, G. and Morello, G.: Congenital Cysts of the Spinal Membranes and Roots, Brit. J. Radiol., *36*, 197, 1963.

Smith, D. T.: Cystic Formations Associated with Human Spinal Nerve Roots, J. Neurosurg., *18*, 654, 1961.

Smith, D. T.: Multiple Meningeal Diverticula (Perineurial Cysts) of the Cervical Region Disclosed by Pantopaque Myelography, J. Neurosurg., *19*, 599, 1962.

Tarlov, I. M.: *Sacral Nerve-Root Cysts: Another Cause of the Sciatic or Cauda Equina Syndrome*, Springfield, Charles C Thomas, 1953.

Teng, P. and Papatheodorou, C.: Spinal Arachnoid Diverticula, Brit. J. Radiol., *39*, 249, 1966.

Teng, P. and Rudner, N.: Multiple Arachnoid Diverticula, A.M.A. Arch. Neurol., *2*, 348, 1960.

Evacuation of Pantopaque After Myelography

When the myelographic examination is completed, the Pantopaque is brought back into the caudal sac by returning the patient to an erect position. The entire canal is then inspected to see if residual droplets are caught in the lateral recesses of the subarachnoid space or in arachnoidal diverticula. If present, these are forced back into the main stream of the subarachnoid space by having the patient cough vigorously so that the droplets rise, come into the midline position, and fall back to the caudal sac (Fig. 84). This maneuver is not always entirely successful.

Inspection of transabdominal lumbar films or turning the patient into a lateral position under the image intensifier permits localization of the needle tip in relationship to the floor of the spinal canal (Fig. 89). With the patient horizontal, the Pantopaque column is centered at the needle tip. The stylet is withdrawn and replaced with the angular adaptor. If the adaptor and plastic tube assembly have been left in place, the tip of the polyethylene tube previously connected to the syringe is fixed to the opening of a sterile test tube taped to the side of the table at a level below that of the vertebral column. Usually, in normal canals Pantopaque starts flowing through the plastic tube spontaneously, relatively slowly at first and with increasing speed as the head of the column gets below the level of the spine (Fig. 66).

When the needle tip is completely immersed, the stream consists entirely of Pantopaque. This can be monitored by observing the flow visually or by means of image intensification fluoroscopy. As the canal empties, the needle bevel becomes partly immersed in Pantopaque and partly in cerebrospinal fluid. The flow changes so that Pantopaque droplets are interspersed with droplets of cerebrospinal fluid. This can be observed through the polyethylene tube. Should flow stop or become hesitant, the myelographer gently rotates the needle tip in place until evacuation resumes.

In most patients it is possible to remove almost all of the Pantopaque quickly and without pain. One gets the impression of a vacuum-cleaner-like action when watching Pantopaque droplets passing the open needle bevel. Difficulty may be encountered with the last droplets because they move with breathing, pulsatile activity, or change in position caused by variations in the configuration of the floor of the canal, so that they

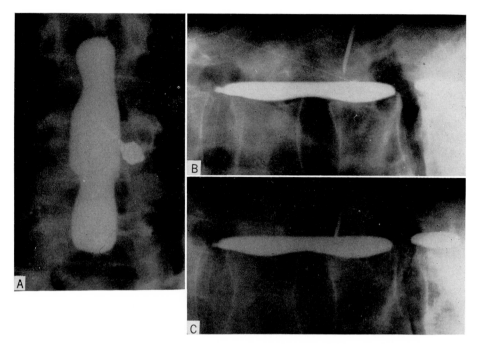

Fig. 89. *A,* Myelogram with 6 ml of Pantopaque, patient in supine position. Cerebrospinal fluid aspirated. *B,* Same patient, transabdominal view. The needle tip is well above the Pantopaque, so that mainly fluid was withdrawn. *C,* Same patient, with needle tip lowered into Pantopaque pool, permitting its aspiration.

cannot be brought to the needle tip. In my experience almost all the Pantopaque can be evacuated even when the needle tip is off center or when at the level of the intervertebral disc (Fig. 90). Theoretically, it should be easier to get Pantopaque out if the needle tip is situated at the hollow of the vertebra and in the midline, but this does not always work out.

Occasionally in order to test the possibility of the production of pain by aspiration, syphonage has been interrupted and a 2-ml syringe inserted into the distal portion of the polyethylene tube. Gentle suction results in further evacuation of the Pantopaque without pain in patients with relatively large spinal canals. However, when the canal is narrow and the fila of the cauda equina are prominent, even very gentle suction produces an exquisitely localized pain. This also occurs in wide canals if a filum is caught in the bevel of the needle.

In some patients with narrow canals or spondylotic spurs causing swelling of the roots of the cauda equina, syphonage is successful until about two-thirds of the contrast material is evacuated. If it is desired to remove the remainder, it is sometimes necessary to withdraw the needle and reinsert it into another interspace. This can be selected by observing the Pantopaque column and choosing the interspace at which the subarachnoid space appears widest (Fig. 91).

Occasionally difficulty is encountered in starting the stream of Pantopaque. This may be caused by entrance of a nerve root into the needle tip, so that it cannot be dislodged. A fold of arachnoid which enters the needle tip produces the same result (Fig. 92). Under these circumstances it is preferable not to work too hard to get flow started but to withdraw the needle and reinsert it at another interspace. It is interesting to note how often patients with relatively narrow lumbar canals have wide thecal sacs at the

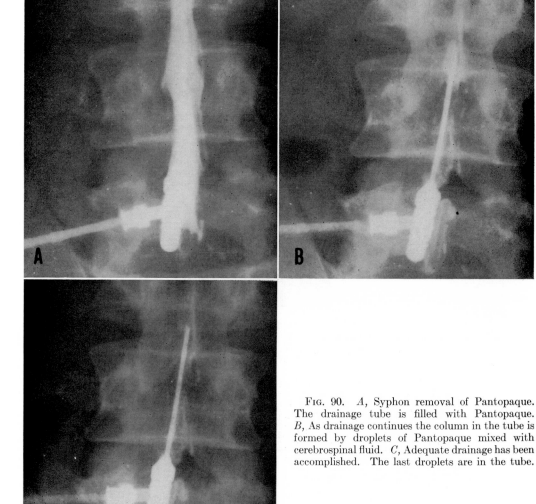

Fig. 90. *A*, Syphon removal of Pantopaque. The drainage tube is filled with Pantopaque. *B*, As drainage continues the column in the tube is formed by droplets of Pantopaque mixed with cerebrospinal fluid. *C*, Adequate drainage has been accomplished. The last droplets are in the tube.

fifth or second lumbar interspaces. If a fifth lumbar interspace tap can be accomplished easily, it is preferable to use this for evacuation of Pantopaque.

In most patients Pantopaque can be removed by means of syphonage quite quickly and painlessly. When difficulty is encountered in aspirating the last droplets, no effort is made to get all out. The procedure requires some delicacy in manipulating the needle tip, but once this is mastered it can be used successfully and with considerable satisfaction. Not only does it work when the needle is accurately placed in the middle of the spinal canal, but it has also proven most satisfying when the needle tip was placed quite laterally. Syphonage has become routine in my practice, and is most helpful in minimizing the painful aspects of myelography.

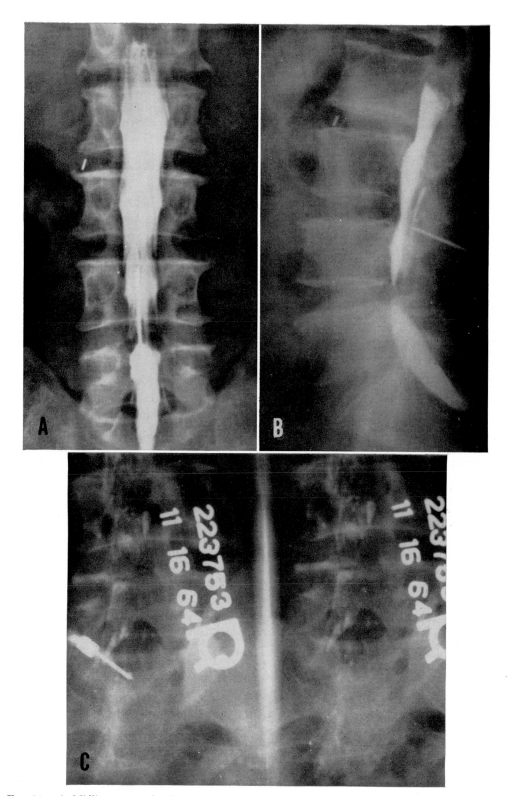

Fig. 91. *A*, Midline tap at the third lumbar interspace in a patient with a narrow canal and a large L4 disc-ridge syndrome, anteroposterior and, *B*, lateral views. Drainage could not be accomplished by gentle suction or syphon. Needle replaced at L5 interspace, *C*, and adequate evacuation was accomplished easily, *D*.

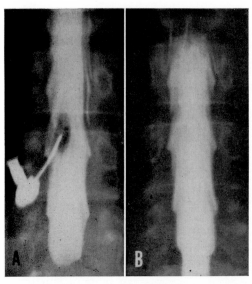

FIG. 92. *A*, The radiolucent shadow at the needle tip is attributed to intrusion of intact arachnoid into the subarachnoid space caused by displacement of the needle tip and subsequent gentle downward pressure to get it back into the canal. This could not be accomplished. When the needle was withdrawn, *B*, the defect vanished. Drainage accomplished after reinsertion at the interspace below.

References

Epstein, B. S.: The Evacuation of Pantopaque from the Lumbar Spinal Canal by Siphon Action, Radiology, *83*, 472, 1964.

Epstein, B. S. and Epstein, J. A.: Myelography Using Image-Intensification Fluoroscopy, Cineradiography, and Siphonage to Remove the Radiopaque, Med. Radiography and Photography, *42*, 9, 1966.

————: Syphonage Technic for Removal of Pantopaque, Acta Radiol., *5*, 1007, 1966.

Kubik, C. S. and Hampton, A. O.: Removal of Iodized Oil by Lumbar Puncture, New England J. Med., *224*, 455, 1941.

Scott, W. C. and Furlow, L. T.: Myelography with Pantopaque and a New Technic for its Removal, Radiology, *43*, 241, 1944.

Subdural Pantopaque

The instillation of Pantopaque into the subdural space in sufficient quantities to give rise to major myelographic defects occurred in only 5 instances in my experience of over 3500 consecutive myelograms. Large subdural placements occur when the needle tip pushes the arachnoid away from the dura, so that the bevel lies mainly in the subdural space. There may be sufficient cerebrospinal fluid present so that a good return flow is obtained, and injection of the contrast material is relatively free. Usually some also enters the subarachnoid space as well, so that a double-barrel configuration appears. When the arachnoid is dissected away from the dura, subdural Pantopaque in sufficient quantity may present as a column which can hardly be distinguished from the subarachnoid space itself. However, after 3 or 4 ml have been injected a rather abrupt cessation of the flow of Pantopaque caudad takes place. If atypical flow is observed, the injection is stopped. The diagnosis can be established by turning the patient on his side and noting the configuration of the column, usually gathered in the superior and lateral subdural spaces. With relatively large quantities of Pantopaque in the subdural space, a rounded appearance at the caudal end of the column sometimes may be mistaken for a rather large midline lesion with obstructive characteristics (Fig. 93). The flow of Pantopaque when the table is tilted is slower than usually observed. However, there were instances when subdural Pantopaque flowed rather freely cephalad and caudad, in some instances reaching the cervical area.

A more characteristic configuration of subdural Pantopaque is that of a thin layer of contrast material around the subdural space (Fig. 94). A very slow flow of Pantopaque is observed both in the cephalad and caudad directions.

When Pantopaque has been delivered into a wide subdural space, it is possible to remove it by syphonage and to continue the examination by replacing the needle one or two interspaces higher (Fig. 93). However, when Pantopaque is in the subdural space in relatively thin layers which extend for considerable distances, it cannot be removed. The examination may have to be abandoned, unless one feels that the problem is of sufficient gravity to warrant an immediate tap at another interspace.

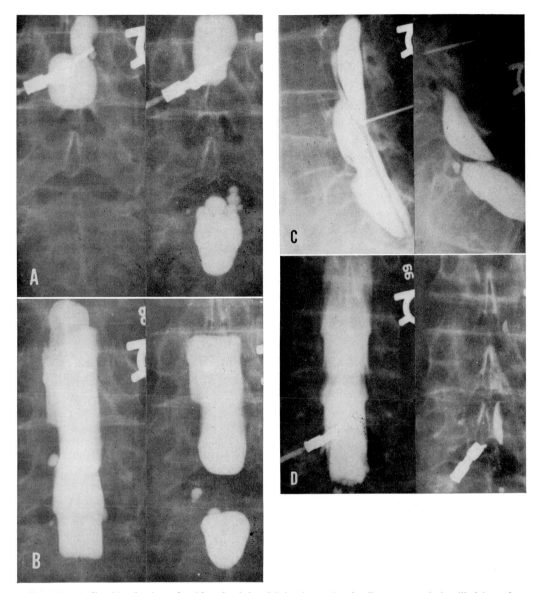

Fig. 93. *A*, Combined subarachnoid and subdural injection. As the Pantopaque is instilled it gathers in a rounded collection. Note that the needle tip is placed laterally. On injecting a bit more, *B*, some Pantopaque descends to the caudal sac, but most remains subdurally. On lateral films, *C*, the needle tip is seen in a high position. The radiolucent line probably is a nerve root. Some of the Pantopaque was aspirated, leaving a collection in the caudal sac, and above it, in the subdural space. It was possible to evacuate almost all the Pantopaque from the subdural space without difficulty. The tap was then repeated at the fourth lumbar interspace and the study continued. After completion, all the Pantopaque was removed except for a bit left in the subdural space *D*. The free flow in the subdural space is unusual, most of the time flow being slow and aspiration from this area difficult.

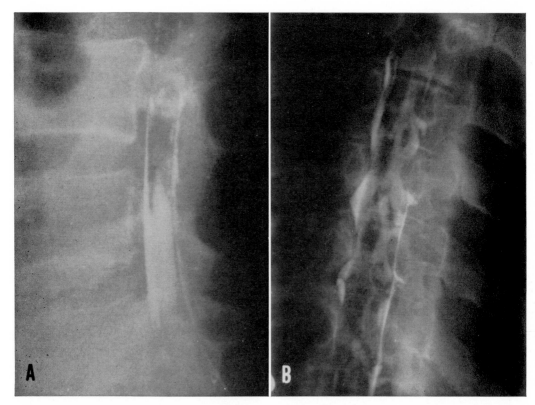

FIG. 94. *A*, Subdural placement of Pantopaque surrounds the lumbar spinal canal and, B, the thoracic spinal canal. Note the thin linear configuration of the column, and the small spicules extending laterally in the thoracic region.

More frequently a small amount of Pantopaque enters the subdural space when the needle tip crosses both the subdural and subarachnoid areas. Occasionally a small amount of Pantopaque enters through the needle perforation, and is visible as a small streak in the dorsal aspect of the spinal canal. These are easy to identify, and usually cause no difficulty.

Ventral subdural intravasation occasionally occurs when the needle point is driven into the floor of the spinal canal. In these instances both epidural and subdural placement is observed. Usually this takes place later in the examination, either when the needle is pushed down inadvertently or when efforts are made to place it close to the floor of the canal for withdrawal of contrast material. Rarely the needle tip is in this position early in the examination, so that the contrast material is injected into the ventral subdural space as well as into the subarachnoid space. The Pantopaque then may gather in an irregular fashion, and possibly be mistaken for arachnoiditis (Fig. 95).

Once in a while the needle tip moves back from the subarachnoid space during myelography. On attempting to return it into the canal the arachnoid is separated and pushed towards the Pantopaque column. A negative defect appears at the needle point. This can be identified on translumbar views, which reveal a depression into the Pantopaque column with the needle tip above the main level of the oil. This possibility can be ascertained by withdrawing the needle. The Pantopaque column then resumes a normal configuration. Replacing the needle at another interspace and removal of the contrast material without leaving any in the

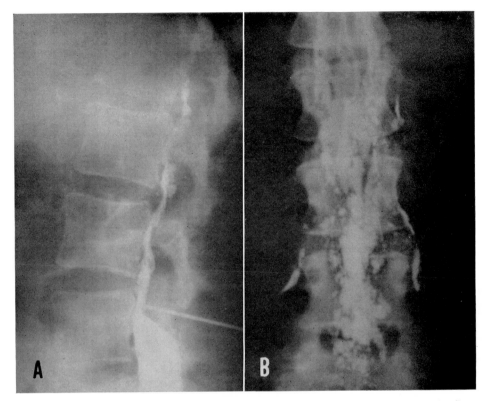

Fig. 95. *A*, Pantopaque enters the subdural space from the ventral aspect of the canal. Some also passes epidurally. *B*, After removal from the subarachnoid space the irregular drop-like contours should not be confused with arachnoiditis.

subdural space indicates that none has entered that region (Fig. 92).

Defects also have been ascribed to lateral placement of the lumbar puncture needle. If this is suspected, the needle should be removed and the examination continued. This can be somewhat troublesome when the needle tip is close to the disc at an interspace where a discal herniation is suspected. If the defect persists after removal of the needle, and one is sure that no subdural cerebrospinal fluid or Pantopaque is present, the myelographic defect can be interpreted in the usual way (Fig. 96).

Epidural Extravasation of Pantopaque

Pantopaque may extravasate if the bevel of the needle tip is so placed that it is partly within the subarachnoid space and partly in either the subdural or the epidural space, or both. Under this circumstance, injection of Pantopaque results in the passage of some into the subarchnoid space, and a considerable amount may enter the epidural space. A pure subdural injection is infrequent, but small amounts do enter fairly often.

With epidural injection, rapid extension of Pantopaque along the outside of the dural sac occurs. The contrast material passes into the peridural areas and along the nerve roots as they go through the respective intervertebral foramina. As a rule, such a mishap is not accompanied by any untoward complication. The Pantopaque remains in the epidural space for a long time, and extends along the nerve roots as far as the midthigh or in the thoracolumbar and cervical areas well out into the flanks or axilla (Fig. 97). Some absorption, however, does occur (Figs. 64, 65). Monitoring of the

10

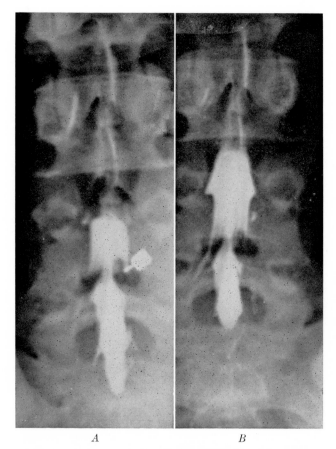

FIG. 96.   *A*, Anteroposterior myelogram showing defect at interspace between fourth and fifth lumbar vertebrae, with needle *in situ*.   The question of needle defect had to be excluded.   *B*, Same case with needle removed.   Defect persisted.   Operation disclosed herniated disc in midline.

examination by image intensification fluoroscopy minimizes this occurrence, because passage of a significant quantity into the epidural space can be detected promptly. The needle is then removed and another lumbar puncture made at a point below or above the original site.   Pantopaque is injected again under image intensification control, and the study may be continued without fear.

Occasionally one finds that even after an easy lumbar puncture and intrathecal injection of Pantopaque, some will flow into the epidural space.   Usually when this occurs, only a small amount extravasates, usually tracking along one or two nerve roots.   This may be incident to some trauma which takes place because the needle *in situ* is jarred as

the patient is moved, and a small laceration occurs.   Even with the needle kept *in situ* it is possible in these patients to evacuate the subarachnoid Pantopaque without difficulty. That left in the epidural space causes no difficulty.

In a review of 85 cases with extradural extravasation, it was noted that in 68 there was a lateral placement of the needle tip. In 2 there was also a considerable subdural instillation and in 6 others a small quantity entered the subdural space.   In the others, the tip was well centered.   In the last 35 of these patients Pantopaque instillation had been made under image intensification control.   The lateral placement of the needle tip was identified, but inasmuch as a ready flow of cerebrospinal fluid into the poly-

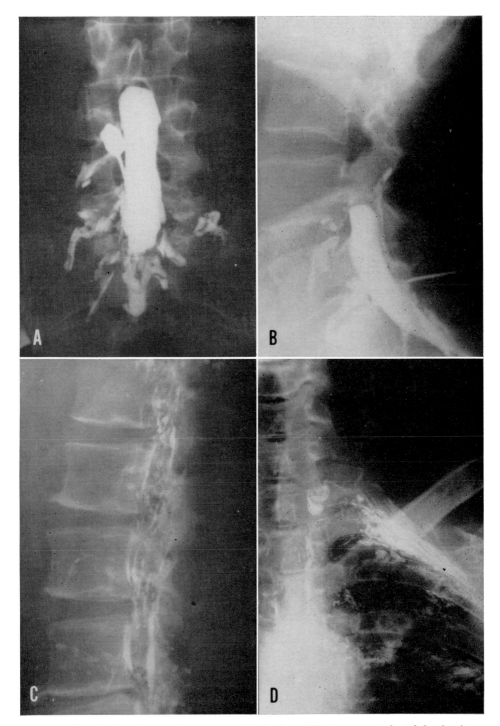

Fig. 97. *A*, Combined epidural and subarachnoid injection of Pantopaque at the 5th lumber interspace with extravasation. *B*, On the lateral view the needle tip is seen so situated that its bevel is just outside the dural sac. *C*, Another patient 1 month after subdural and epidural injection of Pantopaque. The contrast medium extends laterally and dorsally along the nerve roots. *D*, Same patient. The Pantopaque has extended along the brachial plexus. There were no untoward symptoms.

ethylene tube occurred, and the Pantopaque entered the subarachnoid space and dropped down into the caudal sac, the study was continued. In these patients, the Pantopaque appeared in the epidural space slowly. At times this was not noticed until 10 or 15 minutes had passed, and the needle had not been touched. In most of these patients, Pantopaque entered the epidural space on the side on which the needle tip had been inserted and spread cephalad and caudad for about 3 interspaces. Extension of the Pantopaque along the course of the nerve roots extended as far as 5 to 10 cm.

It is of interest that in 45 patients with some extravasation it was possible to recover almost all the Pantopaque from the sub-

arachnoid space using the same needle, by means of syphonage without pain. In 12 of these, syphonage was discontinued during the procedure, and an attempt made to recover the Pantopaque by gentle aspiration with a 2-ml syringe. In almost every one this immediately produced sharply localized pain. On resuming syphonage, it was possible to continue evacuation of the Pantopaque, usually without difficulty. The main problem was keeping the Pantopaque column at the needle tip to permit evacuation of the final droplets. In most cases about 0.5 ml was left in the canal.

Extravasation of Pantopaque also occurs when the needle tip is situated below the level of the anterior aspect of the dural sac.

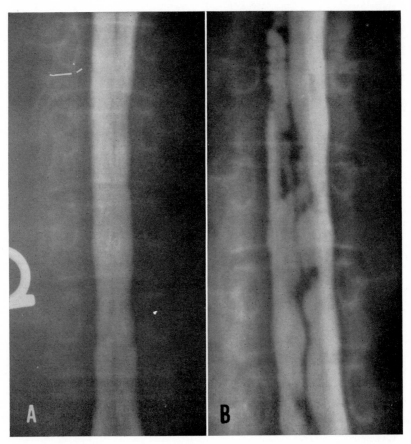

Fig. 98. *A*, A 6-ml myelogram with the patient prone. The column is uniform and the anterior spinal artery is visible. *B*, With the patient supine the column breaks up. This irregular configuration is normal, and should not be mistaken for arachnoiditis, especially when there is a free flow. The midline sinuous radiolucent shadow is probably incident to the septum posticum. (Courtesy Dr. D. Cukier, Hackensack, N. J.)

Here the space available is less than in the dorsal aspect, so that the opaque medium has a more constrained area in which to pass. The globular configuration and poor flow seen in this instance should not be misinterpreted as an indication of arachnoiditis. A somewhat similar appearance occasionally is observed when supine recumbent myelograms are done with relatively small quantities of Pantopaque. Here the flow of Pantopaque is normal, which should clearly differentiate these conditions one from the other (Figs. 95, 98).

Infrequently, a needle tip enters an epidural vein either during the instillation of Pantopaque or later in the examination. We have one instance (Epstein and Epstein, 1965) in which the needle tip entered an

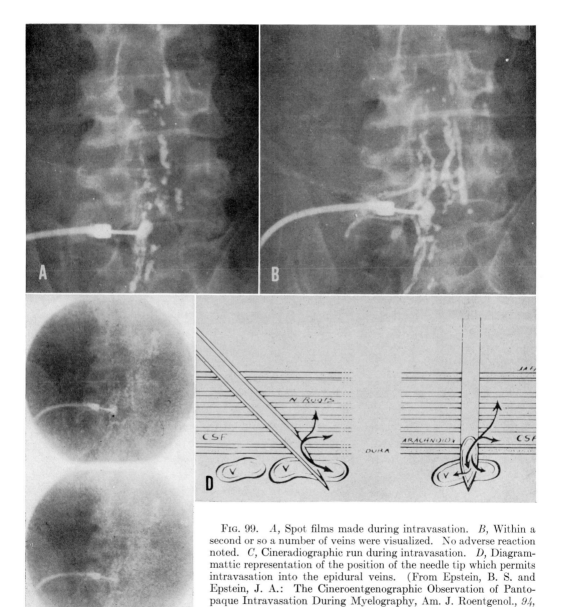

Fig. 99. *A*, Spot films made during intravasation. *B*, Within a second or so a number of veins were visualized. No adverse reaction noted. *C*, Cineradiographic run during intravasation. *D*, Diagrammattic representation of the position of the needle tip which permits intravasation into the epidural veins. (From Epstein, B. S. and Epstein, J. A.: The Cineroentgenographic Observation of Pantopaque Intravasation During Myelography, Am. J. Roentgenol., *94*, 576, 1965, courtesy of Charles C Thomas.)

epidural vein as the patient was being manipulated into the prone position. On the injection of Pantopaque, it was noted that the contrast material flowed into the epidural veins for the height of one to three interspaces, then rapidly passed into lateral branches and entered the inferior vena cava. This "bursting star" appearance was recorded cineradiographically (Fig. 99) and on spot film roentgenograms. Intravasation also may occur when the patient strains violently or coughs during the examination in such a manner that a vessel is torn by a displaced needle tip. No ill effects have been reported from this accident, aside from occasional episodes of minor pulmonary embolism with transient mild pain, slight hemoptosis, cough and mild fever. Pantopaque injected inadvertently into a vertebral body produces the picture of an intraosseous venogram.

Adverse Reactions to Myelography

Adverse sequelae of myelography have been attributed to inflammatory effects of intrathecal injection of positive contrast material. This has been substantiated with Lipiodol, but with Pantopaque it appears that arachnoiditis is a considerably less frequent complication. It is only fair to reflect that arachnoiditis occurs in patients who have had only diagnostic lumbar punctures, spinal anesthesia, intrathecal introduction of medication, or with subarachnoid bleeding. Bleeding into the subarachnoid space with gravitation of the blood into the caudal sac may initiate the development of arachnoiditis. This occurred in one of our patients who had a subarachnoid bleed from an aneurysm of the anterior communicating artery, which was treated successfully by operation. About a year later severe low back pain, with bilateral sciatic and thigh radiation appeared. Myelography disclosed the characteristic pattern of arachnoiditis of the lower lumbar spinal canal. Such an occurrence is infrequent. A relatively large quantity of blood is necessary to have this take place. In most patients who have a bloody tap at lumbar puncture, bleeding probably is due to the needle tip transfixing a small epidural vein as well as the subarachnoid space. This supposition is supported by the fact that most of the time lumbar puncture at another interspace produces clear fluid, or clear fluid may flow if the needle tip is turned.

Howland and Curry (1966) suggested the use of prednisone to avoid inflammatory reactions in the event of a bloody tap. On experimental evidence obtained by injecting blood and Pantopaque mixtures into the subarachnoid space of dogs, they found that their limited studies revealed no evidence of decomposition of the Pantopaque into more toxic products, with particular reference to phenol and iodine. It was suggested that the harmful effects of blood mixed with Pantopaque resulted from a physical phenomenon rather than irritation due to a chemical decomposition product. It may be presumed that if infection occurs it is most likely incident to a break in technic. For this reason, whenever possible, I leave the spinal needle *in situ* with the stylet out, replacing it with the connector and sterile polyethylene tube for instillation. This apparatus is later utilized for syphoning off the Pantopaque.

Schurr, McLaurin and Ingraham (1953) described an intracranial arachnoidal inflammatory reaction after injecting Pantopaque into the subarachnoid space of dogs. Even though the quantities used were greater than those employed clinically, the reaction indicated the desirability for preventing the entrance of Pantopaque into the head. Erickson and VanBaaren (1953) reported a 39-year-old man who expired 15 months after myelography because of an exudative arachnoiditis obstructing the basilar cisterns and the fourth ventricle. Another case of basilar meningitis incident to the entrance of Pantopaque into the cranial cavity was reported by Mason and Raaf (1962). In their patient, 9 ml of Pantopaque was injected without difficulty into the subarachnoid space. The patient became markedly agitated and complained of severe pain in the coccygeal area. About 4 ml were left after 5 ml had been removed. The Pantopaque remained in this position as shown by film 19 days later with the patient in the erect position. Four weeks later the patient became unresponsive and 7 months later he died. Death was attributed to a diffuse aseptic meningitis due to a hypersensitivity, with compression of the brain by the surrounding membrane. Hydrocephalus had developed. A membrane was present over the basilar foramina and the base of the brain. The foramina of Luschka and Magendi were completely obliterated. Cross sections through the cord showed a completely encircling dense fibrous membrane forming a collar about the cord. In the region of the cauda equina there were adhesions between the nerve roots and the meninges.

A fairly common concomitant of myelography is low back pain, occasionally with some aggravated sciatic symptoms, headache and meningismus. These changes may be due to the lumbar puncture itself, and the exact cause of post-spinal tap or myelographic headaches is still unknown. As a rule, these symptoms disappear relatively quickly, but at times headaches are quite disturbing. Delayed reactions with severe headache and cervical stiffness may develop 2 or 3 days or even 10 days after examination. As a rule, the patient is fairly comfortable when lying down, but complains of headache and vertigo when sitting or standing. We have found that keeping the patient recumbent, forcing fluids, and waiting 2 or 3 days usually clears complaints. Recently, Kulick (1966) suggested the use of intrathecal injection of methylprednisone acetate (depo-medrol) as a method for diminishing the untoward effects of spinal puncture for myelography and pneumoencephalography.

Among rare complications which have been reported are extraocular muscle paralysis, as reported by Wright (1949), and

Pantopaque meningitis secondary to hypersensitivity was mentioned by Luce, Leith and Burrage (1951). Taren (1960) reported another patient who had increased intracranial pressure and multiple cranial nerve palsies shortly after myelography. Some of the contrast material had entered the cranium and it was surmised that these events were sequelae of infection of the central nervous system or an unusual sensitivity to the Pantopaque. His patient recovered.

On the other hand, Gass (1963) stated that the fear of retained Pantopaque in the head, especially in small quantities, is not realistic. In my own experiences there have been no instances of which I am aware in which Pantopaque in the cranial cavity was followed by severe or fatal sequalae. Gradual disappearance of Pantopaque from the cranial cavity has been observed (Fig. 63).

Radiopaque emulsions have been used experimentally, but thus far have been found too toxic for clinical application. Teplick, Haskin and Skelley (1968) found that Pantopaque emulsions were irritating to the meninges, and that the degree of irritability was related to the size of the emulsified particles.

References

Bering, Jr., E. A.: Notes on the Retention of Pantopaque in the Subarachnoid Space, Am. J. Surg., *80*, 455, 1950.

Craig, R. L.: Effect of Iodized Poppy-Seed Oil on the Spinal Cord and Meninges, Arch. Neurol. & Psychiat., *48*, 799, 1942.

Davis, F. L.: Effect of Unabsorbed Radiographic Contrast Media on the Central Nervous System, Lancet, *2*, 747, 1956.

Epstein, B. S. and Epstein, J. A.: The Cineroentgenographic Observation of Pantopaque Intravasation during Myelography, Am. J. Roentgenol., *94*, 576, 1965.

Erickson, T. C. and Van Baaren, H. J.: Late Meningeal Reaction to Ethyl Iodophenylundecylate Used in Myelography, J.A.M.A., *153*, 636, 1953.

Fullenlove, T. M.: Venous Intravasation during Myelography, Radiology, *53*, 410, 1949.

Gass, H.: Pantopaque Anterior Basal Cisternography of the Posterior Fossa, Am. J. Roentgenol., *90*, 1197, 1963.

Ginsburg, L. B. and Skorneck, A. B.: Pantopaque Pulmonary Embolism, Am. J. Roentgenol., *73*, 27, 1955.

Globus, J. H. and Straus, I.: Intraspinal Iodolography: Subarachnoid Injection of Iodized Oil as Aid in Detection and Localization of Lesions Compressing Spinal Cord, Arch. Neurol. & Psychiat., *21*, 1331, 1929.

Howland, W. J. and Curry, J. L.: Experimental Studies of Pantopaque Arachnoiditis, Radiology, *87*, 253, 1966.

Hurteau, E. F., Baird, W. C. and Sinclair, E.: Arachnoiditis Following the Use of Iodized Oil, J. Bone & Joint Surg., *36-A*, 393, 1954.

Jones, M. D. and Newton, T. H.: Inadvertent Extra-arachnoid Injections in Myelography, Radiology, *80*, 818, 1963.

Kinkel, C. L.: Entrance of Pantopaque into the Venous System during Myelography, Am. J. Roentgenol., *54*, 230, 1945.

Kulick, S. A.: The Clinical Use of Intrathecal Methylprednisone Acetate Following Pneumoencephalography and Myelography, J. Mt. Sinai Hosp., *33*, 152, 1966.

Luce, J. C., Leith, W. and Burrage, W. S.: Pantopaque Meningitis Due to Hypersensitivity, Radiology, *57*, 878, 1951.

Mason, M. S. and Raaf, J.: Complications of Pantopaque Myelography. Case Report and Review, J. Neurosurg., *19*, 302, 1962.

Schultz, E. H. and Brogdon, H. G.: The Problem of Subdural Placement in Myelography, Radiology, *79*, 91, 1962.

Schultz, E. C. and Miller, J. H.: Intravasation of Opaque Media during Myelography, J. Neurosurg., *18*, 610, 1961.

Schurr, P. H., McLaurin, R. L. and Ingraham, F. D.: Experimental Studies on the Circulation of the Cerebrospinal Fluid. And Methods of Producing Communicating Hydrocephalus in the Dog, J. Neurosurg., *10*, 515, 1953.

Steinbach, H. L. and Hill, W. H.: Pantopaque Embolism during Myelography, Radiology, *56*, 735, 1951.

Taren, J. A.: Unusual Complication Following Pantopaque Myelography, J. Neurosurg., *17*, 323, 1960.

Tarlov, I. M.: Pantopaque Meningitis Disclosed at Operation, J.A.M.A., *129*, 1014, 1945.

Teplick, J. G., Haskin, M. E. and Skelley, J. F.: Total Myelography with Radiopaque Emulsions, Radiology, *90*, 698, 1968.

Wright, E. S.: Extraocular Muscle Paralysis from Spinal Injection of Pantopaque, California Med., *71*, 214, 1949.

Myelography with Water-Soluble Substances

Myelography with water-soluble material is performed with Abrodil (Myelotrast) (monoiodomethane sulfonate). The examination must be preceded by spinal anesthesia, and it cannot be used above the level of the first lumbar or the twelfth thoracic vertebra. A fine needle is used. The patient must be kept quiet and relaxed during the examination to prevent admixture of the contrast medium and the spinal fluid. Following the examination, the patient is kept prone on the tilting table for 1 hour with the thorax elevated and must not be moved until most of the contrast medium has been absorbed. Amundsen, Helsingen and Kristiansen (1963), in a review of 596 lumbar myelographies, mentioned that minor side effects such as headache or transitory leg pain have not been recorded, and that no serious complications have been noted. They had 12 cases in which subdural deposit of Abrodil had no ill effects. They found a considerable increase in the spinal fluid protein content, with or without an increase in cell content in 41 patients, but again no untoward sequelae were noted. Arnell (1948) mentioned that the use of a 35 per cent solution of Perabrodil had been accompanied by shock, indicating the necessity for keeping the concentration down to 20 per cent. Observation of blood pressure showed that there were often moderate sinkings of the pressure after injection of the contrast medium. Lindblom, in 1947, surveyed 721 cases of Abrodil myelography, and complications had been reported in 54. Some of these, such as headache for some days, may have been due to the lumbar puncture and anesthesia. Shock was reported in 32 cases, most of them within 30 minutes. Temporary lumbar pain and leg spasms were reported in 11 cases. Some of these adverse reactions were attributed to over-sensitivity to the contrast agent, or incomplete anesthesia. No lasting meningitic reactions were observed. A study of the effect on the spinal cord of subarachnoid injection of water-soluble contrast material in dogs was reported by Funkquist and Obel (1961). They found that the incidence and severity of spinal cord lesions could be increased by lowering the blood pressure after injection, and by the previous intravenous injection of hypotonic saline solution. Subarachnoid injection of saline solution isotonic with the contrast medium was found to produce the same kind of spinal cord lesions. The reactions were greatest in the pendant portion of the canal, with central necrosis and focal edema the predominant lesions.

There have been occasional reports of patients who have had intrathecal injections of water-soluble contrast agents made by accident. Doroshow, Yoon and Robbins (1962) reported what they considered to be the third case of accidental entry, and the first with a fatal outcome. This followed a translumbar aortogram done in a 31-year-old woman. Clear fluid was obtained from what was believed to be a hydronephrotic sac, but which actually was cerebrospinal fluid. Injection of 7 ml of 50 per cent Hypaque disclosed a myelogram. The needle was withdrawn, reinserted into the abdominal aorta and aortography done. About 45 minutes later, severe lumbar pain and myoclonic constrictions of the lower extremities appeared, and the patient died 2 hours later. At necropsy the brain, spinal cord and site of aortography were normal. Death was attributed to shock following introduction of hypaque into the subarachnoid space. They suggested that because hypaque is hyperbaric the patient should have been sat up and spinal puncture performed to drain off the fluid.

Turner, Fisher and Bernstein (1966) also reported on the intrathecal placement of sodium diatrizoate, and reviewed the literature. Hypaque was found to be a highly toxic and dangerous substance when injected into the subarachnoid space, capable of producing irreparable central nervous system damage, and in large amounts, death. Hypaque used for positive contrast ventriculography is reported as causing progressive and massive cerebral edema. Instillation of hypaque into the cervical spinal canal during vertebral angiography also has been reported, with consequent drop in blood pressure, apnea, cyanosis, pyramidal tract signs (Ederli and co-workers, 1962). O'Malley (1965) observed the effects of intracisternal injection of Abrodil in rabbits, and noted that there were immediate severe physical reactions with muscle spasm, opisthotonus,

tachycardia, and apnea followed by tachypnea. Three of his 36 animals died, and at postmortem examination an inflammatory response was found in the cord meninges. This apparently was not influenced by intracisternal steroid or antihistaminic drug therapy.

References

Amundsen, P., Helsingen, P. and Kristiansen, K.: Evaluation of Lumbar Radiculography ('Myelography') with Water-Soluble Contrast Media, Acta radiol., 1, 659, 1963.

Arnell, S.: Myelography with Water-Soluble Contrast, Acta radiol., Supp. 75, 1948, Stockholm.

————: Myelography with Skiodan, Am. J. Roentgenol., 66, 241, 1951.

Arnell, S. and Lidström, F.: Myelography with Skiodan (Abrodil), Acta radiol., 12, 287, 1931.

Campbell, R. L., Campbell, J. A., Heimburger, R. F., Kalsbeck, J. E. and Mealey, J.: Ventriculography and Myelography with Absorbable Radiopaque Medium, Radiology, 82, 286, 1964.

Davis, F. M., Llewellyn, R. C. and Kirgis, H. D.: Water-Soluble Contrast Myelography using Meglumine Iothalamate (Conray) with Methylprednisone Acetate (Depo-Medrol), Radiology, 90, 705, 1968.

Doroshow, L. W., Yoon, H. Y. and Robbins, M. A.: Intrathecal Injection, an Unusual Complication of Translumbar Aortography, J. Urol., 88, 438, 1962.

Ederli, A., Sassaroli, S. and Spaccarelli, G.: Vertebral Angiography as a Cause of Necrosis of the Cervical Spinal Cord, Brit. J. Radiol., 35, 261, 1962.

Funkquist, B. and Obel, N.: Effect on the Spinal Cord of Subarachnoid Injection of Water-Soluble Contrast Medium. An Experimental Study in Dogs, Acta radiol., 56, 449, 1961.

Harvey, J. P. and Freiberger, R. H.: Myelography with an Absorbable Agent, J. Bone & Joint Surg., 47-A, 397, 1965.

Knutsson, F.: Lumbar Myelography with Water-Soluble Contrast in Cases of Disc Prolapse, Acta orthop., Scandinav., 20, 294, 1951.

Lange, J. and Odegaard, H.: Abrodil Myelography in Herniated Disk in the Lumbar Region, Radiology, 57, 186, 1951.

Lindblom, K.: Complications of Myelography by Abrodil, Acta radiol., 28, 69, 1947.

O'Malley B. P.: Some Observations on Non-Oily Myelographic Media, Clin. Radiol., 16, 405, 1965.

Turner, O., Fisher, C. J. and Bernstein, L. L.: Intrathecal Sodium Diatrizoate, Neurology, 16, 230, 1966.

Gas Myelography

The use of air myelography for the demonstration of the spinal cord is receiving more attention today both abroad and in the United States. Air myelography had been used for the diagnosis of herniated discs (Chamberlain and Young, 1939) (Poppen, 1940). However, it was found that the detail achieved was far less satisfactory than that which could be obtained with positive contrast media. The advantages in visualization of the spinal cord, particularly in the cervical region, was pointed out by Lowman and Finkelstein (1942) who demonstrated that the cord could be clearly identified in the cervical subarachnoid space up to and including the foramen magnum. Prior to that, Van Wagenen (1934) reported on the radiologic localization of spinal subarachnoid block by the use of air myelography.

Recently, new interest has been aroused in air myelography by the work of Roth (1963, 1965), Jirout (1964), Lodin (1966), Westberg (1966), Liliequist (1966), and others who found that they could demonstrate the spinal cord in the thoracic and cervical canal with considerable accuracy, especially enhanced by the use of body section radiography. Conventional radiography can be utilized, particularly in the investigation of the cervical spinal canal.

Several technics are available for air myelography. In one (Liliequist, 1966) the gas is introduced into the suboccipital area by a cisternal tap and air is permitted to flow up into the cervical spinal canal, after the removal of cerebrospinal fluid in fractional amounts. Liliequist's work is directed towards demonstrating the varied appearance of the subarachnoid space in the cervical region.

A two-needle method for introducing gas into the subarachnoid space was recently brought to attention again by Lodin (1966), who used one needle placed in the lumbar subarachnoid space and another into the cisterna magna. The patient is kept in a horizontal position on his side. Lumbar and cisternal punctures are performed, and specimens are taken from the two puncture sites. The patient's head is then lowered, and oxygen is injected continuously through the lumbar needle while the cisternal needle

is kept open. Observation of the flow of fluid from the cisternal needle indicates patency of the subarachnoid space. The oxygen is injected continuously so long as fluid passes from the cisternal needle. When the gas flows from the cisternal needle, it is closed, and Lodin continues to inject oxygen at a pressure of from 250 to 300 ml of water by way of the lumbar needle. He suggests that, in the presence of a subarachnoid block, the upper margin of the block can be identified if the patient is placed in a head-down position and oxygen is injected through the cisternal needle. The lower level is identified by gas injected into the lumbar needle. This double-puncture technic was used in 250 instances, and worked out well in cases with total block as well as in those with constriction of the cerebrospinal fluid space. The procedure was found to be accompanied by only slight discomfort to the patient.

Myelography by the lumbar route alone has been recommended. Roth (1963) performs the examination by completely removing the cerebrospinal fluid from the subarachnoid space in patients without demonstrable block by draining it off with the patient in the sitting position. When the fluid has been completely evacuated, the patient is placed in a horizontal position as for a cervical or lumbar study. He introduces about 10 to 30 ml more of air than fluid removed. The insufflation pressure used is equivalent to 500 ml of water. A sudden rise towards the end of the insufflation indicates that the membranous sac is distending and that further air is not necessary. Preliminary films are followed by tomograms. Lateral films are found most informative. Sagittal views are also helpful. The patient is placed supine on a pad with the head hyperextended so that the air is prevented from escaping into the intracranial spaces. A slow insufflation is preferable, at a rate of about 1 to 2 ml per minute, so that the examination takes from 15 to 20 minutes. Roth notes that the patient has the usual complaints as noted with pneumoencephalography.

The safety of removing cerebrospinal fluid in the presence of a block has been questioned. Evidence from evacuation of the spinal canal for gas myelography, as well as my own experience with syphonage of Pantopaque, indicate that this fear is not entirely valid, but caution is urged nevertheless.

We have not used air myelography to any great extent, except as a relatively routine procedure in the investigation of the cervical spinal canal in patients undergoing lumbar pneumoencephalography. However, with the increased interest in the use of air myelography for the demonstration of atrophy of the spinal cord, or for the characteristic ballooning of the cord occurring with changes in position in patients with syringomyelia or hydromyelia, the procedure undoubtedly will again find favor, but I think in a relatively limited way. One application for air myelography found quite useful is the demonstration of congenital malformations, particularly in the lumbar area in infants and children. In these patients, particularly for the demonstration of meningoceles, air myelography is preferable to positive contrast studies. It has been stated that gas myelography is non-irritating, non-toxic, and does not cause arachnoiditis or cyst formation. However, it is worth recalling that arachnoiditis has been observed after no more than a "routine" spinal tap.

On satisfactory air myelograms, the cord appears as a tubular structure of increased density, with the negative gas shadows both above and beneath (Fig. 100). Movement of the cord takes place when the patient is placed in the face-down or face-up position (Fig. 34). This maneuver may be used to demonstrate the anterior and the posterior surfaces of the cord. The range of movement of the upper cervical cord, particularly in the vicinity of the foramen magnum, exceeds that in the lower cervical region. Liliequist (1966) made measurements of the spinal canal, taking his points from the midline of the vertebral bodies to the corresponding spinal processes, measuring from the pos-terior cortical border of the middle of the vertebral body to the cortical border of the corresponding spinous process. The depth of the subarachnoid space was measured at the same level at right angles to the long axis of the canal. He found that the width of the spinal canal as well as of the subarachnoid space, was somewhat less in females than in males, and ranged between 15 and 20 mm below C1 and C2 for the canal and about 12 to 17 mm for the subarachnoid space.

The thoracic spinal cord usually can be better demonstrated in its anterior aspect, more gas collecting in this portion of the subarachnoid space (Fig. 100). The posterior portion of the thoracic cord is in closer apposition to the roof of the spinal canal, so that the posterior subarachnoid space shows up as a narrower space. This is attributed to the position of the points of attachment and exit of the nerve roots. Lower down in the thoracic canal and in the upper lumbar canal, the normal lumbar bulge can be identified by thickening of the cord, usually towards the anterior wall of the dural sac. Occasionally, the nerve roots themselves can be made out in the lumbar region, so that the filaments of the cauda equina can be identified. The use of transverse cervical myelography with body section radiography for the production of axial sections of the cord was suggested as a valuable supplement to conventional pneumography by Hertzog (1963).

Air myelography, particularly in the cervical region, is becoming an increasingly important tool in what might be termed "closed surgery" of the cervical spinal cord. Rosomoff (1966) utilizes this technic in identifying the cervical cord as the initial step in performing percutaneous chordotomy using a stereotactic micromanipulator for placing a lumbar puncture needle in apposition to the ventral quadrant of the cord. Through this is inserted a stainless steel electrode and a radiofrequency current is applied to produce a permanent spinal lesion. The procedure is performed in the

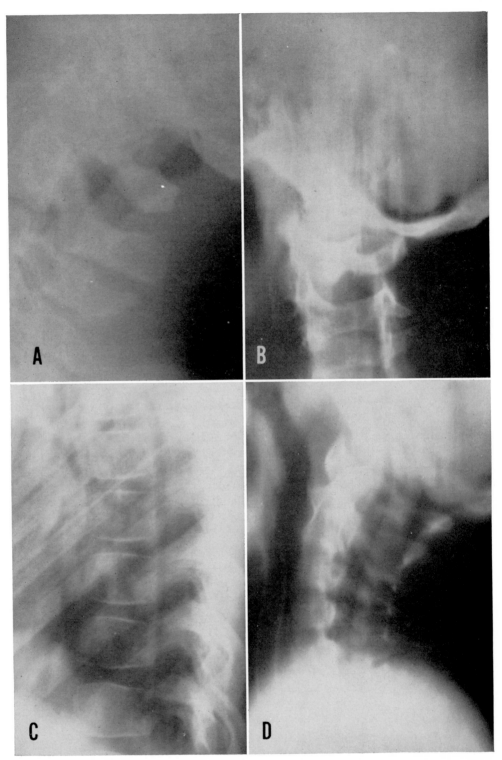

FIG. 100. *A,* The upper cervical cord is visible at the level of the foramen magnum and the upper two cervical vertebrae. Lumbar pneumoencephalogram. *B,* Body section roentgenogram. The air is in the posterior cranial fossa, outlining the cerebellar tonsil. *C,* Lateral thoracic air myelogram outlines the spinal cord. *D,* Same patient, laminagram shows the cerebellar tonsil projecting into the posterior cervical canal and the cervical spinal cord.

department of radiology with the patient awake, using only local anesthesia. The lateral spinothalamic tract is destroyed at the level of the interspace between the first and second cervical vertebrae. Westberg (1966) utilized gas myelography as an aid for percutaneous puncture in the diagnosis of spinal cord cysts.

References

Bonte, G. and Delfosse, C.: Diagnostic des Myelopathies Cervicales d'Origine Discale par la Myelotomographie Gazeuse par Voie Lombaire, Acta radiol., 1, 666, 1963.
Chamberlain, W. E. and Young, B. R.: Air Myelography in the Diagnosis of Intraspinal Lesions Producing Low Back and Sciatic Pain, Radiology, 33, 695, 1939.
————: The Diagnosis of Intervertebral Disk Protrusion by Intraspinal Injection of Air, J.A.M.A., 113, 2022, 1939.
Coggelshall, G. C. and von Storch, T. J. C.: Diagnostic Value of Myelographic Studies of the Caudal Dural Sac, Arch. Neurol. & Psychiat., 31, 611, 1934.
Dandy, W. E.: Ventriculography Following Injection of Air into the Cerebral Ventricles, Ann. Surg., 68, 5, 1918.
————: Roentgenography of the Brain After Injection of Air into the Spinal Canal, Ann. Surg., 70, 397, 1919.
Greenwald, C. M., Eugenio, M., Hughes, C. R. and Gardner, W. J.: The Importance of the Air Shadow of the Cisterna Magna in Encephalographic Diagnosis, Radiology, 71, 695, 1958.
Hertzog, E.: La Tomomyelographie Cervical Haute Transversale, Acta radiol., 1, 721, 1963.
Jacobaeus, H.: On Insufflation of Air into the Spinal Canal for Diagnostic Purposes in Cases of Tumors in the Spinal Canal, Acta med., Scandinav., 55, 555, 1921.
Jirout, J.: Mobility of the Thoracic Spinal Cord under Normal Conditions, Acta radiol., 1, 729, 1963.
Jirout, J., Fischer, J. and Nadvornik, F.: Anatomische und Pneumographische Studien des Hinteren Arachnoidalraumes der Normalen Brustwirbelsäule, Fortschr. Geb. Röntgenstrahlen, 101, 395, 1964.
Liliequist, B.: Gas Myelography in the Cervical Region, Acta radiol., 4, 79, 1966.
Lindgren, E.: Myelographie mit Luft, Nervenarzt, 12, 57, 1939.
————: Myelography with Air, Acta psychiat. & neurol., 14, 385, 1939.
Lodin, H.: Two-Needle Oxygen Myelography, Acta radiol., 4, 62, 1966.
Lowman, R. M. and Finkelstein, A.: Air Myelography for Demonstration of the Cervical Spinal Cord, Radiology, 39, 700, 1942.

Munro, D. and Elkins, C. W.: Two-Needle Oxygen Myelography: A New Technique for Visualization of the Spinal Subarachnoid Space, Surg., Gynecol. & Obst., 75, 729, 1942.
Murtagh, F., Chamberlain, W. E., Scott, M. and Wycis, H. T.: Cervical Air Myelography, Am. J. Roentgenol., 74, 1, 1955.
Poppen, J. L.: The Use of Oxygen in Demonstrating Posterior Herniation of Intervertebral Disks, New England J. Med., 223, 978, 1940.
Rosomoff, H. L., Sheptak, P. and Carroll, F.: Modern Pain Relief: Percutaneous Chordotomy, J.A.M.A., 196, 482, 1966.
Roth, M.: Gas Myelography by the Lumbar Route, Acta radiol., 1, 53, 1963.
————: Caudal End of the Spinal Cord, Acta radiol., 3, 177, 1965.
————: The Caudal End of the Spinal Cord. II. Abnormal Pneumographic Features: Lumbar Intumescence Artery Syndrome and Spinal Dysraphism, Acta radiol., 3, 297, 1965.
Scott, M. and Young, B. R.: Air Myelography in the Diagnosis of Lesions of the Spinal Canal, Arch. Neurol. & Psychiat., 38, 1126, 1937.
Van Wagenen, W. P.: Roentgenological Localization of Spinal Subarachnoid Block by Use of Air in the Subarachnoid Space, Ann. Surg., 99, 939, 1934.
Westberg, G.: Gas Myelography and Percutaneous Puncture in the Diagnosis of Spinal Cord Cysts, Acta radiol., Supp. 252, Stockholm, 1966.
Young, B. R. and Scott, M.: Air Myelography. The Substitution of Air for Lipiodol in Roentgen Visualization of Tumors and Other Structures of the Spinal Canal, Am. J. Roentgenol., 39, 197, 1938.

Strontium-85 Bone Scans

The investigation of metabolic processes in bone by means of radioactive photoscanning has proved useful in the diagnosis of neoplasms in the vertebral column. At present, strontium-85 is used, but investigations with other isotopes such as gallium-68 and fluorine-18 are continuing. Strontium-85 is a monoenergetic gamma emitter (0.513 MEV), with a half life of 64 days. When injected intravenously in a dose of 100 microcuries, it follows the destructive and reparative processes of calcium metabolism in bone. The half-uptake time is about 15 minutes, so that more than 90 per cent of the dose which will eventually reach bone will have done so in about an hour. Only about 20 to 40 per cent of the injected dose enters the bone. That not taken up is excreted in the urine and feces over a longer period of time. Adequate bowel preparation is an important detail in obtaining proper scans. Scans usually are made about 48 hours after injection, when the "signal-to-noise" ratio is diminished.

Strontium is deposited in areas of relatively high metabolic activity, as for example, in the epiphyses, the articular cortex and in new haversian systems of cortical bone. Increased activity is observed at the ends of long bones, especially in adolescents. In young subjects radioactive strontium normally is taken up by immature, poorly mineralized osteoid tissue in growth areas. As calcification proceeds, the rate of strontium deposition diminishes. Older, highly calcified bone shows no uptake.

Radioactive strontium scans are most useful in the identification of small metastatic neoplastic changes, especially when roent-

genograms are "normal." The strontium is deposited in immature osteoid tissue laid down near invading tumor cells. Inasmuch as such osteoid cannot be identified radiologically, it is here that a positive scan may be obtained when there is no demonstrable radiographic change (Fig. 101). With later demineralization of bone, roentgenographic changes appear while the bone scan remains positive. Widespread marrow involvement produces a generalized increased count rate, with obliteration of the normally present gradient seen between static and growing bone. However, once calcification is complete there is little exchange, so that an increased bone density appears on the film and an approximately normal scan is found. Occasionally a bone scan is negative in the presence of extensive tumorous destruction of bone. Biopsy in these patients reveals extensive osteolysis with no evidence of reactive bone formation.

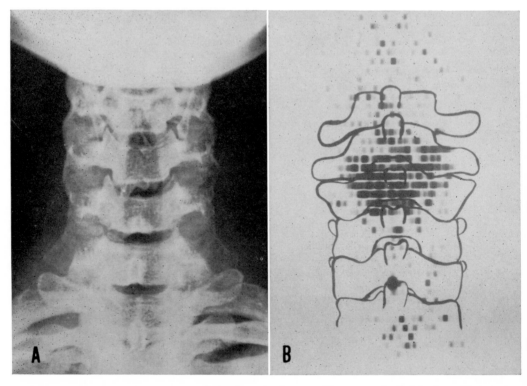

FIG. 101. A, AP roentgenogram, cervical spine, of a 36-year-old woman who had had a radical mastectomy 1 year before. Pain in the lower cervical and upper thoracic region. Plain films were interpreted as normal. B, Strontium scan reveals lesion in the 7th cervical and 1st thoracic vertebrae.

When bone reacts to tumor by both proliferation and destruction, the scan may not be quite as striking, inasmuch as actively metabolizing osteoid tissue is scant. The correlation between immature reactive bone with little change visible radiologically and with marked changes on scans is useful in diagnosis. If an area of osseous involvement is mineralized, failure of a scan to indicate activity may be misleading.

Positive scans also are reported in Paget's disease, osteomyelitis, eosinophilic granulomas, fractures and benign bone tumors. In essence, bone scanning is a nonspecific process, so that other diseases with reactive bone formation also have to be considered. No specific differentiation between primary and metastatic tumors can be made (Charkes and Sklaroff, 1965, 1966).

In estimating the importance of scanning the importance of a meticulous radiologic technic should not be neglected in favor of recovering the error by scanning. In going over several recent positive scans with so-called "negative" roentgenograms it was a little embarrassing to have to point out that the films really were quite positive in some, even though the changes were subtle. In others, the technic could have been considerably improved. After all, there have been some technical advances in radiography of the vertebral column in the past 25 years, and it is not essential that a vertebra be half destroyed before a metastatic process is radiologically demonstrable.

In considering isotopic diagnostic methods, the use of radioactive iodinated human serum albumin intrathecally for the demonstration of spinal block lesions has been used by Perryman, Noble and Bragdon (1958), Dietz, Zeitler and Wolf (1966) and others.

References

Charkes, N. D. and Sklaroff, D. M.: The Radioactive Strontium Photoscan as a Diagnostic Aid in Primary and Metastatic Cancer in Bone, Radio. Clin. North America, 3, 499, 1965.

Charkes, N. D., Sklaroff, D. M. and Young, I.: A Critical Analysis of Strontium Bone Scanning for Detection of Metastatic Cancer, Am. J. Roentgenol., 96, 647, 1966.

Dietz, H., Zeitler, E. and Wolf, R.: Die szinigraphsche Darstellung der Liquorraume mit [131]J-markertem menschlichen Serumalbumin (RIHSA), Fortschr. Röntgenstr., 105, 537, 1966.

Perryman, C. R., Noble, P. R. and Bragdon, F. H.: Myeloscintography: A Useful Procedure for Localization of Spinal Block Lesions, Am. J. Roentgenol., 80, 104, 1958.

Intraosseous Vertebral Plebography

Injection of water-soluble contrast material such as Hypaque into the marrow space of a vertebral body results in passage into the vertebral venous plexuses, which drain into the internal and external venous beds. If concomitant inferior vena caval compression is used, the intervertebral veins and the ascending lumbar veins are opacified. Without caval compression, or concomitant performance of the Valsalva maneuver, the contrast medium extends cephalad and caudad for only a few vertebral levels. Thus, if the caval circulation is retarded flow is definitely more marked cephalad, resulting in far better contrast filling of the channels over the lumbar and lower thoracic spine.

Intraosseous vertebral phlebography has been recommended by Schobinger and Krueger (1963) as being of equal value with myelography in the diagnosis of discal herniations. They also observed that this method could be used for the demonstration of congenital anomalies, adhesive arachnoiditis, intradural tumors and vertebral metastases.

Greitz, Liliequist, and Muller (1962) also found that discal herniations and tumors in the vertebral canal affected the epidural veins. Its application to the demonstration of arteriovenous malformations within the spinal canal, however, was not helpful because the pressure in the efferent veins is much higher than in the surrounding veins. Djindjian, Pansini and Dorland (1963) tried intravertebral phlebography in the diagnosis of discal herniations, angiomas, tumors and injuries of the spinal cord and the vertebral spine. They concluded that the method was not adequate for the confirmation of medullary compression or discal herniation, and that myelography was indispensable. The possibility of danger from intraosseous phlebography was indicated by the report of Gildenhorn, Gildenhorn and Amromin (1960), who found emboli consisting of marrow cells and spicules of bone in pulmonary vessels in a patient who died after injection of contrast medium into the right femur. He mentioned that evidence from various sources indicates that injections into the bone marrow entails certain hazards, as for example dissemination of primary or metastatic tumor cells.

We have not used intraosseous phlebography in the diagnosis of discal lesions or intraspinal lesions. However, it has been helpful in the diagnosis of an occasional hemangioma of the vertebral column.

References

Djindjian, R., Pansini, A. and Dorland, P.: Phlébographie Rachidienne par Voie Trans-épineuse, Acta radiol., *1*, 689, 1963.

Gildenhorn, H. L., Gildenhorn, V. B. and Amromin, G.: Marrow Embolism and Intraosseous Contrast Radiography, J.A.M.A., *173*, 758, 1960.

Greitz, T., Liliequist, B. and Müller, R.: Cervical Vertebral Phlebography, Acta radiol., *57*, 353, 1962.

Isherwood, I.: Spinal Intra-osseous Venography, Clin. Radiol., *13*, 73, 1962.

Schobinger, R. A.: *Intra-osseous Venography*, New York, Grune & Stratton, 1960.

Schobinger, R. A. and Krueger, E. G.: Intraosseous Epidural Venography in the Diagnosis of Surgical Diseases of the Lumbar Spine, Acta radiol., *1*, 763, 1963.

Schobinger, R. A., Krueger, E. G. and Sobel, G. L.: Comparison of Intraosseous Vertebral Venography and Pantopaque Myelography in the Diagnosis of Surgical Conditions of the Lumbar Spine and Nerve Roots, Radiology, *77*, 376, 1961.

Discography

Following experimental work in which he injected red lead into intervertebral discs, Lindblom (1941) studied normal and pathologic discal changes using about 2 ml of 35 per cent Diodrast and 0.5 ml of Novocaine. This was done in order to improve the diagnostic accuracy of myelography, which, in his experience, he had found to be somewhat lacking in this regard. Lindblom noted that normal discs accepted about 0.3 ml of contrast material, while pathologic discs took more.

Normal lumbar discograms disclose two contrast-filled spaces, one along the upper and the other along the lower vertebral margin. These outline the nucleus pulposus, but do not project into the annulus fibrosus. The two layers are joined by an irregular streak of contrast material in the center of the disc, presenting a "collar-button" appearance (Fig. 102). Pathologic discograms reveal varying extent of emergence of the contrast material laterally and towards the floor of the spinal canal (Fig. 103). Fissures extend anteriorly as well, and occasionally such discal herniation is the cause of severe abdominal pain (Lindblom, 1951). Fissures involving the anterosuperior aspect of the respective vertebral bodies are regarded as the cause for the small, and occasionally fairly large, triangular bony separations designated as "limbic bones" (Fig. 378).

The accuracy of the interpretations of lumbar discograms is reportedly dependent on careful assessment of 3 major findings. These include the amount of opaque medium injected, the reproduction of symptoms, and the radiologic appearance of the discal apparatus. Usually a normal disc accepts about 1 ml, but occasionally capacities up to 3 ml have been observed. The mechanism for the production of pain is not clear. Apparently only abnormal discs are supposed to be painful when injected. Peterson (1962) remarked that he had observed cases where only 0.1 ml of contrast medium had caused excruciating back pain. He had also injected a few discs with 1.5 to 2 ml of normal saline solution without pain, and then produced pain by injecting the same disc with contrast medium. Pain was relieved by putting in 2 ml of Novocaine after it had been started by injection of contrast material. Following this, it was possible to further distend the disc with more contrast

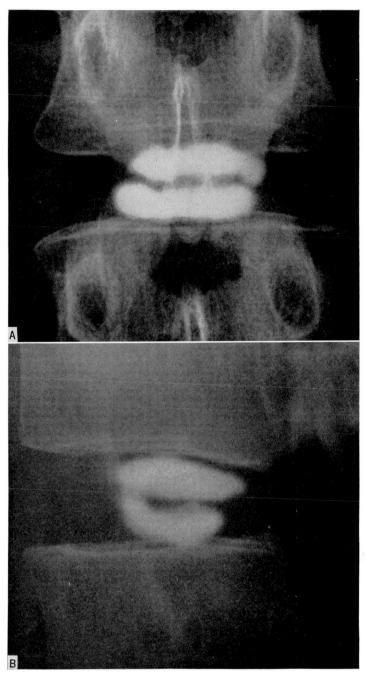

Fig. 102. *A*, Anteroposterior and later (*B*) normal discograms. The contrast material collects in a double disc pattern. (Courtesy of Dr. Ulf Fernström, Acta chirurg. scandinav., Supp. 258, Stockholm, 1960.)

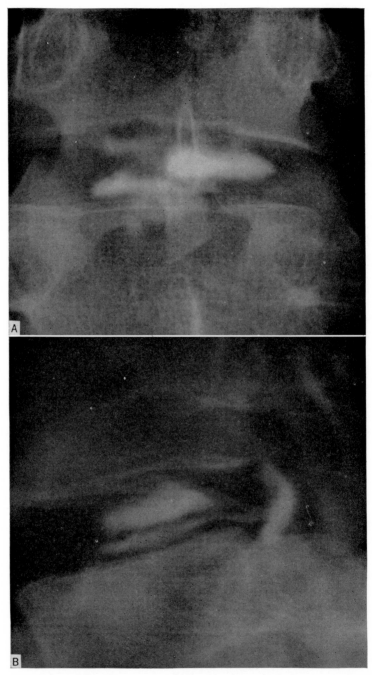

FIG. 103. *A* and *B,* Anteroposterior and lateral discograms in a patient with a herniated lumbar disc. The contrast material extends to the area of herniation. (Courtesy of Dr. Ulf Fernström, Acta chirurg. scandinav., Supp. 258, Stockholm, 1960.)

medium without pain. He believed that this suggested the possibility of irritation of sensory nerve endings within the annulus fibrosus and probably within the posterior longitudinal ligament. Such nerve fibers were first described by von Luschka in 1858 as the nervus sinus vertebralis, and redescribed by Rooke in 1940 as the recurrent lumbar nerve.

Collis and Gardner (1962) preferred lumbar discography to myelography in the routine investigation of intervertebral disc disease. Discograms were classified by them as disclosing normal architecture, or evidence of discal degeneration, protrusion, or extrusion with epidural extension of the contrast material. The latter three were regarded as consistent with herniation. They regarded the pain reaction as important in the interpretation of discal degeneration. Multiple discal degenerations were reported on by Feinberg (1964), who investigated 2320 patients, and injected 6784 disc spaces. Single disc involvement was found in 846, 2 discs in 857, 3 discs in 380 and 4 discs in 32. Negative studies were encountered in 205 patients. A diagnostic accuracy of 99.25 per cent of 1786 patients operated upon was observed by him. However, it was not stated whether or not those with 2, 3 or 4 discal lesions had all levels explored. Collis (1963) observed that 94 per cent of discal herniations could be correctly diagnosed from discograms alone, and an additional 4 per cent located with the aid of pain response to the injection. Collis and Gardner (1961) employed discography and regarded the procedure as very useful in the diagnosis of degenerated discs without herniation and associated with back and leg pain. Plain films were of limited value.

In evaluating discograms, it should be recalled that many patients with discal protrusions and others with discal degeneration are asymptomatic and best left alone. Gardner and his co-workers (1952) had observed that discograms were never normal when an intervertebral disc was narrowed, and the nucleus pulposus was disorganized.

One wonders whether all the multiple discs identified by means of discography require surgical interference, especially in view of the fact that so many patients with multiple discal changes present myelographic evidence of but a single protrusion, and respond well to operation for that lesion alone. A high degree of clinical judgment is required to identify which protrusion is responsible for symptoms and which is unrelated to the patient's complaints.

Cervical discography was advocated by Cloward (1958, 1959), who utilized an anterolateral approach for placement of the needles. Inasmuch as most cervical disc disease occurs in the lower two interspaces, he advocated investigation of these two areas. In his opinion this technic was superior to myelography both in the lumbar and the cervical areas, using the same diagnostic criteria. Again, the question arises whether or not one can rely on the production of pain on injection with Hypaque, the tracking of the contrast material or the amount used. I recently had four instances in which discograms done by a colleague and observed by me were performed first with normal saline solution with no pain at all, then with Hypaque and severe pain, much the same as observed by Peterson (1962). Question has been raised as to whether cervical discography is relevant at all (Sneider, Winslow and Pryor, 1963). Holt (1964) reported on discograms done at 3 cervical interspaces in 50 prison inmates between 21 and 50 years old, and in only 10 disc spaces out of the total of 149 did the contrast material remain within the central confines of the annulus in a normal pattern. He observed no good pattern of pain, and no real correlation in the amount of contrast material used and the degree of pain. Slow injection produced neck spasm, creating intradiscal pressure so that further injections could not be made. I agree with these authors—cervical discography leaves much to be desired and I prefer not to use this procedure.

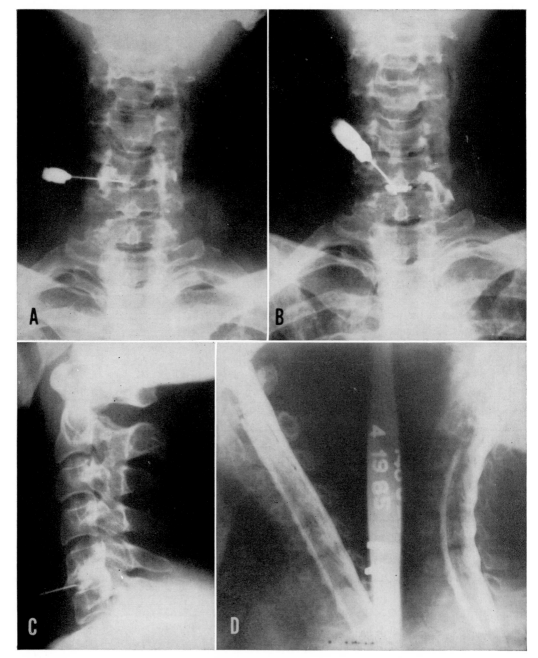

Fig. 104. *A*, Cervical discogram at fifth interspace. Lateral extravasation of Hypaque bilaterally.
B, On injecting the sixth disc extravasation to the left is greater than to the right. *C*, Lateral discogram
with dorsad passage of contrast material. This patient had neck and arm pain when the injections were
made. *D*, Same patient, lateral cervical myelogram is normal. No defects on complete study, including
flexion and extension views, *E*. It was found that the complaints were referable to epicondylitis.

The question as to possible adverse effects of puncturing multiple discs causes some concern. From the reports of Cloward, Fernström, Collis and others it would appear that there is no danger in this procedure. Nevertheless, Butt (1963) mentioned serious complications as being reported in from 0.5 to 1.0 per cent of cases. That infections can occur has been reported by De Seze and Levernieux (1952), Scherbel and Gardner (1960) and Ectors (1959). Earlier observations had indicated that discal trauma might be accompanied by progressive narrowing, superimposed infection and consequent disability (Key and Ford, 1948) (Congdon, 1952). It has been maintained that the small bore of the needle used to penetrate the disc mitigated against the possibility of consequent damage, an opinion supported by many reports in the literature. Another hazard to be considered is the inadvertent instillation of hypaque into the subarachnoid space, which can be quite distressing and dangerous (Collis and Gardner, 1962). Cloward (1963) mentioned that infection of a disc might occur if the esophagus in the neck is perforated.

The main objection to discography as a diagnostic method is that it is limited in its scope, and requires much in the way of manipulation. Results are limited to those intervertebral discs injected. On the other hand, myelography permits investigation of the entire spinal subarachnoid space (Fig. 104). Taken together with the fact that results are difficult to evaluate, I feel that discography is better not done except for a most pressing reason. In my experience, myelography has proven reliable and so well tolerated that I see no need for discography in the diagnosis of discal herniations in the lumbar region. In the cervical area it can be misleading, and I do not use the procedure here at all.

References

Butt, W. P.: Lumbar Discography, J. Canad. A. Radiologists, *14*, 172, 1963.

Cloward, R. B.: Cervical Discography, Acta radiol., *1*, 675, 1963.

Collis, J. S.: *Lumbar Discography*, Springfield, Charles C Thomas, 1963.

Collis, Jr., J. S. and Gardner, W. J.: Lumbar Discography: Analysis of 600 Degenerated Disks and Diagnosis of Degenerative Disk Disease, J.A.M.A., *178*, 67, 1961.

————: Lumbar Discography. An Analysis of 1000 Cases, J. Neurosurg., *19*, 452, 1962.

Congdon, C. C.: Proliferative Lesions Resembling Chordoma Following Puncture of the Nucleus Pulposus in Rabbits, J. Nat. Cancer Inst., *12*, 893, 1952.

Feinberg, S. B.: The Place of Diskography in Radiology as Based on 2,320 Cases, Am. J. Roentgenol., *92*, 1275, 1964.

Fernström, U.: A discographical Study of Ruptured Lumbar Intervertebral Discs, Acta chir. scandinav., Supp. 258, Stockholm, 1960.

Holt, Jr., E. P.: Fallacy of Cervical Discography, J.A.M.A., *88*, 799, 1964.

Meyer, R. R.: Cervical Diskography. A Help or Hindrance in Evaluating Neck, Shoulder, Arm Pain?, Am. J. Roentgenol., *90*, 1208, 1963.

Peterson, H. O.: The Radiologist and Special Procedures, Am. J. Roentgenol., *88*, 18, 1962.

Sneider, S. E., Winslow, O. P. and Pryor, T. H.: Cervical Diskography: Is it Relevant?, J.A.M.A., *185*, 163, 1963.

2

Malformations of the Spinal Column

Occipital Vertebra. The last occipital sclerotome sometimes forms as a partly separate entity. The basilar portion of the occipital bone is formed by fusion of the first three primitive vertebrae, the most caudal of which is referred to as the occipital vertebra, or the pro-atlas. The pro-atlas occurs normally in white rats, in birds and in reptiles as the third (median condyle), and is a separate vertebra interposed between the atlas and the occipital bone. It is, in effect, an extra vertebra not present in man (Wollin, 1963).

The occipital vertebra may appear as a partly separate entity, consisting of an eminence which distorts the periphery of the foramen magnum in a variety of ways. Anteriorly it may appear as a third condyle. Laterally paracondyloid and basilar processes occur. Fused or separate accessory bony elements may be in apposition to or fused with the rim of the foramen magnum and occasionally transverse fissures are noted in the basioccipital bone. Other malformations may appear but are not demonstrable radiologically. Lombardi (1961) includes the ponticulus posticus as one of the variants noted.

Radiographic identification of the various manifestations of occipital vertebra requires meticulous attention to detail, and stereoroentgenographic, laminagraphic and cineradiographic technics can all contribute their share of information. Such examinations demand detailed information and special attention must be given to the investigation of the foramen magnum and the adjacent bony structures (Figs. 105 and 108). The various irregularities occur together or in isolated form. The third condyle usually appears as a bony structure continuous with the anterior rim of the foramen magnum, forming a protrusion from the lowermost aspect of the clivus which terminates in a blunt, rounded surface above the tip of the dens. Usually this is asymptomatic, and is best seen on lateral laminagrams (Fig. 108).

The paracondyloid processes occur as unilateral or bilateral protrusions from the base of the skull, often in association with other bony changes in the rim of the foramen magnum or with atlantoaxial assimilation. Paracondyloid processes project downward from the occipital bone lateral to the condyles, and may fuse with the adjacent vertebrae. Lombardi calls attention to the differentiation between the paramastoid and the paracondyloid processes. The latter originate from the inferior articular apophyses of the occipital vertebra, and are regarded as a congenital variation when larger than normal. When average in size they constitute the points of origin and insertion for the muscles and tendons in that region. The paramastoid processes are located at the posterior borders of the jugular foramina, and are variations observed in animal species.

Scattered bony fragments imbedded in ligamentous tissue may be situated around the periphery of the foramen magnum, and appear mainly above the anterior arch of the atlas in a variable, irregular pattern. A

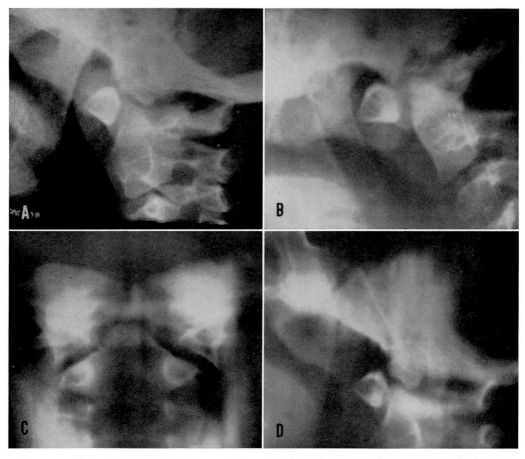

FIG. 105. *A*, Lateral roentgenogram revealing an os odontoideum in a 12-year-old boy who had been injured. The occipital vertebra and attenuation of the dens was discovered at that time. Note the prominent anterior arch of the atlas. *B*, An increased range of motion is permitted in flexion. Note the short, pointed dens. *C*, AP laminagram. The base of the dens is broad. The lateral processes of the atlas are narrow. *D*, Lateral laminagram. An unfused occipital vertebra is seen just inferior to the clivus.

partly formed hypocondylar arch remnant completely or partially united with the anterior rim of the foramen magnum can occasionally be identified, and may simulate a third condyle. Occasionally the neural arch or a transverse process of an occipital vertebra fuses with the rim of the occipital foramen, resulting in a pinched, narrowed opening which can cause cord compression under certain conditions. These deformities, alone or in association with other congenital variations of the cervico-occipital junction including severe dysplasia of the basiocciput, are rare. Unless the space for the cord is compromised or mobility is limited because

of articular changes, such malformations are of little clinical importance.

Atlantoaxial fusion, or assimilation of the atlas and axis, results from maldevelopment of the caudal half of the last occipital and the cranial half of the first cervical sclerotomes. Complete fusion produces circumferential union of the first cervical vertebra with the foramen magnum. Partial fusion results in varying segments of the first cervical vertebra becoming fixed to the foraminal margin, usually the anterior portion of the arch being involved. With complete fusion there are usually no symptoms. Partial fusion, however, may be accompanied by instability of the atlas and axis, abnormal mobility of the dens resulting from lack of fixation of the transverse ligament. Malformation of the foramen magnum may be associated with the varying changes of basilar impression (Fig. 107), which also can produce and exaggerate deformities of the craniocervical junction.

Abnormal ranges of movement can best be seen on lateral roentgenograms in flexion and extension and even better by means of cineradiographic studies. Because of impingement of bony irregularities on adjacent nerves and the spinal cord, a wide range of symptoms may appear, including pain, abnormal attitudes of the head and neck, limitation of movement, weakness of the extremities, ataxia and sensory disturbances. These mimic symptoms of spinal cord degenerative conditions.

Differentiation of an occipital vertebra from atlantoaxial assimilation sometimes is difficult and the conditions may coexist. With atlantoaxial fusion a foramen usually persists on each side between the posterior arch of the fused atlas with the adjacent occipital bone to permit passage of the vertebral artery and first cervical nerve, which retain their normal relations with the atlas and the base of the occipital bone. Atlantooccipital fusion may be accompanied by fusion of two or more cervical segments. Paracondyloid processes often occur on one or both sides of the foramen magnum, narrowing and distorting this area, much the same as with occipital vertebrae. It has been stated that the two can be separated anatomically by observing the disposition of the articular facets. If the joint surfaces of a pro-atlas are projected as planes they will converge caudally as do those of normal occipital condyles. On the other hand, the articular surfaces of an assimilated axis will, if prolonged, extend cranially.

Ossiculum Terminale. This anatomic variant occurs as a separate ossicle which originates from a notochordal remnant in the terminal ligament of the odontoid process. In the normal subject this usually unites at about the age of 6 years. However, when its fusion is incomplete it may persist as a separate bone associated with a shortening and blunting of the dens. It should be distinguished from the "third condyle" which develops on the anterior inner rim of the foramen magnum, and is considered as representative of the body of an occipital vertebra or pro-atlas. Nonunion of the dens with the body of the second cervical vertebra is readily distinguished by the line of demarcation at its base and its occasional displacement or altered configuration.

Among the rarer congenital anomalies in this area are absence of the posterior or anterior arch of the atlas, or absence of the sides of the posterior arch of this structure, with persistence of the medial portion.

BASILAR INVAGINATION, BASILAR IMPRESSION AND PLATYBASIA

These terms are used synonymously so frequently that it has become an almost respectable and acceptable error. Nevertheless, they should be separated and used according to their anatomic counterparts. Platybasia is neither basilar impression nor basilar invagination. By definition, platybasia indicates a flat, broad, wide base, and this term is used by anthropologists for classifying cranial types. Measurement of the basal angle of the skull is made by drawing a line from the foremost point of the foramen magnum to the center of the sella turcica, and from this point to the root of the nose. This angle normally varies from 115 to 150 degrees, and approaches 180 degrees when platybasia is present.

Basilar invagination refers to an indentation of the upper cervical segments into the base of the skull, as if the weight of the cranium causes a sagging of its base against the rigid cervical spine. This results in an arcuate indentation, the base of the skull assuming a convexity directed caudad. Simultaneously, and to more variable extent, the tips of the petrous pyramids become directed upwards. The malformation is asso-

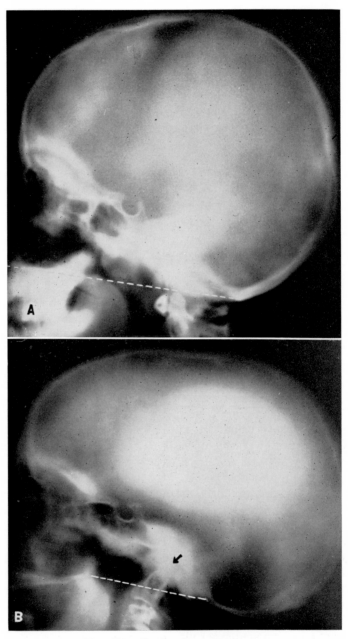

Fig. 106.   *Continued on opposite page.*

ciated with conditions which are associated with bone softening such as osteomalacia, rickets, osteogenesis imperfecta, cleidocranial dysostosis, hyperparathyroidism, the lipoidoses, and quite frequently with Paget's disease (Fig. 106).

Deformity of the margins of the foramen magnum and the base of the skull frequently accompanies bony abnormalities of the cranioverterbal junction. The tip of the dens coming in contact with the anterior rim of the foramen magnum sometimes produces a rounded indentation into the lowermost portion of the clivus. The foramen magnum becomes misshapen and encroached upon because of assimilation of the atlas or the presence of transitional vertebrae. Because of this the tip of the dens projects into the cervical spinal canal just below and at the foramen magnum, thereby narrowing the space available for the medulla oblongata and the proximal cervical spinal cord (Fig. 105).

The incidence of congenital malformation at the occipitocervical junction in patients with basilar impression is frequent. Moreton (1943) reported that in a series of 139 cases 41 had associated cervical anomalies. If it were possible clearly to separate those cases of basilar impression based on congenital malformations from those of acquired origin, the figure would probably be higher. The coexistence of other malformations such as fused vertebrae and spinal neural arch deformities should alert the examiner to investigate the cervicooccipital junction. Laminagrams are most helpful for this purpose.

The diagnosis of basilar invagination and basilar impression is documented further by various linear measurements. Chamberlain (1939) postulated that a line drawn on a true lateral skull roentgenogram from the posterior end of the hard palate to the dorsal margin of the foramen magnum in normal individuals would clear the uppermost tip of the dens. McGregor recommended that a line be drawn from the upper surface of the posterior edge of the hard palate to the most caudal point of the occipital curve on true lateral skull films. When the tip of the dens is 4.5 mm above this line the possibility

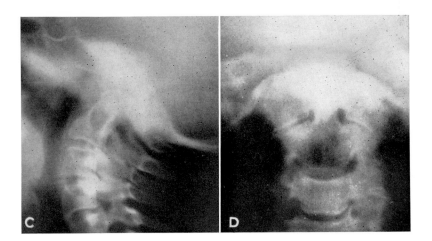

Fig. 106. *A*, Lateral midline laminagram of normal skull. Chamberlain's line is indicated by the dotted white line. *B*, Lateral midline laminagram, basilar invagination. Chamberlain's line passes through the base of the dens. The tip of the dens is displaced upwards (arrow). *C*, Same case, detail showing upward convexity of base. The entire first cervical vertebra is displaced upwards and merges with the basiocciput. *D*, Same case, frontal body section roentgenogram. The occipital condyles and the lateral masses of the first cervical vertebrae are fused. Note the inward projection of the basiocciput.

A

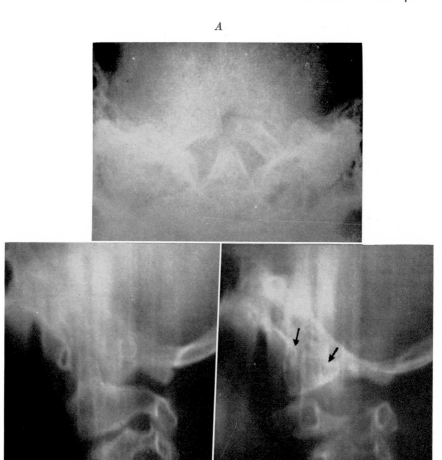

B   *C*

FIG. 107. *A*, Exaggerated Towne's view showing distorted foramen magnum in patient with basilar invagination. The neural arch of the first cervical vertebra is deformed, its right side being fused to the periphery of the foramen magnum, while the left side is separated. *B*, Same case, midline laminagram. The anterior aspect of the first cervical vertebra is high and fused to the foramen magnum. The first neural arch and spinous process likewise are elevated and impressed into the base of the skull. *C*, Same case off-center laminagram. The fused body of the first cervical vertebra with the overlying occipital condyle is in focus (arrows).

of basilar invagination is likely. Bull, Nixon and Pratt (1955) recommended an angle determined by the plane of the hard palate and that of the atlas, a line joining the midpoints of the anterior and posterior arches on lateral films. Angles of 13 degrees or more were regarded as indicating basilar invagination.

Basilar impression or invagination exists without specific symptoms in a rather large proportion of cases. However, when the dens projects sufficiently into the cervical spinal canal, when there is undue mobility of this structure, or when the foramen magnum is sufficiently encroached upon, neurologic changes result either from direct pressure, vascular compression on the adjacent structures or from interference with the cerebrospinal fluid circulation. This may take place regardless of the anatomic cause,

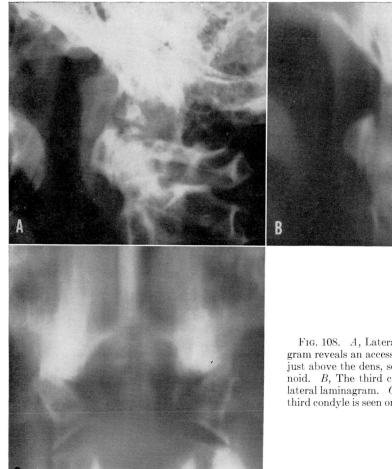
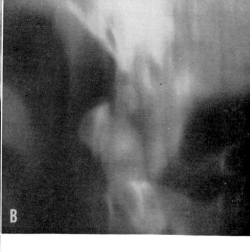

Fig. 108. *A*, Lateral cervical spine roentgenogram reveals an accessory ossicle (third condyle) just above the dens, separate from the basisphenoid. *B*, The third condyle is better seen on a lateral laminagram. *C*, The cap-like shape of the third condyle is seen on this AP laminagram.

and gives rise to perplexing problems simulating syringomyelia, multiple sclerosis or other degenerative demyelinating diseases as well as pictures mimicking tumors of the posterior cranial fossa or the upper cervical spinal canal. Pressure against the cranial nerves or upper cervical nerves may produce paralysis or symptoms referable to cerebellar or medullary compression. In these patients it is most important to make an accurate diagnosis because surgical intervention can do much to relieve their complaints.

As a rule congenital malformations are not difficult to differentiate from fusions of the cervicooccipital junction such as may result from osteomyelitis, tuberculosis, old fractures, advanced arthritis or echinococcus disease. Charcot's disease in this area is rare. The identification of acquired basilar invagination is part of the usual examination of the skull and cervical spine.

Os Odontoideum. A rare developmental anomaly of the axis is the separate odontoid process, the os odontoideum. Its formation may be explained by persistence of a transverse plane of mesenchymal tissue which fails to undergo chondrification. As ossification of cartilage occurs, the persisting mesenchymal tissue cannot withstand the strains caused by movement of the head, so that the cephalad portion of the dens becomes detached from its base, resulting in a divided odontoid process. The dens is divided by a transverse gap, so that the apical segment is without solid support. Depending on the position of the cleft in the dens, the apical portion may articulate with the transverse ligament of the atlas. Movement at the atlanto-axial articulation is exaggerated, and in some instances dislocation results.

The os odontoideum is best demonstrated on lateral films of the atlantooccipital area, and body section roentgenograms at times are essential. The dens is seen as a short, stumpy, sometimes pointed or broadened process which projects upwards from a relatively normal body of the second cervical vertebra. A thin, dense line between the centrum and the dens can be identified. Anterior to the tip of the dens a large, rather prominent, sometimes triangular-shaped overdeveloped anterior arch of the atlas is present. The posterior arch of the atlas may be small. Anterior displacement of the atlas on the axis appears during sharp flexion, sometimes dramatically demonstrated on cineradiographic studies. The degree of such movement varies with the extent of the deformity, being more marked when the height of the dens is diminished. Superior to the shortened dens the os odontoideum is seen separated from the base of the remaining odontoid process by a variable gap. Depending on the extent of forward displacement of the first cervical vertebra, the size of the os odontoideum and the stump of the dens, and the motion between these segments, a varying degree of compromise of the space available for the spinal cord can be anticipated.

Body section roentgenograms are useful for identifying the atypical configuration of the body of the second cervical vertebra and the stump of the dens, particularly the rather triangular configuration of the base of the dens seen in the frontal projection as it rises in a shortened, tapered configuration. Usually the articular surface of the lateral masses of the first and second cervical vertebrae are normal (Fig. 105). The persistent base of the dens is sometimes rather small, at other times large.

The os odontoideum must be differentiated from fractures of the dens with displacement. The demonstration of the atypical anterior arch of the atlas, the presence of the os odontoideum itself and the malformation of the base of the dens serves to differentiate these conditions. With fracture dislocations of the dens the configuration of the displaced dens usually retains a normal configuration.

The third condyle, or os occipitale, corresponds to the body of the occipital vertebra, and appears on lateral skull roentgenograms as a variable extension of the posterior rim of the basisphenoid. It projects downward as a structure broader at its distal end, which bears a cup-like impression for articulation with the tip of the dens. It occurs alone, or together with other anomalies of the cervico-occipital junction. As a rule it produces no symptoms, but when large it may restrict movement of the head.

References

Bolk, L.: Zur Frage der Assimilation des Atlas am Schädel beim Menschen, Anat. Anz., 28, 497, 1906.

Bull, J. W. D., Nixon, W. L. B. and Pratt, R. T. C.: The Radiological Criteria and Familial Occurrence of Primary Basilar Impression, Brain, 78, 229, 1955.

Chamberlain, W. E.: Basilar Impression (Platybasia), Yale J. Biol. & Med., 11, 487, 1939.

Craig, W. M., Walsh, M. N. and Camp, J. D.: Basilar Invagination of Skull—So-called Platybasia, Surg., Gynec. & Obst., 74, 751, 1942.

Custis, D. L. and Verbrugghen, A.: Basilar Impression Resembling Cerebellar Tumor, Arch. Neurol. & Psychiat., 52, 412, 1944.

Davidoff, L. M. and Epstein, B. S.: The Abnormal Pneumoencephalogram, 2nd ed., Philadelphia, Lea & Febiger, 1955.

Hadley, L. A.: Atlanto-Occipital Fusion, Ossiculum Terminale and Occipital Vertebrae as Related to Basilar Impression with Neurological Symptoms, Am. J. Roentgenol., 59, 511, 1948.

Kollman, J.: Variatien am Os Occipitale, besonders in der Umgebung des Foramen Occipitale Magnum, Verhandl. der Anat. Gesellsch., 19, 231, 1905.

Kruyf, E.: Occipital Dysplasia in Infants, Radiology, 85, 501, 1965.

Lichtenstein, B. W.: Cervical Syringomyelia and Syringomyelia-like States Associated with Arnold-Chiari Malformation and Platybasia, Arch. Neurol & Psychiat., 49, 881, 1943.

Lindgren, E.: Roentgenological Views on Basilar Impression, Acta radiol., *22*, 297, 1941.

List, C. F.: Neurological Syndromes Accompanying Developmental Anomalies of Occipital Bone, Atlas and Axis, Arch. Neurol. & Psychiat., *45*, 577, 1941.

Lombardi, G.: The Occipital Vertebra, Am. J. Roentgenol., *86*, 260, 1961.

Malis, L. I., Cohen, I. and Gross, S. W.: Arnold-Chiari Malformation, Arch. Surg., *63*, 783, 1951.

McGregor, M.: Significance of Certain Measurements of the Skull in the Diagnosis of Basilar Impression, Brit. J. Radiol., *21*, 171, 1948.

McRae, D. L.: The Significance of Abnormalities of the Cervical Spine, Am. J. Roentgenol., *84*, 3, 1960.

McRae, D. L. and Barnum, A. S.: Occipitalization of the Atlas, Am. J. Roentgenol., *70*, 23, 1953.

Moreton, R. D.: Basilar Invagination: So-Called Platybasia, Proc. Staff Meeting, Mayo Clin., *18*, 353, 1943.

Ray, B. S.: Platybasia with Involvement of Central Nervous System, Ann. Surg., *116*, 231, 1942.

Saunders, W. A.: Basilar Impression: Position of Normal Odontoid, Radiology, *41*, 589, 1943.

Stephens, R. H.: Platybasia, Surgery, *12*, 943, 1942.

Wollin, D. G.: The Os Odontoideum, J. Bone & Joint Surg., *45-A*, 1459, 1963.

Arnold-Chiari Malformation. The Arnold-Chiari malformation is a deformity of the cerebellum, medulla and the fourth ventricle in which these structures project for varying degrees through the foramen magnum into the upper cervical spinal canal. The condition was reported by Arnold (1894) in a description of a newborn infant with a lumbosacral spina bifida together with a large portion of cerebellum extending downward through the foramen magnum in a tongue-like manner overlying the dorsal aspect of the spinal cord. Chiari (1891) delineated three general types divided according to the extent of displacement of the hindbrain into the cervical spinal canal. In the first the cerebellar tonsils and a variable portion of the inferior lobes of the cerebellum project downward so that the fourth ventricle is not brought below the level of the foramen magnum. This corresponds with the Arnold deformity. The second type is one in which the inferior vermis of the cerebellum and the adjacent lower pons, medulla and fourth ventricle are brought down into the cervical spinal canal, and the

most advanced form; the third type is associated with a herniation of practically the entire cerebellum into a cervical spina bifida and meningocele. The early investigators noted a relatively constant association between the malformation and meningomyelocele and hydrocephalus. Their observations were chiefly of newborn children and infants, in whom the displacement downward was such that the fourth ventricle was brought into the upper spinal canal.

The neuroanatomic complications accompanying the various malformations associated with the Arnold-Chiari malformation were described in considerable detail by Lichtenstein (1942). He pointed out that in many instances of spina bifida an abnormal fixation of the spinal cord was present. This prevented its adequate rostral migration with continued development, and the abnormal fixation in some cases resulted in a wide variety of local and distal neuro-anatomic alterations. Included in this list were a short cauda equina with a low lying conus medullaris, abnormal stretching of the spinal cord above the site of fixation, elongation of the hind brain with displacement of the medulla oblongata into the vertebral canal together with the choroid plexus of the fourth ventricle and parts of the cerebellum, dysplasia of some of the cerebellar folia, and elongation of the lowermost cranial nerves. Impaction against the walls of the foramen magnum produced compression changes in these structures. In addition, stenosis of the aqueduct of Sylvius was noted, together with internal hydrocephalus secondary to obstruction both at the aqueduct of Sylvius and at the fourth ventricle when this structure was impacted into the foramen magnum. Instances of hydromyelia and syringomyelia-like cavitations in the cervical portion of the spinal cord were found, and there was evidence of compression on the anterior spinal arteries and the vertebral systems of veins at the foramen magnum.

Penfield and Coburn (1938) believed that the Arnold-Chiari malformation resulted from traction on the brain stem in embryonic life resulting from fixation of the spinal cord at a meningocele site. Normally the growth of the vertebral column and the spinal cord are equal until about the third month of uterine life, after which the vertebral canal grows more rapidly than the spinal cord. When spina bifida and meningocele are present, the cord may become fixed by the herniation and adhesions at the site of the defect. Traction exerted on the brain stem by the continued growth of the vertebral column pulls the hindbrain down through the foramen magnum. Penfield and Coburn held that this theory was supported by their operative observations that the downward protrusions of the cerebellar tonsils retracted more than 3 cm on being freed from their attachment to the medullary canal. They also noted, as did Russell and Donald (1935), that the spinal nerve roots in the cervical region were found to pass upward to their intervertebral foramina rather than horizontally, and considered this an additional evidence of downward traction on the cerebrospinal axis.

Barry, Pattern and Stewart (1957) regarded the basic cause of the Arnold-Chiari malformation as related to different degrees of overgrowth involving several parts of the neural tube. No need was adduced to postulate traction on the rhombencephalon exerted by means of a structure with as little tensile strength as the embryonic spinal cord. They regarded the hydrocephalus sometimes present as a sequel to the protrusion of the medulla and cerebellum into the spinal canal.

Gardner (1959) postulated that the Arnold-Chiari malformation was related to a congenital failure of permeability of the rhombic roof, thus producing hydrocephalus with a consequent displacement of the tentorium and the hindbrain caudally. Peach (1965) critically reviewed the various theories for the morphogenesis of the Arnold-Chiari malformation, and concluded that the concept that hydrocephalus, mechanical traction on the spinal cord or primary dysgenesis

of the hindbrain could not be upheld. He reviewed the anomalies of the central nervous system present in 20 cases of the Arnold-Chiari malformation. Among these hypoplasia of the tentorium, hydrocephalus, spina bifida, hypoplasia of the falx, craniolacunia, thickening of the interthalamic connexus, anomalies of the septum pellucidum, beaking of the tectum, medullary kinking and microgyria occurred in from 60 to over 90 per cent of his cases. Forking of the sylvian aqueduct, upward herniation of the cerebellum, cyst of the foramen of Magendie, hemivertebrae, hydromyelia and diastematomyelia occurred in from about 15 to 50 per cent. He attributed the Arnold-Chiari malformation to failure of the pontine flexure to develop due to a preceding developmental arrest. The cerebellar component represents, in his opinion, a persistence of the embryonic portion of the intraventricular cerebellum carried down into the cervical canal as a result of the nonproduction of the pontine flexure.

The Arnold-Chiari malformation has often been encountered in association with congenital anomalies at the occipito-cervical junction, such as occipitalized vertebrae and anomalies or failure of fusion of the posterior aspects of the upper cervical segments. Other deformities frequently associated both with the Arnold-Chiari syndrome and meningocele are lacunar skull, congenital and acquired basilar impression and the Klippel-Feil malformation.

The absence of skeletal anomalies in the presence of the Arnold-Chiari malformation is an intriguing occurrence. McConnell and Parker (1938) noted such an occurrence in 5 cases of hydrocephalus without spina bifida or meningocele, and remarked that this cast doubt on the traction theory of the genesis of hindbrain malformation, and that some other mechanism besides traction may be concerned. One of his cases had a normal vertebral column. Reports of Arnold-Chiari malformation without concomitant skeletal changes include, among others, those by Aring (1938), Ogryzlo (1942), Bucy, and Lichtenstein (1945), Epstein (1948) Peach (1964), and Teng and Papatheodorou (1964).

Symptoms associated with the Arnold-Chiari malformation vary greatly. When there is obstruction to the circulation of cerebrospinal fluid because of impingement of the outlets of the fourth ventricle, the outstanding symptoms may be those of hydrocephalus. In others, the clinical picture may be highly suspicious of a cerebellar tumor, with papilledema, vomiting, visual disturbances, and palsies of the cranial nerves. In addition pain may appear in the occipital, suboccipital or high cervical region due to compression of the upper cervical nerve roots. Not infrequently paresthesias appear in the upper extremities, and it has been noted that this pain sometimes can be relieved by stretching or forward flexion of the neck. These symptoms are not constant, but show a definite periodic tendency. Sometimes they are relieved by rest, only to recur after a sudden sneeze or forced movement which may jam the cerebellar tonsils further into the upper cervical spinal canal. Syrinx-like cavitations in the upper cervical spinal cord may produce a picture much like that of syringomyelia, with dissociation of touch and pain and temperature sensibilities over the affected areas. Not infrequently the disease in adults is confused with other neurologic conditions such as multiple sclerosis or various types of degenerative lesions.

Myelography provides the most accurate approach to the diagnosis. The characteristic deformity is produced by the downward protrusion of the cerebellar tonsils, resulting in lobular filling defects in the upper cervical canal. In those instances in which the defect is bilateral a bilobed appearance results, the two arcuate impressions into the Pantopaque column being separated by a vertical central bar (Fig. 109). If one cerebellar tonsil is lower than the other, the defect appears on one side only, or may be asymmetrical. In some instances with pronounced protrusion the defect produced by the herniated tonsils assumes an almost semicircular configuration, with thin lateral columns of Pantopaque extending upwards towards the cisterna magna (Fig. 110).

The lower limit of the filling defect varies. In some it is at the second or third cervical interspace. Advanced downward extension of the cerebellar tonsils as far as the fifth or sixth cervical segment has been described. An unusual example of an atypical filling defect secondary to the Arnold-Chiari malformation was described by Colclough (1950) who reported a case in which the clinical picture simulated that of a herniated cervical disc. According to him, no previous case had been reported where this developmental abnormality presented a history and symptomatology together with myelographic findings consistent with the diagnosis of herniation of a cervical intervertebral disc. The myelographic defects seen in his cases were at the level of the seventh cervical segment.

Good visualization of the cisterna magna can be obtained myelographically. In the presence of the Arnold-Chiari malformation the usual configuration of this cistern is altered by the impingement of the postero-inferior aspect of the cerebellum as it is drawn downward, producing a curvilinear indentation concave caudally. The arcuate or lobulated border produced by some cerebellar herniations may simulate intradural extramedullary tumors such as neurofibromas or meningiomas. This is more likely to occur when the Arnold-Chiari defect presents a curved configuration due to elimination of the central incisura because of the presence of adhesions. However, if Pantopaque is introduced into the cisterna magna the differential diagnosis may be facilitated. The diagnosis of Arnold-Chiari malformation occasionally is made during ventriculography for hydrocephalus in infants. On films made in the inverted position air can be introduced into the fourth ventricle, and demonstration of the caudal angle of this chamber below the foramen magnum is diagnostic. Similar observations made with positive contrast

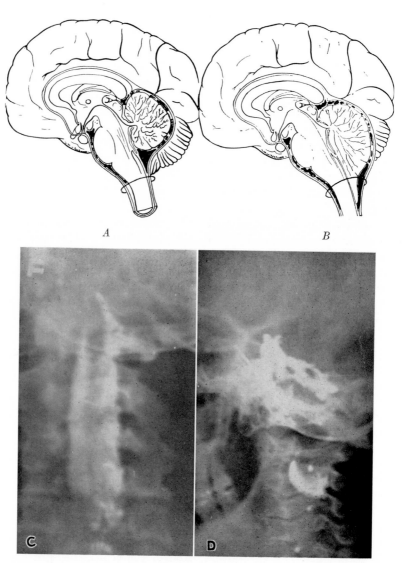

F𝚒𝚐. 109. *A*, Diagram of normal cisterna magna and cisterna pontis. *B*, Diagram of intrusion of Arnold-Chiari malformation into the cisterna magna. *C*, Pantopaque in normal cisterna magna. *D*, Deformity of cisterna magna by Arnold-Chiari malformation. The Pantopaque column is displaced, and at its upper aspect is a semicircular deformity corresponding with the tips of the cerebellar tonsils in the upper cervical spinal canal. (From Epstein, B. S., Am. J. Roentgenol., *59*, 359, 1948.)

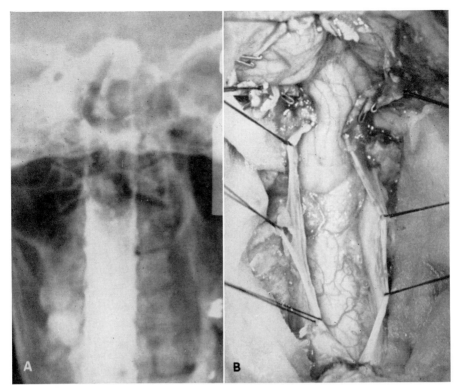

FIG. 110. *A*, Frontal cervical myelogram showing arcuate deformity of head of Pantopaque column at level of second cervical vertebra due to Arnold-Chiari malformation. *B*, Same case as Figure 89-*A*, photograph of Arnold-Chiari malformation *in situ*. (Courtesy of Malis, L. I., Cohen, I. and Gross, S. W., Arch. Surg., *63*, 783, 1951.)

ventriculography permits an even more graphic delineation of the position of the fourth ventricle.

Herniations of the cerebellar tonsils also can be identified on gas myelograms, and should be looked for on lumbar pneumo-encephalograms. The inferior poles of the herniated tonsils appear as rounded densities which may be large enough to fill the space in and below the foramen magnum.

The diagnosis of the Arnold-Chiari malformation, with or without concomitant skeletal malformations, assumes considerable importance in the presence of symptoms which might be relieved surgically.

References

Aring, C. D.: Cerebellar Syndrome in Adults with Malformation of Cerebellum and Brain Stem (Arnold-Chiari Deformity), with Note on Occurrence of "Torpedoes" in Cerebellum. J. Neurol. & Psychiat., *1*, 100, 1938.

Arnold, J.: Myelocyste, Transposition von Gewebskeimen und Sympodie, Beitr. z. path. Anat. u. z. allg. Path., *16*, 1, 1894.

Barry, A., Patten, B. M. and Stewart, B. H.: Possible Factors in the Development of the Arnold-Chiari Malformation, J. Neurosurg., *14*, 285, 1957.

Bucy, P. C. and Lichtenstein, B. W.: Arnold-Chiari Deformity in an Adult, J. Neurosurg., *2*, 245, 1945.

Chiari, H.: Über Veranderungen des Kleinhirns, des Pons, und der Medullar Oblangata in Folge von Congenitaler Hydrocephalie des Grosshirns. Denkschr. d. k. Akad. d. Wissensch. Math.-natur. Kl., *63*, 71, 1895 (quoted by Ogryzlo).

Colclough, J. A.: Simulation of Herniated Cervical Disc by Arnold-Chiari Malformation, Surgery, *28*, 874, 1950.

Epstein, B. S.: Pantopaque Myelography in the Diagnosis of Arnold-Chiari Malformation Without Concomitant Skeletal or Central Nervous System Defects, Am. J. Roentgenol., *59*, 359, 1948.

Lichtenstein, B. W.: Cervical Syringomyelia and Syringomyelia-like States Associated with Arnold-Chiari Deformity and Platybasia, Arch. Neurol. & Psychiat., *49*, 881, 1943.

Liliequist, B.: Encephalography in the Arnold-Chiari Malformation, Acta radiol., *53*, 17, 1960.

Malis, L. I., Cohen, I. and Gross, S. W.: Arnold-Chiari Malformation, Arch. Surg., *63*, 783, 1951.

Marks, J. H. and Livingston, K. E.: Cervical Subarachnoid Space, with Reference to Syringomyelia and Arnold-Chiari Malformation, Radiology, *52*, 63, 1949.

McConnell, A. A. and Parker, H. L.: A Deformity of the Hind-Brain Associated with Internal Hydrocephalus: Its Relation to the Arnold-Chiari Malformation, Brain, *61*, 415, 1938.

Ogryzlo, M. A.: Arnold-Chiari Malformation, Arch. Neurol. & Psychiat., *48*, 30, 1942.

Peach, B.: Arnold-Chiari Malformation with Normal Spine. Arch. Neurol., *10*, 497, 1964.

————: Arnold-Chiari Malformation. Anatomic Features of 20 Cases. Arch. Neurol., *12*, 613, 1965.

Penfield, W. and Coburn, D. F.: Arnold-Chiari Malformation and Treatment, Arch. Neurol. & Psychiat., *40*, 328, 1943.

Russell, D. S. and Donald, C.: Mechanism of Internal Hydrocephalus in Spina Bifida, Brain, *58*, 203, 1935.

Shapiro, R. and Robinson, F.: The Roentgenographic Diagnosis of the Arnold-Chiari Malformation, Am. J. Roentgenol., *73*, 390, 1955.

Swanson, H. S. and Fincher, E. F.: Arnold-Chiari Deformity Without Bony Abnormalities, J. Neurosurg., *6*, 314, 1949.

Teng, P. and Papatheodorou, C.: Arnold-Chiari Malformation with Normal Spine and Cranium. Arch. Neurol., *12*, 622, 1965.

Wickbom, I. and Hanafee, W.: Soft Tissue Masses Immediately Below the Foramen Magnum. Acta radiol., *1*, 647, 1963.

Developmental Anomalies of the Spine

Congenital Absence of the Dens. This infrequent congenital malformation is due to failure of development of the dens. The lateral masses of the first and the body of the second cervical vertebrae retain their normal relationships. The condition frequently remains symptomless, and is not discovered until radiographic examination either discloses the defect incidentally or after trauma has precipitated symptoms. These vary from vague pain at the base of the skull and upper cervical area to sharp neck pain. Weakness of the upper extremities, tingling, hyperesthesia and paresthesia also have been noted. More advanced pressure effects have resulted in quadriparesis. Bladder and bowel symptoms have not been recorded.

The radiographic diagnosis of congenital absence of the dens often is made as an incidental observation in a symptomless patient by the demonstration of a flattened superior surface of the second cervical vertebra. A mound-like bulge sometimes is present in the region corresponding to the base of the absent dens. The relationships between the first and second cervical vertebrae may be otherwise undisturbed, except for an alteration in the range of movement and an exaggerated forward mobility of the head. The open-mouth projection and body section studies in the frontal and lateral projections are best suited for demonstration of this anomaly. While absence of the odontoid process is mostly congenital in origin, an occasional case is reported in which it has been destroyed by tuberculosis (Gwinn and Smith, 1962), and several instances of metastatic tumor involving the dens with marked destruction have been observed in my own experience. Occasionally the odontoid process is hypoplastic, a circumstance which also may be associated with abnormal mobility of the atlanto-axial joint.

References

Fullenlove, T. M.: Congenital Absence of the Odontoid Process, Radiology, *63*, 72, 1954.

Gillman, E.: Congenital Absence of the Odontoid Process of the Axis, J. Bone & Joint Surg., *41-A*, 345, 1959.

Gwinn, J. L. and Smith, J. L.: Acquired and Congenital Absence of the Odontoid Process, Am. J. Roentgenol., *88*, 424, 1962.

Ivie, J. McK.: Congenital Absence of the Odontoid Process, Radiology, *46*, 268, 1946.

Nievergelt, K.: Luxatio atlanto-epistrophica bei Aplasie des Dens epistrophei, Schweiz. med. Wchnschr., *78*, 653, 1948.

Roberts, S. M.: Congenital Absence of the Odontoid Process Resulting in Dislocation of the Atlas on the Axis, J. Bone & Joint Surg., *15*, 988, 1933.

Scannell, R. C.: Congenital Absence of the Odontoid Process, J. Bone & Joint Surg., *27*, 714, 1945.

Schultz, E. H., Jr., Levy, R. W. and Russo, P. E.: Agenesis of the Odontoid Process, Radiology, *67*, 102, 1956.

Weiler, H. G.: Congenital Absence of the Odontoid Process of the Axis with Atlanto-Axial Dislocation, J. Bone & Joint Surg., *24*, 161, 1942.

Congenital Absence of Pedicles and Articular Facets of Cervical Vertebrae. Congenital absence of a pedicle is a relatively infrequent occurrence, and usually is of little clinical importance except from a diagnostic point of view. The condition may be confused with bony changes incident to malignant disease or possibly neurofibromatosis. Erosion due to a dilated and tortuous vertebral artery may simulate an absent pedicle. The deformity is probably the result of an aberration of segmentation arising in the first 8 weeks of fetal life. As a rule the condition is not associated with any specific complaint, but changes in the planes and angles of articulation of the apophyseal joints may result in instability and be associated with pain. The diagnosis is readily made on oblique stereoroentgenograms of the neck. The involved area presents an unusually large intervertebral foramen with no other evidence of adjacent bony distortion. If the deformity is somewhat more advanced, there may be associated changes in the adjacent neural arch, such as absence of the associated lamina or articular processes. The absence of the pedicle also can be seen on anteroposterior films. The pedicles above and beneath the anomalous one usually are normal, but may be slightly smaller or larger than the contralateral pedicles. The shape of the involved intervertebral foramen is ovoid, whereas with a dumbbell tumor it is rounded, and in the presence of a tortuous dilated vertebral artery it tends to be irregular due to extension into the vertebral body (Fig. 480). On myelograms a slight outpouching of the dura mater at the level of the enlarged foramen is present, with no evidence of a mass lesion at this site.

Deficiencies in the transverse processes have also been noted in association with this condition. According to Hadley (1952) this deformity may be multiple, so that several pedicles are absent. Steinback, Boldrey and Sooy (1952) noted that the contralateral lamina in case of congenital absence of the pedicle and superior facet of the seventh cervical vertebra was developed to a greater extent than normal and that this articulated with the posterior surface of the lamina of the suprajacent sixth cervical vertebra. Due to the increase in size of this lamina and the

consequent tilt of the spine, the neural arches of the fifth and seventh cervical vertebrae were in close proximity. In their case the superior articular facet and the posterior portion of the transverse process on the right side of the seventh cervical vertebra were absent, and the anterior or costal portion of the transverse process remained.

Congenital absence of pedicles of the cervical spine are most frequent in the lower three or four segments. Associated anomalies include failure of fusion of the neural arches, partial absence of one of the posterior elements of a neural arch, fused vertebrae and anomalous bodies incident to segmental errors, and myelomeningoceles. Occasionally there appears an instance of failure of development of the neural arch of the first or second cervical vertebra which is partial or complete.

References

Hadley, L. A.: Congenital Absence of Pedicle from the Cervical Vertebrae, Am. J. Roentgenol., *55*, 193, 1946.
————: Tortuosity and Deflection of the Vertebral Artery, Am. J. Roentgenol., *80*, 316, 1958.
Overton, L. M. and Grossman, J. W.: Anatomical Variations in Articulation between Second and Third Cervical Vertebrae, J. Bone & Joint Surg., *34-A*, 155, 1952.
Steinbach, H. L., Boldrey, E. B. and Sooy, F. A.: Congenital Absence of the Pedicle and Superior Facet from a Cervical Vertebra, Radiology, *59*, 838, 1952.
Wilson, C. B. and Norrell, H. A. Jr.: Congenital Absence of a Pedicle in the Cervical Spine, Am. J. Roentgenol., *97*, 639, 1966.
Zatz, L. M., Burgess, P. W. and Hanberry, J. W.: Agenesis of a Pedicle in the Cervical Spine, J. Neurosurg., *20*, 564, 1963.

Klippel-Feil Deformity. This congenital deformity originates in intrauterine life, and usually involves the cervical vertebrae. While the abnormalities described in conjunction with this vary greatly, the malformation is principally one of non-segmentation or fusion of two or more cervical segments. Varying degrees of malformation occur, from partial fusion of two elements to an irregular fusion of the entire cervical spine into one solid bony mass. The number of cervical segments may be normal or diminished, and there are concomitant irregularities in the laminae and spinous processes such as varying degrees of fusion of these structures. While the classical picture of the Klippel-Feil malformation is associated with congenital fusion and a reduction in the number of cervical vertebrae, together with malformation of vertebral bodies, it also appears in a milder form. Here there are a normal number of cervical vertebrae, with fusion of two or more bodies, and as a rule, of their neural arches (Figs. 111 and 112). Remnants of the disc spaces persist, and the intervertebral foramina are small and round. In the classical Klippel-Feil malformation demonstration of the intervertebral foramina is difficult, and these openings are small and irregular. Associated with this may be congenital alterations in the upper ribs, cervical ribs, cervico-occipital fusion and various bizarre types of synostosis. The term has also been used to designate a malformation of the spine consisting of a combination of rachischisis, hemispondylia, block vertebrae and clefts of the neural arches. The involved portions of the spine may be short-ened, kyphotic or scoliotic. The sites of predilection for these changes are the cervicodorsal and dorsolumbar regions (Fig. 111). In its advanced form the Klippel-Feil malformation presents with marked shortening of the neck and extreme extension of the head. At first glance it appears as if there is no neck, but on radiographic examination short, fused bones are seen between the base of the skull and the thoracic spine (Fig. 113). These infants often have severe malformations of the rest of the spine and the occipital area, together with encephaloceles. The condition is referred to as iniencephaly, and usually is associated with visceral as well as skeletal malformations.

Considering the Klippel-Feil deformity as one principally of the cervical spine, a rather typical clinical picture has been worked out. The condition is characterized by shortness of the neck, lowering of the hairline, and limitation of movement of the head (Fig. 111). Other abnormalities include torticollis, facial and cranial asymmetry, a lowered nipple line, syndactylism, club foot, kyphoscoliosis, and occasionally hemivertebrae and hypoplastic lumbar vertebrae. When there is merely synostosis of a couple of cervical

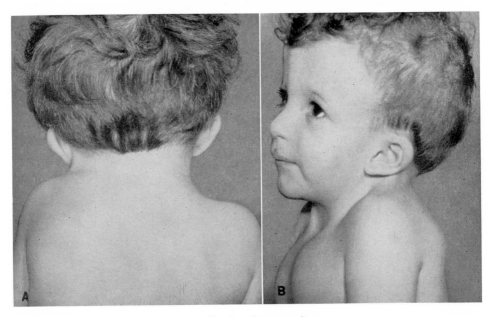

FIG. 111. *Continued on opposite page.*

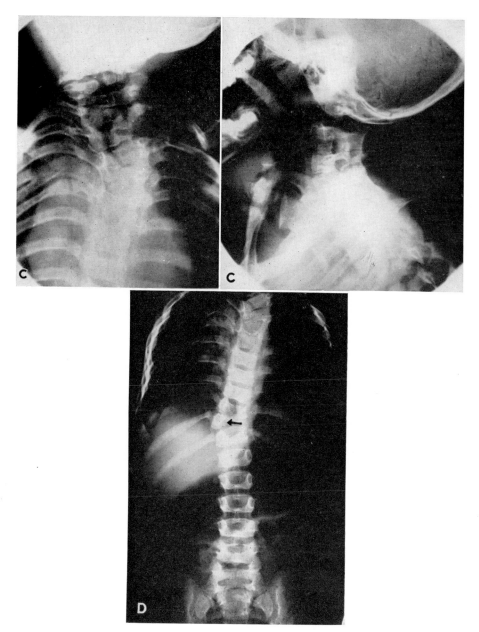

FIG. 111. *A* and *B*, Photographs of child with Klippel-Feil deformity. Note the short neck and the low hair line. *C*, Same case. The cervical vertebrae are deformed and deficient in number. The upper thoracic vertebrae likewise are malformed. *D*, The thoracolumbar spine shows a curvature towards the right. Note the hemivertebrae in the lower dorsal region (arrow).

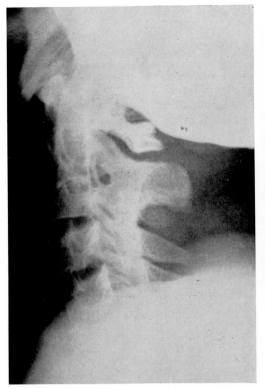

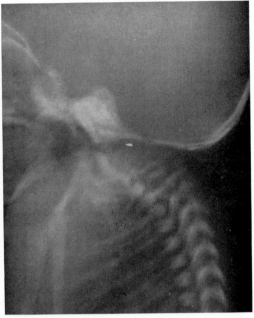

Fig. 113. A newborn infant with hydrocephalus and advanced Klippel-Feil deformity of the cervical spine (iniencephaly).

Fig. 112. Klippel-Feil deformity. The neural arches and vertebral bodies of the second, third and fourth cervical vertebrae are fused.

segments, very little in the way of clinical symptoms follows. In the more marked cases difficulty in swallowing may appear, and in some neurologic manifestations of radiculitis of various cervical nerve roots, basilar impression, defects of the foramen magnum and syringomyelia have been noted. Coexistence of Sprengel's deformity with the Klippel-Feil syndrome has been reported (Furst and Ostrum, 1942), (Erskine, 1946). In this situation a high position or incomplete descent of the scapulae is associated with the vertebral anomaly. Absence of the external auditory meati, deafness and mental deficiency may also be present. One of our patients had a presacral right kidney and malrotation of the colon.

The distorted cervical vertebrae can affect the blood supply to the head, particularly of the vertebral arteries. Sudden changes in the position of the head may cause sufficient transitory change to produce loss of consciousness. The association of the Klippel-Feil malformation with central nervous system disorders indistinguishable from syringomyelia or other degenerative conditions has been commented on, and it has been suggested that the disorder may involve the neurogenic as well as the skeletal structures.

Myelographic investigations in patients with the Klippel-Feil syndrome have disclosed no specific disturbances. In those in whom only block vertebrae were present the flow of Pantopaque was normal. In others, in whom considerable deformity of the cervical vertebrae existed the caliber of the canal reflected the bony changes, and ridge-like defects were observed.

References

Avery, L. W. and Rentfro, C. C.: The Klippel-Feil Syndrome, Arch. Neurol. & Psychiat., 36, 1068, 1936.

Erskine, C. A.: Klippel-Feil Syndrome, Arch. Path., 41, 269, 1946.

Furst, W. and Ostrum, H. W.: Platybasia, Klippel-Feil Syndrome and Sprengel's Deformity, Am. J. Roentgenol., *47*, 588, 1942.

Gray, S. W., Romaine, C. B. and Skandalakis, J. E.: Congenital Fusion of the Cervical Vertebrae. Surg., Gynecol. & Obst., *118*, 373, 1964.

Illingworth, R. S.: Attacks of Unconsciousness in Association with Fused Cervical Vertebrae. Arch. Dis. Childhood, *31*, 8, 1956.

Wycis, H. T.: Lipoma of the Spinal Cord Associated with the Klippel-Feil Syndrome. J. Neurosurg., *10*, 675, 1953.

Block Vertebra. This condition, sometimes called congenital synostosis, involves principally the lumbar vertebrae but also is seen in the cervical and thoracic regions. Rarely fusion of the lower lumbar and the sacral vertebrae is observed at birth, as in one infant seen by us who also had rectal atresia, congenital heart disease and microcephaly. The lesion consists of a partial or complete fusion of two or more segments. This change follows a derangement of embryologic development of the segmental scleromeres, and may be the result of complete chondrification of the dense mesenchymal zone which normally forms the annulus fibrosus. The cartilaginous bodies of the pre-osseous vertebrae become fused and ossify into a solid mass after the periosteal vessels penetrate into the cartilage.

This condition often is identified during x-ray examinations for other conditions, and is asymptomatic. There usually is involvement of two lumbar bodies, as observed in 8 patients. The intervertebral disc may be completely obliterated, or persists as a linear radiolucency partly or completely across the joined vertebral bodies. If the fusion is such that the bodies are about equal in size, the lumbar curve is somewhat straightened (Fig. 114). However, if there is an inequality in the lateral aspects of the involved vertebrae the spine tilts accordingly (Fig. 115).

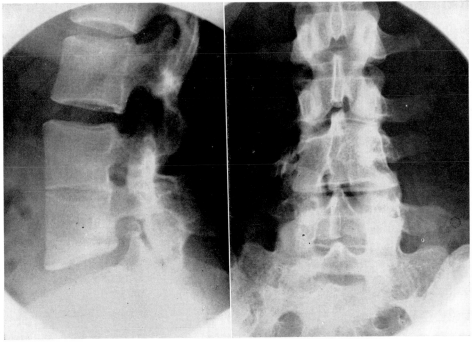

A   *B*

Fig. 114.   *A*, Lateral view showing partly fused third and fourth lumbar vertebral bodies. Note the increased height of the fourth vertebra particularly in its anterior aspect. Some intervertebral disc remains. The intervertebral foramen is diminished in size and the neural arches are partly fused. *B*, Anteroposterior view.   The left lateral aspect of the fourth lumbar vertebra is higher than its right side. The intervertebral disc is wider on the right than on the left side.

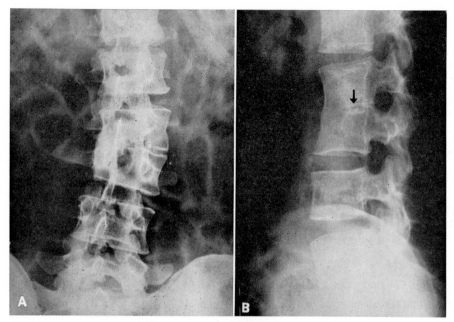

Fig. 115. *A*, Anteroposterior view showing incomplete fusion of second and third lumbar vertebrae, with lateral curvature convex towards the left. Note the persistent intervertebral disc on the left side, while the right is fused. *B*, Same patient, lateral view. The remnant of intervertebral disc is seen at the posterior aspect of the interspace. The lumbar curve is straightened.

The neural arches often are involved, with fusion of the laminae and the spinous processes. Occasionally the pedicles are affected as well, the more cephalad one being large and the caudad one hypoplastic or absent. Rarely an adjacent unfused partly formed vertebral segment is present. The intervertebral foramina become ovoid or bean-shaped in configuration and are diminished in size (Fig. 118).

Block vertebrae in the thoracic region are encountered less often than in the cervical or lumbar spine. Usually two or three segments are affected, more often in the lower thoracic area (Fig. 116). The bodies may be partly or completely united, and the spine tends to be rounded in the vicinity of the involved segments. Occasionally several midthoracic vertebrae are fused, and the vertebral column assumes a straightened appearance in this location. The neural arches are less likely to be involved and the spinous processes remain separated. Concomitant changes in the adjacent ribs, such

as fusion, are sometimes present. The intervertebral foramina tend to be round and smaller than those above and below the involved segments. The condition as a rule is asymptomatic.

Fusion of the cervical vertebrae is regarded by some as a variant of the Klippel-Feil malformation, and as a rule is unassociated with symptoms unless there is significant pressure on the cord or the cervical nerve roots. When two or three vertebral bodies are affected, the alignment of the vertebrae tends to be straightened. The neural arches may be fused, and the involved intervertebral foramina are diminished in size and are rounded. At times one has difficulty in deciding whether or not a patient with such a condition and neck or suboccipital pain can reasonably be diagnosed as having a symptomatic association. Incomplete fusion of one of the involved neural arches may be observed (Fig. 117), and every now and then one of the vertebrae, usually the most cephalad one, appears to be

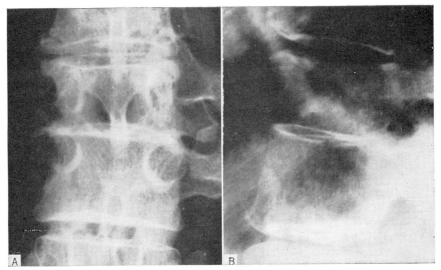

FIG. 116. Fused ninth and tenth thoracic vertebrae. The persistent intervertebral disc is symmetric. Note the disparity in the heights of the vertebrae, the tenth being considerably higher than the ninth.

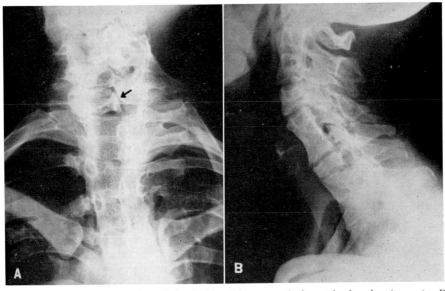

FIG. 117. A, Klippel-Feil deformity. Spina bifida of lower cervical vertebral arches (arrow). B, Same case, lateral view. The bodies of the fifth and sixth cervical vertebrae are fused. The seventh cervical vertebra is partly fused to the first thoracic vertebra, which is fused to the one beneath.

hypoplastic. Cervical vertebral fusion also occurs occasionally as part of other syndromes, as for instance, in the cases of acrocephalosyndactyly reported by Schauerte and St-Aubin (1966).

Failure of growth of one of the involved vertebrae in the lateral or anterior aspects also occurs. In such instances a slight or moderate angulation at the point of deficient growth takes place. The heights of congenital partially or completely fused vertebrae are of approximately proper proportions by measurement in some instances, while in others an increase of from 10 to 20 per cent in height is present, the predominant increase occurring anteriorly (Fig.

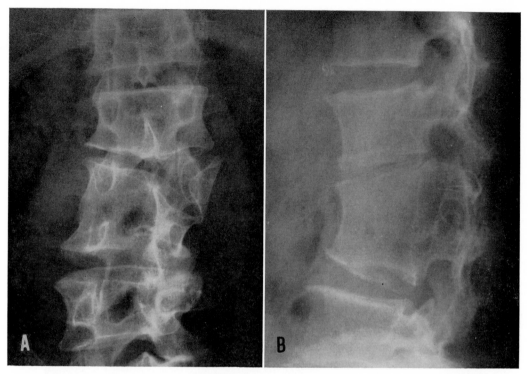

FIG. 118. *A,* The bodies of the 2nd and 3rd lumbar vertebrae are fused. The left pedicle of L2 with its transverse process develops from a separate ossification center, and is divided from the block vertebrae. *B,* Note the diminution in the size of the intervertebral foramen between the fused vertebrae.

114). When asymmetric fusion exists, varying changes in the alignment of the vertebral bodies results in straightening of the usual spinal curves or tilting towards the side of diminished height (Fig. 114). Concomitant malformations occasionally appear, as, for example, an adjacent hemivertebra.

Congenital fusion of the vertebrae must be distinguished from acquired block vertebrae, such as those following trauma. Somewhat similar changes occur after infection of tuberculous or other origin. Patients with rheumatoid arthritis may present synostosis of the cervical vertebrae. Ankylosing spondylitis occasionally results in such marked diminution in the heights of the intervertebral discs that for a moment one thinks of block vertebrae. Senile kyphosis with fusion of the involved vertebral bodies occasionally simulates block vertebrae, as does Scheuermann's disease in its late manifestations. However, the alterations visible at the disc margins, the persistence of disc spaces, evidences of bony overgrowth and paravertebral calcifications help differentiate these conditions. Absence of neural arch abnormalities and irregular configuration of intervertebral foramina also aid in differential diagnosis.

References

Evans, W. A.: Abnormalities of the Vertebral Body, Am. J. Roentgenol., *27*, 801, 1932.

Overton, L. M. and Ghormley, R. K.: Congenital Fusion of the Spine, J. Bone & Joint Surg., *16*, 929, 1934.

Schauerte, E. W. and St-Aubin, P. M.: Progressive Synosteosis in Apert's Syndrome (Acrocephalosyndactyly). Am. J. Roentgenol., *97*, 67, 1966.

Stanislavjevic, S. and St. John, E. G.: Congenital Fusion of Three Lumbar Vertebral Bodies, Radiology, *71*, 425, 1958.

Congenital Lumbar Ribs. This unusual and clinically unimportant condition sometimes is identified on lumbar spine roentgenograms as well as on films taken in the course of investigations unrelated to the vertebral column. They occur more often in females. Lumbar ribs usually present as symmetrical structures which vary in length from a few millimeters to 5 or 6 cm. Instances in which these anomalous ribs are asymmetrical have been described. Lumber ribs usually present well-formed articulations with the transverse processes of the first lumbar vertebra. The osseous structure of the rib is normal bone undistinguishable from those above. Care must be taken in the diagnosis of a lumbar rib to make sure that there is no anomaly of the lumbar vertebrae which would lead to a false count. If there is any question as to a lumbar rib being present, a roentgenogram of the entire spine is required before the diagnosis can be established. The length of the suspected lumbar rib offers no definite clue as to its presence, inasmuch as a normal twelfth rib might be short but otherwise unremarkable.

Sacral Ribs. These are rare. Infrequently tubular, elongated ossicles form in the lateral aspect of the sacrococcygeal area, situated on either side between the first coccygeal and the last sacral vertebrae.

Cervical Ribs. This frequent and sometimes clinically important anomaly represents a progressive development of the embryonic costal processes of the seventh cervical vertebra. The remainder of the cervical spine does not show similar maldevelopment. The radiologic diagnosis of cervical ribs is dependent upon the demonstration of a costal vertebral joint. Cervical ribs develop to a widely varying degree, and present a variety of anomalous configurations. Some terminate sharply a short distance from the joint, others extend as much as 5 to 6 cm parallel to the true first rib. Often the cervical ribs fuse distally with the subjacent first ribs. Anomalous configurations of the distal end of the first and sometimes of the second ribs also occur. Asymmetry of cervical ribs is quite common.

In childhood the costal processes remain ununited until some time between the 4th and 10th years. During the earlier years these are independent of the transverse processes, and should not be interpreted as cervical ribs. The developing costal processes, which lie anteriorly, and the posteriorly situated transverse processes later unite to encircle the foramen transversarium. These foramina are usually not seen on cervical roentgenograms in adults, but may be identified occasionally in children. When cervical ribs exist, they are present at birth. It may be difficult to identify them from normal costal processes, but if their anterior and downward curvatures follow the course of the true ribs one may arrive at a reasonably correct conclusion.

In the x-ray demonstration of cervical ribs it is helpful to tilt the tube towards the head about 10 to 15 degrees to delineate the inferior margin of the suspected cervical rib from the adjacent first rib. Overpenetrated and oblique roentgenograms sometimes help identify an articular space which otherwise might be hidden.

Another anomaly of the seventh cervical transverse processes which at times may assume an importance much the same as cervical ribs is prolongation of the transverse processes.

While cervical ribs are frequently asymptomatic, and often are identified on routine roentgenograms of the chest, the condition nevertheless may be associated with clinical symptoms, notably pain referable to the neck, shoulder or supraclavicular region. This may be accompanied with severe pain extending down the arm following the course of the compressed segments of the brachial plexus. The pain varies considerably in intensity, sometimes being sharp, at other times of a dull, aching nature. Sensory disturbances may be associated with the pain, and if the lesion is such that the vascular structures of the base of the neck are embarrassed, changes referable to such pathologic alteration of the circulation may appear. Surgical intervention is sometimes required for relief of symptoms in severe cases.

References

Adson, A. W. and Coffey, J. R.: Cervical Rib with Methods of Anterior Approach for Relief of Symptoms with Division of Scalenus Anticus Muscle, Ann. Surg., *85*, 839, 1927.

Clare, F. B., Schilp, A. O. and Starr, A. M.: Cervical Rib Causing Gangrene and Necessitating Forearm Amputation, Arch. Surg., *73*, 939, 1956.

Cornwell, W. S. and Ramsey, G. H.: Unusual Bilateral Sacrococcygeal Ossicles, Radiology, *68*, 70, 1957.

Davis, D. B. and King, J. C.: Cervical Rib in Early Life, Am. J. Dis. Child., *56*, 744, 1938.

Eden, K. C.: The Vascular Complications of Cervical Ribs and First Cervical Rib Abnormalities, Brit. J. Surg., *27*, 11, 1939.

Keating, D. R. and Amberg, J. R.: A Source of Potential Error in the Roentgen Diagnosis of Cervical Ribs, Radiology, *62*, 688, 1954.

Samiy, E.: Thrombosis of the Internal Carotid Artery Caused by a Cervical Rib, J. Neurosurg., *12*, 181, 1955.

Simon, S.: Zur Kenntnis der Rippenanomalien im Kindesalter, Röntgenpraxis, *10*, 45, 1938.

Steiner, H. A.: Rib Abnormalities, Radiology, *40*, 175, 1943.

DEVELOPMENTAL ANOMALIES OF THE VERTEBRAL BODIES

Coronal Cleft Vertebrae. Congenital deformities of the vertebral bodies are related to disorders in embryologic development from the notochordal to the mesenchymal state, thence into cartilage, and finally differentiation to bone and intervertebral discs. Aberrations and the consequent deformities occur at any time during the course of growth. Alterations in vascular supply influences growth patterns, and inasmuch as ossification largely depends on blood supply, failure of either the dorsal or ventral distribution is followed by maldevelopment of the affected area. If there is vascular aplasia, the vertebral body fails to ossify and a gibbus deformity results. If the neural arches continue to grow, fusion may take place anterior to the spinal canal, resulting in the appearance of a small dorsal hemivertebra.

When the anterior and posterior ossification centers, usually in the lower thoracic and lumbar vertebrae, persist beyond the usual period a cleft appears in the vertebral body. Radiologically, this is noted on lateral roentgenograms as a zone of radiolucency just behind the midportion of the affected vertebral body. Coronal clefts apparently have not been noted in the cervical or the upper thoracic vertebrae. The condition occurs predominantly in male infants, and has been identified *in utero* (Rowley, 1955) (Fawcett, 1959). Its 9:1 predominance at times permits prediction of the sex of the fetus.

Coronal cleft vertebrae are attributed to persistence of anterior and posterior ossification centers beyond about the 16th week of fetal life (Fig. 119). The division of the ossification center is related to persistence of notochordal remnants. The clefts of cartilage on either side indenting into the midportion of the vertebra are not of abnormal origin. In histologic investigations of two cases Wollin and Elliott (1961) found that one defect was due to a radiolucent axial notochordal rod and the other had lateral clefts filled with cartilage with a core of persistent notochordal cells in the space between the cartilaginous clefts. If normal growth proceeds the cleft vanishes, and by some it is regarded as a normal variant. It is reported to be seen fairly frequently with chondrodystrophia calcificans congenita.

The incidence of coronal cleft vertebrae is infrequent. Eleven were seen by us in the past 8 years, all in newborns. Seven were premature infants. The observation was made incidentally on examinations for fetal respiratory distress in 3. Four had no other anomalies, and had had chest and abdomen roentgenograms for a variety of conditions including possible pneumonia or abdominal disorders. The remaining four had a variety of concomitant congenital defects including congenital heart disease, Pierre-Robin syndrome, cleft palate and supernumerary digits. Cohen, Guido and Neuhauser (1956) found 13 coronal cleft

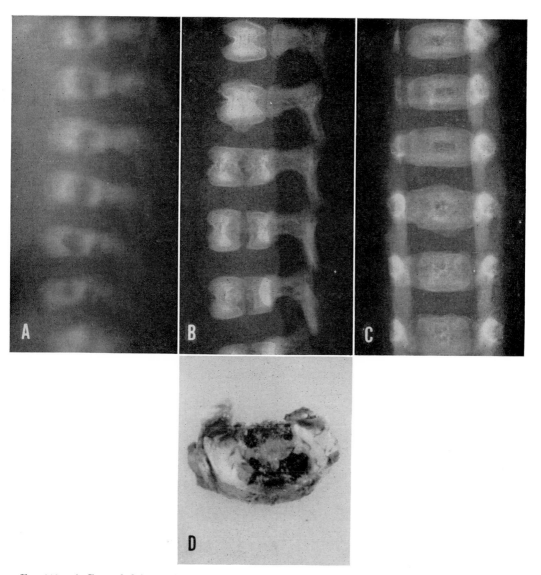

Fig. 119. *A*, Coronal cleft vertebrae in a premature infant. The clefts are ovoid, situated at the junction of the middle and posterior thirds of the centra. *B*, Specimen roentgenogram, coronal cleft vertebrae, lateral. *C*, AP roentgenogram, same specimen. *D*, Craniad surface of horizontally cut vertebra. Cartilage extends from the coronal cleft to both sides. Centers of ossification are seen in front of and behind the cleft.

vertebrae in 200 infants investigated for congenital malformations, while a control group of 200 others picked at random contained 4 with coronal cleft vertebrae. Some degree of meningocele was seen in 4, and 6 others had imperforate anus. In 1 of the 3 cases reported by Wollin and Elliott (1961) a midgut volvulus was present, and another had club feet. This indicates that

identification of coronal cleft vertebrae should alert one to the possibility of other congenital malformations.

The appearance of the coronal cleft varies considerably. In our 11 patients the second and third lumbar vertebrae were involved in 2, the third and fourth lumbar vertebrae in 2, the second, third and fourth lumbar vertebrae in 3, and the lower four lumbar vertebrae in 2. In 2 others the lower three thoracic, and all five lumbar vertebrae presented coronal clefts. As seen on lateral roentgenograms, the cleft appears as a rather indistinct, somewhat irregular division roughly between the middle and posterior thirds of the affected bodies. In 7 there was a somewhat rounded radiolucent defect approximately in the midportion of several of the vertebrae. The width of the cleft is such that it can be readily identified in most cases. In some the cleft appears more like an ovoid rather than a vertical defect in the bone (Fig. 119). Radiographic examination of two specimens removed at necropsy disclosed the same central defect seen during life. The adjacent bony margins of the cleft and the central cord could be well demonstrated. Section of one of the vertebrae disclosed normal cartilage at the periphery of the vertebra, the anterior and posterior centers of ossification and a central bar containing notochordal tissue. Occasionally a vertical streak appears in the vertebrae of older infants (Fig. 120). This bar of increased density probably represent increased calcification in a persistent notochordal streak, and may be the end stage of a coronal cleft vertebrae.

In the 11 cases of coronal cleft vertebrae described here there was one who had a moderate degree of narrowing of the interspace between the third and fourth lumbar vertebra. In all the others the intervertebral discs were normal, and the superior and inferior surfaces of the vertebral bodies presented a normal rounded appearance. The neurocentral synchondroses in 9 were within

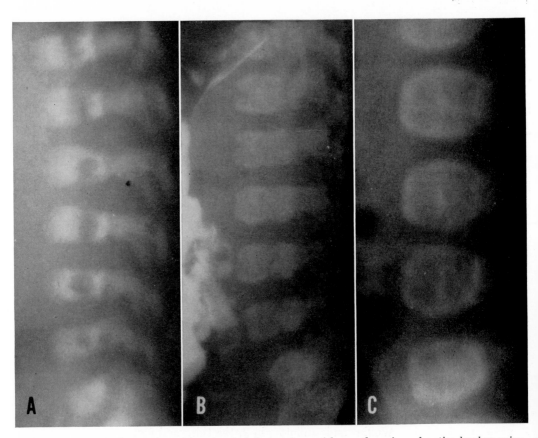

Fig. 120. *A*, Newborn spine with coronal cleft vertebrae of lower thoracic and entire lumbar spine. *B*, Three months later the clefts are closing. *C*, Another patient 6 weeks old with a vertical dense bar in the middle of the vertebrae—probably a calcified notochordal remnant or a fully united coronal cleft.

normal limits as compared with normal newborns (Figs. 47 and 48). In two there was a tapering at the neurocentral synchondroses of the affected vertebrae which I do not think is particularly striking. The sacrum and pelvis were normal in each one. Of some interest in one patient was the presence of a rather prominent venous channel which divided the ossification centers in half, so that on lateral roentgenograms four islands of bone were visible.

There is a tendency for the posterior aspect of the body of a vertebra with a coronal cleft to be smaller than its anterior portion. As a result the adjacent intervertebral disc presents a wider space posteriorly. Should there be some narrowing of the anterior portion of the disc, a V-shaped appearance can be identified (Fig. 119). The individual coronal cleft defects vary from vertebra to vertebra in the same patient. Some segments present complete vertical or ovoid radiolucent bars while others have smaller centrally situated defects (Fig. 121).

Sagittal Cleft Vertebrae. These vertebrae are regarded as abnormalities due to persistence of the ventrodorsal extension of the perichordal sheath, or to failure of fusion of the lateral halves of the vertebral bodies incident to persistence of notochordal tissue (Fig. 12). A wide variety of malformations appear with this structural aberration. In its simplest form a sagittal cleft vertebra is represented by a vertical bar of increased radiolucency visible on anteroposterior roentgenograms, and best identified on body section films. Usually this is associated with some indentation into the upper, the lower, or both surfaces of the affected cen-

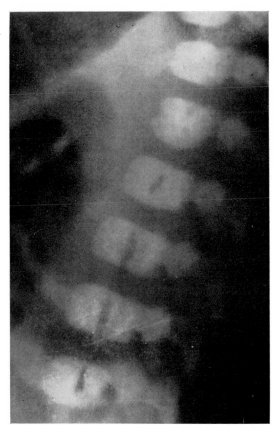

FIG. 121. Coronal cleft defects in a newborn infant. The radiolucent intravertebral bars vary from segment to segment.

trum, with concomitant upward and downward extension of the adjacent vertebrae (Fig. 122). The pedicles may be slightly increased in size, and the interpedicular distance widened somewhat. Minor changes occur in the neural arch.

In more advanced sagittally cleft vertebrae the involved bodies usually are increased in width, and somewhat diminished in height. This change also is most apparent on frontal roentgenograms. On lateral examinations some straightening of the spine in the involved area appears because there usually is some concomitant change in the anterior portion of the vertebra. The pedicles are more widely separated than those above or beneath, and the neural arch may be malformed. The characteristic appear-

ance is one in which the bodies appear as two triangles whose apices face one another (Fig. 123). The intervertebral discs are somewhat narrowed above and beneath, and the vertebral bodies impinge into this cleft. In an occasional instance the sagittal cleft vertebra may be considerably smaller than those above and beneath, so that a local dorsal kyphotic curve appears (Fig. 124). The apices of the facing triangles may be pointed or rounded, and closely approximated or separated appreciably. Thin strands of bone sometimes traverse the cleft.

Sagittal cleft vertebrae are seen in the lumbar and thoracic vertebrae. They usually are not present in the cervical region, unless as part of a widely spread malformation. Multiple sagittal cleft vertebrae are

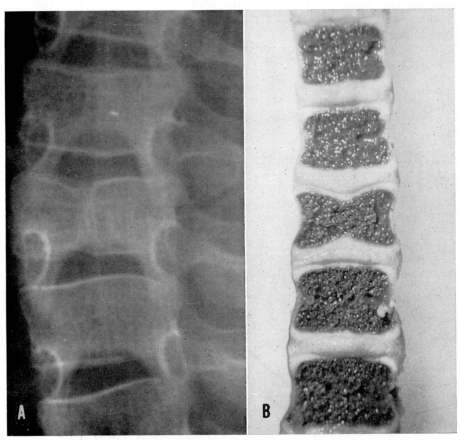

Fig. 122. *A*, Midthoracic sagittally cleft vertebra. The vertebrae above and below present altered configurations corresponding with the indentation in the midportion of the body of the cleft segment. The pedicles of the cleft vertebrae are separated more widely than those of the other segments. *B*, Photograph of specimen, same vertebra.

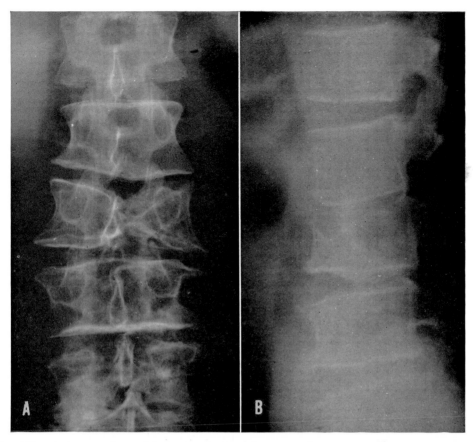

Fig. 123. *A*, A more advanced form of sagittally cleft vertebra ("butterfly vertebra"). The apices of the triangular deformed halves are approximated. The involved segment is widened, and those above and below have accommodated in shape to reflect the altered discs. *B*, The lordotic curve is straightened. The anterior aspect of the "butterfly vertebra" is diminished in height.

not uncommon, especially as part of a generalized change which may also include dysraphic alterations such as meningoceles, myelomeningoceles and diastematomyelia, as well as visceral anomalies involving the mediastinum, the urinary tract and the gastrointestinal tract.

Hemivertebrae. The development of a lateral half of an ossification center with failure of appearance of the opposite side results in a hemivertebra. This usually is situated laterally, the triangular wedge of bone inserted between two vertebrae whose upper and lower margins are deformed to correspond with the inserted wedge. A normal rib may project from the hemivertebra, while that on the contralateral side does

not develop. As a rule, an isolated hemivertebra is uncommon, these malformations tending to occur more often with advanced spinal abnormalities (Fig. 127).

A dorsal hemivertebra is quite uncommon. This results from failure of ossification of the anterior center, probably because of an impaired blood supply. The anterior half is reduced to a fibrous strand, while the dorsal half is triangular in configuration. The posterior wall is in a line continuous with the spinal canal. As a result a rather sharp gibbus deformity appears usually at the thoraco-lumbar junction (Fig. 125). This must be distinguished from the kyphos seen with hypothyroidism, achondroplasia, chondrodystrophy and some other dysplasias

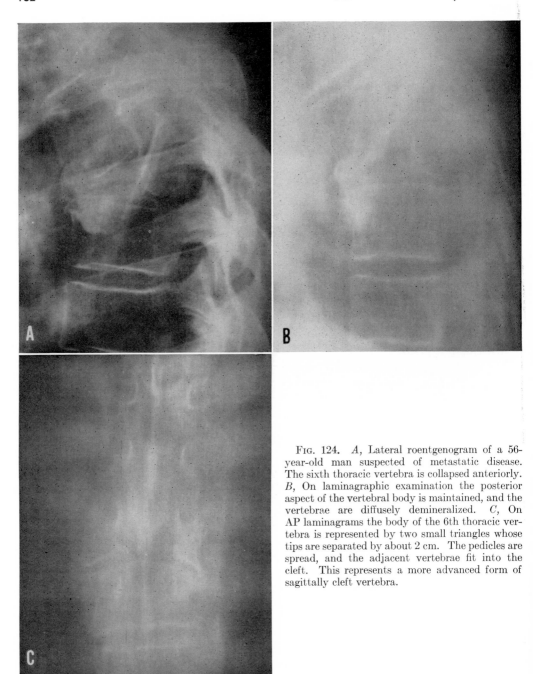

Fig. 124. *A*, Lateral roentgenogram of a 56-year-old man suspected of metastatic disease. The sixth thoracic vertebra is collapsed anteriorly. *B*, On laminagraphic examination the posterior aspect of the vertebral body is maintained, and the vertebrae are diffusely demineralized. *C*, On AP laminagrams the body of the 6th thoracic vertebra is represented by two small triangles whose tips are separated by about 2 cm. The pedicles are spread, and the adjacent vertebrae fit into the cleft. This represents a more advanced form of sagittally cleft vertebra.

such as gargoylism. Theoretically, it is possible for an anterior ossification center to persist and the posterior one to lose its blood supply. I know of no definite instance of a ventral hemivertebra.

The ultimate picture of vertebral body de-velopmental disruption is observed when there is neither pattern nor organization in the malformed spine (Fig. 126). This is attributed to faulty bilateral cranial hemi-metameric shift of the vertebral segments in the early stage of growth of the spine. This

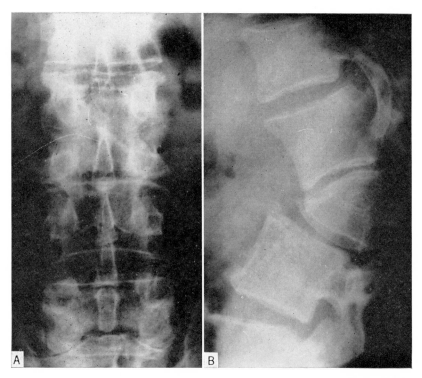

Fig. 125.   A and B, Wedge vertebra, with failure of development of anterior nucleus.
The dorsal hemivertebra produces a gibbus deformity.

shift, occurring on one side, causes an anlage for half a vertebra to remain at the lower as well as at the upper end of the unequally shifted and mismatched vertebrae. In its more advanced form involving most of the spine it is incompatible with life. When localized, it often is associated with other dysraphic malformations.

Asomia. Rarely there is failure of development of an entire vertebral segment, resulting in complete agenesis of one or more vertebrae. This sometimes is seen in stillborn infants with advanced congenital malformations. Agenesis of vertebral bodies was mentioned by Giannini, Borrelli and Greenberg (1948) as a cause of dwarfism. They described a $4\frac{1}{2}$-year-old boy with multiple defects including incomplete development of the thoracic vertebral bodies and complete absence of several segments. In the absence of one or more of the vertebral bodies it is not unusual for the neural arch to

persist (Reinhardt, 1963). Another rare malformation is absence of a centrum with persistence of its neural arch, together with a rudimentary vertebral body which apparently represents persistence of an ossification center more or less parallel to the plane of the suprajacent vertebra (Fig. 128). The affected centra result in a tapered appearance of the vertebral column, a shortening of the lumbar length present and concomitant malformations of the neural arches. Asomia limited to the thoracic spine is rare, and results in a pronounced dorsal kyphosis.

Total absence of the lumbar spine and sacrum is rare. Frantz and Aitken (1967) reported an additional three patients to the 4 previously described by Russel and Aitken (1963), and mentioned that still another had been reported from the University Hospital at Uppsala, Sweden by Dr. Tor Hiertonn. One of their cases came to necropsy. This grave defect is associated

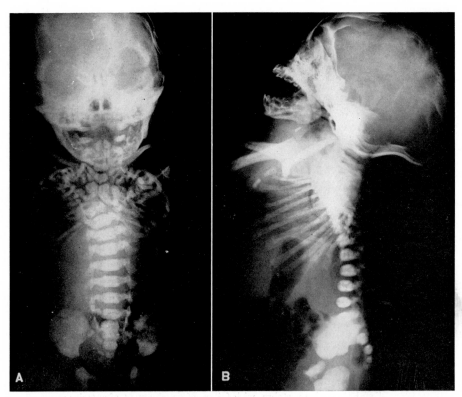

FIG. 126. *A*, Anteroposterior and *B*, lateral views of multiple congenitally malformed dorsal vertebrae. The architecture has been markedly distorted, so that the individual vertebrae and ribs cannot be identified. Note the lacunar skull and the widened lumbar spinal canal (meningocele).

with profound deficiencies including severe deformity and loss of function of the lower limbs, incontinence, a narrow pelvis with the ilia articulating amphiarthrodially, and flexed knees.

Neurenteric Cysts. These appear as a result of failure of proper development of the notochord and endoderm. As the notochord separates from the endoderm there may be areas in which the separation is incomplete, so that a pouch of endoderm is withdrawn from the primitive alimentary tract into the mesosdermal anlage of the vertebral bodies. Such a pouch can then grow to form a mediastinal or intestinal structure which may or may not communicate with the alimentary tract. The column of cells attaching the pouch to the notochord may interfere with proper growth of the vertebral bodies or cause failure of fusion of the neural arches. The combination of malformed ver-

tebrae with a mediastinal mass should immediately suggest the possible existence of a neurenteric cyst (Fig. 127).

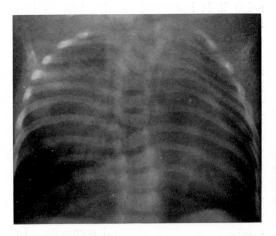

FIG. 127. Multiple vertebral anomalies, including hemivertebrae. The opacity in the right chest is produced by a neurenteric cyst.

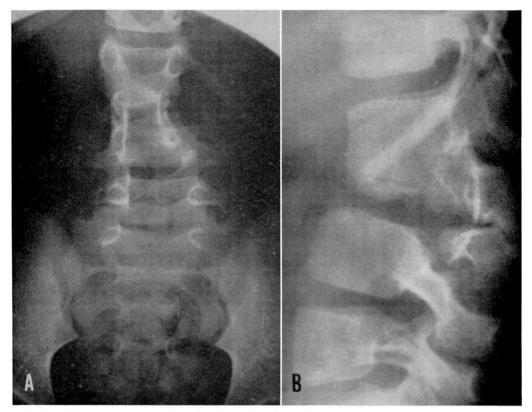

FIG. 128. *A*, AP lumbar spine with vestigial 2nd lumbar vertebra which still has a neural arch. *B*, Lateral view shows a small bar of bone immediately beneath L 2. A separate neural arch with a good-sized spinous process articulates with that of L 2. This was considered as asomia.

A neurenteric cyst presents a wall lined with cells which resemble a segment of the foregut. It may be connected by means of a stalk to the meninges or the spinal cord. Occasional congenital intraspinal enterogenous cysts have been reported (Scoville *et al.*, 1963) (Dorsey and Tabrisky, 1966). The usual spinal changes associated with neurenteric cysts are malformed vertebrae, particularly cleft segments, and deformities of the neural arches and a widened canal. If the cysts communicate with the gastrointestinal tract, gas and fluid levels appear within the cyst. Occasionally calcifications are present in the cyst, which can also displace the esophagus.

"Wedged" Vertebra. The term "wedged" vertebra refers to that condition in which only a single half of a vertebral body is present, a true hemivertebra. This is attributed to a defect in ossification of the cartilaginous body in early fetal life, and has been ascribed by Junghanns to a local deficiency in blood supply in the affected half. At first the developing half maintains a relatively cuboidal configuration, but with further growth and strain the change in pressure results in a triangular, wedge-like configuration with the apex directed medially. The term also may be applied to some of the instances of sagittal cleft vertebrae mentioned above, particularly those with advanced and multiple malformations (Fig. 127).

References

Bentley, J. F. R. and Smith, J. R.: Developmental Posterior Enteric Remnants and Spinal Malformations. The Split Notochord Syndrome, Arch. Dis. Childhood, *35*, 76, 1960.

Cave, P.: "Butterfly Vertebrae," Brit. J. Radiol., *31*, 503, 1958.

Cohen, J., Guido, C. and Neuhauser, E. B. D.: A Significant Variant in the Ossification Centers of the Vertebral Bodies, Am. J. Roentgenol., *76*, 469, 1956.

Dorsey, J. F. and Tabrisky, J.: Intraspinal and Mediastinal Foregut Cyst Compressing the Spinal Cord, J. Neurosurg., *24*, 563, 1966.

Ehrenhaft, J. L.: Development of the Vertebral Column as Related to Certain Congenital and Pathological Changes, Surg., Gynec. & Obst., *76*, 282, 1943.

Fallon, M., Gordon, A. R. G. and Lendru, A. C.: Mediastinal Cysts of Foregut Origin Associated with Vertebral Anomalies, Brit. J. Surg., *41*, 520, 1954.

Fawcitt, J.: Some Radiological Aspects of Congenital Anomalies of the Spine in Childhood and Infancy, Proc. Royal Soc. Med., *52*, 331, 1959.

Fischer, F. J. and Vandemark, R. E.: Sagittal Cleft (Butterfly) Vertebra, J. Bone & Joint Surg., *27*, 695, 1945.

Frantz, C. H. and Aitken, G. T.: Complete Absence of the Lumbar Spine and Sacrum, J. Bone & Joint Surg., *49-A*, 1531, 1967.

Giannini, M. J., Borrelli, F. J. and Greenberg, W. H.: Agenesis of the Vertebral Bodies—A Cause of Dwarfism, Am. J. Roentgenol., *59*, 705, 1948.

Gjorup, P. A.: Dorsal Hemivertebra, Acta orthop. Scandinav., *35*, 117, 1964.

Gleeson, J. A. and Stovin, P. G. I.: Mediastinal Enterogenous Cysts Associated with Vertebral Anomalies, Clinical Radiology, *12*, 41, 1961.

Knuttson, F.: Die frontale Wirbelkörperspalte, Acta radiol., *21*, 597, 1940.

March, H. C.: A Vertebral Anomaly: Probable Persistent Neurocentral Synchondrosis, Am. J. Roentgenol., *52*, 408, 1944.

Neuhauser, E. B. D., Harris, G. B. C. and Berrett, A.: Roentgenographic Features of Neurenteric Cysts, Am. J. Roentgenol., *79*, 235, 1958.

Pedersen, H.: Mediastinal Enterogenous Cyst with Spinal Malformations, Acta paediatrica Scandinavica, *54*, 392, 1965.

Reinhardt, K.: Asoma an der Lendenwirbelsaule, Fortschr. Röntgenstr., *99*, 197, 1963.

Rowley, K. A.: Coronal Cleft Vertebrae, J. Fac. Radiologists, *6*, 267, 1955.

Russell, H. E. and Aitken, G. T.: Congenital Absence of the Sacrum and Lumbar Vertebrae with Prosthetic Management, J. Bone & Joint Surg., *45-A*, 501, 1963.

Schmorl, G. and Junghanns, H.: *The Human Spine in Health and Disease*, New York, Grune & Stratton, 1959.

Scoville, W. B., Manlapaz, J. S., Otis, R. D. and Cabieses, F.: Intraspinal Enterogenous Cyst, J. Neurosurg., *20*, 704, 1963.

Veeneklaas, G. M. H.: Pathogeneis of Intrathoracic Gastrogenic Cysts, Am. J. Dis. Child., *83*, 500, 1952.

Windeyer, B. W.: Chordoma, Proc. Royal Soc. Med., *52*, 1088, 1959.

Wollin, D. G. and Elliott, G. B.: Coronal Cleft Vertebrae and Persistent Notochordal Derivatives of Infancy, J. Canad. A. Radiologists, *12*, 78, 1961.

Cleft Spinous Processes. This is a common vertebral anomaly and often is unassociated with specific complaints. Its mildest form is a lack of fusion of the neural arches of one or several vertebrae. The most common location is the fifth lumbar neural arch, and the first sacral segment is next. The coexistence of both lesions is not uncommon. One often observes a variable degree of lack of fusion of the dorsal plate of the lower sacrum, varying from a small cleft in the distal portion of the bone extending over one or two segments to an almost complete lack of fusion represented by a central radiolucent streak extending for the entire length of the sacrum (Fig. 129).

Statistics as to the incidence of failure of fusion of the upper sacrum and the fifth lumbar neural arch vary. Southworth and Bersack (1950) reported that of 550 patients with anomalies of the lumbosacral vertebrae most had little or no symptoms referable to the low back. Spina bifida occulta was present in 18.2 per cent; 2.2 per cent of these occurred in the lumbar spine and 16.0 per cent involved the sacrum. They analyzed the defects in the neural arches and found that of the lumbar defects only one was to the left of the midline. Of the sacral defects 3 were to the right, 2 to the left of the midline, and 1 bilateral. The vast majority of the defects were central in location. Dittrich (1938) reported that 5 per cent of all spines examined roentgenologically presented spina bifida occulta, a figure close to that reported by Breck, Hillsman and Basom (1944), who reported an incidence of 6 per cent in a series of 450 cases. However, Friedman, Fischer and Van Demark (1946) reported an incidence of 36 cases of spina bifida occulta in a review of the cases of 100 soldiers. My own experience coincides with the last authors' insofar

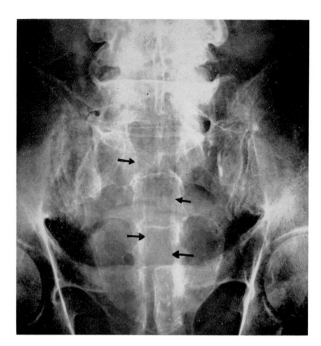

Fig. 129. Failure of fusion of the dorsal plate of the sacrum extending from the first to the last sacral segment (arrows).

as frequency of occurrence is concerned. It is not at all infrequent in the course of routine gastrointestinal or genitourinary examinations to encounter an unsuspected and symptomless cleft spinous process of the fifth lumbar vertebra, the first sacral segment of the lower dorsal aspect of the sacrum. Combinations of these three are frequent, and together with them atypical formation of the articular processes between the fourth and fifth and fifth lumbar and first sacral segments is not uncommon.

In addition to cleft spinous processes in the regions named above occasional instances are noted of lack of fusion of the spinous processes of the lower thoracic and upper lumbar vertebrae (Fig. 130). Similar changes appear in the spinous processes of the first and seventh cervical and first and second thoracic vertebrae. These less frequent examples portray the embryologic change more faithfully in that the lesion is represented by a thin radiolucent cleft in the spinous process of the affected vertebra. The range of variation in the appearance of

the laminae and pedicles of these vertebrae is less than in the fifth lumbar or first sacral segments. Cleft spinous processes in these regions follow the pattern of fusion of the laminae in the midline to form the spinous process. The laminae fuse at about the first year of life and their development is completed during adolescence. The spinous process is capped at about this time by an apophysis which calcifies completely and fuses with the main mass of the spinous process at about the 24th or 25th year of life. This additional apophysis sometimes fails to unite with the spinous process, and the structure appears as a rather oval calcific shadow overlying the defect in the involved neural arch. This too sometimes assumes an anomalous appearance and grows to a fairly large hook-shaped bone. An instance of this rather rare anomaly associated with considerable back pain is shown in Figure 131.

While most patients with lumbar cleft spinous processes have no specific complaints, certain cases are accompanied by

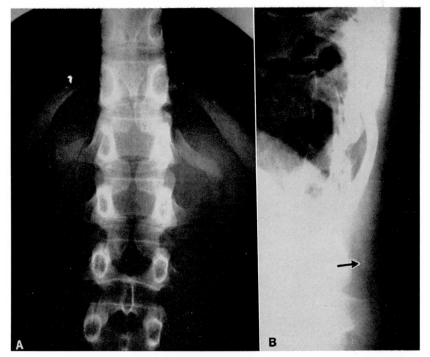

FIG. 130. *A*, Incomplete fusion of the neural arches of the first, second and third lumbar vertebrae, with absence of spinous processes. Bilateral lumbar ribs. *B*, Same case, lateral view. The spinous processes are missing. A rudimentary ossicle is seen above the normally developed spinous process of the third lumbar vertebra (arrow).

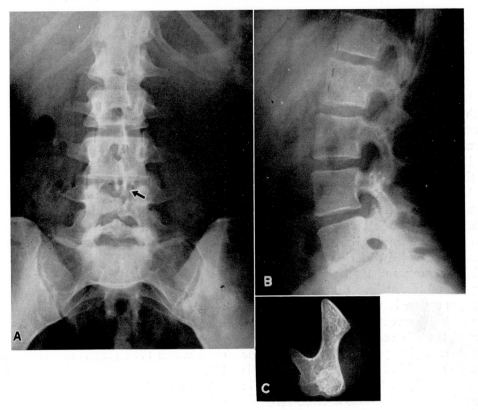

FIG. 131. *A,* Anteroposterior view of lumbar spine. Incomplete fusion of the spinous process of the fourth lumbar vertebra. Just above this cleft is a linear ossicle (arrow) directed towards the left of the midline. *B*, Same case, lateral view. The ossicle can be seen just above the base of the spinous process of the fourth lumbar vertebra. *C*, Same case, operative specimen. The ossicle was anchored to the dura by firm adhesive bands.

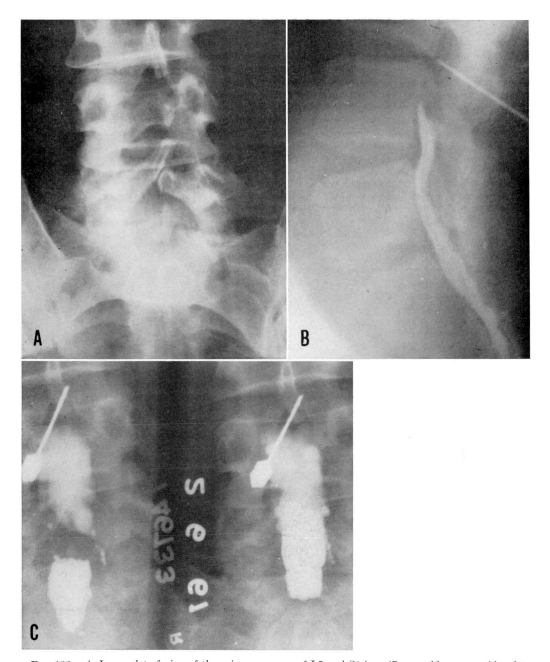

Fig. 132. *A*, Incomplete fusion of the spinous process of L5 and S1 in a 47-year-old man considered to have a herniated disc. *B*, Myelography reveals partial block at the L5 level, which on lateral examination, *C*, is produced by heavy overgrowth of the fifth neural arch. The spinal canal is narrowed. At operation the defect was found to be due to pressure from the neural arch which compressed the cauda equina. Relief followed decompression.

low back pain. These are difficult to evaluate, and the defect should not be held as the responsible factor until all other possibilities have been excluded (Fig. 132).

An interesting series was published by Jelsma and Ploetner (1953), who reported a group of 18 patients with low back pain radiating to the hips, and sometimes to both

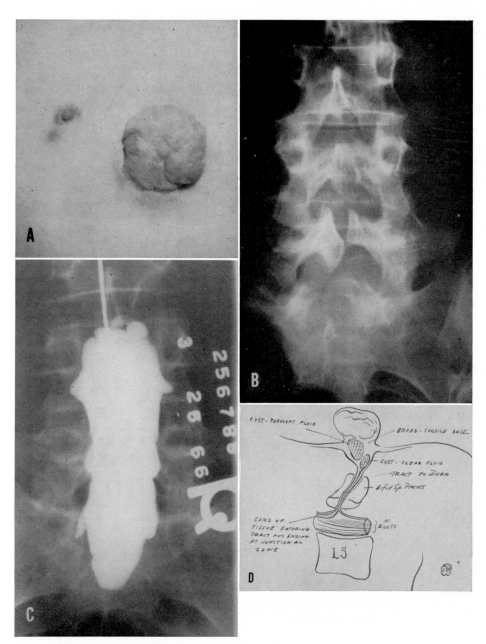

Fig. 133. *A*, A lipomatous mass is present over the lower lumbar spine in a 47-year-old woman with weakness of both lower extremities. *B*, AP roentgenograms reveal incomplete fusion of the neural arches of L5 and S1. *C*, Myelography reveals the canal to be wide, and the axillary pouches are directed horizontally, indicating a shortened filum terminale with traction. The conus was identified at L2. *D*, At operation a meningocele was found beneath the lipoma. This communicated with a tract through the bifid spinous process to the dura, entered the dura and terminated in a thick junctional zone with a heavy filum terminale.

legs or to one leg. While this pain was sometimes recurrent, it often was continuous over a period of years and could be aggravated by bending. Usually no reflex or sensory changes were noted. Operation disclosed a mass of fibrous or fibrolipomatous tissue, often with a constricting mass of fibrous tissue involving the dura. At times fibrosis involving the sheaths of the emerging nerve roots was encountered. They did not observe cord involvement by traction on the filum terminale. None of their cases showed any evidence of myelodysplasia, and the bony defects were minimal. Apparently the pain was produced by a traction mechanism in which the dense fibrous tissue extended from the dura to an insertion where the posterior spinous processes ordinarily would have appeared, and there the fibrous bands become attached to the lumbar fascia of the back.

Occasionally an ununited spinous process may be the clue to a more serious neuroanatomic defect, especially if accompanied by some seemingly minor disturbance such as a cutaneous dimple, a bit of hair over the lower spine, a subcutaneous lipoma or telangiectatic patch (Fig. 133). Should the bifid spinous process also be associated with congenital malformations elsewhere in the spine, or with gait disturbances, limping, stumbling, or with deformities of the feet such as high arches or clawing of the toes, the possibility of a tight filum terminale with tethering of the conus medullaris deserves further consideration, and myelography can be important in establishing this diagnosis. Progressive neurologic deficiencies of the lower extremities and urinary difficulties also appear with involvement of the conus. The myelographic change to be anticipated is a low position of the conus as demonstrated on air myelograms, or by positive contrast myelography. With the latter procedure the position of the anterior spinal artery is helpful in establishing the location of the conus, and the filum terminale sometimes can be identified as well. It appears that identifidation of the filum terminale can

be better accomplished with the patient supine when positive contrast examination is made (Fig. 134). A horizontal position of the axillary pouches is an important indication of a tethered conus and cauda equina (Fig. 133C).

References

Breck, L. W., Hillsman, J. W. and Basom, W. C.: Lumbosacral Roentgenograms, Ann. Surg., *120*, 88, 1944.

Dittrich, R. J.: Roentgenologic Aspects of Spina Bifida Occulta, Am. J. Roentgenol., *39*. 937, 1938.

Friedman, M. M., Fisher, F. J. and Van Demark, R. E.: Lumbosacral Roentgenograms, Am. J. Roentgenol., 55, 292, 1946.

James, C. C. M. and Lassman, L. P.: Spinal Dysraphism. The Diagnosis and Treatment of Progressive Lesions in Spina Bifida Occulata. J. Bone & Joint Surg., *44-B*, 828, 1962.

Jelsma, F. and Ploetner, E. J.: Painful Spina Bifida Occulta, J. Neurosurg., *10*, 19, 1953.

Love, J. G., Daly, D. D. and Harris, L. E.: Tight Filum Terminale, J.A.M.A., *176*, 31, 1961.

Southworth, J. D. and Bersack, S. R.: Anomalies of Lumbosacral Vertebrae, Am. J. Roentgenol., *64*, 624, 1950.

Diastematomyelia. This infrequent malformation of the spinal cord represents a dysraphic developmental error of growth of the neural plate and the neurenteric canal. In vertebrates the neurenteric canal is a minute connection between the amniotic cavity and the yolk sac. It passes through the primitive node, which migrates caudally as the neural plate evolves into the spinal cord. At no time in its development is the cord duplicated, so that diatematomyelia does not represent a twinning, or actual double development, of the cord. Persistence of a connection between the dorsal aspect of an ectopic or accessory neurenteric canal is followed by malformations of the cord, the vertebrae and the neural arches. Similar communications between the ventral aspect of the neurenteric canal results in various malformations dependent on the open area. Enterogenous cysts may follow persistence of the midportion, duplication of the bowel from persistence of the ventral portion alone, while if the terminal segments

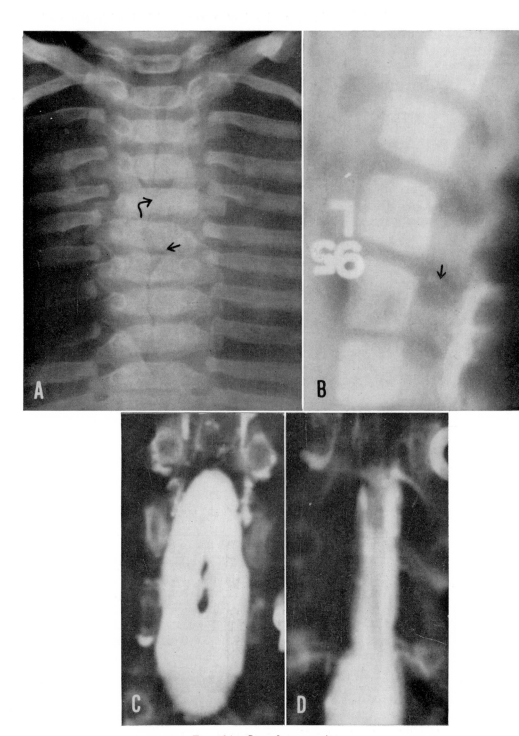

FIG. 134. *Legend on opposite page.*

persists, a wide variety of lesions such as cutaneous vascular malformations and sinuses, dermoids or teratomas may occur singly or in combination. If both the dorsal and ventral portions of an accessory neurenteric canal persists, various combinations of vertebral and visceral malformations can occur. The basic embryologic defect occurs at the 4th week of gestation, when the neural tube is being formed.

The term "diastematomyelia" indicates the presence of a fissure of the spinal cord. The spur formation often observed in the middle of the defect is attributed to the formation of a central fused pedicle resulting from abnormal growth of the underlying malformed vertebra, which, in the process of growth as a bifid structure, laid down a rudimentary pair of pedicles. When calcified, the central spur is a reliable index to the correct diagnosis. In some instances the spur is fibrous or cartilaginous, and hence cannot be identified on plain spinal roentgenograms. The bifurcation of the cord, which may extend over several segments, cannot be estimated from the position of the spur. Occasionally body section roentgenograms are useful in delineating a spur (Fig. 134).

Diastematomyelia is encountered in either sex from fetal life to old age. In most cases there are pronounced associated anomalies of vertebral bodies and the neural arches, and in some meningocele or myelomeninogocele is found. Death from infection of these structures may occur in early life. The lesions occur anywhere in the dorsal or lumbar spine but appear to be most frequent in the lower dorsal or upper lumbar regions. Instances have been encountered in the mid-dorsal and lower lumbar areas. Splitting of the spinal cord occurs in varying degrees from an abortive doubling with no clinical or radiologic manifestations to division of the cord into parallel structures. In marked cases there may even be doubling of the lower spinal column (Pickles, 1949). The divided spinal cord may be contained within a single dural sheath. In such a situation the midline spur usually is absent. If each half of the divided cord is inside its own dural covering, a spur usually is present. The possibility of symptoms referable to the cord are greater in the latter instance, because of tethering of the cord and failure of its normal ascent or because of pressure on one side or the other of the divided cord. Such effects usually present themselves early in life, although they can first become apparent later on (James and Lassman, 1964). When the cord is doubled, the length involved may be greater than the extent of the associated vertebral anomaly. As a rule the cord is united above and below its split por-

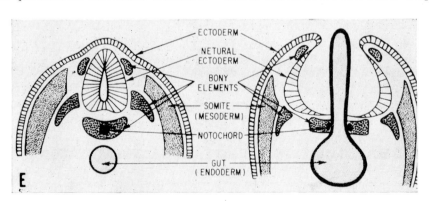

Fig. 134. *A,* Thoracic diastematomyelia with spur at T4 and 5 level (arrows). *B,* Lateral laminagram, lumbar spine of another patient with spur projecting dorsad. *C,* Myelogram of patient with lumbar diastematomyelia. The central defect is produced by the spur. The conus is low in position and the filum terminale is heavy, *D. E,* Diagram of embryologic basis for splitting of the cord. (*B,* courtesy of G. Moore, New Zealand) (*C,* courtesy of J. Bull, Queen Square Hospital, London) (*E,* courtesy of P. E. Sheptak and A. F. Susen, Am. J. Dis. Child., *113,* 210, 1967.)

tion. While the split portions usually are separated, at times they lie close to one another.

The split in the cord in itself is asymptomatic, adverse effects resulting from the associated vertebral malformations and the tethering of the cord. While the identification of spinal dysraphism often is suggested by the presence of midline cutaneous changes, James and Lassman (1962) found that external manifestations might be lacking, and that the diagnosis was facilitated by detection of changes in gait, various deformities of the feet, and later on trophic ulceration, incontinence and paraplegia. In such instances the identification of even minor malformations of the lumbar neural arches can be most helpful. Tethering of the cord during the growth period also takes place because of fibrous bands extending from the subcutaneous tissues into the intradural space in patients with defects in the neural arches, intraspinal lipomas and dermoids or neurofibromas as well as from diastematomyelic spurs. The lesions may be intradural as well as extradural extending into the thecal space, so that relief can be obtained only if the cause of the tethering is identified by opening the dura at operation.

Roentgenographic examination of the spine in diastematomyelia discloses fairly characteristic changes. These consist of a wide variety of malformations of the vertebral bodies, including hemivertebrae, unsegmented and hypoplastic vertebral bodies, narrow intervertebral spaces, kyphosis and scoliosis. The neural arches may be malformed, and failure of fusion of the neural arches is frequent. The interpedicular spaces in the involved areas are widened. The pedicles retain average configurations, although sometimes they are flat and thin. The condition is often diagnosed by the demonstration of a spur which protrudes from below upwards between the split spinal cord or cauda equina as a bony septum up to 1.5 cm in length. It occurs as a rather spindle-shape or oval bony density in an area with malformed vertebral bodies and neural arches. This spur may be attached to the dorsal aspect of the underlying vertebral body with its apex directed into the lumen of the canal. While usually single, it sometimes is multiple. The bony spur may be absent, and in its place a band of connective tissue which sometimes contains cartilage protrudes between the divided segments of the spinal cord. This connective tissue septum may be quite long, and within it a bony spicule may be present.

Pantopaque myelography is helpful in diagnosing diastematomyelia, particularly if the characteristic spur is absent. In such cases the myelograms disclose a radiotransparent midline linear shadow pointing towards the existence of an unsuspected cartilaginous or fibrous septum. Associated with this may be irregularities in the Pantopaque column secondary to arachnoidal adhesions. Tethering of the cord is identified by caudal displacement of the conus and the anterior spinal artery (Fig. 134).

References

Blight, A. S.: Diastematomyelia, Clin. Radiol., *12*, 158, 1961.

Bremer, J. L.: Dorsal Intestinal Fistula; Accessory Neurenteric Canal; Diastematomyelia, Arch. Path., *54* 132, 1952.

Cohen, J. and Sledge, C. B.: Diastematomyelia, Am. J. Dis. Child., *100*, 257, 1960.

Cowie, T. N.: Diastematomyelia with Vertebral Column Defects, Brit. J. Radiol., *24*, 156, 1951.

————: Diastematomyelia. Tomography in Diagnosis, Brit. J. Radiol., *25*, 263, 1952.

Freeman, L. W.: Late Symptoms from Diastematomyelia, J. Neurosurg., *18*, 538, 1961.

Gryspeerdt, G. L.: Myelographic Assessment of Occult Forms of Spinal Dysraphism, Acta Radiol., *1*, (N. S.) 702, 1963.

Herren, R. Y. and Edwards, J. E.: Diplomyelia (Duplication of the Spinal Cord), Arch. Path., *30*, 1203, 1940.

James, C. C. M. and Lassman, L. P.: Diastematomyelia, Arch. Dis. Childhood, *33*, 536, 1958.

————: Spinal Dysraphism. The Diagnosis and Treatment of Progressive Lesions in Spina Bifida Occulta, J. Bone & Joint Surg., *44-B*, 828, 1962.

————: Diastematomyelia, Arch. Dis. Childhood, *39*, 125, 1964.

Liliequist, B.: Diastematomyelia. Report of a Case Examined by Gas Myelography, Acta Radiol., *3*, 497, 1966.

Matson, D. D., Woods, R. P., Campbell, J. B. and Ingraham, F. D.: Diastematomyelia (Congenital Clefts of the Spinal Cord), Pediatrics, *6*, 98, 1950.

Maxwell, H. and Bucy, P. C.: Diastematomyelia, J. Neuropath. & Exper. Neurol., *5*, 165, 1946.

Neuhauser, E. B. D., Wittenborg, M. H. and Dehlinger, K.: Diastematomyelia, Radiology, *54*, 659, 1950.

Perret, G.: Diagnosis and Treatment of Diastematomyelia, Surg., Gynecol. & Obst., *105*, 69, 1957.

Pickles, W.: Duplication of Spinal Cord (Diplomyelia), J. Neurosurg, *6*, 324, 1949.

Rhaney, K. and Barclay, G. P. T.: Enterogenous Cysts and Congenital Diverticula of the Alimentary Canal with Abnormalities of the Vertebral Column and Spinal Cord, J. Path. & Bact., *77*, 457, 1959.

Walker, A. E.: Dilatation of Vertebral Canal with Congenital Anomalies of Spinal Cord, Am. J. Roentgenol., *52*, 571, 1944.

Spina Bifida Cystica (Meningocele, Myelomeningocele and Hydromyelomeningocele). Protrusion of the meninges through a cranial or vertebral defect, with the spinal cord resting in its normal position within the spinal canal, is regarded as a meningocele. Both the dura mater and the arachnoid form the wall, and the sac is filled with cerebrospinal fluid. The underlying embryologic defect is one which involves the mesodermal structures only. Usually the spinal cord is normal, and terminates at its accustomed position at the second lumbar level, but at times it is adherent to the spinal canal with the nerves emerging perpendicularly so that the cauda equina is absent.

When the embryological error is principally mesodermal, and is associated with a concomitant defect in ectodermal development, a myelomeningocele or hydromyelomeningocele appears. Here the neural tube has remained approximated to the ectoderm for some distance while most of it has closed off. The nerve roots in the involved area are directed downwards to reach their intervertebral foramina, or are integrated into the wall of the sac and are covered by thin, glistening silky integument. The surface layer may be intact (Fig. 135) or raw and ulcerated, presenting a central zona vasculosa surrounded by a semitransparent membranous remnant of meninges and skin. The spinal cord proximal to the lesion often

is deformed, presenting a wide variety of lesions including hydromyelia, diastematomyelia, syringomyelia, or cysts. Hydromyelomeningocele infers concomitant hydromyelia, the cord dorsally placed, adherent to the roof of the lesion, and the nerve trunks directed ventrally to emerge through the intervertebral foramina. The nerve roots may be free or incorporated into the wall of the sac.

With gross maldevelopment of the neural ectoderm and associated mesodermal defect, the cord lies exposed as a malformed structure on the surface, with abnormal formation of the adjacent meninges and skin, and advanced neural arch defects are present. The term "rachischisis" implies such an advanced defect, involving either the entire vertebral column or localized to one area, usually lumber or thoracolumbar (Fig. 136).

While in most patients with meningoceles other anomalies are not present, those with myelomeningoceles usually present concomitant defects in the central nervous system, the gastrointestinal and urinary tracts, or the appendicular skeleton. Among these are included lacunar skull, the Arnold-Chiari malformation, aqueductal lesions, congenital dislocation of the hips, various defects in the upper and lower extremities, and mediastinal and pulmonary malformations as well as rib anomalies.

The existence of a bifid spine is not absolutely necessary for the development of a meningocele. This is particularly true in the cervico-thoracic and sacral regions where protrusion may occur through an intervertebral foramen or an incompletely developed sacrum, with absence of its anterior component and protrusion of the hernial sac into the chest or pelvis.

Meningoceles occur most frequently in the lumbar and lumbosacral regions. The incidence of cervical and thoracic meningoceles is less frequent, and high cervical occipital meningoceles are even less common. In a series of 385 cases reported by Moore (1905) 23 per cent were sacral, 34 per cent lumbar, 29 per cent lumbosacral, 4.5 per cent

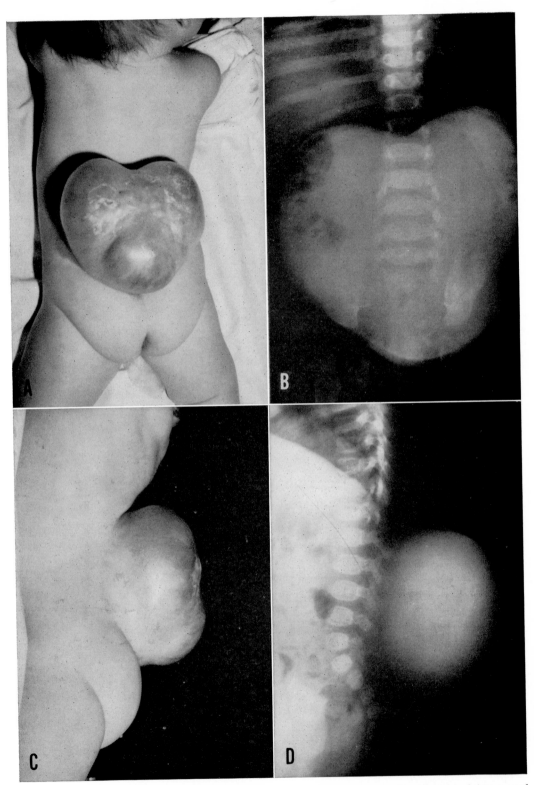

FIG. 135. *A*, Large lumbar myelomeningocele. *B*, Roentgenogram reveals defect involving neural arches of the lumbar spine. *C*, Lateral view of meningocele and *D*, lateral lumbar spine roentgenogram discloses normal vertebral bodies.

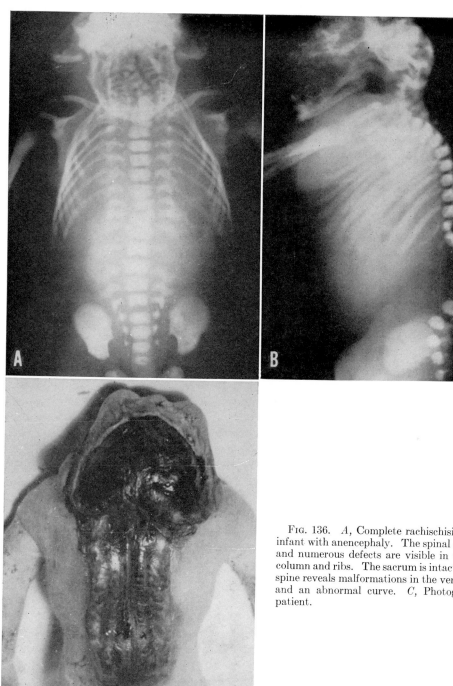

Fig. 136. *A*, Complete rachischisis in newborn infant with anencephaly. The spinal canal is wide, and numerous defects are visible in the vertebral column and ribs. The sacrum is intact. *B*, Lateral spine reveals malformations in the vertebral bodies and an abnormal curve. *C*, Photograph of the patient.

thoracic, 9.5 per cent cervical and 2 patients had occipital meningoceles.

Usually the diagnosis of meningocele or myelomeningocele is fairly obvious. The bony defects are best demonstrable radiologically. In most instances of uncomplicated meningocele or myelomeningocele of the lumbar, sacral or lumbosacral regions one encounters varying degrees of spreading of the pedicles beneath the protruding sac. The area involved may be only one or two vertebrae, or more commonly the pedicles of several vertebral segments are involved. The spreading is arranged in a fusiform fashion, the widest portion of the interpedicular area being at the middle of the lesion. Immediately above and beneath the interpedicular spaces approach normal as the upper and lower extremes of the defect are

reached, unless concomitant vertebral anomalies exist (Fig. 137). Associated with this is maldevelopment of the neural arches, the laminae and spinous processes being absent or malformed. The neck of the protruding meningocele does not necessarily correspond to the area of maximum widening of the interpedicular spaces. As a rule this region is considerably wider than the anatomic neck of the sac.

The pedicles may be relatively flattened, but more often retain a rather attenuated but still circular appearance. One gets the impression that the vertebral body is seen through the sac in better detail than the segments in which the neural arches are intact. In some cases the intervertebral discs spaces are relatively well maintained and the vertebral bodies are well formed. The con-

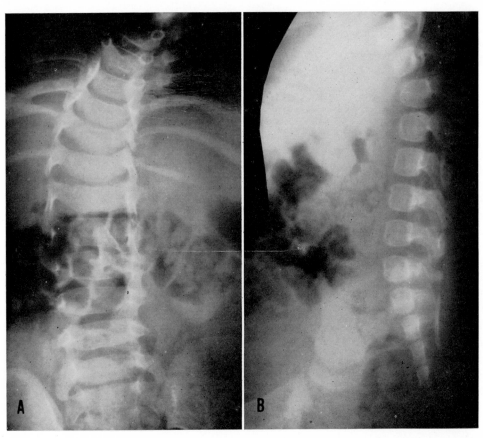

Fig. 137. *A*, Large myelomeningocele involving the lower thoracic and the lumbar vertebrae. The neural arches are spread and the pedicles are widely separated. *B*, On the lateral film the vertebral bodies are somewhat square in configuration, but an angulation is present at the 11th and 12th thoracic segments.

currence of congenital malformations of the vertebral bodies and changes in alignment is common.

On lateral views the soft tissue components and osseous contents of the protruding sac can be demonstrated, and are helpful in recording configuration and size. The sac may also be seen on the anteroposterior views overlying the spine as a faintly radio-opaque shadow with a smooth outline. A radiologic diagnosis of meningocele *in utero* might be postulated if roentgenograms show a curvature of the lumbodorsal area convex dorsally, or if defects in the vertebral column are seen.

Information as to the position of the spinal cord and the capacity of the subarachnoid space is best obtained by means of myelography. Positive contrast myelograms permit identification of downward displacement of the conus and of the configuration of the fluid-containing portions of the involved area. Gas myelography is regarded as preferable for these purposes inasmuch as it is non-irritating, is absorbed readily and less likely to result in arachnoiditis or cyst formation (Swedberg, 1963). If concomitant Arnold-Chiari malformation is suspected, identification of the position of the fourth ventricle in relation to the foramen magnum and upper cervical spinal canal can be obtained by means of gas or positive contrast ventriculography.

In the less frequently encountered meningoceles and myelomeningoceles of the cervical and thoracic regions, a similar type of defect of the neural arches is noted, but as a rule the changes is less marked. It is hard to determine even with roentgenograms whether a meningocele protrudes from a defect in the posteroinferior aspect of the occipital bone, or from an associated anomaly of the neural arches of the first and second cervical vertebrae. We have encountered instances in which defects were present in the neural arches of the upper cervical segments together with maldevelopment of the inferior aspect of the occipital bone. In other cases the lesion protruded from a circular defect in the middle of the lower portion of the occipital bone. In both circumstances, the external appearance of the hernial sac was very much the same.

The concurrence of lacunar skull with the meningoceles and meningomyeloceles is frequent. The lacunation disappears within a few months if a shunting procedure is successful in halting concomitant hydrocephalus. This does not imply that the lacunar deformity is associated with increased intracranial pressure.

Intrathoracic meningoceles are uncommon lesions characterized by protrusion of a sac of dura through an enlarged intervertebral foramen into the thorax, displacing the posterior aspect of the parietal pleura anteriorly. In configuration and extent they are rather similar to hourglass tumors, and their association with neurofibroma is relatively frequent. It is presumed that intrathoracic meningoceles arise from a primary dural defect associated with hypoplasia of adjacent bone. Congenital mesodermal aberration affects both the dura and the vertebra, and because about two thirds of the reported cases of intrathoracic meningoceles have been associated with vertebral anomalies a common origin is postulated. Intrathoracic meningoceles without concomitant neurofibromatosis has been reported, but in these cases vertebral defects also have been noted.

Intrathoracic meningoceles occur as unilateral, and sometimes as bilateral lesions. The diagnosis is facilitated by the identification of associated spinal deformities such as kyphosis, scoliosis, vertebral erosions, enlarged intervertebral foramina, or scalloping of the adjacent vertebral bodies and ribs. Other malformations such as fused vertebrae or hemivertebrae with aplasia of the corresponding ribs also occur. An intrathoracic meningocele should be suspected when a mediastinal tumor is associated with neurofibromatosis or spinal anomalies.

It has been observed that in some cases of intrathoracic meningocele the amount of cerebrospinal fluid which can be removed is unusually large. The diagnosis can be established with certainty by means of myelography. Pneumomyelography is particularly applicable, the demonstration of air entering the thoracic sac being of basic diagnostic significance. Similar observations also are possible with Pantopaque. Unless clearly indicated by the patient's condition, surgery is considered inadvisable because of the danger of secondary infection.

References

Bunner, R.: Lateral Intrathoracic Meningocele, Acta radiol., *51*, 1, 1959.

Cmyral, R.: Über ein Fall von intrathoracaler bilateraler Meningocele, Radiol. Austriaca, *5*, 23, 1952.

Cross, G. O., Raevis, J. R. and Saunders, W. W.: Lateral Intrathoracic Meningocele, J. Neurosurg., *6*, 423, 1949.

Early, C. B. and Sayers, M. P.: Pantopaque Ventriculography in Infants with Myelomeningocele, J. Neurosurg., *22*, 474, 1965.

Graf, R. A., Smith, J. H., Flocks, R. H. and van Epps, E. F.: Urinary Tract Changes Associated with Spina Bifida and Myelomeningocele, Am. J. Roentgenol., *92*, 255, 1964.

LaVielle, C. J. and Campbell, D. A.: Neurofibromatosis and Intrathoracic Meningocele, Radiology, *70*, 63, 1958.

Mendelson, H. I. and Kay, E. B.: Intrathoracic Meningocele, J. Thoracic Surg., *18*, 124, 1949.

Moore, J. E.: Spina Bifida. With Report of Three Hundred and Eighty-Four Cases Treated by Excision, Surg., Gynecol. & Obst., *1*, 137, 1905.

Nanson, E. M.: Thoracic Meningocele Associated with Neurofibromatosis, J. Thoracic Surg., *33*, 650, 1957.

Papatheodorou, C. A. and Teng, P.: Air-Pantopaque Ventriculography in Congenital Hydrocephalus and Myelomeningocele, Am. J. Roentgenol., *91*, 647, 1964.

Rubin, S. and Stralemeyer, E. H.: Intrathoracic Meningocele, Radiology, *58*, 552, 1952.

Swedberg, M.: Meningocele and Myelomeningocele Studied by Gas Myelography, Acta radiol., *1*, 796, 1963.

YaDeau, R. E., Clagett, O. T. and Divertie, M. B.: Intrathoracic Meningocele, J. Thoracic and Cardiovasc. Surg., *49*, 202, 1965.

Anterior Sacral Meningocele. This is a relatively infrequent congenital anomaly, usually associated with absence of part of the sacrum producing a curvilinear, sometimes semicircular defect in either the right or left lateral halves (Fig. 138). Projecting from this is a sac-like intrapelvic protrusion containing cerebrospinal fluid. Symptoms may be produced by pressure of the tumor on the pelvic viscera. Neurologic deficits are incurred by involvement of the sacral segments, and a bizarre and most interesting symptom is the development of headache from intermittent increases in intracranial pressure by direct hydraulic action (Brown and Powell, 1945). Rarely agenesis of the lower sacrum is bilateral rather than unilateral.

In addition to the plain films, which in themselves may be diagnostic, further information may be obtained by myelograms in which air or Pantopaque can be demonstrated entering the meningocele. Occasionally partial sacral agenesis produces a rather similar bony defect without a meningeal sac but with a bizarre intrasacral terminal sac.

References

Brown, M. H. and Powell, L. D.: Anterior Sacral Meningocele, J. Neurosurg., *2*, 535, 1945.

Calihan, R. J.: Anterior Sacral Meningocele, Radiology, *58*, 104, 1952.

Leigh, T. F. and Rogers, J. V., Jr.: Anterior Sacral Meningocele, Am. J. Roentgenol., *71*, 906, 1954.

Rowlands, B. C.: Anterior Sacral Meningocele, Brit. J. Surg., *43*, 301, 1955.

Schurr, P. H.: Sacral Extradural Cyst. J. Bone & Joint Surg., *37-B*, 601, 1955.

Intrasacral (Occult) Meningocele refers to a widening of the distal end of the dural sac, with or without gross maldevelopment of the adjacent bone other than a variable widening of the sacral canal. The diagnosis is usually established myelographically. The caudal sac, instead of showing a pointed distal end, widens out into a spherical or cylindrical bag enclosed within the sacrum, sometimes demonstrable on lateral roentgenograms as a thinning of its dorsal aspect at approximately the second, third and fourth segments. The sac usually is connected with the spinal subarachnoid space by a channel of variable size. In several cases which we have observed the channel

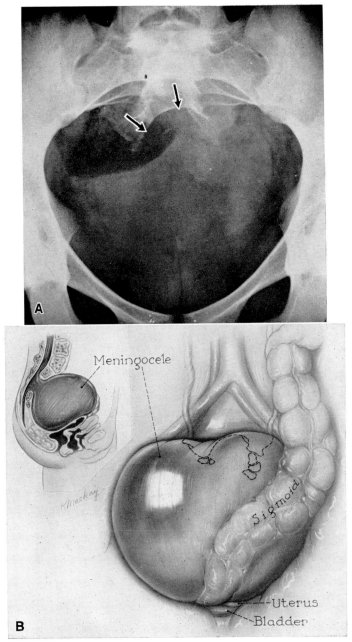

Fig. 138.   *A*, Anterior sacral meningocele, with crescent deformity of the sacrum and adjacent soft tissue mass (arrows).   *B*, Same case.   (From Leigh, T. F. and Rogers, J. V., Jr., Am. J. Roentgenol, *71*, 808, 1954.)

leading into the meningocele was quite narrow (Fig. 139).

Occult, or intrasacral, meningocele often is asymptomatic, but also has been associated with backaches and sacral nerve pain, urinary incontinence and various neurologic defects. Physical examination as a rule does not disclose a mass in this vicinity, but a congenital lipoma may be observed just beneath the skin or in the deeper structures.

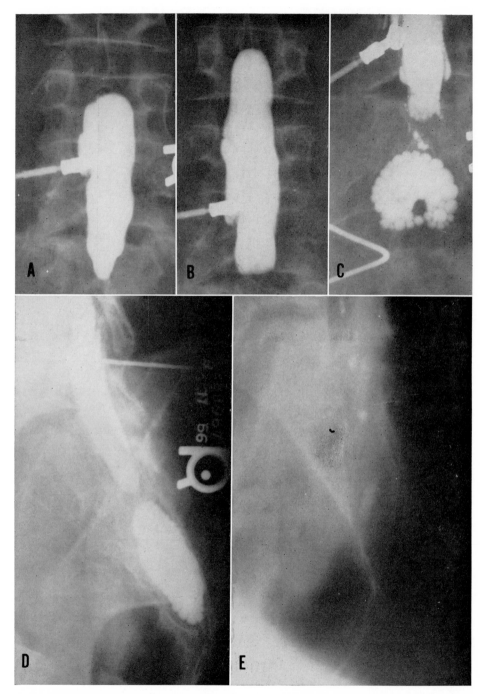

Fig. 139. *A*, Pantopaque introduced into the 4th lumbar interspace at first presents a normally tapered caudal sac and *B*, flows smoothly. *C*, Later in the examination an intrasacral meningocele fills through a narrow channel. The cavity in the sacrum involves the upper three segments *D*, On reviewing the plain films, and better seen on laminagrams, *E*, a bony defect within the sacrum corresponding to the fluid filled sac is demonstrable. No symptoms were attributed to this malformation. The study was done for a cervical root problem.

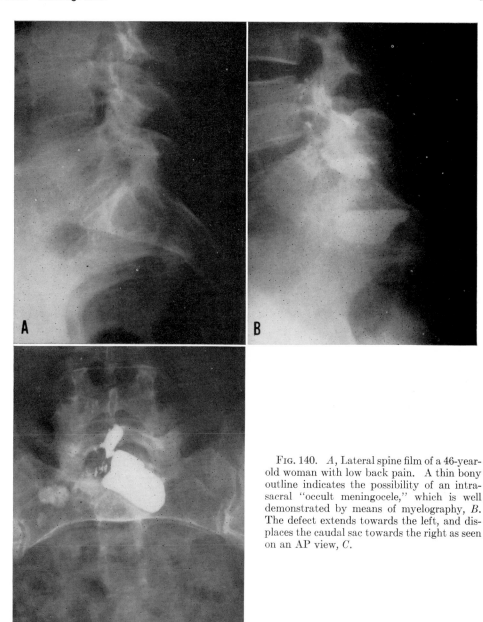

Fig. 140. *A*, Lateral spine film of a 46-year-old woman with low back pain. A thin bony outline indicates the possibility of an intrasacral "occult meningocele," which is well demonstrated by means of myelography, *B*. The defect extends towards the left, and displaces the caudal sac towards the right as seen on an AP view, *C*.

Pool (1952) described traction effects on the spinal cord and local signs produced by occult sacral meningoceles in adults, and relief followed surgical intervention. At operation the sac was found to be lined with arachnoid, with nerve roots incorporated in its wall. Communications with the spinal canal was by way of a narrow neck. One of his cases had an associated lipoma. The others had no lipoma, dermal sinus or aberrant cord. The filum terminale merged with the dura, forming the upper end of the meningocele. This was so taut that any traction resulted in a visible stretching effect.

This condition should be differentiated from the small outpouching sometimes ob-

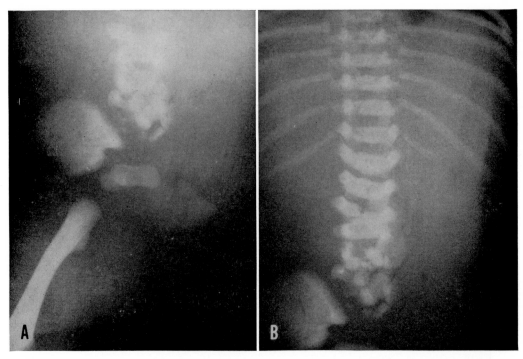

Fig. 141. *A*, Congenital absence of the left half of the sacrum and the left lower extremity. The lumbo-sacral spine is "mixed up," and marked variations are seen in the sacrum as well. The cervical and the thoracic vertebrae, *B*, were intact.

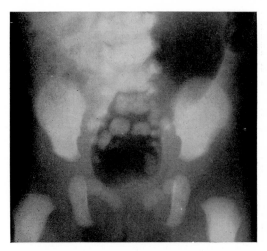

Fig. 142. Disorganized formation of sacrum with dysgenesis of lower segments. The iliac bones also are anomalous. This baby had an obstruction to the sigmoid deemed neurogenic, and expired after a spontaneous pneumoperitoneum appeared.

served on myelograms along the courses of the lower lumbar and first sacral nerve roots. These present themselves laterally as oval or sometimes circular shadows about a centimeter or so in diameter, usually located close to the axillary pouches and are considered to be arachnoidal diverticula. Occasionally one of these may become large enough to approximate an occult meningocele (Fig. 140).

AGENESIS, DYSGENESIS AND DYSPLASIAS OF THE SACRUM AND COCCYX

Complete agenesis of the sacrum is an infrequent condition, recognized clinically by narrowing of the pelvis and shortening of the intergluteal fold because of absence of the sacrum and approximation of the iliac bones. Atrophy and dimpling of the buttocks are prominent, and the muscles of the lower extremities become atrophied. Muscular deficiency becomes prominent with growth. Concomitant defects are frequent, including vertebral, genitourinary and gastrointestinal tract anomalies, dislocation of the hips, club

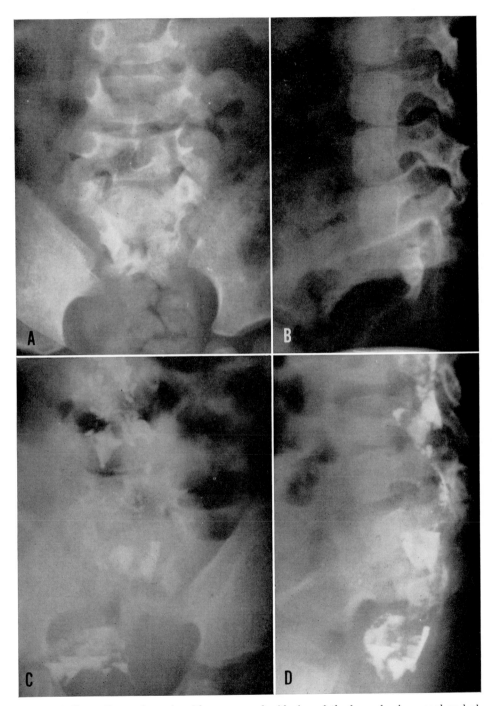

Fig. 143. *A*, Large lipomeningocele with pronounced widening of the lower lumbar canal and almost complete sacral agenesis in a 22-month-old girl with a cord bladder, paresis of both legs and delayed onset of walking. Note the approximation of the iliac bones. On lateral films, *B*, the short, stumpy residual of the sacrum is seen. Myelographic examination, *C* and *D*, reveal widening of the canal and a large intra-pelvic sacral meningocele.

feet, rib synostosis and congenital subluxations of the knees. Radiologic diagnosis is established readily by noting the absence of the entire sacrum or a major portion of this bone, identification of other skeletal and visceral malformations should be pursued. Rarely half of the pelvis also fails to develop, associated with malformation of the ipsilateral limb (Fig. 141).

Partial agenesis of the sacrum and coccyx, dysgenesis, is far more frequent. It is an important diagnostic point, especially in the recognition of associated anomalies of the anorectal region and the urinary tract. The formation of the vertebral column, the rectum and the lower urinary tract during the 5th to about the 8th week of gestation explains the frequency of concomitant malformations in these regions. In a review of 25 consecutive infant patients with sacral dysgenesis, it was found that 13 had imperforate anus, and of these 8 had either rectovaginal or rectovesical fistulae (Fig. 142). A wide variety of other anomalies existed, including congenital cardiac malformations in 4, kidney malformations in 4, and hydrocephalus, duodenal and ileal stenosis and atresia, tracheo-esophageal fistuala, micro-

cephaly, myelomeningocele, lipomeningocele, various forms of cleft vertebrae singly or in combination (Fig. 143). In a group of 10 patients over 8 years of age concomitant kidney anomalies were present in 3. One had both ovaries in bilateral inguinal hernias, and 2 had been operated upon in infancy for rectal stenosis.

Dysgenesis of the sacrum presents in a wide variety of structural changes (Fig. 144). The segments may be deficient, asymmetrically formed, fused in a variety of bizarre patterns, or absent. The defects may be more prominent on one side than on the other. Sagittal clefts occasionally are prominent in the upper sacrum, with the sacral segments separated in the midline widely, in addition to being malformed.

With sacrococcygeal dysgenesis the extent of the malformation is less striking. The lower coccygeal segments may be fused and deviated to one side or the other. Minor irregularities in fusion in the distal sacral segments exist, and the coccyx sometimes is absent, or if present, elongated and deviated away from the sacral defect. In these patients the possibility of concomitant urinary tract malformations should be investigated.

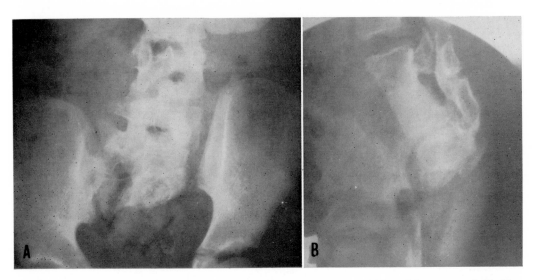

Fig. 144. *A,* Partial dysgenesis of the left side of the sacrum in a 7-year-old girl with a neurogenic bladder. Previous operation during infancy for imperforate anus. *B,* Lateral films reveal fusion of the lower lumbar segments and the malformed sacrum.

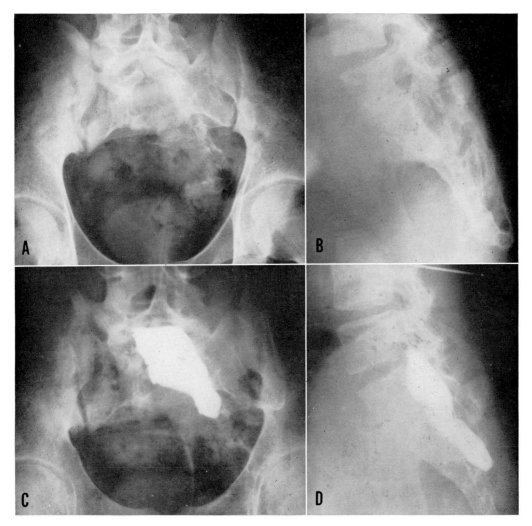

FIG. 145. *A*, AP view of the sacrum of a 15-year-old boy with sphincteric disturbances. There is a curvilinear defect in the right lateral aspect of the sacrum and failure of fusion of the spinous process of S1. The rest of the sacrum deviates sharply to the left. On lateral examination, *B*, the sacral canal is widened. Myelography, *C* and *D*, reveals a wide intrasacral malformation, but no extension beyond the bony confines.

Myelographic investigations in patients with partial agenesis of the sacrum disclose a variety of malformations, particularly intrasacral meningoceles. In some the defect on one side of the sacrum may be sharply delineated, so that the possibility of a sacral meningocele has to be considered. This is best investigated myelographically, although a clinical hint as to its presence can be obtained by identification of a pelvic mass (Fig. 145).

References

Abbott, K. H., Retter, R. H. and Leimbach, W. H.: The Role of Perineural Sacral Cysts in the Sciatic and Sacrococcygeal Syndromes, J. Neurosurg., *14*, 5, 1957.

Alexander, E., Jr. and Mashold, B. S. Jr.: Agenesis of the Sacrococcygeal Region, J. Neurosurg., *13*, 507, 1956.

Berdon, W. E., Hochberg, B., Baker, D. H., Grossman, H. and Santulli, T. V.: The Association of Lumbosacral Spine and Genitourinary Anomalies with Imperforate Anus, Am. J. Roentgenol., *98*, 181, 1966.

Blumel, J. Evans, E. B. and Eggers, G. W. N.: Partial and Complete Agenesis of Malformation of the Sacrum with Associated Anomalies, J. Bone & Joint Surg., *41-A*, 497, 1959.

Dassel, P. M.: Agenesis of the Sacrum and Coccyx, Am. J. Roentgenol., *85*, 697, 1961.

Del Duca, V., Davis, E. V. and Barroway, J. N.: Congenital Absence of the Sacrum and Coccyx, J. Bone & Joint Surg., *33-A*, 248, 1951.

Freeman, B.: Congenital Absence of Sacrum and Coccyx, Brit. J. Surg., *37*, 299, 1950.

Grand, M., Eichenfeld, S. and Jacobson, H. G.: Sacral Aplasia (Agenesis), Radiology, *74*, 611, 1960.

Herlinger, H.: Radiological Investigation of a Case of Sacrococcygeal Agenesis, Brit. J. Radiol., *37*, 376, 1964.

Pirkey, E. L. and Purcell, J. H.: Agenesis of Lumbosacral Vertebrae, Radiology, *69*, 726, 1957.

Schurr, P. H.: Sacral Extradural Cyst: An Uncommon Cause of Low Back Pain, J. Bone & Joint Surg., *37-B*, 601, 1955.

Sutton, D.: Sacral Cysts, Acta radiol., *1*, 787, 1963.

Williams, D. I. and Nixon, H. H.: Agenesis of the Sacrum, Surg., Gynec. & Obst., *105*, 84, 1957.

Dermal Sinuses. Pilonidal sinuses are included among the manifestations of dysraphism. They may be accompanied by other congenital vertebral malformations or intraspinal masses such as dermoids or lipomas. Occasionally, multiple dermal sinuses occur, sometimes associated with a variety on concomitant lesions (Fig. 146). The presence of a dimple or sinus opening, sometimes with a hair protruding from the crater, is observed most often in the lower lumbar, the sacral and the coccygeal regions. However, similar lesions occur elsewhere, particularly in the cervical and upper thoracic regions. With superimposed infection meningitis must be recognized as a complication, particularly with recurrent episodes. Relief can be obtained only on identification of the entire lesion and subsequent eradication. Cervical pilonidal sinuses extending into the posterior cranial fossa associated with infection or an epidermoid can present the signs and symptoms of a posterior fossa tumor. The intraspinal extensions of pilonidal sinuses also present the possibility of the symptom complex associated with tethering of the conus. Myelographic investigation is important in the determination of such a disturbance.

References

Clifton, E. E. and Rydell, J. R.: Congenital Dermal (Pilonidal) Sinus with Dural Connection, J. Neurosurg., *4*, 276, 1947.

Garceau, H. J.: Filum Terminale Syndrome, J. Bone & Joint Surg., *35-A*, 711, 1953.

Kooistra, H. P.: Pilonidal Sinuses Occurring Over Higher Spinal Segments, Surgery, *11*, 63, 1942.

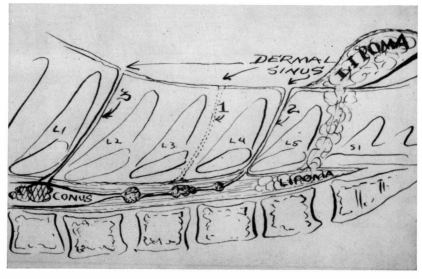

FIG. 146. Line drawing showing a variety of lesions associated with dermal sinuses. (From Epstein, J. A.: Tumors of the Spinal Cord in Infancy and Childhood, New York State J. Med., *65*, 2439, 1965.)

Lichtenstein, B. W.: "Spinal Dysraphism." Spina Bifida and Myelodysplasia, Arch. Neurol. & Psychiat., *44*, 792, 1940.

Matson, D. D. and Jerva, M. J.: Recurrent Meningitis Associated with Congenital Lumbosacral Dermal Sinus Tract. J. Neurosurg., *25*, 288, 1966.

Iliac Horns. In 1946 Fong reported a condition which he designated as iliac horns, represented by symmetrical bilaterally placed protrusions from the posterior surfaces of the iliac bone adjacent to the sacroiliac joints. His case occurred in a 27-year-old woman. The processes measured approximately 2.5 cm in diameter, and projected laterally and anteriorly for a distance of about 3 cm. He was unable to explain their etiology. This was later clarified by the work of Roeckerath (1951) who considered this deformity indicative of a hereditary dysplasia, associated in some of his cases with hypoplasia of the iliac bones, protrusion of the acetabulae, coxa valga, dysplasias of the knee joints, elbows, feet, arms, hands and shoulder girdles and particularly of the nails. Anomalies of pigmentation of the iris also were seen. His work was confirmed by Cotette and Pfandler (1952) who reported on the radiologic and genetic aspects of this condition in a family comprising 51 subjects of four generations. They included spinal changes such as increased lumbar lordotic and cervical curvatures among the radiologic alterations.

References

Chawla, S. and Bery, K.: Iliac Horns with Arthrodysplasia and Dystrophy of the Nails—Fong-Lesion, J. Canadian Assn. Radiol., *15*, 60, 1964.

Cotett, P. and Pfändler, U.: Dysplasia Osseuse et Unguéale Héréditaire, Acta radiol., *37*, 111, 1952.

Fong, E. E.: "Iliac Horns" (Symmetrical Bilateral Central Posterior Iliac Processes), Radiology, *47*, 517, 1946.

Roeckerath, W.: Hereditäre Osteo-Onycho-Dysplasie. Fortschr. Röntgenstra., *75*, 700, 1951.

Congenital Torticollis. Hulbert (1950) reviewed 100 cases of torticollis and 117 cases of sternomastoid tumors. These were subdivided into postural and muscular groups· Congenital postural torticollis is present at birth and is not associated with sternomastoid tumor. The condition is transient and does not require operation for relief. Congenital muscular torticollis may be preceded by a sternomastoid tumor which is evident in about 20 per cent of cases on physical examination. Most of these respond spontaneously and leave no deformity. Excision in childhood is inadvisable. There are no definite associated skeletal changes in the cervical spine with either condition.

References

Hulbert, K. F.: Congenital Torticollis, J. Bone & Joint Surg., *32-B*, 50, 1950.

Congenital Rotation of the Spinal Cord. Morely (1953) reported a case in a paraplegic patient in whom the spinal cord at the level of the eighth and ninth thoracic vertebrae was found to be rotated about 60 degrees. The nerve roots were coiled half way around the cord above and below, with the dorsal root ganglion displaced into the canal. The left nerve root emerged from the right canal, and the right nerve root passed through the left canal. There were no roentgenographic changes associated with this condition.

References

Morely, T. P.: Congenital Rotation of Spinal Cord, J. Neurosurg., *10*, 690, 1953.

Spinal Curvatures. The term scoliosis refers to lateral curvatures of the spine. Much depends on proper identification and management of these deformities. The clinical acumen and good judgment of the responsible physician often determines whether a patient undergoes one form of treatment or another, or indeed no treatment at all. Radiologic investigations must be accurate and the progress of the condition under continuous observation to help in preventing progression to a distressing and disabling malformation in some instances.

The classification of scoliosis takes into account curvatures of known and unknown etiology. Accordingly, they are designed as due to congenital abnormalities such as osteochondrodystrophy, vertebral malformations such as, for example, hemivertebrae, or neurofibromatosis. Among other known causes are poliomyelitis, the various myopathies and neuropathies which result in muscular weaknesses and imbalances, and structural causes such as deformities which follow thoracoplasty. The larger group, of unknown origin, is referred to as the idiopathic group. Some question has been raised as to a possible relationship between the myopathic and the idiopathic groups. A physiologic form also is recognized.

The concept of primary and secondary curves as stressed by Cobb (1960) is basic to the understanding of scoliosis problems. Following Ferguson's teaching, he points out that a primary curve is one produced by a deforming factor or force. A secondary curve is regarded as the result of involuntary muscular action to center the head on the pelvis as best as possible.

The normal spine as seen laterally presents four normal curves. The sacral and thoracic curves are concave anteriorly and the cervical and lumbar curves are concave posteriorly. The sacrum, being a fixed structure incapable of movement, presents a structural curve which Cobb regarded as a primary curve. The thoracic vertebrae, being partly movable, has elements of both the primary (structural, fixed) curve and the secondary (functional) curves. The cervical and lumbar portions of the spine are capable of changing their configurations by bending, rotation or angulation. This permits the appearance of flexible, correctible curves which are regarded as functional (secondary) curves. Lateral curves are not normally present, but may form during motion, and then straighten out. In this sense, they are regarded as functional lateral curves. Some degree of this type of movement is present in the lower thoracic spine.

Normally the vertebral bodies are verti-

cally aligned on a central axis, and are symmetrically formed. No changes in the configuration of the individual vertebrae are observed when the individual bends or moves. The alteration in the configuration of the spine is accomplished by the action of the intervertebral discs and the normal range of motion of the various vertebral segments. The presence of vertebral wedging and rotation is of primary importance in the identification of a structural curve. The angulation and position of the vertebrae likewise are extremely significant. Cobb is of the opinion that the terms "primary curve" and "secondary curve" might better be replaced by the designations "structural' and "functional" curve. Those with major structural changes can then be designated as major structural curves, those with minor structural changes as minor structural curves. Combined structural-functional curves are those which possess both structural and functional elements which the patient can correct when erect.

Physiologic scoliosis was investigated by Farkas (1941), who reported that measurements of the twelve thoracic and five lumbar vertebrae of 21 normal spines and 1 scoliotic spine in patients from 6 to 86 years old showed that the postnatal development of a normal spine became asymmetric at about the age of 6 years and progressed with advancing age. This asymmetry occurred in the vertebral bodies and pedicles as well as in the arches. The most striking feature was a dorsoventral elongation of the vertebral bodies. In the upper thoracic region this occurred predominantly on the left side, while in the lower thoracic region it was more prominent on the right side. In the lumbar region this change was again present on the left side. Lengthening of the pedicles on the side of the elongation and broadening of the pedicles on the opposite side was noted. Deviation of the neural arches and broadening of the pedicles opposite the side of the elongation were present. He felt that in physiologic scoliosis, contrary to the findings in pathologic scoliosis, wedging of the vertebrae was of only minor importance. He ascribed the cause of physiologic scoliosis to the human gait, which forces the spine into a threefold curve changing alternately at every step.

Idiopathic scoliosis accounts for 80 to 90 per cent of cases and may be familial in origin. Relatively few of these patients require surgical correction. The curvature of the spine is lateral. The primary curve is that which persists with the patient in forward flexion, and occurs anywhere in the spine. Compensatory curves are those above and below the primary curve, and usually straighten out in flexion. In lumbar scoliosis the primary curve is such that no compensatory curve forms below, so that only two are present. Cervical curves are uncommon.

Infantile idiopathic scoliosis makes up an important group. This condition begins before the 2nd or 3rd year, and is either resolving or progressive in its course. In the former group the curvature diminishes as the child grows, or the curve remains relatively unchanged. No treatment is required. With the progressive form of infantile idiopathic scoliosis the curvature usually is in the thoracic region with the convexity toward the left side. The condition supposedly is more frequent in males, and may progress rapidly to severe deformities or dwarfism. Idiopathic scoliosis also appears in juvenile or adolescent youngsters as a more rapidly progressive deformity. It has been stated that the lower the curve, the better the outlook for the patient. Progression of the curvature is possible up until the time the vertebrae cease to grow. A relationship to the appearance of the iliac apophyses has been noted, vertebral growth ending when these appear. After this time the curves do not progress much. Curvatures of the thoracic spine also occur toward the right side, but supposedly are later in onset. The factors which appear to influence the prognosis include the length of the curve, the degree of vertebral rotation at the apex, the age of onset and the rapidity of deterioration.

In idiopathic scoliosis a more complex deformity exists, consisting of lateral deviation of the spine with rotation of the vertebrae. As a rule, the curves present with idiopathic scoliosis are multiple. A single major curve accompanied by one or two compensatory curves is observed fairly frequently, the curves compensating for the spinal vertical alignment. Single major curves are more likely to cause structural deformities. Idiopathic scoliosis may involve the lumbar spine alone beginning at about 10 years of age and continuing to adolescence. This type, as a rule, is innocuous, but may be followed by degenerative hypertrophic changes of a painful nature later in life. Involvement of the thoracolumbar region alone is infrequent. This curvature usually develops during adolescence, and may be deforming. It requires careful observation. Scoliosis limited to the dorsal spine may be severe and rapidly progressive, requiring expert evaluation and management. It occurs mainly in girls from 5 to 8 years of age.

Opinion is still divided as to whether the lateral deviation or the rotation of the vertebrae is the initial deformity, whether these two changes are independent of each other, or whether they are the natural concomitants of some underlying cause. According to Thomas (1947) it is generally assumed that rotation is secondary to lateral deviation. The latter element is always accompanied by some rotation except in the mildest grades, while with more severe curvatures the degree of rotation is more pronounced. No constant ratio exists between these two components. The rotational defect appears to be the more resistant to correction. Knuttson (1966) believed that unequal growth at the paired neurocentral junctions leads to rotation of the vertebral body out of its relationship to the vertebral column. Progression of scoliosis which follows can then be explained by the continuous growth of the vertebral bodies.

The structural changes in the vertebrae responsible for this change in alignment is principally the development of a wedge-like deformity of the vertebral body. Accompanying this, and much more difficult to explain are the rotational defects of the involved vertebrae which appear as the lateral deviation develops. The rotation occurs on a vertical axis situated somewhere behind its spinous process. Rotary displacement may be recognized roentgenologically by the lateral displacement of the spinous process and by the general asymmetry of the shadows of the pedicles in relation to the corresponding vertebral bodies. The pedicles on the convex side of the deformity are placed medially away from the lateral borders of the bodies on that side, while the pedicles on the concave side become less distinct and in some advanced cases may disappear from view entirely. The neural arches of the rotated vertebrae likewise become deformed, and the articular facets on the concave side are thrown out of alignment with those on the convex side, with consequent locking of the vertebrae in their rotated position.

The most deforming curves originate early in life. It has been noted that scoliosis appearing later in adolescence usually has a better prognosis. The curvature usually ceases to progress about 1 year before ossification is complete. According to Ponseti and Friedman (1950) a rapid increase in the curve as noted on serial roentgenograms is of poor prognostic significance. James (1951) stated that only 5 to 10 per cent of idiopathic curves become severe enough to require correction and fusion.

Arkin (1949) believed that wedging can best be explained by unilateral epiphyseal arrest. This had also been brought out experimentally by Bisgard and Musselman (1940), who produced scoliosis by destroying only one side of a growing vertebra, so that wedge-shaped vertebral bodies and lateral deviations of the spine were produced. Experimental scoliosis was also studied by Nachlas and Borden (1950), who produced a human-like type of scoliosis in dogs by experiments which controlled epiphyseal growth with piano wire staples. The deform-

ities were progressive even after the staples had been removed. Compensatory thoracic spine curves appeared in several animals. The relationship of the growing epiphysis to scoliosis was brought out by Haas (1939) who in dog experiments was able to produce kyphosis and scoliosis by injuring the cartilaginous vertebral plates. He concluded that the growth in the length of vertebrae occurs in a manner similar to growth in length of long bones, namely, by a proliferation at the cartilage end plate with no interstitial growth within the body. Somerville (1952) reported that so-called structural scoliosis was the result of failures of growth of the posterior elements of a segment of the spine. He presented the results of experiments in young rabbits in which trauma to the laminae and spinous processes was followed by curvature of the spine.

Radiologic investigations of the spine in cases of scoliosis should include films which visualize the spine from the level of the iliac crests up to the cervical region. These studies should be made with the patient in the supine, the sitting, and in the erect positions. In the event of a significant degree of curvature, further studies may be made with the patient seated with a 2- to 3-inch block under each buttock. Additional studies may be required with the patient erect, first with the right and then with the left foot elevated by a 2- to 3-inch block as deemed necessary. The study should be augmented by lateral films as well as cone-down studies of the lumbosacral articulation in the anteroposterior and lateral views. Repeated examinations for changes in the scoliosis angles should be made at from 3- to 6-month intervals. The scoliosis angles may be identified as shown in Figure 147. A chart may then be prepared in which the degree of wedging, rotation, angulation and the position of the vertebrae is recorded according to date, utilizing the same points of reference for each study as developed by Cobb (1948), whose "Outline for the Study of Scoliosis" should be read carefully in the original. Kilfoyle, Foley

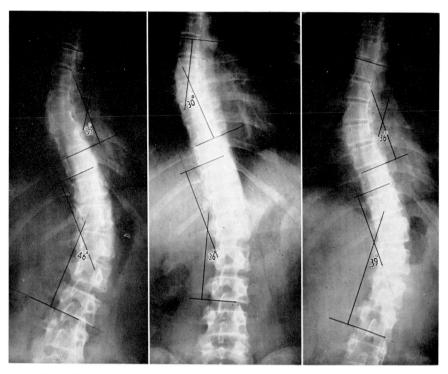

Fig. 147. *A*, Scoliosis study, erect posture. *B*, Same case, supine position.
C, Same case as *A* and *B*, sitting position.

and Norton (1965) stressed the importance of the relationship of the head to the spine. Scoliosis was regarded as balanced when, with the patient's head erect and his shoulders level, both were centered over a level pelvis, whatever the deformity was between the pelvis and shoulders. Partial balance exists when the curvature is associated with pelvic obliquity, the center of gravity still falling between the ischial tuberosities when the patient is sitting, and between the feet when erect. A state of imbalance is reached when the obliquity and the curvature is such that the center of gravity is so far lateral that the patient is unable to stand or sit without support.

Paralytic scoliosis following poliomyelitis may appear within a few months after the acute episode, and be rapidly progressive. It may also be slow in development, appearing several years after the original disease. According to Cobb this group makes up 30 to 50 per cent of all cases requiring fusion, and is one of the more serious complications of the disease, requiring prolonged and expert management. Fortunately, this complication has diminished with the advent of current preventative measures.

The weakening of spinal muscles by poliomyelitis results in structural and postural imbalances causing a wide variety of spinal curvatures. The superficial longitudinal muscle group controls extension, while the deep oblique and transverse groups affect rotary movement. Both groups participate in lateral flexion. The extraspinal muscles also participate in the establishment of normal posture, and departures from their normal action because of poliomyelitis as well as changes in the alignment of the pelvis contribute to the development of spinal curvatures. Poliomyelitis first causes paralytic effects, followed by scoliosis. Functionally the paralytic spine has increased mobility with a high degree of flexibility and compressibility, with resultant loss of the thoracic kyphosis and lumbar lordosis and translatory shift of the vertebrae. With relatively mild disturbances, a generalized relatively slight thoracolumbar "C" curve develops which improves on recumbency. More advanced changes produce practically a collapse of muscular tone, with extensive, mobile thoracolumbar curvatures which include rotational deformities as well. As a rule a primary curve appears first, which is fixed and usually the most pronounced. Sometimes a double curve appears.

Radiologically the involved vertebrae reflect the positional and nutritional changes incident to lack of movement and muscle tone. The bodies assume a somewhat clouded and demineralized appearance. The discs diminish in size, and are distorted in conformity with the changed vertebral bodies. Minute calcific flecks or somewhat large calcareous deposits may appear in the discs. The time required for these changes is variable, and years may go by before the final effects are attained. During this course the curvatures may change considerably.

Unusual forms of scoliosis have been reported because of weakness of the spinal muscles occurring in conditions such as pseudohypertrophic muscular dystrophy arachnodactyly, progressive muscular dystrophies and dystonia musculorum deformans.

Scoliosis also may follow empyema, the concavity of the spinal curvature being directed towards the site of the empyema, with relatively little or no rotation of the vertebral bodies (Selig and Arnheim, 1939). Such changes can follow thoracoplasty, in which case the convexity occurs towards the resected ribs. The vertebrae in these instances develop little or no structural change, and the deformity may be corrected surgically by removing a portion of the thoracic wall, which may release the pull of a pleural scar. Bisgard (1934) pointed out that such realignment of the vertebrae would be impossible in the presence of significant structural changes in the vertebral bodies.

Intensive radiation therapy directed over the spine also can produce scoliosis by suppressing vertebral epiphyseal growth. Arkin and Simon (1950) were able to produce structural scoliosis in rabbits by irradiating the vertebrae asymmetrically, resulting in wedging of the bodies whith the lesser height towards the irradiated side. Arkin, Pack, Ransohoff and Simon (1950) reported a case in a 13-year-old schoolgirl who had been treated during infancy for pigmented diffuse nevi on which melanotic tumors had developed, which were later excised. When 19 months old, the patient was treated for a Wilms' tumor by means of preoperative x-ray therapy, nephrectomy and postoperative irradiation. Scoliosis appeared at the age of 9 years and by the age of 13 the curves were seen to follow exactly the fields of irradiation with the wedging directed towards the irradiated sides. They noted that in addition to the insufficiency of growth in the vertebral bodies, similar changes occurred in the twelfth left rib, a left lumbar transverse process and the left ilium, all of which had been included in the field of treatment.

The effects of irradiation on the growing spine were summarized by Neuhauser, Wittenborg, Berman and Cohen in 1952, who reported on 45 patients who had received x-ray therapy over the spine. Thirty-four of these patients were living and had been observed over a period averaging $6\frac{1}{2}$ years. Postmortem examinations were available on 11 patients. The significant changes in these were nonspecific growth retardation and irregularity of ossification of the epiphyseal cartilages. These authors noted that scoliosis is only rarely produced if the spine received uniform irradiation.

Scoliosis and Spinal Cord Disease. In a review of 2000 cases of scoliosis of all types Ruhlin and Albert (1941) found 7 with symptoms referable to the central nervous system. Three of these patients had rachitic scoliosis, 3 congenital scoliosis and 1 was of doubtful origin, associated with neurofibromatosis. In no instance was cord involvement observed in paralytic or habitual types of scoliosis. The paralytic signs developed regardless of the direction of the primary curve, but all of the curves involved were in the cervicothoracic region and were sharply angulated.

In comparison with these changes in which the nervous system damage was due to the scoliosis, one may cite the cases reported by Boldrey, Adams and Brown (1949) in which scoliosis appeared as a manifestation of disease of the cervicothoracic portion of the spinal cord. They reported 10 such cases in which scoliosis was the first or an early principal sign. Included in this group were cystic lesions of the cord, angioma, spinal varix, adhesions and extramedullary tumor. They mentioned that of a total of 60 consecutive surgically proven spinal cord lesions moderate to pronounced scoliosis was demonstrable in 15, with the convexity usually towards the side of the lesion where this was demonstrable. Williams and Stevens (1953) were of the opinion that any child with idiopathic scoliosis should have careful neurologic examination, and cited the case of an 8-year-old boy with gradual curvature of the spine, frequent stumbling and back pain, enuresis and progressive constipation in whom the plain roentgenograms were normal and myelograms revealed a block at the level of the tenth dorsal vertebra. Operation disclosed an ependymoma.

Paraplegia complicating scoliosis has been noted in occasional cases and has been considered as due to the unequal growth of the dura and the spinal column in a tight dural canal. The cause for the paralysis is the inability of a tight dura to accommodate itself to such growth (Kleinberg, 1951). In a review of 41 cases McKenzie and Dewar (1949) noted that the paralysis appeared during the period of rapid growth at a time when the scoliosis, if not controlled by treatment, is suddenly and markedly increased. At operation in their cases a linear thickening of the dura was noted which extended across the neural canal obliquely, compressing the cord. One patient had a spur of bone compressing the cord. The treatment in such cases is surgical. Myelography is of prime importance in establishing the site of compression, which is usually close to the apex of the curve. Most of the cases of this nature observed by the authors were idiopathic scoliosis, but others have been associated with rickets, poliomyelitis and neurofibromatosis.

References

Arkin, A. M.: Mechanism of Structural Changes in Scoliosis, New York State J. Med., *49*, 495, 1949.
————: Mechanism of Structural Changes in Scoliosis, J. Bone & Joint Surg., *31-A*, 519, 1949.
————: Prophylaxis of Scoliosis, J. Bone & Joint Surg., *34-A*, 47, 1952.
Arkin, A. M., Pack, G. T., Ransohoff, N. S., and Simon N.: Radiation-induced Scoliosis, J. Bone & Joint Surg., *32-A*, 401, 1950.
Arkin, A. M. and Simon, N.: Radiation Scoliosis, J. Bone & Joint Surg., *32-A*, 396, 1950.
Bisgard, J. D.: Thoracogenic Scoliosis, Arch. Surg., *29*, 417, 1934.
Bisgard, J. D. and Musselman, M. M.: Scoliosis, Surg., Gynec. & Obst., *70*, 1029, 1940.
Boldrey, E., Adams, J. E. and Brown, H. A.: Scoliosis as a Manifestation of Disease of the Cerviocothoracic Portion of the Spinal Cord, Arch. Neurol. & Psychiat., *61*, 528, 1949.
Cobb, J. R.: Study of Scoliosis, American Academy of Orthopaedic Surgeons, Instructional Course Lectures, *5*, 261, 1948.
————: The Problem of the Primary Curve, J. Bone & Joint Surg., *42-A*, 1413, 1960.
Colonna, P. C. and Vom Saal, F. A.: Study of Paralytic Scoliosis Based on Five Hundred Cases of Poliomyelitis, J. Bone & Joint Surg., *23*, 355, 1941.
Epstein, B. S. and Abramson, J. L.: Roentgenologic Changes in the Bones in Cases of Pseuodhypertrophic Muscular Dystrophy, Arch. Neurol. & Psychiat., *46*, 868, 1941.
Farkas, A.: Physiological Scoliosis, J. Bone & Joint Surg., *23*, 607, 1941.
————: Paralytic Scoliosis, J. Bone & Joint Surg., *25*, 581, 1943.
George, K. and Rippstein, J.: A Comparative Study of the Two Popular Methods of Measuring Scoliotic Deformity of the Spine, J. Bone & Joint Surg., *43-A*, 809, 1961.
Gucker, T., III.: Experiences with Poliomyelitis Scoliosis After Fusion and Correction, J. Bone & Joint Surg., *38-A*, 1281, 1956.
Girdany, B. and Danowski, T. S.: Muscular Dystrophy, Am. J. Dis. Child., *91*, 339, 1956.
Haas, S. L.: Experimental Production of Scoliosis, J. Bone & Joint Surg., *21*, 963, 1939.
James, J. I. P.: Two Curve Patterns in Idiopathic Structural Scoliosis, J. Bone & Joint Surg., *33-B*, 399, 1951.

————: Idiopathic Scoliosis, J. Bone & Joint Surg., *36-B*, 36, 1954.

————: Paralytic Scoliosis, J. Bone & Joint Surg., *38-B*, 660, 1956.

James, J. I. P., Lloyd-Roberts, G. C. and Pilcher, M. F.: Infantile Structural Scoliosis, J. Bone & Joint Surg., *41-B*, 719, 1959.

Kilfoyle, R. M., Foley, J. F. and Norton, P. L.: Spine and Pelvic Deformity in Childhood and Adolescent Paraplegia, J. Bone & Joint Surg., *47-A*, 659, 1965.

Kleinberg, S.: Scoliosis with Paraplegia, J. Bone & Joint Surg., *33-A*, 225, 1951.

Knuttson, F.: Vertebral Genesis of Idiopathic Scoliosis in Children, Acta radiol., *4*, 395, 1966.

Mayer, L.: Further Studies of Fixed Paralytic Pelvic Obliquity, J. Bone & Joint Surg., *18*, 87, 1936.

McKenzie, K. G. and Deward, F. P.: Scoliosis with Paraplegia, J. Bone & Joint Surg., *31-B*, 162, 1949.

Nachlas, I. W. and Borden, J. N.: Experimental Scoliosis—the Role of the Epiphysis, Surg., Gynec. & Obst., *90*, 672, 1950.

Neuhauser, E. B. D., Wittenborg, M. H., Berman, C. Z. and Cohen, J.: Irradiation Effects of Roentgen Therapy on Growing Spine, Radiology, *59*, 637, 1952.

Parker, A. S. and Hare, H. F.: Arachnodactyly, Radiology, *45*, 220, 1945.

Ponseti, I. and Friedman, B.: Prognosis in Idiopathic Scoliosis, J. Bone & Joint Surg., *32-A*, 381, 1950.

Risser, J. C.: Scoliosis: Past and Present, J. Bone & Joint Surg., *46-A*, 167, 1964.

Roaf, R.: Paralytic Scoliosis, J. Bone & Joint Surg., *38-B*, 640, 1956.

————: Vertebral Growth and its Mechanical Control, J. Bone & Joint Surg., *42-B*, 40, 1960.

Ruhlin, C. W. and Albert, S.: Scoliosis Complicated by Spinal-Cord Involvement, J. Bone & Joint Surg., *23*, 877, 1941.

Scott, J. C. and Morgan, T. H.: The Natural History and Prognosis of Infantile Idiopathic Scoliosis, J. Bone & Joint Surg., *37-B*, 400, 1955.

Selig, S. and Arnheim, E.: Scoliosis Following Empyema, Arch. Surg., *39*, 789, 1939.

Somerville, E. W.: Rotational Lordosis; Development of the Single Curve, J. Bone & Joint Surg., *34-B*, 421, 1952.

Thomas, G. E.: Idiopathic Scoliosis, J. Bone & Joint Surg., *29*, 907, 1947.

Williams, J. M. and Stevens, H.: Recognition of Surgically Treatable Neurologic Disorders of Childhood, J.A.M.A., *151*, 455, 1953.

Kyphoscoliosis and kyphosis are characterized by angular or curvilinear deformity of the spine. The convexity is directed dorsally or dorsolaterally, and occurs most frequently in the thoracic region. A large variety of pathologic states may be responsible for this malformation. It is most commonly due to faulty posture, generalized weakness, poliomyelitis, congenital deformities, neurofibromatosis and occupational diseases. Ferguson (1955) postulated that persistence of the anterior vascular grooves in the thoracic vertebrae results in weakening of the involved segments, which then undergo anterior wedging, resulting in kyphosis. Usually the grooves disappear by the time a child is 6 years old, so that this mechanism comes into play in children from 6 to 10 years of age. Association of a uniformly rounded kyphos involving all the lumbar vertebrae with myelomeningocele was observed by Barson (1965). The vertebral bodies are wedged, with rounded anterior surfaces. Scoliosis accompanies this condition when other congenital defects such as hemivertebrae of unilateral fusion of vertebral bodies or ribs also are present. With advanced defects, which extend to involve the lower thoracic and the sacral areas as well, the meninges present as a sac containing nervous tissue, and paraplegia and other neurologic deficits are found. Various forms of osteoporosis, arthritis, rickets, Paget's disease, acromegaly, hyperparathyroidism, may be causative factors. All of these produce more or less smooth curves which vary in degree from a mild dorsal convexity to an almost semicircular configuration. An angular kyphosis is usually incident to tuberculosis, syphilis, malignant disease, congenital anomalies of vertebral column or compression fractures. These will be discussed under their respective headings. Rachitic kyphoscoliosis with spinal cord compression was reported by Ponsold (1935). Angular kyphosis of nontuberculous origin is relatively rare. According to Gulledge and Brav (1950) only 41 such cases have been described in the literature.

Kyphosis and kyphoscoliosis both may be associated with paraplegia due to compression of the spinal cord because of the angular deformity of the respective vertebrae or because of protrusion of bony spurs or fibrous bands into the spinal canal (McKenzie and Dewar, 1949). These lesions may be identified by means of myelography, and the demonstration of block is of great diagnostic importance (Kleinberg and Kaplan, 1952).

The development of other complications such as cor pulmonale (Samuelson, 1952) and (Steinberg, 1966), atelectasis, emphysema and bronchitis (Hertzog and Manz, 1943), and compression of the pulmonary vessels and mediastinum have been mentioned (Chapman, Dill and Graybiel, 1939) and (Kerwin, 1942). The presence of esophageal ulcers with kyphoscoliosis was reported by Haubrich (1953) and with hiatal hernia by Kassem, Green and Fraenkel (1965).

Lordosis. In this condition there is an exaggerated convexity of the lumbar spine directed anteriorly. This may be produced by weakness of the back muscles from any cause such as poliomyelitis or muscular dystrophy, or it may result as a compensation for a kyphotic curve. Lordosis may also be associated with enlargement of the abdomen such as may occur with obesity, pregnancy, ascites or hepatosplenomegaly. An exaggerated form of lumbar lordosis may sometimes be observed in achondroplastic dwarfs and cretins. Probably the most frequent cause of lordosis is simply poor posture.

The radiologic changes associated with these various conditions are discussed under their specific headings. In those cases of lordosis in which there is only the element of poor posture or relaxation of muscular support, no gross changes in the vertebral bodies or their interspaces can be seen.

References

Barson, A. J.: Radiological Studies of Spina Bifida Cystica. The Phenomenon of Congenital Lumbar Kyphosis. Brit. J. Radiol., *38*, 294, 1965.

Bingold, A. C.: Congenital Kyphosis, J. Bone & Joint Surg., *35-B*, 579, 1953.

Chapman, E. M., Dill, D. B. and Graybiel, A.: Decrease in Functional Capacity of Lungs and Heart Resulting from Deformities of the Chest, Medicine, *18*, 167, 1939.

Ferguson, A. B., Jr.: Symposium on Pediatric Orthopedics: Dorsal Wedging Round Back in Preadolescents, Pediat. Clin. North America, *2*, 951, 1955.

Gulledge, W. H. and Brav, E. A.: Non-Tuberculous Thoracic Kyphosis with Paraplegia, J. Bone & Joint Surg., *32-A*, 192, 1950.

Hanson, R.: Some Anomalies, Deformities and Diseased Conditions of the Vertebrae During Their Different Stages of Development, Acta chirurg. Scandinav., *60*, 309, 1926.

Haubrich, R.: Über das Ulcus oseophagi bei schwerer Kyphoscoliose, Fortschr. Röntgenstr., *78*, 419, 1953.

Hertzog, A. J. and Manz, W. R.: Right-sided Hypertrophy (Cor Pulmonale) Caused by Chest Deformity, Am. Heart J., *25*, 399, 1943.

James, J. I. P.: Kyphoscoliosis, J. Bone & Joint Surg., *37-B*, 414, 1955.

Kassem, N. Y., Groen, J. J. and Fraenkel, M.: Spinal Deformities and Oesophageal Hiatus Hernia, Lancet, *1*, 887–889, 1965.

Kerwin, A. J.: Pulmonocardiac Failure as a Result of Spinal Deformity, Arch. Int. Med., *69*, 560, 1942.

Kleinberg, S. and Kaplan, A.: Scoliosis Complicated by Paraplegia, J. Bone & Joint Surg., *34-A*, 162, 1952.

Ponsold, E.: Lesions of Spinal Cord after Rachitic Kyphoscoliosis, Arch. f. Psychiat., *103*, 299, 1935.

Samuelson, S.: Cor Pulmonale Resultng from Deformities of Chest, Acta med. Scandinav., *142*, 399, 1952.

Somerville, E. W.: Rotational Lordosis. The Development of the Single Curve, J. Bone & Joint Surg., *34-B*, 421, 1952.

Steinberg, I.: Cor Pulmonale in Kyphoscoliosis. Am. J. Roentgenol., *97*, 658, 1966.

3

Diseases of Congenital, Endocrine or Metabolic Origin

Congenital Disorders

OSTEOCHONDRODYSTROPHY (Morquio-Brailsford's Disease)

The nomenclature applied to this familial condition often causes confusion. Among these designations are familial osseous dystrophy (the term first used by Morquio), chondrodysplasia, familial osteochondrodystrophy, dyschondroplasia foetalis, ecchondrodysplasia, osteodystrophia fibrosa, atypical achondroplasia, osteochondrodystrophy deformans, eccentrochondrodysplasia, spondyloepiphyseal dysplasia congenita and Morquio-Ullrich's disease (Jacobsen, 1939) (Langer and Carey, 1966). Maroteaux and Lamy (1965) include Morquio's disease with osteodystrophies associated with abnormal excretion of mucopolysaccharides in the urine. Keratosulfate is found in the urine of patients with Morquio's disease. The other osteodystrophies with metabolic disorders of the acid mucopolysaccharides include Hurler's disease, polydystrophic oligophrenia and polydystrophic dwarfism, each with a specific mucopolysaccharide in the urine.

Rubin (1964) included Morquio's disease among the modeling errors of the epiphysis, postulating a metabolic defect selectively affecting articular cartilage but not growing cartilage or ossification of the epiphyseal nuclei. He suggested that the term "spondylo-epiphyseal dysplasia" be used for Morquio's disease as best fitting the skeletal dysplasia encountered. However, Langer and Carey (1966) did not favor this because changes are not limited to the spine and the epiphyses alone. They preferred the designation "KS mucopolysaccharidosis of Morquio" as combining the biochemical and eponymic attributes. It seems that the term "Morquio's disease" is the one most in use, and it probably will continue so for the present.

Morquio's disease is transmitted by the autosomal recessive mode, and consanguinity is frequently involved. The usual picture is that of an infant who is apparently normal at birth, and develops well until about 2 or 3 years. At this time growth may slow down, and dwarfism with malformations of the trunk and extremities begins to appear, associated with progressive weakness. The disorder becomes evident at about 4 or 5 years of age, when difficulties in walking and deformities of the spine are noted by the parents. In this connection it is interesting to note that the original case described by Wheeldon (1920) was first seen at the age of 22 months, and later was reported again by Pohl (1939) at the age of 22 years. The full-blown appearance is that of a markedly shortened and deformed individual, usually of normal mentality, with a short neck and trunk, kyphosis and deformities of the arms and legs, including the hands and feet. The chest is deepened and flattened, and the sternum is prominent. The muscular weakness produces alterations in gait and stance. The joints are large, and have a peculiar hypermobility and laxity, so that the patient stands with hips and knees flexed in a crouching position, with the pelvis tilted forward and the head sunken between the shoulders.

The variability in the changes associated with osteochondrodystrophy was stressed by Brailsford (1952), who divided such cases into four groups. The first was that in which the disease was evident *in utero* or shortly after birth. The second group was that in which the active phase of the condition appeared to cease before puberty, giving rise to a moderate generalized form with marked shortening of the limb bones and pressure deformities of the extremities and the long bones and vertebral bodies. His third group was one with changes confined chiefly to the spine and hip joints, and less frequently to the knees. In the fourth group changes were confined to the vertebral column, with no irregularity or growth disturbances visible in other parts of the skeleton.

Osteochondrodystrophy is characterized by hyperplasia of cartilage growth accompanied by osteoporotic deformities of the skeleton which probably are incident to disuse. Radiologically this is manifested by shortening and distortion of the various bones of the extremities, with non-union and distortion of the epiphyses and delayed ossification. The joint surfaces become widened and the articular surfaces are irregular, flattened and eroded. The acetabular and glenoid fossae are shallow and irregular. The vertebral bodies rarely are involved in the sense that cartilaginous rests occur in their bony substance. However, Russo (1943) reported a case of a 26-year-old dwarf seen in the 7th month of pregnancy in whom radiologic examination of the vertebral bodies disclosed numerous areas of translucency which he considered to be due to islands of cartilage which had failed to calcify.

The radiologic changes evident in the spine are among the important ones associated with osteochondrodystrophy. In its

most developed form there is practically complete involvement of the vertebral column, the characteristic change being a pronounced flattening and widening of the respective vertebral bodies (Fig. 148). In their anterior aspects the vertebrae present a peculiar tongue-like elongation of the central portion of the body. The superior and inferior articular surfaces of the vertebral bodies may be quite roughened, and anterior wedging of varying degrees is frequently observed. Multiple centers of ossification appear at the apophyseal rings, which later unite. These deformities of the vertebral bodies result in varying degrees of kyphosis, some of which are of an advanced nature. Occasionally the deformity is so great that a marked kyphosis with gibbus formation results. It may appear as if the vertebral bodies at the thoracolumbar junction had been squeezed out of line over the small vertebral body at the apex of the curve. These kyphotic disturbances are frequently accompanied by lateral curvatures of the thoracic and lumbar vertebral column. In the cervicothoracic region these changes cause shortening of the neck. The intervertebral discs may remain relatively normal, but sometimes are considerably thickened. The odontoid process of the second cervical vertebra is hypoplastic, or may be absent. The posterior arch of the first cervical vertebra indents the occipital bone, resulting in a deformity which may be regarded as a form of basilar impression.

Little has been written concerning the neurologic changes caused by alterations in the configurations of the spinal canal incident to the architectural variations caused by Morquio's disease. Donath and Vogl (1925, 1927) indicated that the spinal cord itself was unaffected by the basic cartilaginous disorder which produced the vertebral changes. They stressed as a matter of practical importance the fact that the consequent shortness of the pedicles due to the premature synostosis of the centers of ossification of the body with those of the lamina led to a considerable narrowing of the entire spinal the various conditions with platyspondyly can undoubtedly be diminished by emphasis on demonstration of corneal and dental abnormalities, and especially by identification of abnormal urinary polysaccharides. Maroteaux and Lamy (1965) mention that with children there is also increase in the chondroitin sulfate A (or C) fraction as well as keratosulfate in the urine. From a radiologic point of view it is important to keep in mind that the extraspinal manifestations of Morquio's disease may be variable, and here caution must be exercised to exclude other disease entities.

References

Brailsford, J. F.: Chondro-osteo-dystrophy, Am. J. Surg., 7, 401, 1929.
————: Chondro-osteo-dystrophy. J. Bone & Joint Surg., 34-B, 53, 1952.
Crawford, T. A.: Morquio's Disease, Arch. Dis. Childhood, 14, 70, 1939.
Donath, J. and Vogl, A.: Untersuchungen über den chondrodystrophischen Zwerguchs, Wien. Arch. f. inn. Med., 10, 1, 1925.
Einhorn, N. H., Moore, J. R. and Rowntree, L. G.: Osteochondrodystrophia Deformans (Morquio's Disease), Am. J. Dis. Child., 61, 776, 1941.
Fairbank, H. A. T.: Chondro-Osteodystrophy, Morquio-Brailsford Type, J. Bone &Joint Surg., 31-B, 291, 1949.
Farrell, M. J., Maloney, J. D. and Yakovlev, P. I.: Morquio's Disease Associated with Mental Defect, Arch. Neurol. & Psychiat., 48, 456, 1942.
Feldman, N. and Daveport, M. E.: Osteochondrodystrophia Deformans (Morquio-Brailsford Disease), Arch. Dis. Childhood, 26, 279, 1951.
Jacobsen, A. W.: Hereditary Osteochondrodystrophia Deformans, J.A.M.A., 113, 121, 1939.
Langer, L. O. and Carey, L. S.: The Roentgenographic Features of the KS Mucopolysaccaridosis of Morquio (Morquio-Brailsford's Disease), Am. J. Roentgenol., 97, 1, 1966.
Maroteaux, P. and Lamy, M.: Hurler's Disease, Morquio's Disease, and Related Mucopolysaccharidoses, J. Pediat., 67, 312, 1965.
Morquio, L.: Dystrophie Osseuse Familiale, Arch. de méd. des enf., 32, 129, 1929.
Pohl, J. F.: Chondro-osteodystrophy (Morquio's Disease). Progressive Kyphosis from Congenital Wedge-shaped Vertebrae. J. Bone & Joint Surg., 21, 187, 1929.
Robins, M. M., Stevens, H. F. and Linker, A.: Morquio's Disease; an Abnormality of Mucopolysaccharide Metabolism, J. Pediat., 62, 881, 1963.
Vestermark, S.: Osteochondrodystrophia Deformans with Mucopolysaccharidosis, Arch. Dis. Childhood, 40, 106, 1965.
Wheeldon, T. F.: Achondroplasia, Am. J. Dis. Child., 19, 1, 1920.
Zellweger, H., Ponseti, I. V., Pedrini, V., Stamler, F. S. and von Norden, G. K.: Morquio-Ullrich's Disease, J. Pediat., 59, 549, 1961.

Spondyloepiphyseal Dysplasia Tarda is one of the conditions which must be separated from Morquio's disease. This, too, is a familial condition transmitted as a sex-linked recessive trait. Characteristically patients with spondyloepiphysial dysplasia tarda present with a short trunk but with relatively normal arms and legs. The extent of the platyspondyly is not as striking as observed with Morquio's disease, and the intervertebral discs are not as widened. The extent of the tongue-like protrusions observed are distinctly less than those noted with Morquio's disease (Fig. 149). The vertebral bodies also are less deformed, although considerable variation in structure occurs. A rather specific change occurs in the superior and inferior surfaces of the dorsolumbar vertebrae. This presents as a dense protrusion occupying the posterior portion of the end plates. The anterior portions of the vertebral bodies remain flattened, or even are slightly wedged. These changes were noted by Langer (1964) in adults, and in childhood and adolescence by Poker, Finby and Archibald (1965). An associated change which can be helpful is the demonstration of flattening of the intercondyloid notches at the distal ends of the femurs. Apparently no abnormal excretion of mucopolysaccharides has been observed in these patients.

From a clinical point of view there is a vast difference between the deformed patient with Morquio's disease and the rather short but otherwise not particularly striking appearance of patients with spondyloepiphyseal dysplasia tarda. The skull, pelvis and small bones in these patients are usually normal.

References

Langer, L. O., Jr.: Spondyloepiphysial Dysplasia Tarda. Hereditary Chondrodysplasia with Characteristic Vertebral Configuration in the Adult. Radiology, 82, 833, 1964.

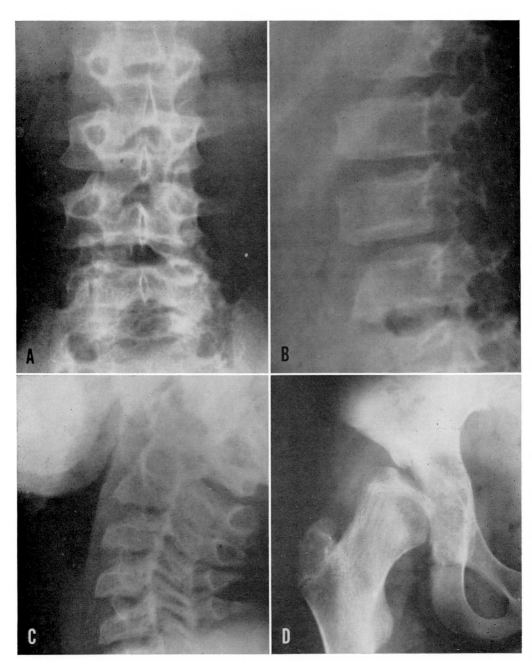

Fig. 149.   *A*, AP roentgenogram of the lumbar spine in a 13-year-old boy with spondylo-epiphyseal dysplasia tarda.   The vertebral bodies are flattened, and diminished in height.   The intervertebral discs are relatively wide, and there is a tendency towards a tongue-like deformity of several of the lumbar vertebrae, *B*. A sharpening of the anterior inferior aspect of the body of L4 is present.   Note the mound-like configuration of the posterior superior aspect of L2 and 3.   *C*, Lateral roentgenogram of the cervical spine shows the dens to be hypoplastic and the vertebrae flattened and elongated.   The intervertebral discs are wide.   In this patient a disturbance in the formation of the hip, *D*, and of the distal ends of the femurs also was present.

and tilted together. The development of the wrist epiphyses is delayed. The metacarpels tend to be bottle-shaped and the phalanges cylindrical. The spade-like appearance of the hand is due to the shortening of the bones, which also present pointed ends, particularly at the proximal aspect of the metacarpals and the distal ends of the phalanges.

The lower extremities are affected less extensively. The acetabular sockets may be shallow, and the proximal ends of the femurs rather thin. The distal ends of the femurs are apt to be normal, but genu valgum is often present. No flaring of the ends of the bones is present in Hurler's disease, and the pointed appearance noted helps in differentiating this from conditions such as achondroplasia. Moderate coxa vara or coxa valga deformities may be present, and the femoral heads sometimes are flattened and present irregularities in their articular surfaces. If kyphotic changes are mild and the lower extremities are not grossly shortened, dwarfism is not apparent.

Changes in the facial bones reflect the flattened nasal structures and heavy supraorbital ridges. The bump at the junction of the coronal and sagittal sutures may be moderately prominent, and the sella turcica elongated and widened. The ribs present a thinning and constriction of their proximal portions, with gradual flaring distal to this site (Fig. 150). This change is more apparent in the lower ribs. Thickening of the sternal ends of the clavicles and shortening of these bones is sometimes rather prominent.

Caffey (1952) reported changes like rickets or hyperparathyroidism in the long bones in the early stages of Hurler's disease which disappeared spontaneously. This osteoporotic phase may have been overlooked previously because x-ray examinations were not available at early stages. In his 2 cases followed over a period from 15 to 24 months, thoracolumbar kyphosis did not appear, but other manifestations of Hurler's disease became prominent.

Patients with Hurler's disease usually die early in life or soon after adolescence from heart failure or respiratory ailments.

References

Caffey, J.: Gargoylism (Hunter-Hurler Disease, Dysostosis Multiplex, Lipochondrodystrophy), Am. J. Roentgenol., 67, 715, 1952.

Ellis, R. W. B., Sheldon, W. and Capon, N. B.: Gargoylism (Chondro-osteodystrophy, Corneal Opacities, Hepatosplenomegaly and Mental Deficiency), Quart. J. Med., 5, 119, 1936.

Dorfman, A.: Heritable Diseases of Connective Tissue: the Hurler Syndrome in *The Metabolic Basis of Inherited Disease*, 2nd ed. Edited by Stanbury, J. B., Wyngaarden, J. B. and Fredrickson, D. S. New York, McGraw-Hill, pp. 963–994, 1966.

Berggord, I. and Bearn, A. G.: The Hurler Syndrome. A Biochemical and Clinical Study. Am. J. Med., 39, 221, 1965.

Horrigan, W. D. and Baker, D. H.: Gargoylism: a Review of the Roentgen Skull Changes with a Description of a New Finding. Am. J. Roentgenol., 86, 473, 1961.

Jervis, G. A.: Gargoylism (Lipochondrodystrophy), Arch. Neurol. & Psychiat., 63, 681, 1950.

Magee, K. R.: Leptomeningeal Changes Associated with Lipochondrodystrophy, Arch. Neurol. & Psychiat., 63, 282, 1950.

Maroteaux, P. and Lamy, M.: Hurler's Disease, Morquio's Disease, and Related Mucopolysaccharidoses, J. Pediat., 67, 312, 1965.

McKusick, V. A.: Heritable Disorders of Connective Tissue: the Hurler Syndrome, J. Chron. Dis., 3, 360, 1956.

Sanfillipo, S. J., Podosin, R., Langer, L. and Good, R. A.: Mental Retardation Associated with Acid Mucopolysacchariduria (Heparitin Sulfate Type), J. Pediat., 63, 837, 1963.

PLATYSPONDYLY WITH OTHER CHONDRODYSPLASIAS

The appearance of platyspondyly in Morquio's disease, particularly in its full-blown form, together with the clinical picture, usually permits an accurate diagnosis. However, platyspondyly also occurs in a variety of other chondrodysplasias. In Hurler's disease the biconvex configuration of the involved vertebrae, the associated kyphosis and the anteriorly projecting beak of the midportions of the lower thoracic and upper lumbar involved vertebrae are readily distinguished from the flattened vertebrae of Morquio's disease. The clinical picture usually permits such a differentiation to be made as readily because the appearance of a patient with Hurler's disease, particularly the facies, which has prompted the designation of "gargoylism" is striking. Spondyloepiphysial dysplasia tarda is a little more difficult to distinguish because the flattening of the vertebrae sometimes is rather prominent. However, the bony bump in the posterior aspect of the upper and lower surfaces of the affected vertebrae, the absence of associated skeletal changes and the appearance of the patient, permits ready differentiation. Multiple epiphysial dysplasia sometimes presents a rather prominent degree of platyspondyly, but more often the changes are moderate and may be more like those seen with Scheuermann's disease. Usually the spine is within normal limits with multiple epiphysial dysplasia. Achondroplasia, particularly in infancy, often is associated with marked flattening of the vertebrae and widening of the intervertebral disc spaces. At this age the vertebral changes with Morquio's disease are likely to be less striking, and the skeletal changes in the pelvis and hips as well as in the extremities in patients with achondroplasia differ considerably from those with Morquio's disease. Mention should also be made that isolated flattening of one or several vertebrae should not be confused with the platyspondyly associated with the various chondrodystrophies. Instances of pronounced flattening of one or more vertebrae appear with eosinophilic granuloma, with the various lymphomas and metastatic disease of other malignant origin, with osteoporosis and after trauma. These usually are readily recognized and differentiated from chondrodystrophic platyspondyly, but differential diagnosis between isolated vertebral flattening sometimes is difficult.

Kyphoscoliosis with tongue-like projections from the anterior aspect of the vertebrae have been observed with Ehlers-Danlos syndrome (Macfarlane, 1959). Another rare condition in which chondrodysplasia occurs is chondroectodermal dysplasia (Ellis-

van Creveld syndrome). In this condition the limbs are shortened, polydactyly and syndactyly appear, and there is hypoplasia of the nails, teeth, and sometimes of the hair. The spine, however, is not affected. A rare condition sometimes misdiagnosed as Morquio's disease or Hurler's disease is Leri's pleonosteosis, a genetically transmitted condition involving mainly the connective tissues with symptoms referable to the cutaneous, skeletal and optic systems. In the cases described by Rukvina, Falls, Holt and Block (1959) the vertebrae presented changes of interest in that overgrowth of bone was manifested by increase in the heights of the pedicles and overgrowth of the vertebral bodies, suggesting the changes occasionally seen with acromegaly.

Maroteau and Lamy (1965) refer to two other conditions associated with metabolic disorders of the acid mucopolysaccharides, in addition to Hurler's disease. In the disorder in which heparitin sulfate is present in the urine, and which is associated with marked mental deterioration, the designation polydystrophic oligophrenia is suggested. The vertebrae here usually are ovoid in configuration, and may present an anterior spur. However, the changes are not as striking as seen with Morquio's disease. The other condition is polydystrophic dwarfism, associated with excretion of chondroitin sulfate B. Here the skeletal changes are more striking. The patient presents dwarfism involving the trunk and the limbs, with genu valgum, lumbar kyphosis and anterior sternal protrusion. The vertebrae are flattened somewhat, but not to the extent observed with Morquio's disease. A kyphos appears at the thoracolumbar junction with wedging of these segments. The posterior aspects of the vertebral bodies are concave, and the posterior arcs are deepened.

Thoracolumbar kyphosis with wedging, hypoplasia and posterior displacement of the vertebral bodies has been observed with defective metaphyseal ossification without concomitant metabolic changes in the urine and the blood. Kozlowski and Budzinska

(1966) refer to 2 cases of combined metaphyseal and epiphyseal dysostosis with dwarfism recognized early in life, and later developed crippling deformities of the spine and limbs. They stressed the difficulties encountered in classifying enchondral dysostoses.

References

Alvarez-Borja, A.: Ellis-Van Creveld Syndrome, Pediatrics, *26*, 301, 1960.

Ellis, W. B. and Andrew, J. D.: Chondroectodermal Dysplasia, J. Bone & Joint Surg., *44-B*, 626, 1962.

Kozlowski, K. and Budzinska, A.: Combined Metaphyseal and Epiphyseal Dysostosis. Am. J. Roentgenol., *97*, 21, 1966.

Lane, J. W.: Roentgenographic Manifestations of the Cartilaginous Dysplasias, Am. J. Med. Sci., *240*, 636, 1960.

Langer, L. O.: The Radiographic Manifestations of the HS-Mucopolysaccharidosis of Sanfillipo, Ann. radiol., *7*, 315, 1964.

Macfarlane, I. L.: Case of Ehlers-Danlos Syndrome Presenting Certain Unusual Features, J. Bone & Joint Surg., *41-B*, 541, 1959.

Maroteaux, P., Lamy, M. and Bernard, J.: La dysplasia Spondylo-épiphysaire Tardive: Description Clinique et Radiologique, Presse méd., *65*, 1205, 1957.

Rubin, P.: *Dynamic Classification of Bone Dysplasias.* Chicago, Year Book Medical Publishers, Inc., 1964.

Rukavina, J. G., Falls, H. F., Holt, J. F. and Block, W. D.: Leri's Pleonosteosis, J. Bone & Joint Surg., *41-A*, 397, 1959.

Sanfillipo, S. J., Podosin, R., Langer, L. and Good, R. A.: Mental Retardation Associated with Acid Mucopolysachariduria (heparatin-sulfate type). J. Pediat., *63*, 837, 1963.

Smith, H. L. and Hand, A. M.: Chondroectodermal Dysplasia (Ellis-van Creveld syndrome). Pediatrics, *21*, 298, 1958.

Walls, W. L., Altman, D. H. and Winslow, O. P.: Chondroectodermal Dysplasia (Ellis-van Creveld Syndrome), J. Dis. Childhood, *98*, 242, 1959.

HEREDITARY MULTIPLE EXOSTOSES (DIAPHYSICAL ACLASIA, HEREDITARY DEFORMING DYSCHONDROPLASIA).

This is a hereditary disturbance in the nature of a mesodermal dysplasia which is progressive from infancy to adolescence. The condition affects principally the growing ends of bone, but manifests itself in any bone formed in cartilage. It may become apparent during adolescence, when rapidly progressing growth is accompanied by sudden progression in the size of some of the exostoses, making them apparent to the patient for the first time.

The exostoses are unilateral or bilateral, and occur as single lesions or in multitudes. Most of the time the distribution is asymmetric. The most common bones affected are the femurs and tibias, the upper portions of the humeri, the fibulas, the radius and ulna. Involvement of the pelvis, the clavicles, sternum, mandibles and ribs is less frequent. Exostoses projecting from the middle of the bone shafts are uncommon. Shortening of the growth of a long bone may produce visible deformity, such as Madelung's deformity of the forearm and wrist. Malignant degeneration is reported in about 5 per cent of patients with this disease.

While infrequent, vertebral involvement with multiple exostoses has been recognized. A case with an exostosis within the spinal canal was reported by Ochsner and Rothstein (1907). Involvement of the vertebrae with exostoses usually occurs in the neural arches. In themselves, these lesions are not of particular significance, but if they should be directed towards the spinal canal compression of the cord or nerve roots may follow. The vertebral bodies are rarely affected. Slepian and Hamby (1951) found 19 cases in which neurologic complications were directly related to an encroaching osteochondral exostosis. Out of the 15 cases in which the sex was stated, 14 were males. The spinal cord was involved in 10 cases. These authors reported 2 additional cases, 1 with a broad-based osteochondroma over the fifth and sixth cervical vertebrae, in which myelography revealed a complete block. Laminectomy showed the canal to be narrowed in the anteroposterior diameter, with elevation of the dura and displacement of the thecal sac to the right by a grumous bony growth.

Involvement of the spinous and transverse processes of the vertebrae is uncommon (Fig. 151). In these areas pressure from a

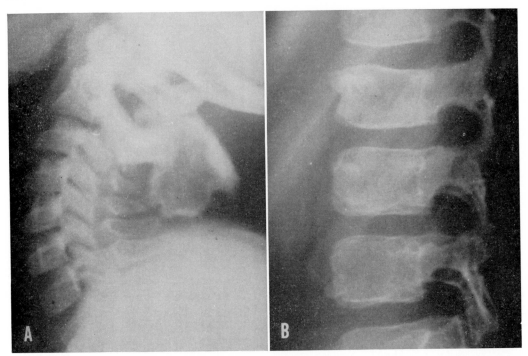

Fig. 151. *A,* Large exostosis of the second cervical spinous process in a 6-year-old boy with hereditary multiple exostoses. The patient had neck pain with limitation of motion. *B,* Another patient, a 12-year-old boy without symptoms, with hereditary multiple exostoses with small projections from the anterior portion of several of the lumbar vertebrae.

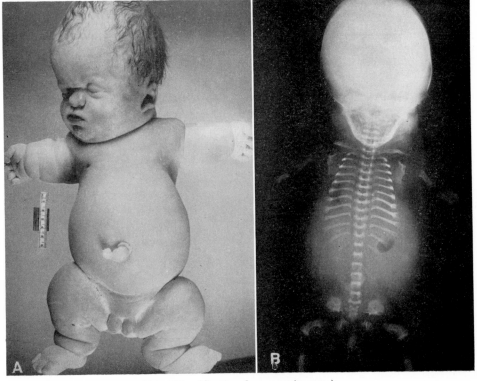

Fig. 152. (*Continued on opposite page.*)

large exostosis is known to produce local pain or to impinge on adjacent nerve trunks.

References

Abel, I.: Chondrodysplasia, Arch. Surg., *41*, 213, 1940.

Fairbank, H. A. T.: Dyschondroplasia; Metaphyseal Dysostosis, J. Bone & Joint Surg., *30-B*, 339, 1948.

Kierulf, E.: Dyschondroplasia, Acta radiol., *32*, 169, 1949.

Larson, N. E., Dodge, H. W., Jr., Rushton, J. G. and Dahlin, D. C.: Hereditary Multiple Exostoses with Compression of the Spinal Cord, Proc. Staff Meeting, Mayo Clin., *32*, 728, 1957.

Slepian, A. and Hamby, W. B.: Neurologic Complications Associated with Hereditary Deforming Chondrodysplasia, J. Neurosurg., *8*, 529, 1951.

ACHONDROPLASIA (Micromelia, Chondrodystrophia Fetalis, Chondrodystrophy)

Achondroplasia is the commonest and most ancient known form of dwarfism. The condition is transmitted by a dominant mutant gene and is familial, although many sporadic cases are known to exist. Most achondroplastic infants are still-born or die soon after birth. Those which survive, however, are apt to be of normal inteligence, and as a group are active and quite vigorous. The dwarfism is of the short limb type, associated with a large head, small face with a prognathous chin, an exaggerated lumbar

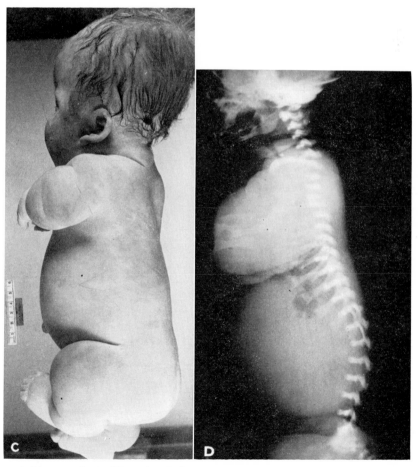

Fig. 152. *A*, Photograph of stillborn female fetus with achondroplasia. *B*, Same case. Anteroposterior roentgenogram. Note the short limbs and small pelvic and shoulder girdle development, and the large head. The spine is straight. *C*, Same case. Photograph of infant in lateral position. *D*, Same case. Lateral roentgenogram. A dorsal curvature is present at the thoracolumbar junction. The vertebral bodies are flat and the intervertebral discs are markedly enlarged. Deficient ossification of the pedicles and laminae is present.

lordosis and prominent buttocks. The lips are thick and the tongue tends to protrude. The bridge of the nose is flattened. The movements of the limbs are limited, and the patient's gait is waddling and duck-like. Females are afflicted more often than males. In many the hands present a "trident" appearance, being broad and short, with a spreading of the second and third from the fourth and fifth digits.

Achondroplasia represents a dysplasia which is incident to an inborn error in the growth and development of cartilage, with retardation and irregularity of cartilaginous osseous growth. Unossified islands of cartilage persist at the epiphyseal ends. The columns of cells in the provisional zone of enchondral calcification remain short, and are irregular and uneven in length. Because periosteal bone growth remains normal, the long bones thicken while longitudinal growth is retarded. This results in broad, short limbs with cupped, irregularly spurred or jagged ends and wedge-shaped imperfections. The shafts of the long bones retain a fairly normal width, but the ends are flared and during the period of growth there is an indented appearance of the widened metaphyseal end, while the epiphysis is smaller and rounded. The skull shows normal growth of bones originating in membrane, while those derived from cartilage are delayed. Thus the head is disproportionately enlarged in the calvarium, while the base is small. A triangular configuration results, with a small sella turcica and foramen magnum. The ribs are shortened, with flared distal ends. The short tubular bones of the hands and feet are shortened, thick and present cupped growth zones.

Changes in the spine are apparent at birth, and are as striking as those seen in

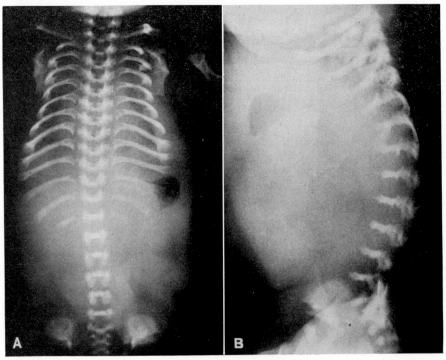

Fig. 153. *A*, Anteroposterior roentgenogram of newborn infant with achondroplasia. Note the widened intervertebral spaces and the poor development of the vertebrae. *B*, Same case as *A*, lateral view. The spine presents a thoracolumbar dorsad curvature, with flat vertebral bodies and markedly enlarged intervertebral discs. Note the tongue-like protrusions at the anterior aspects of the lumbar vertebrae. (See opposite page for Figure 153*C* and *D*.)

the arms and legs. The outstanding change is a marked thinning of the vertebral bodies, with disproportionately widened intervertebral discs. These radiolucent spaces are due to unossified cartilage at the vertebral epiphyseal plates, which radiologically are indistinguishable from the intervertebral discs. Not infrequently small linear, tongue-like projections appear from the anterior aspect of the ossified vertebral bodies. A well-defined convexity is seen at the lower thoracic and lumbar spine (Figs. 152, 153). As the child grows, the long kyphotic curve is replaced with a lumbar lordosis which may become so marked that the sacrum assumes a horizontal position. Because of delayed enchondral growth at the neurocentral junctions, growth of the pedicles is impaired with the result that the dorsoventral diameter of the spinal canal is narrowed.

As growth proceeds the vertebral bodies increase in size, to the extent that in some adult achondroplasts the bodies appear relatively well formed, while the pedicles are shortened so that the intervertebral foramina present an elongated, narrow configuration. In younger individuals some wedging may be present anteriorly and the anterior angles of the vertebral bodies are rounded (Fig. 154). A slight kyphos is then present at the thoracolumbar junction, while a prominent lordosis is seen in the lumbosacral area. The posterior walls of the vertebrae are relatively increased in height, and they present a rather sharp concave appearance. The fifth lumbar vertebra becomes wedged between the iliac bones (Fig. 155). The narrowing of the spinal canal is a most significant change, and accounts for the fact that relatively minor disturbances in the intervertebral discs such as minor protrusions, may have catastrophic results. Multiple decompressive laminectomies may be required to provide relief. The development of a dorsolumbar kyphosis sometimes pro-

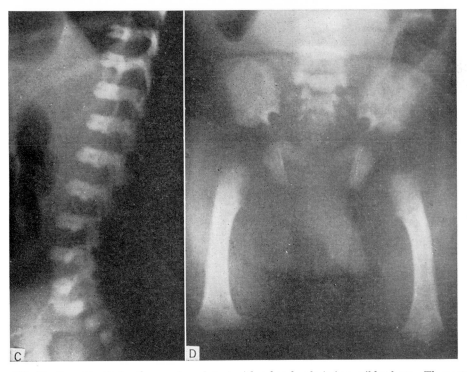

Fig. 153. (Continued.) C, Another newborn infant with achondroplasia in a milder form. The vertebral bodies are larger than in the patient represented in A and B. The intervertebral spaces are wide. D, Same patient as C. The pelvis, hips and femurs show the characteristic osseous and joint changes.

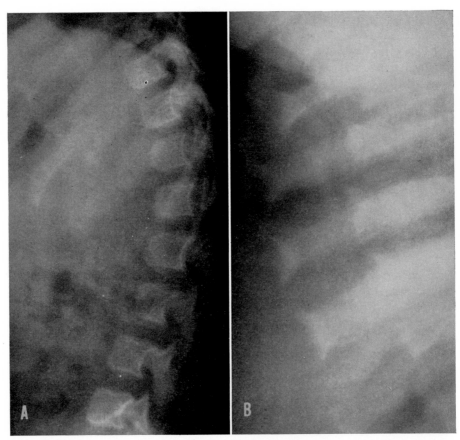

Fig. 154. *A*, Thoracolumbar spine of a child with achondroplasia. A moderate kyphosis is present. The dorsal surfaces of the vertebral bodies are scalloped. The anterior margins are round, particularly at the apex of the curve. The intervertebral foramina are elongated and indented by the discs. *B*, The costochondral junctions of the ribs are flared, shortened and heavily calcified.

ceeds until a gibbus is formed, predisposing to neurologic complications. Vogl and Osborne (1949) suggested that orthopedic measures be instituted before the upright position is assumed in an effort to compensate for a dorsolumbar kyphosis before a gibbus forms.

Myelographic examination in patients with achondroplasia is rendered difficult by the technical factors encountered in obtaining a good flow of cerebrospinal fluid. Even with the needle accurately placed one obtains only a few drops of fluid. Instillation is best performed under image intensification fluoroscopy. Observation of the entering flow of positive contrast material reveals first its accumulation in the deepened concavities of the dorsal aspects of the vertebral

bodies, then a slow trickle to either side until successive lakes separated by horizontal radiolucencies are observed (Fig. 156). Only a small quantity is required to get a good filling of the entire lumbar canal, a good indication of the reduced capacity of the subarachnoid space. Removal of the Pantopaque usually is difficult. It is helpful to place the patient erect and to get drainage from the lowest interspace which can be entered. Complete block sometimes is encountered when minimal discal protrusions are present (Fig. 157). Similarly, subluxation of one vertebra on another can produce cord compression (Spillane, 1952). Neurologic sequelae are most frequent in the lumbar region.

The sacrum in achondroplastic dwarfs is

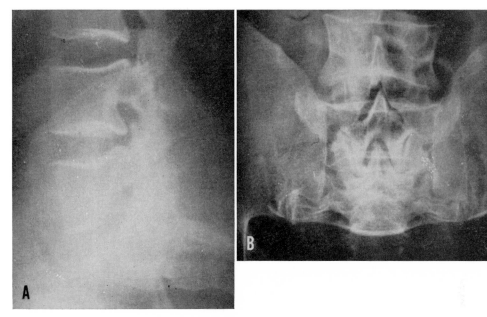

Fig. 155. *A*, Lower lumbar spine of an adult achondroplast. The sacrum is almost horizontal and the lumbar lordotic curve is straightened. The discs are wide and biconvex. The intervertebral foramina are elongated, narrow and constricted at their midportions by the prominent discs and the elevations of the posterosuperior and postero-inferior lips of the vertebral bodies. *B*, AP view of the lumbosacral junction shows the fifth lumbar vertebra buried deep between the iliac bones. The sacrum is small and the sacroiliac joints are closely positioned because of the small size of the upper sacrum.

narrow, and articulates low on the iliac bones. The fifth lumbar vertebra, caught between the ilia, presents a characteristically marked narrowing of the interpedicular spaces (Fig. 155). The sciatic notches are elongated and slit-like, and the iliac bones are squared off. The configuration of the pelvic inlet has been likened to that of a champagne glass, a factor which usually results in cesarean section being necessary for delivery of achondroplastic mothers. The sacrum becomes rotated on a transverse axis, displacing the hip joints backwards, thereby resulting in increased prominence of the buttocks.

About 30 per cent of achondroplastic dwarfs have a thoracolumbar kyphosis which varies from a mild arcuate curve to a severely angulated gibbus. The vertebrae at the apex of the kyphos are wedged, a change usually noted in the lowermost two thoracic and uppermost two lumbar vertebrae. The vertebrae above and below articu-late with the wedged bodies, which may present an elongated, tongue-like projection anteriorly at the apex of the curve. Compressive changes of the cord and cauda equina are likely to occur, with slowly progressive neurologic deficits.

In differential diagnosis Morquio's disease is excluded by the platyspondyly observed in that condition. In addition, the broad spatulate hand seen with Morquio's disease differs from the trident hand associated with achondroplasia. The skull in achondroplastic dwarfs presents a characteristic broadened calvarium and narrowed base, together with relatively small upper cervical vertebrae, a tendency to basilar invagination and a small foramen magnum. In Morquio's disease the skull is relatively normal, although hypoplasia of the dens is often present. With Hurler's disease the skull is large, and the sella often elongated. The length of the long bones in Morquio's disease is considerably greater than those in achon-

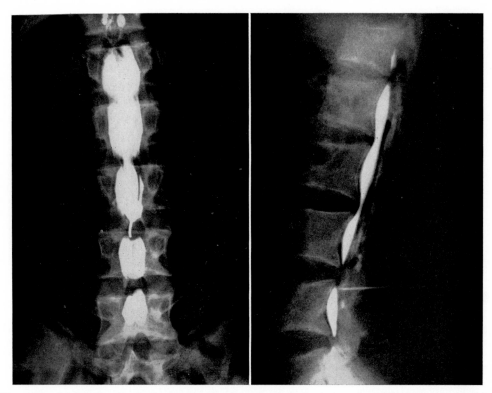

FIG. 156. Adult achondroplastic dwarf with severe back and sciatic pain. Spinal tap accomplished with difficulty. Transverse defects present at each level, with the column interrupted by protrusion of the discs. This, together with heavy neural arches, hypertrophied ligamenta flava and the narrow canal produced severe cauda equina and nerve root pressure. Relief of symptoms followed multiple decompressive laminectomies (courtesy of Dr. Joseph A. Epstein).

droplastic dwarfs, while both present changes in the articular ends. In Hurler's disease the tongue-like protrusion in the lowermost thoracic and upper lumbar vertebrae together with the sharp angular gibbus at the thoracolumbar junction can readily be differentiated from the platyspondyly of Morquio's disease and the narrowed spinal canal seen in older patients with achondroplasia. In infancy the universally narrowed and elongated vertebral bodies and markedly widened intervertebral spaces of achondroplastics, together with the shortened limbs projecting at right angles from the body, are easily identified. With spondyloepiphyseal dysplasia the vertebral bodies are flattened and elongated, and often present a prominent bony bump at the midportion or posterior portion of the superior and inferior surfaces which serves to identify this condition. The

changes in the long bones here, too, are less striking than those with Morquio's disease, Hurler's disease or achondroplasia.

In the various osteochondrodystrophies instances occur in which the changes are not entirely characteristic, yet point towards one or another of these conditions. These are referred to as the "tarda" forms, and often tax one's diagnostic acumen. Osteochondrodystrophy involving mainly the thorax, with shortening of the ribs resulting in a small immobile thorax is another rare condition (Pirnar and Neuhauser, 1966). Variable involvement of the skeleton occurs, and the skull and spine are relatively normal. These infants usually are prone to respiratory difficulties, and do not survive very long. One case seen by us had a deformity of the ribs, and this patient had cuboidal vertebrae. This patient was 3 years old

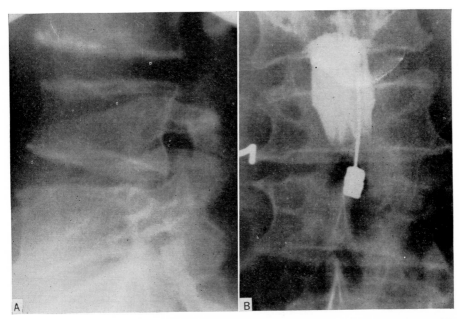

Fig. 157. *A*, Adult male achondroplastic dwarf with intense radicular pain. The intervertebral foramina as seen on the lateral film are elongated and narrowed. The pedicles and laminae are heavy. The vertebral bodies are flattened. *B*, Myelogram shows a complete block at the third lumbar interspace. A relatively small herniated disc was found at operation. The canal was small, so that even a small intrusion caused a complete block.

and when he was seen by us he was in good health (Fig. 158).

Pseudoachondroplastic forms of spondylo-epiphyseal dysplasia and of multiple epiphyseal dysplasia have been reported. In these patients the bony shortening and marked irregularities of the growing ends simulate achondroplasia, but the configuration of the vertebrae serves to help identify these conditions. In the pseudoachondroplastic form of spondylo-epiphyseal dysplasia the vertebral bodies present the typical flattened appearance, while with multiple epiphyseal dysplasia the vertebral bodies remain normal or show some changes along the annular apophyses. Neither of these have narrowing of the sagittal diameter of the spinal canal. Scoliosis does not appear in achondroplasia or spondyloepiphyseal dysplasia, but may occur together with hemivertebrae in multiple epiphyseal dysplasia.

Diastrophic dwarfism, previously regarded as an atypical form of achondroplasia, presents generalized osseous developmental anomalies consisting of dwarfism, clubfoot deformity and scoliosis. Deformity of the external ears and cleft palate also is present. This is a short-limbed form of dwarfism, which is hereditary and associated with normal mentality. Early progressive scoliosis, sometimes combined with kyphosis is present, together with limitation of mobility and a tendency to dislocation of various joints, most often the hips. The sacrum is sharply tilted backwards. The metaphyses and epiphyses of the long bones are shortened and widened. Flattening of the humeral heads corresponding to widening of the glenoid fossae is observed, while the distal humeri are grossly and irregularly deformed in most cases. The forearms are short, and the proximal epiphyses of the radii and ulnae are deformed as well. The vertebrae maintain a fairly normal configuration, and platyspondyly is not present. The interpedicular spaces and heights of the pedicles remain normal but may be diminished in

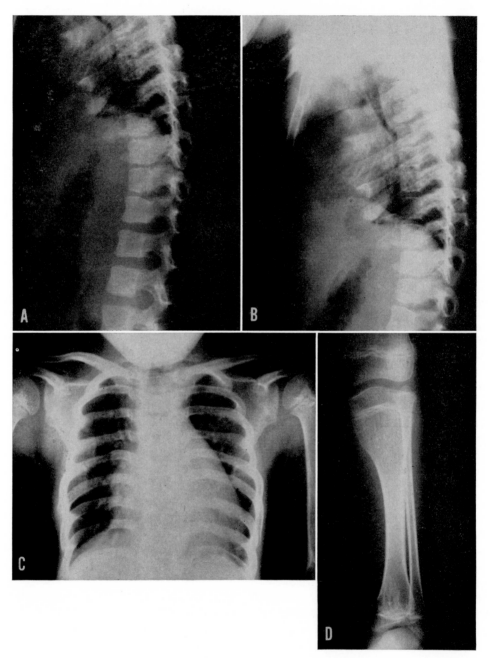

Fig. 158. *A*, Infant with osteochondrodystrophy affecting the ribs and extremities particularly. The vertebrae are rather elongated. The ribs are markedly shortened, *B*, with prominent costochondral junctions. The thorax, *C*, is small. The legs, *D*, present broadening of the metaphyseal ends of the long bones and slight epiphyseal irregularities. The fibula appears out of proportion to the size of the tibia.

the lumbar region. With weight bearing scoliosis becomes quite prominent. Langer (1965) mentioned a patient with kyphosis of the upper cervical spine, and dislocation of the second on the third cervical vertebra. The long axis of the dens was parallel to the foramen magnum in this patient. The skull remains normal, with no alteration of its base. Adults with this condition are strikingly deformed.

References

Burkhart, J. M., Burke, E. C. and Kelly, P. J.: The Chondrodystrophies. Proc. Staff Meet., Mayo Clin., *40*, 481, 1965.

Caffey, J.: Achondroplasia of Pelvis and Lumbosacral Spine, Am. J. Roentgenol., *80*, 449, 1968.

Duvoisin, R. C. and Yahr, M. D.: Compressive Spinal Cord and Root Syndromes in Achondroplastic Dwarfs. Neurology, *12*, 203, 1962.

Epstein, J. A. and Malis, L. I.: Compression of Spinal Cord and Cauda Equina in Achondroplastic Dwarfs, Neurology, *5*, 875, 1955.

Fairbank H. A.T.: Achondroplasia, J. Bone & Joint Surg., *31-B*, 600, 1949.

Hancock, D. O. and Phillips, D. G.: Spinal Compression in Achondroplasia, Paraplegia, *3*, 23, 1965.

Langer, L. O., Jr.: Diastrophic Dwarfism in Early Infancy, Am. J. Roentgenol., *90*, 399, 1965.

Pirnar, T. and Neuhauser, E. B. D.: Asphyxiating Thoracic Dystrophy of the Newborn. Am. J. Roentgenol., *98*, 358, 1966.

Rubin, P.: *Dynamic Classification of Bone Dysplasias*, Chicago, Year Book Medical Publishers, Inc., 1964.

Schreiber, F. and Rosenthal, H.: Paraplegia from Ruptured Lumbar Discs in Achondroplastic Dwarfs, J. Neurosurg., *9*, 648, 1952.

Spillane, J. D.: Achondroplasia, J. Neurol., Neurosurg. & Psychiat., *15*, 246, 1952.

Taybi, H.: Diastrophic Dwarfism, Radiology, *80*, 1, 1963.

Osteogenesis Imperfecta

Osteogenesis imperfecta is a fairly common familial, hereditary disturbance of mesenchymal development which produces a marked alteration in bone characterized by softening and brittleness in varying proportions. There is a failure in the ability to form bone matrix, the disease representing a form of osteoporosis.

Other names applied to this condition are idiopathic fragilitas ossium, osteopsathyrosis, brittle bones with blue sclerae, osteosclerosis, osteitis parenchymatosa chronica, dystrophia periostalsis, periosteal aplasia and periosteal dysplasia. Brailsford suggested that all these terms be dropped, and the term osteogenesis imperfecta be extended to include fetal, infantile, adolescent and adult types (1943). Chont (1941) had also suggested a revision of nomenclature to include two forms of the disease: osteoporosis imperfecta congenita, all cases of which either die *in utero* or are born with the disease, constituting thereby a fetal and infantile variety. The second major classification would be osteogenesis imperfecta tarda occurring in infants apparently normal at birth and in whom the disease occurs early in life, usually in the 2nd year. This group could be subdivided into a hereditary group with blue sclerae and non-hereditary group which may or may not have blue sclerae. Caniggia, Stuart and Guideri (1958) regard as valid the unitary concept of fetal and adult forms of osteogenesis imperfecta in the genetic, pathogenetic and histopathologic domains. They recommend that the term fragilitas ossium hereditaria, Typus Vrolick, or osteogenesis imperfecta Vrolick type, or Vrolick's disease be used to indicate the congenital fetal form of the disease. The adult type can be referred to as osteogenesis imperfecta Ekman-Lobstein type, or Ekman-Lobstein disease.

Fairbank (1948) in a report of 12 cases of osteogenesis imperfecta mentioned 3 types, the first being the thick bone type with severe bony changes particularly in the ribs, together with stunted limbs such as may be seen with achondroplasia. The second type presented slender fragile bones with osteoporosis of the entire skeleton. In this type the vertebral bodies may be translucent, shallow, spread and biconcave with biconvex intervertebral discs. A third type, which he mentioned as very rare, presents pronounced honeycombing of the bones of a progressive nature. He termed this osteogenesis imperfecta cystica. Rosenbaum (1944) questioned whether there was any difference in the type of osteogenesis imperfecta in which intra-uterine fractures occurred or in which only post-natal fractures occurred. He reported cases of the 2 types in the same family, tending to disprove the duality of the syndromes. There does not appear to be sufficient evidence to warrant the division of this disease into 2 specific categories. The evidence appears to point towards the existence of several forms of the same disease. Some become manifest during intra-uterine life; others appear to be milder in the extent of osseous change. The prognosis when the disease is manifest early in life is not as good as when later development of osteogenesis imperfecta occurs.

There are marked variations in the severity of the disease. The usual picture is one of a short, poorly nourished individual of normal intelligence with many bony deformities associated with multiple fractures, some of which appear practically spontaneously. The skull tends to be triangular in shape, and dental development is retarded. Excessive mobility of the joints is due to relaxation of the articular capsules and restraining ligaments, together with poor muscular development. The presence of blue sclerae is considered requisite for the hereditary type of the disease, but is not always present. Deafness, a fairly frequent accompaniment, is attributed to ankylosis of the ossicles. In more advanced cases, actual involvement of the bones of the middle ear exists.

The pathologic changes associated with osteogenesis imperfecta are imperfect formation and calcification of the bony trabeculae. Islands of cartilage are seen, especially beneath the periosteum, in which imperfectly calcified osteoid trabeculae replace normal bone. The periosteum may be thickened, beneath which the bone is discontinuous and fragmentary. The medullary content is in part fibroid, lymphoid or fatty. Studies by Fairbank (1948) indicated that there may be a great variation in the development of the osteoblasts. He pointed out that while a deficiency in the number of osteoblasts had been stressed, his studies showed that in

number they may be quite numerous although the formation of bone was deficient. Knaggs (1926) had mentioned before that a deficiency in osteoblasts was common, and that formation of cartilage cells from the periosteum instead of the osteoblast is the most characteristic pathologic change.

Prepartum diagnosis of osteogenesis imperfecta occasionally can be made from abdominal roentgenograms. The limbs of the fetus present a slender appearance, and fractures can be identified. In others the wrinkled appearance of the bones, particularly of the ribs, is diagnostic.

Roentgenologic examination of the extremities in some cases with intrauterine or fetal osteogenesis imperfecta reveals a marked wrinkled appearance of the long bones. These are short and relatively stumpy, with practically no distinguishing marks between the cortex and medullary canal. Some subperiosteal thickening may be present, giving rise to irregular, rather scalloped peripheries of the tubular bones. These also show numerous radiopaque bands due to the bending over of the softened bone. Deformities are marked, some of the bones presenting almost right angle configurations in the middle of their shafts, others appearing to be collapsed upon themselves in an irregular accordion-like fashion. The ribs may be markedly involved and the thoracic cavity greatly compressed because of the marked softening and irregularities of the ribs. It is interesting to note that this change is most marked in the portion of the thoracic cage occupied by the lungs. The infradiaphragmatic ribs usually are kept more or less in position by the underlying liver, spleen and other abdominal viscera. (Fig. 159).

In stillborn infants with osteogenesis imperfecta the skull bones are practically invisible except for the base. The scalp covers membranous bone almost equally soft, so that considerable deformity is present. Occasionally better calcification exists with numerous interlacing linear markings of bone interspersed irregularly in the vault. In

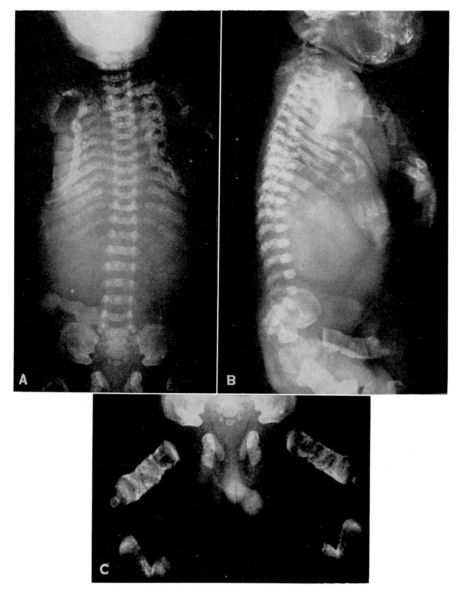

Fig. 159. A, Anteroposterior roentgenogram of stillborn infant with osteogenesis imperfecta. Note the wrinkled appearance of the ribs, and the inward collapse of the supradiaphragmatic costal structures. The vertebral column is quite straight. B, Same case, lateral view. Note the dorsal convexity at the thoracolumbar junction, and the anterior wedging of the lower thoracic and upper lumbar vertebrae. Ossification appears adequate. C, Same case, illustrating the marked deformity of the lower extremities.

infants who survive the cranium is thin, and the shape of the skull maintained. Rarely some hyperostosis appears. Basilar invagination develops later in life in some patients. Other cases of osteogenesis imperfecta of the intra-uterine and fetal type present changes which are much less marked. Frac-

ture lines are sharply visible and there may be considerable displacement of the bony fragments. Angular deformities of the long bones, particularly the femurs and legs, are frequent. The degree of deformity of the ribs may be less marked, and rather than presenting an irregular crenated type of bony deformity the long bones thin and slender.

As maturity is reached the disease may take one of two roads. In some individuals the development of bone slowly proceeds in a more or less normal fashion so that by the time adolescence is reached and growth stops, the bony structures are deformed, thin, but still capable of carrying the weight of the child. Further growth is accompanied by less and less deformity, and these individuals may reach maturity and be symptomless. It is even possible for some of these patients to go through life without the diagnosis being definitely established, inasmuch as symptoms are so few as to make medical attention unnecessary in early life when the disease might have been more easily recognized. Other individuals show marked deficiency in development of bone, and the bones may present a tubular appearance. The cortex and medullary canals are relatively well differentiated but the bones are soft and deformities and fractures occur frequently. The patient often is stunted and deformed because of multiple fractures and consequent malformations of the spine and extremities. The skull is large, with poor dentition. Odontogenesis imperfecta, recognizable on transillumination by the opalescent amber appearance of the teeth occurs with osteogenesis imperfecta, but also appears without skeletal disease. The teeth are small, crumble easily, and their root canals and pulp chambers are small or absent. The lamina dura is not altered.

The appearance of the vertebral column in patients with osteogenesis imperfecta is variable. Spinal curvatures are frequent. The vertebrae become softened, with resultant compression and widening of the bodies and ballooning of the intervertebral discs. In the more advanced cases compressive action on the spine produces pronounced flattening of the vertebrae which assume the appearance of a thin biconvex lens. It has been noted that occasionally the vertebral bodies at the lower lumbar levels are somewhat increased in height in patients who have the greatest extent of spinal compressive change. The vertebrae are demineralized, the compact bone being considerably thinned and the cancellous bone reduced in volume so that the trabecular spaces are widened. The remaining trabeculae, however, are quite well calcified.

Observations in a case of intra-uterine osteogenesis imperfecta were made by postmortem roentgenograms of the skeleton immediately after the delivery of the stillborn fetus, and in these the vertebral column was of particular interest (Fig. 159). The alignment of the vertebral bodies was about normal for the fetus at term, insofar as the cervical and thoracic spine was concerned. The lumbosacral curve was slightly more developed than usual. In the anteroposterior view, the vertebral column was quite straight. The middle cervical segments presented a definite anterior wedging of the vertebral bodies while posteriorly these bodies maintained their height. The thoracic spine showed a definite decrease in the height of the vertebral bodies together with a proportionate increase in the width of the intervertebral spaces. The superior and inferior aspects of the respective vertebral bodies were quite straight and parallel to each other. The thoracolumbar junction was of interest in that there was a rather abrupt wedging of the anterior aspect of the bodies of the eleventh and twelfth dorsal vertebrae, and to a lesser degree of the anterior aspect of the body of the first lumbar vertebra. The other lumbar vertebrae were rather small but otherwise well formed. The anterior and posterior venous channels entering the vertebral bodies were not identifiable. The neural arches presented the same type of wrinkled appearance as was noted in the markedly altered long bones. However, the interpedicular spaces and the pedicles were not visibly disturbed.

Another case of osteogenesis imperfecta in a newborn infant presented a considerably different appearance of the vertebral bodies. In this patient the bones did not show the accordion-pleated wrinkling noted in the previous case. The medullary canals were fairly well identified and the fracture lines in

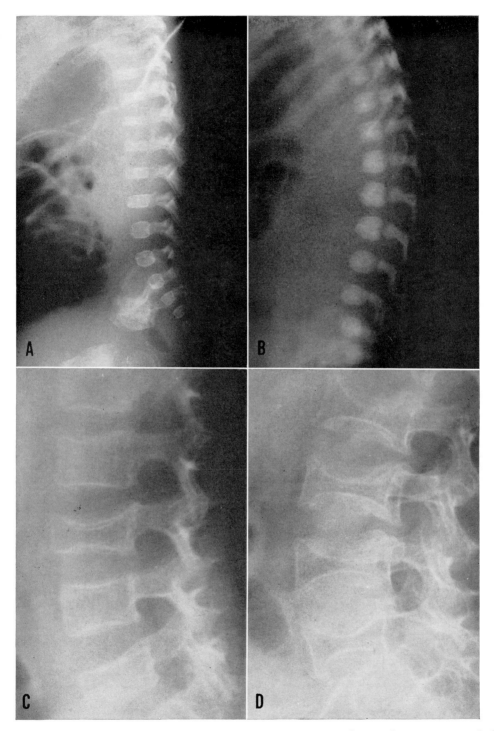

Fig. 160. *A*, One-month-old infant with osteogenesis imperfecta. The vertebrae are symmetrically flattened. The discs are wide. A slight irregularity can be demonstrated along the anterior margins of some of the vertebrae. *B*, Another infant in whom the vertebral bodies are relatively intact. A slight dorsal curve is present at the thoracolumbar junction. The skull and extremities presented classical changes. *C*, A 4-year-old patient with partial collapse of the third lumbar vertebra and lesser indentations in the others. The discs are wide. *D*, Another 7-year-old child with extensive changes. The discs are wide and biconvex, the vertebral bodies are reduced to lens-like biconcave structures.

the arms and legs were sharply demarcated. A definite narrowing of the bodies of the thoracic vertebrae was noted. The intervertebral spaces were markedly increased in height. The vertebral column was well aligned in the anteroposterior view, while in the lateral view a slight but fairly definite tendency towards a dorsal roundness in the thoracolumbar region could be demonstrated. The thinness of the vertebral bodies was greatest in the thoracic spine, while in the lumbar spine the vertebral bodies returned to an almost normal height. The vascular indentations of the anterior and dorsal aspects of the vertebral bodies were inconspicuous but could be faintly made out in the lumbar segments (Fig. 160A and B).

With advancing growth the height of the vertebral bodies increases and their bony density improves. However, when the disease is markedly advanced, demineralization of the vertebral bodies is so pronounced that the structures are virtually indistinguishable on the roentgenogram. In such cases the vertebral bodies become reduced to a fraction of their normal height and assume biconvex deformities associated with enlargement and biconcave configurations of the intervertebral discs. Continued observation of such a patient showed a marked improvement in the density of the flattened and deformed vertebral bodies over a period of years, so that when the condition was apparently healed the deformity of the vertebral bodies was quite marked, although the bony densities had returned to a fairly normal state. In this case the vertebrae presented marked broadening and flattening, with increased densities of the margins of the vertebral bodies. There also was an associated spreading of the interpedicular distances both in the thoracic and lumbar segments, considered part of the picture of spreading of the vertebral bodies associated with the softening accompanying osteogenesis imperfecta (Fig. 160C and D).

Osteogenesis imperfecta with a relatively latent clinical course may be associated with

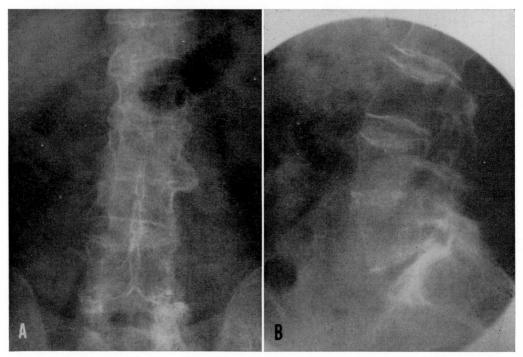

Fig. 161. A, AP lumbar spine in a 55-year-old woman with osteogenesis imperfecta. Diffuse demineralization of bone is present, with prominent spurring along the lateral margin on the left. B, Lateral film again shows the diffuse bone loss. The discs are varied, some being wide and others narrow.

a lesser degree of biconvex deformity of the vertebral bodies. In such cases, the length of the pedicles of the lumbar vertebrae as seen in the lateral view appeared to be increased, with a consequent widening of the spinal canal. It is worth mentioning that in 1 case the child's mother was known to have had osteogenesis imperfecta, and that roentgenologic examination of her spine showed no deformity.

These patients can reach adult life and are capable of almost normal activity. The spine in one such individual (Fig. 161) revealed a moderate thoracolumbar scoliosis, with diffuse demineralization of the vertebral bodies. Some intervertebral discs were narrowed, but others revealed a widened biconvex configuration. Moderate spondylotic hyperplastic overgrowth was visible.

A most unusual and infrequent change reported is hyperplastic callus formation enveloping some of the long bones in long, parallel, irregular multiple strands. This usually appears in the femur or humerus, and may be associated with trauma. It has not been observed in the vertebral column.

The diagnosis of osteogenesis imperfecta can be made *in utero* when the characteristic wrinkling and shortening of the limbs and the flattened vertebral bodies and widened intervertebral discs are present. The shortness of the limbs may momentarily suggest the possibility of achondroplasia, but the striking radiologic differences quickly resolve this difficulty. The cystic form of the disease is rare, and in the few cases reported is associated with deformities and bending of bone at an early age (Fairbank, 1948, 1951), dating from birth and increases with age.

References

Bickel, W. H., Ghormley, R. K. and Camp, J. D.: Osteogenesis Imperfecta, Radiology, *40*, 145, 1943.

Brailsford, J. F.: Osteogenesis Imperfecta, Brit. J. Radiol., *16*, 129, 1943.

Caniggia, A., Stuart, C. and Guideri, R.: Fragilitas Ossium Hereditaria Tarda. Ekman-Lobstein Disease, Acta med. Scandinav., Supp. 340, Stockholm, 1958.

Chont, L. K.: Osteogenesis Imperfecta, Am. J. Roentgenol., *45*, 850, 1941.

Colonna, P. C.: Osteogenesis Imperfecta, Am. J. Surg., *15*, 336, 1932.

Fairbank, H. A. T.: Osteogenesis Imperfecta and Osteogenesis Imperfecta Cystica, J. Bone & Joint Surg., *30-B*, 164, 1948.

————: Atlas of General Affections of the Skeleton, Edinburgh, E. & S. Livingstone, Ltd., 1951.

————: Hyperplastic Callus Formation, With or Without Evidence of a Fracture, in Osteogenesis Imperfecta: With an Account of the Histology by S. L. Baker, Brit. J. Surg., *36*, 1, 1948.

Frerking, H. W. and Zink, O. C.: Osteogenesis Imperfecta Diagnosed in Utero, Am. J. Roentgenol., *67*, 103, 1952.

Key, J. A.: Brittle Bones and Blue Sclerae; Hereditary Hypoplasia of Mesenchyme, Arch. Surg., *13*, 523, 1926.

Knaggs, R. L.: Osteogenesis Imperfecta, Brit. J. Surg., *11*, 737, 1924.

Levin, E. J.: Osteogenesis Imperfecta in the Adult, Am. J. Roentgenol., *91*, 973, 1964.

Riesenman, F. R. and Yater, W. M.: Osteogenesis Imperfecta, Arch. Int. Med., *67*, 950, 1941.

Rosenbaum, S.: Osteogenesis Imperfecta and Osteopsathyrosis, J. Pediat., *25*, 161, 1944.

Schwartz, E.: Hypercallosis in Osteogenesis Imperfecta, Am. J. Roentgenol., *85*, 645, 1964.

Zander, G. S. F.: Osteogenesis Imperfecta Tarda with Platyspondylosis, Acta radiol., *21*, 53, 1940.

CLEIDOCRANIAL DYSOSTOSIS

The exact developmental error responsible for cleidocranial dysostosis is presumed to be one of mesenchymal development involving bone originating in membrane, particularly the cranium and the clavicles. Changes also appear in the pelvis, particularly in the pubic region, where deficient ossification results in a separation of the midline synchrondrosis. Deficient ossification of the skull bones results in multiple and prominent wormian bones. In infants and children the fontanelles remain widely open, and there is delayed ossification of the frontal, parietal and occipital bones. A circular bony defect is sometimes present in the midfrontal region. The palate is high, the facial bones and paranasal sinuses are small, and deficient dentition with persistent deciduous teeth can be observed. The clavicles may be involved asymmetrically, and usually the distal thirds are absent, although several fragments may persist. The defect varies from complete absence to a small defect which simulates fracture.

In the spine there often is failure of fusion of the neural arches. The bodies of the vertebrae are occasionally wedged and biconvex in configuration. The thorax may be quite slender due to unusual mobility of the shoulders because of the clavicular deficiencies.

References

Brocher, J. E.: Konstitutionell bedingte Veränderungen des Wirbelbogens. Fortschr. Geb. Röntgenstr., *92*, 363, 1960.
Salmon, D. D.: Hereditary Cleidocranial Dysostosis. Radiology, *42*, 391, 1944.
Thoms, J.: Cleidocranial Dysostosis, Acta radiol., *50*, 514, 1958.

OSTEOPETROSIS (Albers-Schönberg's disease, marble bones, chalk bones, osteosclerosis fragilis generalisata and osteopetrosis generalisata)

This disease is of familial nature and has been encountered in all decades of life from intra-uterine life to the eighth decade. Consanguinity of parents has been noted. Its cause is unknown. It affects both sexes equally, and its severity may vary markedly from patient to patient. In some, particularly those with the disease *in utero* or during the first year of life, progression is rapid, with complete involvement of the entire skeletal system, anemia, optic atrophy, retarded growth and fatal outcome within a relatively short time. Others present a more attenuated form and the diagnosis may be established in the course of roentgenologic examinations made for other purposes. The disease is characterized to some degree by activity and remissions, or there may be complete cessation of the developmental error. Schulte (1951) divided Albers-Schönberg disease into three groups, including a malignant form of osteosclerosis in children with brittle bones and anemia, a benign form without anemia but bone sclerosis and weakness, and osteosclerosis with neither fractures nor anemia.

The anemia associated with osteopetrosis is ascribed to myelophthisis caused by encroachment on the marrow cavity. Metaplasia of extramedullary hematopoietic centers accounts for enlargement of the liver, spleen and lymph nodes. With extensive skull involvement constriction of the optic foramina and the auditory canals produces symptoms referable to the cranial nerves affected. However, it is remarkable that even when the skull is extensively altered relatively few cranial nerve deficiencies are noted in some patients. In spite of the apparent hardness of the bones, spontaneous fractures are not uncommon, and cases sometimes are first observed as a result of fractures produced by slight trauma.

The osseous dysplasia of osteopetrosis is characterized by persistence of the dense primary spongiosa, while chondro-osseous formation proceeds normally. There is overgrowth and persistence of excess enchondral and periosteal bone, with failure of the osteoclastic resorptive process. While it usually is considered that diminished numbers or absence of osteoclasts is an important factor, Enticknap (1954) observed that in a patient seen by him both osteoblastic and osteoclastic activity were undiminished. Engfeldt and his co-workers (1954) demonstrated that normal bone resorbed by osteoclastic activity was replaced by immature bone which did not progress to normal bone. The involvement of cortical and cancellous bone is the same, and there is no difference in the process in bone originating from cartilage or membrane. The long bones assume a peculiar expanded plug-like configuration at their distal ends, while the shafts present a bone within bone appearance. This also occurs in the ribs. The markedly increased density of the cranium, particularly the base, is associated with constriction of the basilar foramina. The pelvis presents parallel rows of increased density at the ilial epiphyses as growth proceeds.

The configuration of the vertebrae in infants is relatively normal, aside from a tendency to rounding of the margins and a deepened indentation for the anterior and posterior veins. The heights of the vertebrae are not disturbed and the intervertebral discs are well maintained. The neurocentral synchondroses are not visibly altered, and the neural arches are well formed. The spinous and transverse processes are increased and dense. The ribs are of average length, but expand distally and end in a straight, widened configuration (Fig. 162). Radiographic examination discloses a marked increase in the density of the upper and lower plates, with a relatively lucent zone sometimes present and at other times an almost uniform density. The notching of the vascular channels in the anterior and posterior aspects of the vertebral bodies often is accentuated.

Adults with osteopetrosis present a so-called "sandwich" appearance of the vertebral bodies. This appearance varies considerably, even in the same patient. In some, the upper and lower aspects of the vertebral bodies are uniformly dense, and the vertebrae otherwise are normal in appearance. There may be a relatively smooth, parallel configuration of these osteopetrotic zones, which extend from the posterior portions of the bodies almost up to the anterior margins. In other patients the sclerotic plates assume a rectangular appearance, with discontinuity anteriorly and posteriorly corresponding to the middle of the respective centra. A radiolucent zone sometimes separates the dense from the normal appearing bone. Involvement of the vertebrae may show dissimilar configuration of the endovertebral sclerotic process in the same patient (Fig. 163). Occasionally the sclerotic zone within a vertebral body is cuboidal in configuration. The overall configuration of the respective vertebrae is not grossly disturbed. The sacrum is involved in a rather similar fashion, with sclerotic changes most marked adjacent to the sacro-iliac joints.

While the radiologic picture of osteopetro-

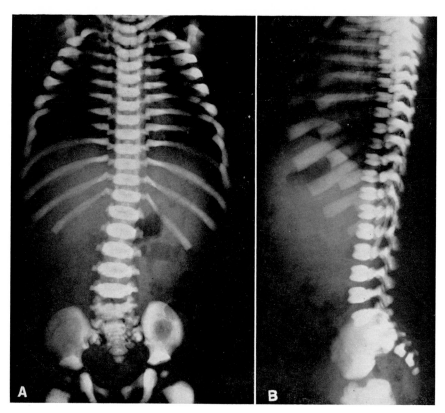

FIG. 162. Anteroposterior and lateral roentgenograms of infant with osteopetrosis.

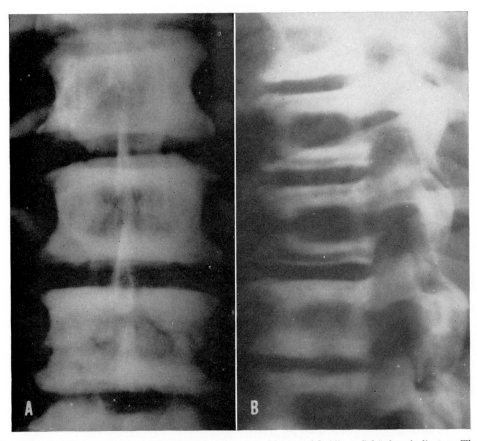

Fig. 163. *A*, AP view of upper lumbar spine in a 35-year-old man with Albers-Schönberg's disease. The increased bone formation beneath the epiphyseal plates and the radiolucent centra are characteristic. Lateral examination shows the bone-within-bone configuration. Note the discontinuity in the vicinity of the anterior and posterior vascular grooves.

sis is one of great density, the true nature of the osseous structures does not conform with this impression of hardness. The bone itself varies from a granite-like density to a consistency like that of chalk. Striking variations in density occur in various areas in the same patient. In adults it is not infrequent to discover the disease incidentally, an observation which emphasizes the differences between the early and late manifestations of the disease.

Osteopetrosis can readily be identified in infancy when the condition is advanced. In doubtful cases it may be wise to delay before coming to a conclusion. Conditions also to be considered include heavy metal deposits, which do not produce the same

pattern of bone change. Fluorosis spares the skull and involves mainly growth centers, produces ligamentous calcification and mottled teeth. Myelosclerosis results in a more diffuse, reticular pattern of endosteal sclerosis. Metastatic osteosclerotic lesions are distributed in an irregular manner, and none of the entities mentioned present the sandwich-like configuration noted with adult osteopetrosis. The "rugger-jersey" appearance seen with hyperparathyroidism should be differentiated without difficulty.

References

Albers-Schönberg, H.: Röntgenbilder einer Seltenen Knochenerkrankung, Munchen. med. Wchnschr., *51*, 365, 1904.

Callender, G. R., Jr. and Miyakawa, G.: Osteopetosis in an Adult, J. Bone & Joint Surg., *35-A*, 204, 1953.

Cassidy, W. J., Allman, F. C. and Keefe, G. J.: Osteopetrosis, Arch. Int. Med., *82*, 140, 1948.

Clifton, W. M., Frank, A. and Freeman, S.: Osteopetrosis (Marble Bones), Am. J. Dis. Child., *56*, 1020, 1936.

Engfeldt, B., Engström, A. and Zetterström, R.: Biophysical Studies on Bone Tissue; Osteopetrosis (Marble Bone Disease), Acta paediat., *43*, 152, 1954.

Engfeldt, B., Karlberg, P. and Zetterström, R.: Studies on the Skeletal Changes and on the Etiology of the Anaemia in Osteopetrosis, Acta path. et microbiol. Scandinav., *36*, 10, 1955.

Enticknap, J. B.: Albers-Schönberg Disease (Marble Bones), J. Bone & Joint Surg., *36-B*, 123, 1954.

Fairbanks, H. A. T.: Osteopetrosis; Osteopetrosis Generalisata, Marble Bones: Albers-Schönberg's Disease, Osteosclerosis Fragilitans Generalisata J. Bone & Joint Surg., *30-B*, 339, 1948.

Hasenhuttl, K.: Osteopetrosis, J. Bone & Joint Surg., *44-A*, 359, 1962.

Hinkel, C. L. and Beiler, D. D.: Osteopetrosis in Adults, Am. J. Roentgenol., *74*, 46, 1955.

Jenkinson, E. L., Pfisterer, W. H., Latteier, K. K. and Martin, M.: Prenatal Diagnosis of Osteopetrosis, Am. J. Roentgenol., *49*, 455, 1943.

Klintworth, G. K.: The Neurologic Manifestations of Osteopetrosis (Albers-Schönberg's Disease), Neurology, *13*, 512, 1963.

Lott, G. and Klein, E.: Osteopetrosis, Am. J. Roentgenol., *94*, 616, 1965.

McPeak, C. N.: Osteopetrosis, Am. J. Roentgenol., *36*, 816, 1936.

Pines, B. and Lederer, M.: Osteopetrosis, Albers-Schönberg's Disease, Am. J. Path., *23*, 775, 1947.

Schulte, K.: Marmorknochenerkrankung nach Albers-Schönberg, Fortschr. Röntgenstr., *75*, 720, 1951.

Seigman, E. L. and Kilby, W. L.: Osteopetrosis, Am. J. Roentgenol., *63*, 865, 1950.

FIBROUS DYSPLASIA (Fibrocystic Disease of Bone, Fibro-osseous Dysplasia)

Although brought into prominence by the report of Albright, Butler, Hampton and Smith (1937) as a syndrome characterized by osteitis fibrosa disseminata, areas of pigmentation and endocrine dysfunction with precocious puberty in females, this condition has been recognized as a separate entity for a considerably longer time. Albright and Reifenstein (1948) mentioned that in a review of von Recklinghausen's original monograph (1891) a number of conditions which certainly were not hyperparathyroidism were encountered. They believed that 2 out of the 3 cases in the monograph which had been considered examples of hyperparathyroidism reflected the syndrome described by Albright and his co-workers. Albright commented that "as far as the bone manifestation of the syndrome are concerned, von Recklinghausen preceded the author and his colleagues by forty-two years." Albright and Reifenstein agreed with Jaffe and Lichtenstein (1942) that the term best applicable to this condition is simply fibrous dysplasia, omitting the word "polyostotic" in order to include cases confined to one bony lesion. These can be referred to as monostotic fibrous dysplasia. If multiple bones are affected with no evidence of endocrine changes, the term polyostotic fibrous dysplasia can be applied. In instances with extensive bone lesions together with endocrine changes, the designation of fibrous dysplasia with endocrine manifestations can be used, or one might employ the term "Albright's disease" as suggested by Jaffe (1958).

Fibrous dysplasia is a condition of unknown etiology, and has no familial or hereditary background. It is far more associated with relatively limited skeletal and skin changes than with the form attended by endocrine changes. It occurs in a 2 or 3 to 1 proportion in females, and often comes to light early in life. There is some question as to whether or not the condition is congenital. The association of skin changes with skeletal manifestations is not constant, and indeed may be absent. When present it does not follow the distribution of the bone lesions. The tan pigmentation is caused by melanin in the basal cells of the epidermis, sometimes in the granulosa but also occasionally in the corium layer. While sexual precocity is more apt to appear in females, it may also rarely occur in males. The bone lesions tend to stabilize as the patient grows older, and the sexual precocity recedes. Indeed, some instances are known in which female patients have given birth to normal children.

In its completely developed form, fibrous dysplasia affects multiple bones which have a marked tendency to be unilateral in their distribution, although both sides of the body may be affected. The patient presents brown, unelevated pigmented areas of the skin which are usually on the same side of the body as the bony lesion. This is accompanied in females with an endocrine dysfuntion characterized by precocious puberty. The most common grouping of bone involvement is one leg associated with lesions in the pelvis and skull together with scattered lesions in the metatarsal and phalangeal bones. The femurs and humeri also frequently are affected as well as the small bones of the hand. As a rule the proximal portions are more involved. The pelvis, tarsal and carpal bones, the sternum and mandible are affected less frequently, and the vertebrae are seldom involved. The affected bones present considerable widening of the medullary canal with thinned cortices. The medullary canal is attacked by a thick white rubbery fibrous tissue which contains zones of scattered hyalin cartilage. The normal bony architecture of both the cortex and the medulla becomes disrupted by a dense fibrous tissue replacement with many fusiform spindle cells containing pale staining nuclei and a vague cytoplasmic outline. The fibrous tissue may contain small trabeculae of primitive metaplastic bone. Occasional small cysts containing amber fluid are present. The transition from pathologic to normal bone is often abrupt. The abnormal tissue has a gritty character due to spicules of primitive bone (Fairbank, 1950; Russell and Chandler, 1950). Laboratory findings are usually of little help. The blood calcium and phosphorus are normal. The phosphatase value varies considerably, and in some cases is increased. At times no single study, be it clinical, radiologic, operative or pathologic can sharply and accurately differentiate fibrous dysplasia from bone cysts or giant cell tumors.

The onset of this condition is usually insidious. First indications may be brought about by a fracture following a slight trauma or by a fairly rapidly appearing deformity of an extremity secondary to a local enlargement of the bone. A considerable asymmetry of the face or body also appears later in the disease. Pain and stiffness are less common initial symptoms. The skull changes of fibrous dysplasia may progress to the point where the disease assumes the proportions of leontiasis ossia with gross deformity of the face.

Fibrous dysplasia is regarded by Lichtenstein and Jaffe (1942) as a congenital developmental anomaly. Schlumberger (1946) was of the opinion that this was a true dystrophy in which the tendency of the mesenchyme to normal ossification is blocked or prevented by a fundamental local disturbance yet to be demonstrated. Albright and Reifenstein held that there probably is an endocrine disturbance related to a neurologic or embryologic defect disturbing the afferent impulses to the anterior lobe of the pituitary gland. Neller (1941) believed that polyostotic fibrous dysplasia was due to multiple embryonic defects, stating that the simultaneous involvement of the many different regions was evidence against a defect in a single system. The coexistence of other congenital defects with fibrous dysplasia has been reported by Stauffer, Arbuckle and Aegerter (1941) and by Coleman (1939). It appears that no one theory has accounted for the multiple manifestations of fibrous dysplasia of bone as associated with cutaneous and endocrine disturbances.

The radiologic changes in the long bones reflects the widening of the medullary canals and thinning of the cortex. Single or multilocular cysts occur together with various deformities incident to fractures and bending, changes induced by the softening of the bone. In some instances a characteristic ground glass appearance of the medullary cavity is observed, a change apparent more often in younger patients. In older people the cystic changes may become more pronounced, grotesquely deforming the bones and producing multiloculated cystic areas. Changes in the skull may simulate those of Paget's disease, and sometimes the two conditions are misdiagnosed one for the other. This situation can be avoided by due attention to the more characteristic manifestations of Paget's disease in the long bones, pelvis and spine.

Involvement of the vertebral column is rare. A review of the literature indicates only sporadic examples of such change. Albright and Reifenstein (1948) mentioned a case in which the entire spine was involved, while in another only the cervical vertebrae were affected. Spinal involvement was observed in 2 cases reported by Furst and

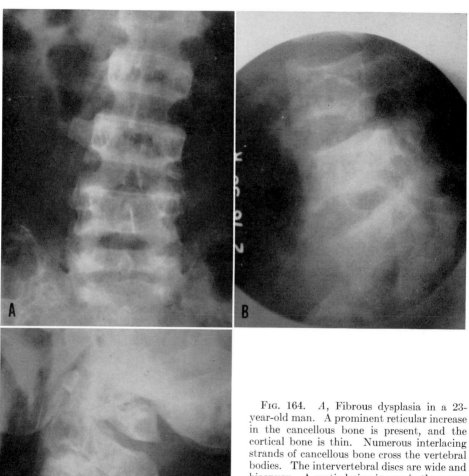

Fig. 164. *A*, Fibrous dysplasia in a 23-year-old man. A prominent reticular increase in the cancellous bone is present, and the cortical bone is thin. Numerous interlacing strands of cancellous bone cross the vertebral bodies. The intervertebral discs are wide and biconvex. A cystic lesion is seen in the upper right iliac bone. On the lateral examination, *B*, the bulging discs are again seen. Some prominent vertical striations are also visible. *C*, The cervical spine is normally aligned. Sclerotic changes are present in the 3rd and 4th cervical vertebrae. Changes also are seen in the occipital bone.

Shapiro (1943), and in 2 of the cases reported by Dockerty, Ghormley, Kennedy and Pugh (1945). Other single instances were recorded by Warrick (1949) and by Schlumberger (1946).

I have had the opportunity of following a young man with this condition from the age of 18 to 24 years. In addition to the classical changes in his extremities and the skin pigmentation, he had extensive involvement of his entire spine which remained relatively constant in appearance. The changes consisted mainly of a thinning of cortical bone, loss of trabecular markings and somewhat widened intervertebral discs. The cervical vertebral bodies were somewhat increased in density, with slight narrowing of their anterior aspects. A slight forward shift of the fifth on the sixth cervical vertebra was present, probably due to the increased lordotic cervical curve. The bodies of the thoracic and lumbar vertebrae had diminished density, and there were numerous vertical striations traversing the medullary spaces. The superior and inferior surfaces presented a biconcave appearance. The neural arches were somewhat demineralized but not deformed. In this patient the fifth lumbar vertebra was sacralized, sinking deeply into the superior surface of the sacrum. The transverse processes of the fourth lumbar vertebra were lower than the iliac crests and were directed upwards (Fig. 164). This was probably due to progressive softening of the bone and the strains of standing and walking. At no time did this patient complain of spinal pain, nor was there any indication of central nervous system irritation. Rosencrantz (1965) reported an 18-year-old male patient who developed paraplegia incident to wedging of thoracic vertebra producing a gibbus deformity.

In differential diagnosis the vertebral changes are not helpful. The conditions to be considered include, in general, bone cysts, enchondromas, non-ossifying fibromas, hyperparathyroidism, neurofibromatosis and enchondromatosis. The lipoid granulomatoses also might be included. The possibility of malignant degeneration, while infrequent, should be kept in mind (Schwartz and Alpert, 1964).

References

Albright, F., Butler, A. M., Hampton, A. O. and Smith, P. H.: Syndrome Characterized by Osteitis Fibrosa Disseminata, New England J. Med., *216*, 727, 1937.

Albright, F. and Reifenstein, E. C., Jr.: *Parathyroid Glands and Metabolic Bone Disease*, Baltimore, The Williams & Wilkins Co., 1948.

Coleman, M.: Osteitis Fibrosa Disseminata, Brit. J. Surg., *26*, 705, 1939.

Daves, M. L. and Yardley, J. H.: Fibrous Dysplasia of Bone, Am. J. Med. Sci., *234*, 590, 1957.

Dockerty, M. B., Ghormley, R. K., Kennedy, R. L. J. and Pugh, D. G.: Albright's Syndrome, Arch. Int. Med., *75*, 357, 1945.

Fairbank, H. A. T.: Fibrocystic Disease of Bone, J. Bone & Joint Surg., *32-B*, 403, 1950.

Furst, N. J. and Shapiro, R.: Polyostotic Fibrous Dysplasia, Radiology, *40*, 501, 1943.

Harris, W. H., Dudley, H. R., Jr. and Barry, R. J.: The Natural History of Fibrous Dysplasia, J. Bone & Joint Surg., *44-A*, 207, 1962.

Jaffe, H. L.: *Tumors and Tumorous Conditions of the Bones and Joints*, Philadelphia, Lea & Febiger, 1958.

Jaffe, H. L. and Lichtenstein, L.: Non-Osteogenic Fibroma of Bone, Am. J. Path., *18*, 205, 1942.

Lichtenstein, L.: Polyostotic Fibrous Dysplasia, Arch. Surg., *36*, 874, 1938.

Neller, J. L.: Osteitis Fibrosa Cystica (Albright), Am. J. Dis. Child., *61*, 590, 1941.

Proffutt, J. N., McSwain, B. and Kalmon, E. H., Jr.: Fibrous Dysplasia of Bone, Ann. Surg., *130*, 881, 1949.

Reed, R. J.: Fibrous Dysplasia of Bone, Arch. Path., *75*, 480, 1963.

Rosencrantz, M. A.: A Case of Fibrous Dysplasia (Jaffe-Lichtenstein) with Vertebral Fracture and Compression of the Spinal Cord, Acta orthop. Scandinav., *36*, 435, 1965.

Rosendahl-Jensen, S.: Fibrous Dysplasia of the Vertebral Column, Acta chir. Scandinav., *3*, 490, 1956.

Russell, L. W. and Chandler, F. A.: Fibrous Dysplasia of Bone, J. Bone & Joint Surg., *32-A*, 323, 1950.

Schlumberger, H. G.: Fibrous Dysplasia of Single Bones (Monostotic Fibrous Dysplasia), Military Surgeon, *99*, 504, 1946.

Schwartz, D. T. and Alpert, M.: The Malignant Transformation of Fibrous Dysplasia, Am. J. Med. Sci., *247*, 1, 1964.

Stauffer, H. M., Arbuckle, R. K. and Aegerter, E. E.: Polyostotic Fibrous Dysplasia with Cutaneous Pigmentation and Congenital Arteriovenous Aneurysms, J. Bone & Joint Surg., *23*, 323, 1941.

Warrick, C. K.: Polyostotic Fibrous Dysplasia, J. Bone & Joint Surg., *31-B*, 175, 1949.

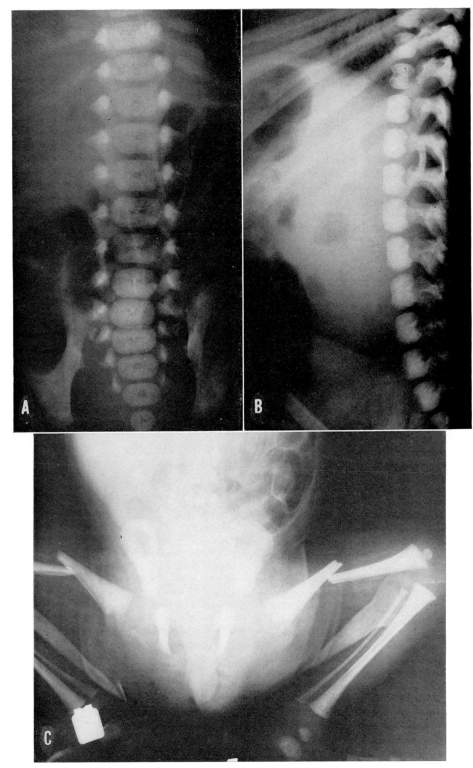

FIG. 165. *A*, AP thoracolumbar spine in a newborn infant with arthrogryposis. *B*, The increase in the height of the vertebral bodies is more apparent on the lateral film. *C*, Characteristic changes in the legs and the hip, knee and ankle joints.

ARTHROGRYPOSIS MULTIPLEX CONGENITA (Amyoplasia Congenita,, congenital multiple or rigid joints, arthromyodysplastic syndrome)

This term is used to designate multiple contractures of the joints, the term literally meaning crooked or bent joints. The disease is of a hereditary familial nature and the characteristic changes are present in newborn infants. Two instances were reported in which the diagnosis was suggested on roentgenograms made before delivery in women with mild hydramnios by the peculiar stick-like extension of the legs on the femurs (Epstein, 1961). Mild forms of the disease are consistent with long, normal life.

The changes in the joints are primarily of a non-articular nature. The primary pathologic condition is an atrophy and fatty replacement of the involved muscles with thickening of the periarticular structures and multiple contractures. An abnormality in anterior horn cells in the spinal cord and a denervation atrophy of muscle has been reported. The affected extremities assume an appearance which has been referred to as resembling a "stuffed sausage." As a rule, the involvement is symmetric, involving both the upper and lower extremities. Associated deformities such as myelo-meningocele, hypoplasia of the jaw, congenital malformations of the hands and feet, disturbances of pigmentation of the skin and hair, and congenital deafness have been reported.

The bony structures of the extremities characteristically present an elongated thinned-out appearance with adequate markings differentiating the medullary canal from the cortex. In 2 of our cases pathologic fractures occurred in the shafts of the bone, in 1 a concomitant of delivery. In another case, the femurs showed evidences of fractures in utero with healing, while the bones of the legs presented a slender appearance with a considerable degree of bowing secondary to softening of the bones. Bilateral club-feet was observed in 3 of the 4 patients, together with congenital strictures of the wrist joints in 2 of these.

Involvement of the spine is manifested by a lateral curvature attributed to a change in muscle pull. No vertebral changes are seen, especially in the mild form of this condition. Rarely the vertebral bodies become narrow and elongated. The discs are not disturbed. In one patient, a newborn who died within a few hours, there were fractures of the long extremities, which were thin and long, with fixed joints. The vertebrae (Fig. 165) were elongated and narrow.

References

Banker, B. Q., Victor, M. and Adams, R. D.: Arthrogryposis Multiplex Due to Congenital Muscular Dystrophy, Brain, 80, 319, 1957.

Epstein, B. S.: Radiographic Identification of Arthrogryposis Multiplex Congenita in Utero, Radiology, 77, 108, 1961.

Hillman, J. W. and Johnson, J. T. H.: Arthrogryposis Multiplex Congenita in Twins, J. Bone & Joint Surg., 34-A, 211, 1952.

Katzeff, M.: Arthrogryposis Multiplex Congenita, Arch. Surg., 46, 673, 1943.

Mead, N. M., Lithgow, W. C. and Sweeney, H. J.: Arthrogryposis Multiplex Congenita, J. Bone & Joint Surg., 40-A, 1285, 1958.

OSTEOPOIKILOSIS (osteopathia condensans disseminata, osteopoecilia, osteitis condensans disseminata, spotted bones)

This is a hereditary disease of mesenchymal disturbance characterized by the presence of multiple small round or ovoid foci of increased density scattered throughout the skeletal system, affecting chiefly the long bones and the pelvis. Involvement of the skull is rare. These small increased bony concentrations are much like small osteomas and microscopically consist of densely packed bony tissue (Hinson, 1939).

In most cases the disease was discovered incidentally and was not accompanied by symptoms referable to the islands of condensed bone. However, congenital anomalies associated with osteopoikilosis have been described, an example of which is coarctation of the aorta (Phalen and Ghormley, 1943).

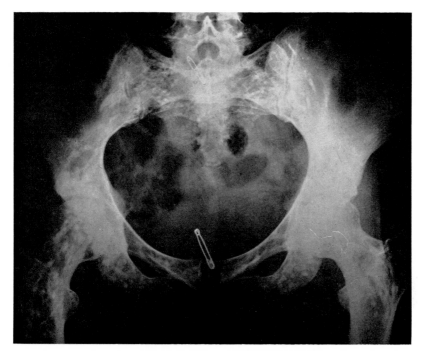

FIG. 166.   Osteopoikilosis in an adult female patient.

The spine is rarely involved in this condition. Published reports indicate only an occasional island in the lower lumbar spine or in the sacrum. In the case observed by us, a considerable involvement of the sacrum was observed together with similar involvement in the pelvis, and both upper femurs. In addition, islands of compact bone were demonstrable in the fourth and fifth lumbar vertebrae. These were rather conspicuous in the transverse processes and neural arches (Fig. 166).

The multiple dense spots are within the cancellous bone. These appear as circular or ovoid shadows with their long axes usually parallel to the long axis of the affected bone. No such deposits have been observed in the cortex.

References

Albers-Schönberg, H.: Eine seltene, bisher nicht bekannte Strukturanomalie des Skelettes. Fortschr. Röntgenstr., *23*, 174, 1915.

Archer, C. M. and Fox, K. W.: Osteopoikilosis, Radiology, *47*, 279, 1946.

Bloom, A. R.: Osteopoecilia, Am. J. Surg., *22*, 239, 1933.

Fairbank, H. A. T.: Osteopoikilosis, J. Bone & Joint Surg., *30-B*, 544, 1948.

Harmston, G. J.: Osteopathia Condensans Disseminata, Radiology, *66*, 556, 1956.

Hinson, A.: Familial Osteopoikilosis, Am. J. Surg., *45*, 566, 1939.

Phalen, G. S. and Ghormley, R. K.: Osteopathia Condensans Disseminata Associated with Coarctation of the Aorta, J. Bone & Joint Surg., *25*, 693, 1943.

Thompson, R. H., Hoover, R. and Fulton, H. F.: Osteopoikilosis, Am. J. Roentgenol., *49*, 603, 1943.

OSTEOPATHIA STRIATA (Voorhoeve's disease)

This is an unusual affliction characterized by vertical striation of the skeleton, particularly the metaphyses of the long bones. It is a disease of unknown origin and probably congenital in nature. It has been suggested that oseopathia striata is related to osteopoikilosis (Hurt, 1953) and dyschondroplasia (Voorhoeve, 1924), the three disorders being variants of the same fundamental error. However, Fairbank (1950) hesitated to accept this view. There are no definite symptoms referable to this dysplasia of bone, except that the patients sometimes complain of vague aches and pains. The outstanding radiologic change includes vertical striations in all of the bones except the skull and clavicles. The striation as a rule affects the shafts of the long bones, appearing as dense lines parallel to the long axis. The thickness of the striations may vary considerably and the bone between various clusters of striated change may be osteoporotic. The striation may or may not extend to adjacent epiphyses. The epiphyses are sometimes mottled with dense and clear spots. The spine is involved infrequently. In 1 of the cases reported by Fairbank, coarse vertical striations were present in the vertebral bodies.

References

Fairbank, H. A. T.: Osteopathia Striata, J. Bone & Joint Surg., *32-B*, 117, 1950.
Hurt, R. L.: Osteopathia Striata—Voorhoeve's Disease, J. Bone & Joint Surg., *35-B*, 89, 1953.
Voorhoeve, M.: L'Image Radiologique Non Encore Déscrite d'une Anomalie du Squelette. Acta radiol., *3*, 407, 1924.

DYSPLASIA EPIPHYSIALIS PUNCTATA (punctate epiphyseal dysplasia; chondroangiopathia calcarea seu punctata; chondrodystrophia calcificans congenita; chondrodystrophia punctata; chondrodystrophia calcificans congenita [Conradi's Disease], stippled epiphyses)

This condition is a rare disorder of infancy of unknown origin, and may be familial. It occurs in about 1 in 500,000 births, and is perhaps more frequent in premature infants. The prognosis is poor, few surviving beyond 2 years. Nevertheless, instances have been recorded in which the patients reached adolescence or beyond this age. In some, no definite symptoms are observed, but more often associated changes such as shortened extremities, dry scaly skin, contractures of joints in flexion, syndactylism, congenital cataracts, microcephaly, oxycephaly, mental

retardation, cleft palate or congenital cardiac defects have been present. Haymes and Wanger (1951) reported stippled epiphyses in an achondroplastic dwarf.

The disease involves the cartilaginous portions of the epiphyses. The disturbances of calcification simulate those of chondrodystrophia fetalis, representing a congenital enchondral disturbance of ossification. As a result the long bones are shortened, with thick bowed shafts and wide irregular metaphyseal ends. However, the long bones may retain a normal tubular configuration, and the stippling be confined only to the epiphyses and the adjacent articular structures. The signs common to the disease include micromelia, rhizomelia, cataracts and stippled epiphyses. The nasal bridge is flat, but the skull itself is not affected.

The characteristic lesion is stippling of the various epiphyses, as if they were ossifying from multiple centers. The spots vary considerably in size and number and may extend to the soft tissues outside the involved joints in advanced cases. Anatomically there is disturbance of vascularization with spotty, mucoid degeneration of the epiphyses, as a result of which the hyalin cartilage becomes fragmented. Each fragment in turn may serve as a site for the formation of additional cartilage which ossifies and becomes connected by intervening cartilaginous bands. When the infant survives the formation of bone from cartilage slowly returns to normal and the islands of stippled density disappear. Bones which apparently were unaffected later in life may show malformations like those of chondrodystrophy. Licht and Jesiotr (1957) reported an atypical relatively symptomless manifestation of the disease in a 24-year-old man in whom the vertebrae were flattened and contained numerous areas of increased density due to spotty calcific deposits located principally in the anterior aspects of the bodies arranged in two symmetric lines opposite the pedicles.

The vertebrae participate in this generalized affection of enchondral calcification. Involvement of the sacrum often is prominent. As a result, stippling of the bodies appears, which follows the same tendency to vanish if the child survives. In some instances an atypical form of ossification of the vertebral bodies has been described, consisting of a coronal cleft of chondroid tissue on either side of which is stippling and disturbed ossification. Instances in which the vertebral bodies were deformed because of structural weakness also are known, occurring principally in youngsters who had survived well beyond 1 year. With extensive involvement this has been observed in infancy as well. The changes bear some resemblance to those of Scheuermann's disease. Disturbances in the ossification of the cervical vertebrae occasionally are followed by changes in the usual lordotic curve. Persistence of stippling into adolescence also occurs.

The coronal cleft type of deformity is attributed to the persistence of an anterior and posterior ossification center which failed to unite, presumably because of enchondral disturbance. Calcific flecks in the intervertebral discs result from occasional deposits of ossifying tissue in these structures during the period of growth. With survival, there is the same tendency to resumption of a normal growth pattern.

In some patients with a relatively mild form of achondroplasia the epiphyses assume a stippled appearance which might be confused with chondrodystrophia calcificans congenita. These individuals may also have the more characteristic changes in the spine, such as flattened vertebrae and particularly narrowing of the spinal canal. Stippled epiphyses occasionally appear in patients with short limbs and normal vertebrae, or with vertebrae showing irregularities at the anteroinferior and anterosuperior angles such as seen with Scheuermann's disease. The spinal canal is normal here, and the interpedicular spaces are average. This pseudoachondroplastic form of punctate epiphyseal dysplasia is observed in patients who survive longer, and who may be normal at birth, with changes in the extremities first coming to attention at about the age of 4 or 5 years. The fine stippling noted with the dysplasia under discussion can readily be distinguished from that observed with hypothyroidism, which is coarser and associated with the other changes incident to the latter condition. The stippled epiphyses observed with chondrodystrophia calcificans congenita can also be easily differentiated from the punctate changes present with osteopoikilosis.

References

Allansmith, M. and Senz, E.: Chondrodystrophic Congenita Punctata (Conradi's Disease), Am. J. Dis. Child., *100*, 109, 1960.

Brogdon, B. G. and Crow, N. E.: Chondrodystrophia Calcificans Congenita, Am. J. Roentgenol., *80*, 443, 1958.

Cohen, J., Currarino, G. and Neuhauser, E. B. D.: A Significant Variation in the Ossification Centers of the Vertebral Bodies, Am. J. Roentgenol., *76*, 469, 1956.

Fairbank, H. A. T.: Dysplasia Epiphysialis Punctata, J. Bone & Joint Surg., *31-B*, 114, 1949.

Haynes, E. R. and Wangner, W. F.: Chondroangiopathia Calcarea seu Punctata, Radiology, *57*, 547, 1951.

Hillard, C.: Chondro-Osseous Dystrophy with Punctate Epiphyseal Dysplasia, Brit. J. Radiol., *16* 144, 1943.

Josephson, B. M. and Oriatti, M. D.: Chondrodystrophia Calcificans Congenita, Pediatrics, *28*, 425, 1961.

Kaser, H.: Chondrodystrophia Calcificans Congenita, Schweitz. med. Wchnschr., *87* 676, 1957.

Licht, J. and Jesiotr, M.: Chondroangiopathia Calcarea seu Punctata (Chondrodystrophia Calcificans Congenita): An Atypical Stationary Form of the Disease, Am. J. Roentgenol., *78*, 493, 1957.

Maitland, D. G.: Punctate Epiphyseal Dysplasia, Brit. J. Radiol., *12*, 91, 1939.

Maudsley, R. H.: Dysplasia Epiphysialis Multiplex, J. Bone & Joint Surg., *37-B*, 228, 1955.

McCullough, J. A. L. and Sutherland, C. G.: Epiphyseal Dysplasia Punticularis (Stippled Epiphyses), Radiology, *34*, 131, 1940.

Mosekilde, E.: "Stippled Epiphyses" in Newborn and in Infants, Acta radiol., *37*, 291, 1952.

Paul, L. W.: Punctate Epiphyseal Dysplasia, Am. J. Roentgenol., *71*, 941, 1954.

Raap, G.: Chondrodystrophia Calcificans Congenita, Am. J. Roentgenol., *49*, 77, 1943.

Savignac, E. M.: Chondrodystrophia Calcificans Congenita, Radiology, *58*, 415, 1952.

Sheach, J. M. and Middlemiss, J. H.: Dysplasia Epiphysialis Punctata, Brit. J. Radiol., *29*, 111, 1956.

Epiphysial Dysplasia Multiplex

This occurs as a rare, possibly familial congenital anomaly which involves several or many epiphyses, principally those of the hips, shoulders, ankles, and less often the hands and feet. The condition is discovered when difficulty in walking, pain and stiffness of the various joints brings the patient to his physician. The patients usually are short, and have thick broad fingers and hands as well as other joint deformities. The radiologic changes are most evident in the growing epiphyses of the long bones, where flattening, irregularity of ossification and distortion of the bone ends are most evident. A characteristic change which sometimes suggests the diagnosis is a deficiency of the lateral aspect of the distal tibial epiphyses, resulting in an irregular articular surface which is obliquely directed downwards and medially. The slanted appearance of the distal end of the tibia and the associated bony overgrowth of the subjacent astragalus is bilateral. Other joints also are affected, and arthritic changes are apparent later in life, especially in the weight-bearing joints. The carpal and tarsal bones are hypoplastic. Delay in the ossification of the epiphyses occurs bilaterally, and these structures also are hypoplastic.

Changes in the spine are not a particularly striking part of this condition. Irregularities like those seen with Scheuermann's disease, narrowing of the intervertebral discs and wedging and irregularities of the surfaces of the vertebral bodies in the thoracic region have been observed.

References

Christensen, W. R., Lin, R. K. and Berghout, J.: Dysplasia Epiphysialis Multiplex, Am. J. Roentgenol., *74*, 1059, 1955.

Fairbank, H. A. T.: Generalized Disease of Skeleton. Proc. Royal Soc. Med., *28*, 1611, 1935.
————: Dysplasia Epiphysialis Multiplex, Brit. J. Surg., *34*, 225, 1947.

Gram, P. B., Fleming, J. L., Frame, B. and Fine, G.: Metaphyseal Chondrodysplasia of Jansen, J. Bone & Joint Surg., *41-A*, 951, 1959.

Jansen, M.: Über atypische Chondrodystrophie (Achondroplasie) und über eine noch nicht beschriebene angeborene Wachstumstorung des Knochensystems: Metaphysäre Dysostosis, Ztschr. f. orthop. Chir., *61*, 253, 1934.

Leeds, N. E.: Epiphysial Dysplasia Multiplex, Am. J. Roentgenol., *84*, 506, 1960.

Waugh, W.: Dysplasia Epiphysialis Multiplex in Three Sisters, J. Bone & Joint Surg., *34-B*, 82 1952.

Progressive Diaphyseal Dysplasia

The disease, also known as Engelmann's disease and osteopathia hyperostotica (sclerotisans) multiplex infantalis is characterized by a progressive symmetrical thickening of the shafts of the long bones, associated with retarded growth and weakness. Particularly affected are the humeral and the femoral shafts and the bones of the forearms and legs. The vault and the base of the skull may show a diffuse thickening which sometimes reaches considerable proportions.

Cortical thickening of the long bones involves mainly the shafts, with little change at the metaphyseal or epiphyseal ends. In some the entire shaft of the bone is affected, so that there is a cylindrical configuration without the usual localized spindle-shaped swelling limited to the diaphyses. The disease is incident to excessive periosteal activity, and the bulging sclerotic shafts of the long bones are usually symmetric. Endosteal overactivity also appears, with thickening of bone encroaching on the medullary cavity. The surfaces of the bone become irregular. As the patient grows older, the density of the involved bone increases.

Involvement of the pelvis and spine is unusual in Engelmann's disease. Occasional reports of vertebral involvement are seen, as, for instance, in the case reported by Mottram and Hill (1965). They followed a patient over a $12\frac{1}{2}$-year period, and noted that on the last examination, when the child was 14 years old, a "bone within bone" appearance of the vertebral bodies had appeared. Some flattening of vertebral bodies was noted by Lennon and coworkers (1961).

References

Bingold, A. C.: Engelmann's Disease; Osteopathia Hyperostotica (Sclerotisans) Multiplex Infantalis; Progressive Diaphyseal Dysplasia. Brit. J. Surg., *37*, 266, 1960.

Mottram, M. E. and Hill, H. A.: Diaphyseal Dysplasia, Am. J. Roentgenol., *95*, 162, 1965.

Neuhauser, E. B. D., Schwachman, H., Wittenborg, M. and Cohen, J.: Progressive Diaphyseal Dysplasia, Radiology, *51*, 11, 1948.

Lennon, E. A., Schechter, M. M. and Hornabrook, R. W.: Engelmann's Disease, J. Bone & Joint Surg., *43-B*, 273, 1961.

METAPHYSEAL DYSPLASIA (Pyle's syndrome)

This is a rare familial condition characterized by clubbing of the metaphyseal ends of the long bones, which assume a widened, somewhat tapered appearance with thinning of the cortex proximally and distally. The long bones may become bowed, and transverse lines of increased density are observed crossing the widened areas. The origin of this condition is unknown. The thinning renders them susceptible to fractures and stress deformities. In the cases reported by Feld, Switzer, Dexter and Langer (1955) incomplete pneumatization of the paranasal sinuses and thickening of the dorsum sellae with a small sella turcica were observed. These authors also noted that the vertebral bodies in one of their cases presented some lengthening in the anteroposterior diameter. Kowins (1954) described marked hyperostosis involving the facial bones and the base of the skull, prognathism and deficient dentition. The spine in his cases revealed some loss of the normal dorsal and lumbar curves. Caffey (1961) mentions a 12-year-old boy who had sclerosis and flattening of all the vertebral bodies.

References

Bakwin, H. and Krida, A.: Familial Metaphyseal Dysplasia, Am. J. Dis. Child., *53*, 1521, 1937.

Caffey, J.: *Pediatric X-ray Diagnosis*, Chicago, Year Book Medical Publishers, Inc., 1967.

Feld, H., Switzer, R. A., Dexter, M. W. and Langer, E. M.: Familial Metaphyseal Dysplasia, Radiology, *65*, 206, 1955.

Hormel, M. B., Gershon-Cohen, J. and Jones, D. T.: Familial Metaphyseal Dysplasia, Am. J. Roentgenol., *70*, 413, 1953.

Jackson, W. P. U., Albright, F., Drewry, G., Hanelin, J. and Rubin, M. I.: Metaphyseal Dysplasia, Epiphyseal Dysplasia, Diaphyseal Dysplasia and Related Conditions, Arch. Int. Med., *94*, 871, 1954.

Jackson, W. P. U., Hanelin, J. and Albright, F.: Metaphyseal Dysplasia, Epiphyseal Dysplasia, Diaphyseal Dysplasia and Related Conditions, Arch. Int. Med., *94*, 886, 1954.

Kowins, C.: Familial Metaphyseal Dysplasia (Pyle's Disease), Brit. J. Radiol., *27*, 670, 1954.

Pyle, E.: Case of Unusual Bone Development, J. Bone & Joint Surg., *13*, 874, 1931.

Taybi, H.: Generalized Skeletal Dysplasia with Multiple Anomalies. A Note on Pyle's Disease, Am. J. Roentgenol., *88*, 450, 1962.

METAPHYSEAL DYSOSTOSIS

This is another derangement of metaphyseal ossification which involves the long bones. The normal bone is replaced by irregular masses of calcified epiphyseal cartilage, and the disturbed endochondral bone formation results in shortening of the limbs, while the configuration of the trunk is not affected to the same extent. There is a significant genetic element in the transmission of this condition, as indicated in the recent report of involvement of 18 individuals in a single family (Stickler and co-workers, 1962). The epiphyseal changes simulate those seen in rickets, and confusion with vitamin-D resistant rickets can be anticipated. Miller and Paul (1964) point out that the junction of the epiphysis and metaphysis is indistinct in vitamin D resistant rickets, while in metaphyseal dysostosis the margins of bone and cartilage are irregular but quite sharply marginated. The metaphyseal fragmentation likewise is considerably more advanced in the presence of metaphyseal dysostosis. The shafts of the long bones present changes suggestive of osteomalacia (Daeschner and co-workers, 1960). Vertebral involvement in a $12\frac{1}{2}$-year-old male patient was observed by Schmidt and his co-workers (1963). They described the presence of a dorsolumbar kyphosis with generalized osteoporosis. Platyspondyly of the thoracic vertebral bodies was noted, and the lumbar bodies were deformed, with anterior protuberance of their median portions. In most instances, however, the spine and skull are not affected, although some hypoplasia of the pelvis may be present.

A milder form of this disturbance was described by Schmid (1949). Combined metaphyseal and epiphyseal dysostosis was reported in 2 patients by Kozlowski and Budzinska (1966).

References

Daeschner, C. W., Singleton, E. B., Hill, L. L. and Dodge, W. F.: Metaphyseal Dysostosis, J. Pediat., *57*, 844, 1960.

Kozlowski, K. and Budzinska, A.: Combined Metaphyseal and Epiphyseal Dysostosis. Am. J. Roentgenol., *97*, 21, 1966.

Miller, S. M. and Paul. L. W.: Roentgen Observations in Familial Metaphyseal Dysostosis, Radiology, *83*, 665, 1964.

Rosenbloom, A. L. and Smith, D. W.: The Natural History of Metaphyseal Dysostosis, J. Pediat., *66*, 857, 1965.

Schmid, F.: Beitrag zur Dysostosis Enchondralis Metaphysaria. Monatschr. f. Kinderh., *97*, 393, 1949.

Schmidt, B. J., Beçak, W., Beçak, M. L., Soibelman, I., Queiroz, A. da S., Lorga, A. P., Secaf, F., Antonio, C. F. and Carvalho, A. de A.: Metaphyseal Dysostosis, J. Pediat., *63*, 106, 1963.

MARFAN'S SYNDROME (Hyperchondroplasia, arachnodactyly)

The underlying defect in Marfan's syndrome is unknown. The basic lesion is excessive hyperplasia of cartilage, and consequent overgrowth of the tubular bones. However, the concomitant lesions in the cardiovascular system and the ocular abnormalities indicate that some mesenchymal disorder exists. The classical clinical picture of a thin, tall individual with long, tapering fingers who moves awkwardly and appears older than his chronological age is well known. These people usually also have a high arched palate, large ears and lenticular disturbances. Aortic aneurysms occur frequently, and rupture may lead to early death. Radiographic examination of the limbs are in accord with the elongated, thin bony structures. The skull usually is normal. The pelvis may present some hypoplasia of the iliac bones.

The full spectrum of Marfan's disease is not encountered constantly. Wilner and Finby (1964) caution against using the term arachnodactyly as synonymous with Marfan's syndrome, pointing out that the complete picture was present in but 4 of their 18 patients.

While the trunk in patients with Marfan's syndrome appears unremarkable, changes are noted in the vertebrae which are in accord with the generalized increase in the length of the various bones. The vertebral bodies are elongated, presenting a tall appearance. The pedicles are long, so that the width of the spinal canal is increased, while the interpedicular spaces are not conspicuously altered. Increased indentations into the dorsal aspect of the vertebral bodies has been observed. As a consequence of the laxity of the ligamentous and muscular structures scoliosis is frequently noted, together with varying roundness of the thoracic dorsal curve. The intervertebral discs are narrowed, and irregularities in the apposing surfaces of the vertebral bodies can be identified (Fig. 167).

Nelson (1958) called attention to the presence of other congenital defects, including spina bifida, congenital fusion and underdevelopment of the spinous processes. In 2 patients out of 5 seen by me, additional vertebral changes included congenital fusion of the second and third cervical vertebrae in one and a sagitally cleft vertebra in another. Narrowing of the pedicles and widening of the interpedicular spaces of a haphazard nature, with increase in the depth or width of the spinal canal or both also can be seen.

References

Nelson, J. D.: The Marfan Syndrome, with Special Reference to Congenital Enlargement of the Spinal Canal. Brit. J. Radiol., *31*, 561, 1958.

Wilner, H. I. and Finby, N.: Skeletal Manifestations in the Marfan Syndrome. J.A.M.A., *187*, 490, 1964.

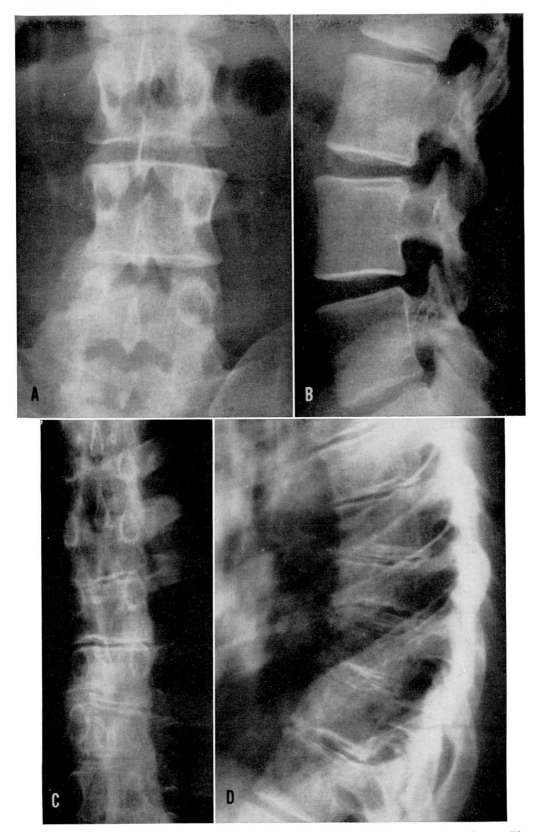

Fig. 167. *A*, AP roentgenogram of the lumbar spine in a 23-year-old man with Marfan's syndrome. The vertical bodies are elongated. The increase in height is better seen on the lateral view, *B*. The thoracic spine presents irregularities and narrowing of the midthoracic discs and a mild dorsum rotundum, *C* and *D*. The midthoracic vertebrae are moderately narrowed in comparison with the other segments, particularly the lumbar vertebrae. A mild scalloping is seen dorsally in the midlumbar segments, *B*.

INFANTILE CORTICAL HYPEROSTOSIS
(Caffey's disease)

In 1945 Caffey and Silverman reported on a syndrome which they designated as infantile cortical hyperostosis. The condition is of unknown etiology, and usually manifests itself in infancy by a thickening of the periosteum in the shafts of the long bones of the arms and legs, the short bones of the hand, the clavicles, and particularly the mandibles. Similar changes have been observed in the ribs. No involvement of the vertebral column has been reported, aside from the observation made by MacLeod, Douglas and Mahaffy (1965) of a "double contour" of the lower dorsal and upper lumbar vertebrae in a 4-month-old male patient.

In the cases observed by us no changes other than those reported in the literature were observed.

References

Barba, W. P., II. and Freriks, D. J.: The Familial Occurrence of Infantile Cortical Hyperostosis in Utero, J. Pediat., *42*, 141, 1953.

Caffey, J. and Silverman, W. A.: Infantile Cortical Hyperostosis, Am. J. Roentgenol., *54*, 1, 1945.

Cayler G. C. and Peterson, C. A.: Infantile Cortical Hyperostosis, J. Dis. Childhood, *91*, 119, 1956.

MacLeod, W., Douglas, D. M. and Mahaffy, R. G.: Infantile Cortical Hyperostosis, Clin. Radiol., *16*, 269, 1965.

Walley, J. A.: A Case of Infantile Cortical Hyperostosis Affecting Only the Clavicle and Scapula, J. Bone & Joint Surg., *35-B*, 427, 1953.

DOWN'S SYNDROME (Mongolism, trisomy 21 anomaly)

The relationship between chromosomal abnormalities and Down's syndrome was first demonstrated by Lejeune (1959). These patients have a total of 47 rather than 46 chromosomes. The extra chromosome is a small, acrocentric chromosome, either number 21 or 22, and the affected infant is trisomic for this chromosome. The condition arises as an error in the distribution of chromosomes at the time of cell division, either as a translocation or a nondisjunction phenomenon. The risk for this is greatly increased in older mothers. The understanding of chromosomal aberrations in the development of congenital defects has clarified to an appreciable extent understanding of certain conditions (Table 1).

TABLE 1. DIFFERENTIAL DIAGNOSIS OF CHROMOSOMAL DEFECTS. (From Singleton, E. B., Rosenberg, H. S. and Yang, S-J., The Radiographic Manifestations of Chromosomal Abnormalities, Radiol. Clin. North America, *2*, 281, 1964.)

I. Congenital defects

  A. Sex chromosomes

    1. Chromatin-positive phenotypic male
      *a. Klinefelter's syndrome—47 XXY
      b. True hermaphrodite—46 XX
      c. Female pseudohermaphrodite—46 XX

    2. Chromatin-negative phenotypic female
      *a. Turner's syndrome—45 XO
      b. Male pseudohermaphrodite—46 XY
      c. Testicular feminization—46 SY

    3. Miscellaneous
      *a. Triplo X ("Superfemale")—47 XXX
      *b. Multiple X syndromes—XXXX, XXY, etc.
      *c. Mosaics

  B. Somatic chromosomes
    *1. Trisomy, 21–22, mongolism—47
    *2. Trisomy, 13–15–47
    *3. Trisomy, 16–18–47

II. Acquired defects
  A. Chronic granulocytic leukemia.

* The true chromosomal abnormalities are indicated by asterisks.

A mongoloid infant usually is small at birth, and in about one-fifth of cases is premature. The skull is small, with poor development of the occipital region. The palpebral fissures slant upwards and outwards, and the eyes do not appear properly set into the orbits. The tongue protrudes, the neck is broad and the shoulders sloping. The hands are short, with broad stubby fingers and a shortened, incurved fifth finger with the second phalanx rudimentary in about half the patients. There is a high, arched configuration to the roof of the mouth, and the cribriform plate is high in the cranial cavity. The development of the paranasal sinuses is retarded. The calvarium is thin, and the sphenoid bone rotated upwards and backwards in relation to the clivus. The nasal bridge is depressed, and the ears appear crumpled. While in its complete form a mongoloid infant can be identified fairly accurately, the diagnosis is by no means easily established in many cases.

Concomitant cardiovascular defects include atrial and ventricular septal defects and persistent atrioventricular canal. Gastrointestinal congenital anomalies also are frequent, including duodenal atresia, esophageal atresia, malrotation of the bowel, and annular pancreas. The association of leukemia with Down's syndrome also is in excess to that observed in the normal population.

In the first year of life identification of changes in the hips and pelvis are helpful in diagnosis. Caffey and Ross (1956) reported a triad consisting of flaring of the iliac wings, flattening of the acetabular roofs and tapering of the ischia as being characteristic of mongolism. The iliac index, determined as the sum of the acetabular angle and the iliac angle, was regarded as the most sensitive indication. The normal iliac index in newborns varies from 69 to 97 degrees, while in mongoloid infants the range is from 49 to 87 degrees, with an average of 62 degrees. Astley (1963) regards the diagnosis of mongolism as likely if the iliac index is less than 60 degrees, and that the infant most likely is normal if the index is over 78 degrees.

Skeletal maturation is often delayed in mongolism. The protruding tongue and drooling from the mouth usually are present in more advanced cases. The condition usually terminates in death before adolescence. The children are usually small for their age, are mentally retarded and have poorly developed musculature so that lack of coordination soon becomes evident.

Changes in the spine are rather subtle. As a result of poor muscular tone scoliosis becomes evident, and in some patients with large protuberant abdomens a moderate dorsal convexity appears. Forward displacement of the atlantooccipital joint together with an abnormally thin and small

atlas was noted by Spitzer, Rabinowitch and Wybar (1961) in 9 of their 29 mongoloid patients from 8 to 49 years old. An increase in the height of the vertebral bodies, together with a decrease in their anteroposterior diameters and a broad concavity of the anterior margins (Fig. 168) was noted by Rabinowitz and Mosely (1964). Martel and Tishler (1966) attributed displacement and increased mobility of the atlas to a possible malformation or aplasia of the transverse ligament. In 14 out of 79 patients they observed Scheuermann-like lesions in the cervical and dorsolumbar spine in young adults, but not in children.

TURNER'S SYNDROME

Another disorder associated with chromosomal defects is Turner's syndrome. The karyotype pattern consists of 45 chromosomes, an XO type—a monosomy defect. This occurs in females with dysgenesis of the gonads and the external genitalia, and is accompanied by primary amenorrhea, minimal sexual development, short stature, and increased pituitary excretion of follicle-stimulating hormone. There is marked variation in the associated clinical picture. Some patients are almost normal, others are grossly abnormal with subnormal intelligence, webbing of the neck, a tendency to short stature and epiphyseal dysplasia. Diminished mineralization of bone which is quite advanced in older patients is another concomitant of Turner's syndrome. Congenital cardiac deformities occur in about 20 per cent of these patients, the most common being coarctation of the aorta. Other changes appear in the wrists and fingers, with angulation of the distal ends of the radii and relative shortening of the fourth metacarpals. The knees present a vara-type deformity of the tibias with depression and medial prominence of the proximal tibial epiphyses. There is relative elongation and bowing of the fibulae. The maturation of the carpal centers is normal up until about 15 years of age, and the centers appear at

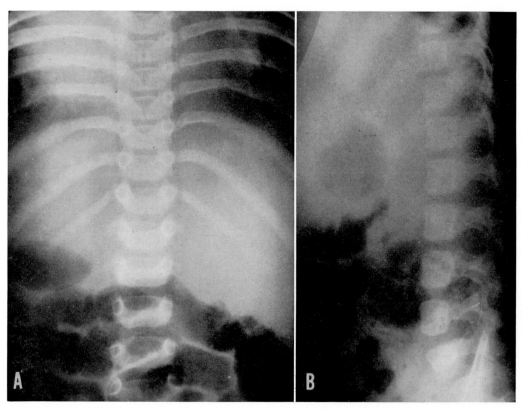

FIG. 168. *A*, AP film of the thoracolumbar spine in a 6-month-old male infant with Down's disease. Aside from a rather ovoid configuration of the bodies no specific change is seen. On the lateral study, *B*, elongation of the vertebral bodies becomes visible. The vertebrae are narrow, especially the fifth lumbar segment.

the usual time. Fusion of the epiphyses, however, may be delayed.

A "positive metacarpal sign" is associated with shortening of the fourth and fifth metacarpals. This is determined by a line drawn tangential to the distal ends of the heads of the fourth and fifth metacarpals. A positive metacarpal sign is considered present when the line passes through the head of the third metacarpal. When the line is tangential to the head of the third metacarpal, the sign is considered borderline. Keats and Burns (1964) regard the occurrence of a positive metacarpal sign as significant if it is seen in only one generation. However, when it appears in more than one generation in the same family, no endocrine significance is attached to it.

Changes in the spine in Turner's disease include scoliosis, irregularities in the apposing surfaces of the vertebral bodies, demineralized vertebrae, and a variety of relatively minor congenital defects including fusion of two upper cervical vertebrae, hypoplasia of the first cervical vertebra and diminution in the size of its posterior arch. The vertebral bodies present a squared-off appearance. The intervertebral discs, particularly in the thoracic spine, may be somewhat narrowed posteriorly (Fig. 169). Sclerotic changes along the sacro-iliac joints also are present occasionally.

Turner's syndrome has also been described in male patients, accompanied by gonadal dysgenesis, sexual infantilism, short stature and various somatic abnormalities. Mental retardation, renal and ocular defects and cardiovascular malformations occur. It is

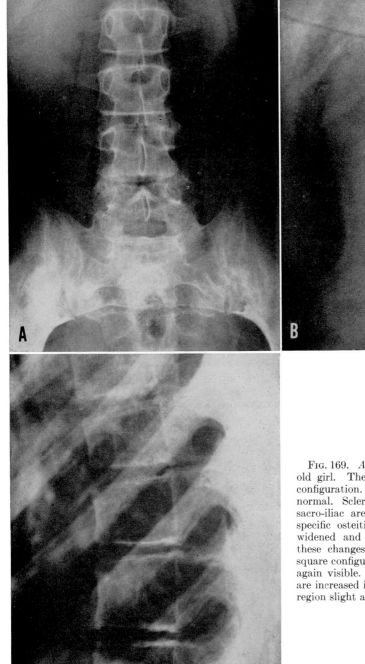

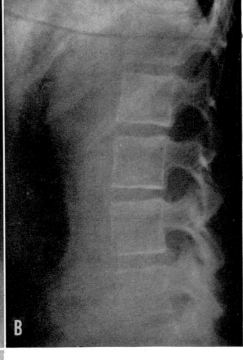

Fig. 169. *A*, Turner's syndrome in a 16-year-old girl. The vertebral bodies are cuboid in configuration. The intervertebral discs are normal. Sclerotic changes are seen in the right sacro-iliac area, probably incident to a nonspecific osteitis. The left sacro-iliac joint is widened and irregular. The significance of these changes is open to question. *B*, The square configuration of the lumbar vertebrae is again visible. *C*, The thoracic vertebrae also are increased in height, but in the midthoracic region slight anterior wedging is present.

of interest that coarctation is infrequent in males with Turner's syndrome. The spine changes are much the same as seen in females (Meyerson and Gwinup, 1965).

Increase in the heights of the vertebral bodies and vertebral fusions also have been reported in the trisomy 18 syndrome (Ozonoff, Steinbach and Mamunes, 1964).

References

Benda, C. E.: *Mongolism and Cretinism*, New York, Grune & Stratton, 1949.

Caffey, J. and Ross, S.: Mongolism (Mongoloid Deficiency) During Early Infancy—Some Newly Recognized Diagnostic Changes in the Pelvic Bones. Pediatrics, *17*, 642, 1956.

Finby, N. and Archibald, R. M.: Skeletal Abnormalities Associated with Gonadal Dysgenesis, Am. J. Roentgenol., *89*, 1222, 1963.

Keats, T. E. and Burns, T. W.: The radiographic Manifestations of Gonadal Dysgenesis. Radiol. Clin. North America, *2*, 297, 1964.

Martel, W. and Tishler, J. M.: Observations on the Spine in Mongoloidism. Am. J. Roentgenol., *97*, 630, 1966.

Meyerson, L. and Gwinup, G.: Turner's Syndrome in the Male, Arch. Int. Med., *116*, 125, 1965.

Miller, R. W.: Down's Syndrome (Mongolism), Other Congenital Malformations and Cancers Among the Sibs of Leukemic Children, New England J. Med., *268*, 393, 1963.

Ozonoff, M. B., Steinbach, H. L. and Mamunes, P.: The Trisomy 18 Syndrome, Am. J. Roentgenol., *91*, 618, 1964.

Rabinowitz, J. G. and Moseley, J. E.: The Lateral Lumbar Spine in Down's Syndrome, Radiology, *83*, 74, 1964.

Singleton, E. B., Rosenberg, H. S. and Yang, S-J.: The Radiographic Manifestations of Chromosomal Abnormalities, Radiol. Clin. North America, *2*, 281, 1964.

Spitzer, R., Rabinowitch, J. Y. and Wybar, K. C.: A Study of the Abnormalities of the Skull, Teeth and Lenses in Mongolism, Canad. M.A.J., *84*, 567, 1961.

MELORHEOSTOSIS

This is a rare bony disturbance characterized by an unusual distribution of hyperostosis dispersed along the sides of bones of the limbs comparable to tallow dripping down a candle. It is usually confined to a single limb, with the hyperostosis selecting only one side of the bone. Limitation of the movements of the joints of the affected limb

has been observed in about half the reported cases (Fairbanks, 1948). Scleroderma, with fibrosis and thickening of the muscles and other soft tissues may be responsible for this stiffness. Involvement of the spine is rare. Carpender, Baker, Perry and Outland (1943) reported an 18-year-old female in whom the lateral aspects of the vertebral bodies extending from the seventh thoracic to the first lumbar vertebrae showed the striations characteristic of melorheostosis. Masserini (1944) also noted vertebral involvement with a dense, patchy well circumscribed type of deposit of compact bone in the vertebral bodies without distortion or symptoms.

References

Carpender, J. W. J., Baker, D. R., Perry, S. P. and Outland, T.: Melorheostosis, Am. J. Roentgenol., *49*, 398, 1943.

Fairbank, H. A. T.: Melorheostosis, J. Bone & Joint Surg., *30-B*, 533, Z1948.

Kraft, E.: Pathology of Monomelic Flowing Hyperostosis or Melorheostosis, Radiology, *20*, 47, 1933.

Spiegel, M. B. and Koiransky, G. H.: Melorheostosis Léri, Am. J. Roentgenol., *64*, 789, 1950.

MULTIPLE ENCHONDROMATOSIS (Ollier's disease, dyschondroplasia)

Multiple enchondromatosis is a non-hereditary developmental error characterized by multiple cartilaginous enchondroses which represent portions of epiphyseal plates which failed to develop into normal bone and had become incorporated into mature bone. These enchondromatous deposits are seen mainly in the long bones, and may cause expansion and consequent gross deformities. Occasionally exostoses are present. With the onset of puberty growth of the enchondromas terminates and calcification within the lesions results in an irregularly stippled radiolucent pattern. Dyschondroplasia with multiple hemangiomas is designated as Maffucci's syndrome. The disease rarely affects the vertebral column, but I have noted two instances in which small radiolucencies were observed in the transverse processes of a lumbar vertebra.

References

Carleton, A., Elkington, J. St. C., Greenfield, J. G. and Robb-Smith, A. H. T.: Maffucci's Syndrome (Dyschondroplasia with Hemangiomata), Quart. J. Med., *11*, 203, 1942.

Cohn, I.: Dyschondroplasia, Ann. Surg., *123*, 673, 1946.

Murray, A. M. and Cruickshank, B.: Dyschondroplasia, J. Bone & Joint Surg., *42-B*, 344, 1960.

Krause, G. R.: Dyschondroplasia with Hemangiomata (Maffucci's Syndrome), Am. J. Roentgenol., *52*, 620, 1944.

Kuzma, J. F. and King, J. M.: Dyschondroplasia with Hemangiomatosis (Maffucci's Syndrome), Arch. Path., *46*, 74, 1948.

Strang, C. and Rannie, I.: Dyschondroplasia with Haemangiomata (Maffucci's Syndrome), J. Bone & Joint Surg., *32-B*, 376, 1950.

TUBEROUS SCLEROSIS

This condition is considered a congenital hamartial ectodermoses, one of a group which includes von Recklinghausen's neurofibromatosis, Sturge-Weber syndrome and Hippel-Lindau's disease. The underlying potato-like growths vary in size from 0.5 to 3.0 cm in diameter. These occur most frequently in the cerebral hemispheres, although other parts of the central nervous system may be involved. The masses project into the ventricles from immediately beneath the ependyma, and calcification may occur within them. The pyramidal cells and glia are most affected. The condition is associated with epilepsy, mental deficiency, adenoma sebaceum, congenital tumors of the eye and many visceral organs. In some the endocranial lesions dominates the picture, while in others the visceral tumors are responsible for the patient's complaints. Involvement of the skeleton is infrequent.

Radiologic changes include diffuse and widely varying skeletal manifestations of cystic, sclerotic or combined lesions. These occur as periosteal thickening, fragmentation of cortical layers of bone, sclerotic mottling of the skull, rarefied changes in the skull, and cyst formations in the terminal phalanges. The vertebrae may contain multiple sclerotic foci scattered through the whole of the spine and pelvis, including the neural arches. These can be confused with osteoplastic metastatic lesions. Occasionally a cystic rarefaction appears in a vertebral body.

References

Ackermann, A. J.: Pulmonary and Osseous Manifestations of Tuberous Sclerosis, Am. J. Roentgenol., *51*, 315, 1944.

Ashby, D. W. and Ramage, D.: Lesions of the Vertebrae and Innominate Bones in Tuberous Sclerosis, Brit. J. Radiol., *30*, 274, 1957.

Gottlieb, J. S. and Lavine, G. R.: Tuberous Sclerosis with Unusual Lesions of the Bones, Arch. Neurol. & Psychiat., *33*, 379, 1935.

Holt, J. F. and Dickerson, W. W.: Osseous Lesions of Tuberous Sclerosis, Radiology, *58*, 1, 1952.

Whitaker, P. H.: Radiological Manifestations of Tuberous Sclerosis, Brit. J. Radiol., *32*, 152, 1959.

PROGERIA (Werner's Syndrome)

This is a condition of premature old age and represents a rare form of senilism which has a rapid onset, with retention of normal intelligence and without a perceptible cause. Loss of hair, short stature, a small bird-like face, shrivelling of the nails, congenital cataracts and emaciation, together with a loss of subcutaneous fat and precocious arteriosclerosis (Moehleg, 1946) are prominent. Roentgenologic examinations usually reveal diffuse osteoporosis with swelling of the epiphyses and no change in the centers of ossification. Scleroderma together with hypoplasia of the terminal phalanges of the hands and feet may occur. The skull may be rather large with slightly separated suture lines. Very little is mentioned about the spine in these rare cases. Talbot, Butler, Pratt, MacLachlan and Tannheimer (1945) reported a case in which they had carried out metabolic studies during the year preceding death from coronary thrombosis at $7\frac{1}{2}$ years in a case of progeria. Roentgenograms of the spine in this patient showed an unusual degree of anterior notching in the lateral views. At necropsy no cause for the condition could be ascertained. Tanenbaum (1965) mentions spondylotic deformities of the spine as being present.

References

Jacobson, H. G., Rifkin, H. and Zuckerman, F. D.: Werner's Syndrome, Radiology, *74*, 373, 1960.
Moehlig, R. C.: Progeria with Nanism and Congenital Cataracts, J.A.M.A., *132*, 640, 1946.
Rosenthal, I. M., Bronstein, I. P., Dallenbach, F. D., Pruzansky, S. and Rosenwald, A. K.: Progeria, Pediatrics, *18*, 565, 1956.
Talbot, N. B., Butler, A. M., Pratt, E. L., McClachlan, E. A. and Tannheimer, J.: Progeria, Am. J. Dis. Child., *69*, 267, 1945.
Tanenbaum, M. H.: Werner's Syndrome. Progeria of the Adult, Arch. Int. Med., *116*, 499, 1965.

HYPOPHOSPHATASIA

Hypophosphatasia is a familial condition inherited as an autosomal recessive trait, characterized mainly by rachitic-like deformities in children, associated with low serum and tissue alkaline phosphatase activity and defective bone formation. Hypercalcemia and renal damage are often present. The presence of phosphoethanolamine in the urine and plasma are significant diagnostic signs. The disease may begin *in utero*, and manifests itself in neonatal life or later. In the newborn severe deformities of the extremities are present, together with soft skeletal structures and a globular skull which has markedly deficient ossification. The calcification of the skeleton likewise is scanty, the ends of the bones showing widely separated areas corresponding to the bony deficiencies. Multiple fractures occur. Infants so afflicted rarely survive.

When the disease appears after an initial period of apparent normalcy, symptoms of anorexia, vomiting, hypotonia and failure to thrive develop, together with cyanosis and convulsions. In these patients the joint structures are prominent, the skull enlarged and rachitic-like changes are present in the epiphyses and costochondral junctions. If the patient survives, the skeletal changes interfere with walking and standing, and craniostenosis appears. In children in whom the onset of hypophosphatasia takes place after about 18 months of age similar bony changes are present, and the development of the child is retarded. Craniostenosis is less frequent as a later manifestation.

Dentition is deficient in both groups. The pathologic changes have been described as resembling osteogenesis imperfecta in the newborn, while in older patients there is resemblance to rickets. The cause of death is usually renal failure. In those who survive residual and sometimes prominent skeletal deformities persist.

The vertebral column of newborns with hypophosphatasia partakes in the marked failure of ossification. In those who survive deficient calcification is manifested by delayed and irregular bone formation, while still later relatively minor vertebral malformations with intact bodies and occasionally dorsolumbar angulations are present.

References

Bonucci, E. and Agostinelli, O.: Radiological and Microradiographic Features in a Case of Congenital Hypophosphatasia, Radiol. Clin. Biol., *35*, 80, 1966.
Currarino, G., Neuhauser, E. B. D., Reyersbach, G. C. and Sobel, E. H.: Hypophosphatasia, Am. J. Roentgenol., *78*, 392, 1957.
James, W. and Moule, B.: Hypophosphatasia, Clin. Radiol., *17*, 368, 1966.
Rathbun, J. C.: "Hypophosphatasia," New Developmental Anomaly, Am. J. Dis. Child., *75*, 822, 1948.

Endocrine Disturbances

PRIMARY HYPERPARATHYROIDISM

Albright and Reifenstein (1948) defined primary hyperparathyroidism as a condition in which excess parathyroid hormone is manufactured. The parathyroid glands usually exist as four discrete structures, two beneath the inferior aspect of each lobe of the thyroid. The underlying pathologic change may be either a diffuse hypertrophy of all the parathyroid tissue or the development of single or multiple adenomas. A small number of malignant parathyroid tumors associated with hyperparathyroidism also have been reported (Gentile, Skinner and Ashburn, 1941; Meyer and Ragens, 1943; Stephenson 1950; Barnes, 1961). Certain chemical findings are characteristic of hyperparathyroidism. These include increased serum calcium and decreased inorganic phosphorus, excessive excretion of calcium and inorganic phosphorus in the urine, and in those cases in which the skeletal system is extensively involved, an increased serum alkaline phosphatase content. Hypercalciuria may be a less prominent indication of hyperparathyroidism because it does not take place if filtration through the glomeruli is impaired, as occurs in many patients with this condition. Hypercalciuria also appears with renal calculi even if parathyroid activity is normal. Because of the increased excretion of calcium, calcium phosphate and oxalate stones are frequently present. Conversely, the presence of kidney stones should bring to mind the possibility of hyperparathyroidism. The effect of hyperparathyroidism on the kidney represents the greatest danger to the patient, first because of renal tubular damage causing dehydration and electrolyte abnormalities and then because of irreversible effects of hypercalcemia, hypercalciuria and nephrocalcinosis in producing glomerular insufficiency. The effect of hyperparathyroidism on bone is sometimes spectacular, but subtle changes are more frequent and in many instances no visible osseous changes can be identified.

Hyperparathyroidism influences the phosphate metabolism by lowering the renal threshold for the excretion of phosphorus in the urine. This in turn is accompanied by a fall in the blood serum phosphate. The serum calcium increases in order to keep the relationship between the serum calcium and phosphorus constant, thereby mobilizing calcium phosphate from the bone with consequent hypercalciuria.

The original description of osteitis fibrosa was made by von Recklinghausen, who considered the change a primary disease of the skeleton. The association of osteitis fibrosa with a parathyroid tumor was noted in 1904 by Askanazy (Snapper, 1949) and experimental evidence of the influence of the parathyroid glands on calcium metabolism was reported by Erdheim (1907). Erdheim believed that the hyperplasia of these glands

was a compensatory mechanism to permit calcium mobilization from the skeleton replacing calcium lost in the urine and stool. In 1926 Mandl reported the first case successfully operated upon for the removal of a parathyroid tumor. Mandl had transplanted four parathyroid glands from a moribund patient to a patient who preoperatively showed extensive osteitis fibrosa. This was done to test Erdheim's concept that parathyroid hyperplasia was a compensatory mechanism. Following the operation the patient became worse, whereupon Mandl not only removed the transplanted glands, but explored the patient's mediastinum and removed the offending parathyroid tumor. Operation was followed by a rapid cessation of clinical symptoms and return of the blood calcium to a normal level. The first case in this country of hyperparathyroid tumor with surgical removal of a lesion from the mediastinum was described by Hannon, Shorr, McClellan and DuBois (1930). The monograph by Shelling summarized all available data up to 1935.

In hyperplasia of the parathyroids the growth is mainly of the clear cells. With adenomas the chief, or principal, cells multiply in acinar formations, with intervening areas of degeneration and small cyst formations. The presence of a small tumor of clear cells surrounded by a shell of normal parathyroid tissue is considered quite characteristic of an adenoma. The pathologic changes were described in detail by Castleman and Mallory (1935).

The clinical picture of hyperparathyroidism apparently is the same no matter whether the clear cells or the chief cells predominate. It is currently considered that the water clear cells of the parathyroid glands represent the stage of greatest hormonal activity. The chief, or principal, cells indicate a resting stage. Young chief cells, which are water clear transitional chief cells, are regarded as possibly being activated principal cells. The eosinophilic cells found in the parathyroid glands have no known endocrine activity. In a review of 63 cases,

Black (1948) encountered single adenomas in 56 cases, multiple adenomas in 3, and diffuse primary hyperplasia in 4. Generalized osteitis fibrosa cystica was present in less than 40 per cent of his cases. Thirty-five per cent had renal complications, but no evident bone disease, and 20 per cent had bone changes without renal complications. About 20 per cent had both renal and bone disturbances. He considered the urinary changes more frequent and more important than the bony complications.

Hyperparathyroidism occurs in either sex, but is rather more frequent in females of middle age. However, cases have been observed in children and elderly individuals. Familial instances have been reported (Schachner and co-workers, 1966). The condition may exist in a subclinical form for several years, becoming evident only when manifestations secondary to demineralization of bone results in weakening of these structures, with consequent deformities and pathologic fractures. Coburn (1944) reported such a case followed for 15 years. The patients may also develop a peculiar, and sometimes profound, muscular atonicity due to hypercalcemia. Anorexia, nausea, vomiting and abdominal pain may be noted. With the maintenance of hypercalciuria the urine may be supersaturated with calcium phosphate and stones appear. These sometimes become quite large and responsible for impaired renal function. Another type of deposition of calcium is so-called metastatic calcification, in which lime salt is laid down in various organs, especially the kidneys, and less often the heart, the lungs, and sometimes the corpora cavernosa and the mucosa of the gastrointestinal tract. When the kidneys are considerably infiltrated with such calcification, the lime salt deposits can be identified on roentgenograms as nephrocalcinosis. The difficulties in establishing a diagnosis of hyperparathyroidism on biospy material alone was stressed by Black and Ackerman (1950), who believed that the characteristic roentgenographic and chemical changes were also required to make the diag-

nosis. Secondary hyperparathyroidism due to renal disease may so simulate primary hyperparathyroidism that the two are indistinguishable.

The clinical picture of hyperparathyroidism may be one which has to be differentiated from others which in part produce similar details. For instance, nephrocalcinosis may be seen with chronic pyelonephritis or glomerulonephritis, which in turn often results in the indistinguishable secondary form of hyperparathyroidism. Other causes for nephrosclerosis which are more readily distinguished include vitamin D intoxication, hyperchloremic acidosis, sarcoidosis, idiopathic hypercalcuria, excessive osteolytic activity such as may be associated with multiple myeloma or extensive bone metastases, bone tuberculosis or the milk-alkali syndrome observed in patients with peptic ulcers undergoing rigorous treatment. The association and persistence of peptic ulcers in patients with hyperparathyroidism alone or as part of multiple endocrine adenomas is worthy of special note, since some of the resistant patients may have hyperparathyroidism without the more readily detectable features. Hypertension with hyperparathyroidism is related to the underlying renal damage. The association of pancreatitis with hyperparathyroidism was regarded as more than coincidental by Turchi and his co-workers (1962).

The skeletal changes in hyperparathyroidism are caused by osteoclastic activity which produces rapid decalcification, leading to osteitis fibrosa, a nonspecific reaction to rapid demineralization. Cyst formation, and brown giant cell tumors, the so-called osteoclastomas, are found. The increased parathormone causes proliferation of osteoclasts in the bone marrow, with erosion of trabeculae followed by decalcification and osteitis fibrosa. The rise in blood and urinary calcium is a result of the bony disturbance. Because of the increased phosphate excretion by the kidneys, hypophosphatemia develops. The rise in phosphate renal excretion is due to excess parathyroid hormone. Whether this hyperphosphaturia is simply due to increased glomerular filtration or to decreased phosphate resorption in the renal tubules, or to a combination of both conditions is still undecided. No agreement has been reached as to whether a decreased phosphate reabsorption is due to a direct parathyroid hormone influence on the tubules, or whether hypercalcemia irrespective of its cause can decrease tubular reabsorption of phosphates. There is reason to believe that the demineralization in hyperparathyroidism may depend on still unknown mechanisms.

From a roentgenologic viewpoint, hyperparathyroidism is accompanied by a diffuse form of osteoporosis which may involve the entire skeleton. In those areas in which bone resorption is most pronounced the cortex of the bone is thinned out, presenting a scalloped appearance. Adjacent thereto the bones may be expanded, with numerous connecting areas of radiolucency presenting at times an almost web-like appearance. Considerable deformity of the long bones secondary to softening and pathologic fractures is not infrequent. The skull may show a miliary form of decalcification and occasionally this assumes a fairly sharply delimited appearance resembling osteitis circumscripta. The demineralization of the skeletal structures may proceed fairly rapidly, and in the most advanced forms there are large cyst-like regions of demineralization crisscrossed by residual bands of fibrous tissue. In other instances of hyperparathyroidism the cortex of the bone presents numerous small sharply circumscribed areas of decalcification, which later become confluent with ill-defined borders. The lamina dura around the teeth disappear but exceptions to this are not uncommon. Another helpful sign is ungual tuft resorption, and more often subperiosteal decalcification with small vertical spicules of bone produces a palisade formation (Pugh, 1952). This also occurs with secondary hyperparathyroidism, as does trabecular resorption of spongy bone at areas of stress such as the symphysis pubis and the distal ends of the clavicles.

In several cases of hyperparathyroidism which we have observed in adults who had been bedridden for several years, in addition to the cystic changes in the bones there was marked sharpening and pointing of the distal ends of the radius and ulna and of the small bones of the hands, with marked dislocations of these structures because of complete loss of articular structures.

Roentgenologic manifestations of hyperparathyroidism in the spine appear in a variety of patterns. The more common form is the one in which the osteoporosis is pronounced (Fig. 170). Demineralization of the vertebral column results in the formation of a variable dorsolumbar or dorsal kyphosis with shortening of the height of the patient and a forward protrusion of his head and neck. The vertebral bodies may collapse in a uniform fashion so that the normal height of the affected vertebral body is reduced, leaving the articular surfaces relatively smooth and the intervertebral spaces about average. This occurs usually in the dorsal spine, and may be accompanied by changes in the adjacent ribs (Fig. 170). In the lumbar spine the osteoporosis may be manifested by a progressively more marked biconcave appearance of the vertebral bodies, and a consequent biconvex increase in the height of the intervertebral discs. With softening the protrusion of nucleus pulposus into the vertebral bodies may become quite prominent, with little bony reaction around the herniated nuclear material. While neither change described above is characteristic of hyperparathyroidism, that possibility must be kept in mind and further evidence sought both clinically and in radiographic studies of other skeletal structures and the kidneys.

Another less frequent form of spine involvement with hyperparathyroidism is that of a reticular web-like change with relatively sharply defined lacunae together with cyst-like lesions of varying sizes and configurations. In 1 of the cases observed by us this was particularly prominent in the cervico-

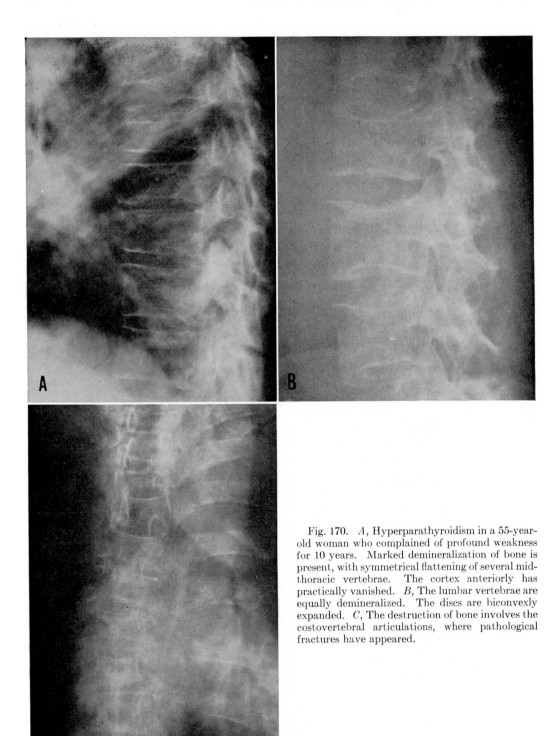

Fig. 170. *A*, Hyperparathyroidism in a 55-year-old woman who complained of profound weakness for 10 years. Marked demineralization of bone is present, with symmetrical flattening of several mid-thoracic vertebrae. The cortex anteriorly has practically vanished. *B*, The lumbar vertebrae are equally demineralized. The discs are biconvexly expanded. *C*, The destruction of bone involves the costovertebral articulations, where pathological fractures have appeared.

dorsal region, with similar alterations in the adjacent ribs (Fig. 171). The bones of the extremities in this patient had normal density but contained numerous small and moderately large sharply circumscribed cysts. There was a diffuse collapse of the body of the seventh cervical vertebra. Interspersed in the other osteoporotic cervical segments were numerous small fairly sharply defined islands of dense bone. In this patient it was also of interest that the softening of the ribs had apparently lowered the thoracic inlet so that the first and second dorsal vertebrae were clearly outlined above the first rib shadows.

Hyperparathyroidism may cause decalcification of the sacrum and practically complete obliteration of the sacro-iliac joints. The width of the sacrum may become narrowed as a consequence of pressure of both iliac bones.

Diffuse osteosclerotic punctate changes appear within osteoporotic vertebrae. Irregularities appear in the superior and inferior surfaces, together with wedging and exaggerated thoracic kyphotic and lumbar lordotic curves. In advanced cases erosive changes are occasionally found in the spinous processes, particularly in the cervical

spine. The tips become pointed and subcortical erosions are seen along the shafts (Fig. 172). Similar changes are found in the apophyseal joints, more often in the lumbar region.

Osteosclerotic banded changes at the upper and lower aspects of the vertebral bodies were reported by Crawford and his co-workers (1955) in patients with uremia, and also with secondary hyperparathyroidism of renal origin. This is referred to as the "rugger jersey sign," and is seen mainly in the thoracic and lumbar vertebrae (Fig. 173). It is not entirely specific, because somewhat similar changes appear with other conditions, notably osteopetrosis in adults and idiopathic hypercalcemia in infancy. Vaughan and Walters (1963) pointed out that such changes may result from a hypercalcemic state before the epiphyses are closed as well as with the osteosclerosis which occurs in some patients with uremia. They point out that the vertebral sclerosis due to uremia presents narrow and ill-defined translucent zones, while in hypercalcemia the sclerotic area is well-defined and presumably represents bone formed during the hypercalcemic episode. In osteopetrosis the width

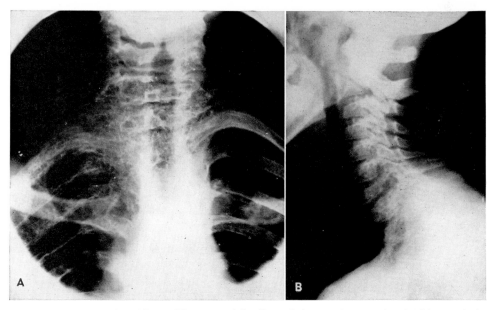

Fig. 171. Hyperparathyroidism. The upper right ribs and the vertebrae are involved in a reticular osteoporotic pattern, which extends to the neural arches as well.

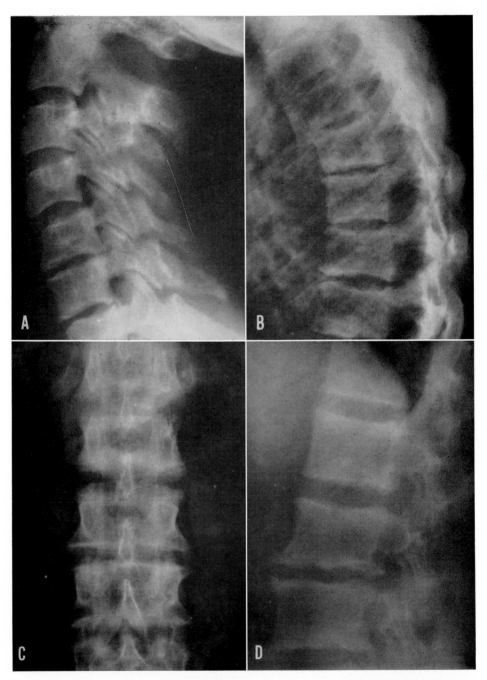

Fig. 172. *A*, Lateral cervical spine in a 51-year-old woman with hyperparathyroidism. The vertebrae are demineralized. The spinous processes of C3, 4 and 5 are slender and present erosive changes along their cortical margins. *B*, A mild dorsum rotundum is present, with diffuse patchy osseous demineralization and flattened discs. However, the discal contours are biconvex. *C*, The lumbar spine is demineralized as well, with sclerotic changes involving the upper and lower margins of the first lumbar vertebra. This patient had been diagnosed as arthritis for a year before a chest film disclosed classical changes in the distal ends of the clavicles. A skeletal survey revealed advanced bony changes in the skull, hands, and to a lesser extent in the extremities. The kidneys functioned well but contained miliary calcareous deposits. Diagnosis verified at operation.

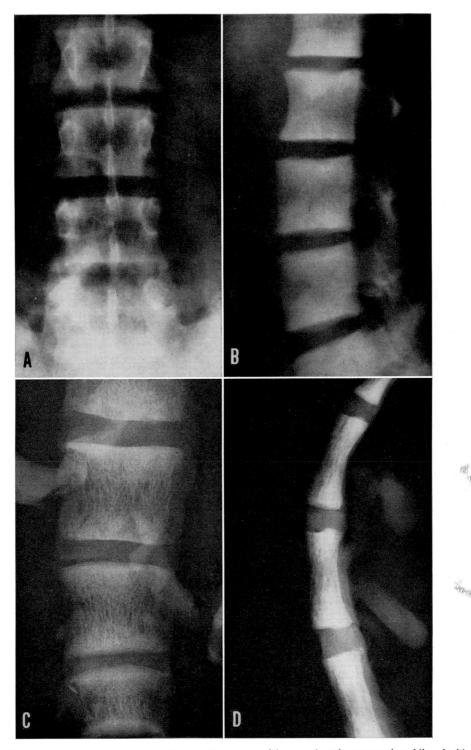

Fig. 173. *A*, AP lumbar spine in a 39-year-old woman with secondary hyperparathyroidism incident to renal disease. The vertebrae are intact. The upper margins are sclerotic, the centra are demineralized. The "rugger jersey" appearance of the upper and lower aspects of the vertebrae is better seen on the lateral view, *B*. *C* and *D*, roentgenograms of lumbar spine specimens taken at necropsy.

of the sclerotic area varies with the severity of the condition (Fig. 163). The appearance of the hands is helpful in diagnosis, inasmuch as with uremia no change appears while with secondary hyperparathyroidism the characteristic subperiosteal palisading is striking.

Chondrocalcinosis has been observed with hyperparathyroidism, but is not regarded as characteristic (Vix, 1964). The condition is characterized by the presence of calcium pyrophosphate crystals in the synovial fluid. Currey and his co-workers (1966) found no gross metabolic abnormality in most patients with chondrocalcinosis, but an appreciable minority had either gout or hyperparathyroidism. Calcifications are found in the knees, elbows, shoulders, the wrist and hand, the symphysis pubis and the ligaments adjacent to the intervertebral discs (Fig. 174). Calcifications appear in the menisci and other joint cartilage. Vertebral chondrocalcinosis is more likely to be seen in the cervical and lumbar regions (Zitnan and Sit'aj, 1963).

SECONDARY HYPERPARATHYROIDISM

Under secondary hyperparathyroidism are included conditions which result in parathyroid hyperplasia with formation of excess parathyroid hormone. It may occur with or without the characteristic chemical or bony changes, and with histologically normal glands (Soffer and Cohen, 1943). Chief among these conditions is chronic renal disease, leading to the designation of the disorder as renal osteodystrophy. Such renal disease follows primary urinary tract disturbances such as chronic glomerular nephritis, pyelonephritis and nephrosis. Congenital malformations of the kidneys such as polycystic kidneys and renal hypogenesis also are causative. Other urinary tract disturbances including obstructions due to urethral valves, prostatic hypertrophy, urethral strictures and bladder neck or ureteral strictures may also be responsible. A rare cause of secondary hyperparathyroidism is the primary renal tubular disorder called Fanconi's syndrome, with acidosis, hyper

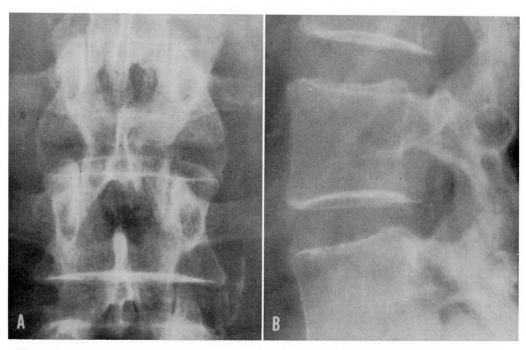

FIG. 174. A, AP and lateral, B, roentgenograms of the lumbar vertebrae in a 68-year-old man with chondrocalcinosis. The calcifications are prominent along the lateral margins of the intervertebral disc between L2 and 3. The patient was diabetic, and had no indications of other metabolic disease.

chloremia, glucosuria and an abnormal excretion of organic acids in the urine with a low serum phosphorus content. Secondary hyperparathyroidism is associated with dietary calcium deprivation, pregnancy, lactation, rickets and osteomalacia. Idiopathic hypercalcuria is another form of so-called vitamin D–resistant rickets, with increased calcium excretion of unknown etiology.

Renal insufficiency may be accompanied by abnormal serum phosphate and nonprotein nitrogen retention, and normal or slightly diminished serum calcium content. A high serum phosphatase level is present, as well as acidosis. Hyperplasia of the parathyroids follows the low serum calcium content which compensates for the elevated phosphate in the blood. The parathyroids in such patients either remain average in size or increase markedly in bulk (Castleman and Mallory, 1935). There is an increase in the number of normal-sized chief cells, with no mitotic activity. Diminution or absence of intercellular fatty tissue appears, and there is a higher glycogen content than observed with parathyroid hypertrophy or adenomas. Such a hyperplastic gland, as occurs with secondary hyperparathyroidism, can increase its parathyroid hormone productive capacity because of glandular tissue replacing the normal intercellular fat.

Secondary osteonephropathy may exhibit pronounced bone changes, particularly in children. These individuals are deficient in growth, resulting in the picture of renal dwarfism, renal nanism. The epiphyses present a marked degree of widening, with irregularities of their margins which resemble advanced rickets, leading to the designation of "renal rickets."

It has been suggested by Albright and his co-workers and by Snapper that this term be discarded. Albright pointed out that the epiphyseal lesions of renal rickets are quite unlike those seen with true rickets, and that hyperparathyroidism with osteitis fibrosa generalisata uncomplicated by kidney damage is not associated with epiphyseal lesions in children. A pronounced degree of osteoporosis of the entire skeletal system may be observed, with a translucency of bones much more pronounced than usually present with rickets. Subperiosteal elevation occurs in the ends of the long bones and in the hands and feet. The epiphyses remain open for an unusually long time even if the patient reaches adolescence or adult age (Cancelmo and Bromer, 1951).

In the case illustrated here (Fig. 175) the patient was a 19-month-old boy with congenital obstruction at the vesical neck. This had remained untreated for more than a year because his parents refused to heed medical advice. The child was admitted with acute urinary retention, with a urea nitrogen content of the blood varying between 85 and 100 mg per cent, a blood calcium of 10, alkaline phosphatase of 6 and an inorganic phosphorus content of 6.1 mg per cent. This patient presented a classical picture of renal osteodystrophy, with subperiosteal absorption at the distal ends of the humerus and forearms, an irregular appearance of the resorptive bone at the distal ends of the clavicles and generalized stunted growth. The lamina dura of his teeth were deficient, but the skull itself showed no gross change.

Roentgenographic examination revealed the spinal column to be normally aligned. The vertebrae were of normal height, as were the intervertebral discs. The vertebral bodies presented a reticular decalcification immediately beneath their superior and inferior surfaces. To some degree this change was present along the anterior and posterior aspects of the vertebral bodies. We had available for comparison roentgenograms when the patient was 6 months of age, when the skeletal changes were minimal, being limited to the epiphyses. Apparently the time necessary for pronounced bony changes to develop in this patient had been a year or less.

Renal osteodystrophies in adults also present prominent bone changes. These do not occur at the ends of the long bones because the epiphyses are united. The condition

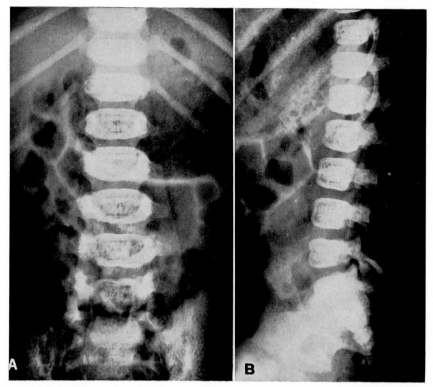

Fig. 175. Renal osteodystrophy due to congenital obstruction at the vesicle neck of a 19-month-old boy. The vertebral bodies present a dense core around which is a layer of radiolucent structure, which in turn is enveloped in a thin dense periphery of cortical bone.

may manifest itself as metastatic calcinosis, with deposits in the soft tissues, and Mönckeberg's form of medial arteriosclerosis, together with a varying degree of osteoporsis and other bone changes much the same as in primary hyperparathyroidism. Dreskin and Fox (1950) reported a 27-year-old man with chronic renal disease since childhood with osteoporosis, parathyroid hyperplasia and metastatic calcification. The unique feature in this case was the predominant enlargement of one parathyroid gland simulating a palpable adenoma. The bones, including the vertebrae, showed islands of hematopoiesis, but the major portion of the marrow space was occupied by large numbers of irregular trabeculae of cross-fibrillar bone lying in a fibrous matrix. The spongiosa showed predominantly osteoblastic new bone formation with rows of plump osteoblasts aligned along the trabeculae, and the spicules had moderately wide osteoid margins. There was no apparent delay in calcium salt deposition in the osteoid material. Osteoclastic activity was seen also, with multinucleated osteoclasts lying in wide lacunar spaces. This lytic process was accompanied by deposition of new bone. The cortices were thin throughout, with enlarged lacunar spaces containing fibrous tissue. Here, too, new bone was being laid down. The fibrous tissue was vascular and moderately dense, and there was no evidence of inflammatory reaction.

Increased density of the upper and lower aspects of the vertebral bodies, the "rugger jersey sign," appears with chronic renal disease and secondary hyperparathyroidism (Fig. 173).

References

Albright, F. and Reifenstein, E. C., Jr.: *Parathyroid Glands and Metabolic Bone Disease*, Baltimore, The Williams & Wilkins Co., 1948.

Albright, F., Drake, T. G. and Sulkowitch, H.: Renal Osteitis Fibrosa Cystica, Bull. Johns Hopkins Hosp., *60*, 377, 1937.

Barnes, B. A.: Carcinoma of the Parathyroid Glands, J.A.M.A., *178*, 556, 1961.

Bartlett, N. L. and Cochran, D. Q.: Reparative Processes in Primary Hyperparathyroidism, Radiol. Clin. North America, *2*, 261, 1964.

Beveridge, B., Vaughan, B. F. and Walters, M. N. I.: Primary Hyperparathyroidism and Secondary Renal Failure with Osteosclerosis, J. Fac. Radiologists, *10*, 197, 1959.

Bywaters, E. G. L., Dixon, A. St. J., and Scott, J. T.: Joint Lesions of Hyperparathyroidism, Ann. Rheum. Dis., *22*, 171, 1963.

Crawford, T., Dent, C. E., Lucas, P., Martin, N. H. and Nassim, J. R.: Osteosclerosis Associated with Renal Failure, Lancet, *2*, 981, 1954.

Cancelmo, J. J. and Bromer, R. S.: Osteonephropathy in Children, Am. J. Roentgenol., *65*, 889, 1951.

Castleman, B. and Mallory, T. B.: Pathology of Parathyroid Glands in Hyperparathyroidism. Am. J. Path., *11*, 1, 1935.

Cronqvist, S.: Renal Osteonephropathy, Acta radiol., *55*, 17, 1961.

Currey, H. L. F., Key, J. J., Mason, R. M. and Swettenham, K. V.: Significance of Radiological Calcification of Joint Cartilage, Ann. Rheum. Dis., *25*, 295, 1966.

Dreskin, E. A. and Fox, T. A.: Adult Renal Osteitis Fibrosa with Metastatic Calcification and Hyperplasia of One Parathyroid Gland, Arch. Int. Med., *86*, 533, 1950.

Fletcher, R. F., Jones, J. H. and Morgan, D. B.: Bone Disease in Chronic Renal Failure, Quart. J. Med., *32*, 321, 1963.

Follis, R. H. and Jackson, D. A.: Renal Osteomalacia and Osteitis Fibrosa in Adults, Bull. Johns Hopkins Hosp., *72*, 232, 1943.

Gatzimos, C. D., Schulz, D. M. and Newnum, R. L.: Cystinosis (Lignac-Fanconi Disease), Am. J. Path., *31*, 791, 1955.

Mieher, W. C., Jr., Thibaudeau, Y. and Frame, B.: Primary Hyperparathyroidism. Arch. Int. Med., *107*, 361, 1961.

Nathanson, L. and Slobodkin, M.: Acromio-Clavicular Changes in Primary and Secondary Hyperparathyroidism, Radiology, *55*, 30, 1950.

Pugh, D. H.: Subperiosteal Resorption of Bone, Am. J. Roentgenol., *66*, 577, 1951.

Rogers, H. M.: Parathyroid Adenoma and Hypertrophy of Parathyroid Glands, J.A.M.A., *130*, 22, 1946.

Schachner, S. H., Riley, T. R., Old, J. W., Taft, D. A. and Hamwi, G. J.: Familial Hyperparathyroidism, Arch. Int. Med., *117*, 417, 1966.

Schlaeger, R., LeMay, M. and Wermer, P.: Upper Gastro-Intestinal Tract Alterations in Adenomatosis of the Endocrine Glands, Radiology, *75*, 517, 1960.

Scott, J. T., Dixon, A. St. J. and Bywaters, E. G. L.: Association of Hyperuricaemia and Gout with Hyperparathyroidism, Brit. M. J., *1*, 1070, 1964.

Steinbach, H. L., Gordon, G. S., Eisenberg, E., Crane, J. T., Silverman, S. and Goldman, L.: Primary Hyperparathyroidism; A Correlation of Roentgen, Clinical and Pathologic Features. Am. J. Roentgenol., *86*, 329, 1961.

Stephenson M. U.: Malignant Tumors of the Parathyroid Glands, Arch. Surg., *60*, 247, 1950.

Templeton, A. W., Jaconette, J. R. and Ormond, R. S.: Localized Osteosclerosis in Hyperparathyroidism, Radiology, *78*, 955, 1962.

Turchi, J. J., Flandreau, R. H., Forte, A. L., French, G. N. and Ludwig, G. D.: Hyperparathyroidism and Pancreatitis, J.A.M.A., *180*, 799, 1962.

Twigg, H. C., Zvaifler, N. J. and Nelson, C. W.: Chondrocalcinosis, Radiology, *82*, 655, 1964.

Vaughan, B. F. and Walters, M. N. I.: Sclerotic Banded Vertebrae (Rugger Jersey Sign), J. Coll. Radiol. Australasia, *7*, 87, 1963.

Valvassori, G. E. and Pierce, R. H.: Osteosclerosis in Chronic Uremia, Radiology, *82*, 385, 1964.

Vix, V. A.: Articular and Fibrocartilaginous Calcification in Hyperparathyroidism: Associated Hyperuricemia, Radiology, *83*, 468, 1964.

Wolf, H. L. and Denko, K. J. V.: Osteosclerosis in Chronic Renal Disease, Am. J. Med. Sci., *235*, 33, 1958.

Zvaifler, N. J., Reefe, W. E. and Black, R. L.: Articular Manifestations in Primary Hyperparathyroidism. Arth. & Rheum., *5*, 237, 1962.

Zitman, D. and Sit'aj, S.: Chondrocalcinosis Articularis, Ann. Rheum. Dis., *22*, 142, 1963.

Zimmerman, H. B.: Osteosclerosis in Chronic Renal Disease: Report of 4 Cases Associated with Secondary Hyperparathyroidism, Am. J. Roentgenol., *88*, 1152, 1962.

HYPOPARATHYROIDISM

This condition is due to a deficient production of parathyroid hormone, usually due to glandular injury or accidental removal in the course of thyroid surgery. Rare cases of idiopathic hypoparathyroidism occurring without known reason have been described. Hypoparathyroidism is associated with tetany, characterized by muscular cramps, carpopedal spasm, convulsions and laryngeal stridor. Cataracts are also frequently present. Calcification in the basal ganglia of the brain, which Albright and Reifenstein regard as evidence that the change in hypoparathyroidism is in the direction of supersaturation of body fluids with calcium phosphate, may be seen on skull roentgenograms. However, such calcifications are not necessarily pathognomonic of hypoparathyroidism. Hypoparathyroidism is associated with hypocalcemia and hyperphosphatemia.

There are no changes in the spinal column which are attributed specifically to this condition.

References

Harrison, H. E.: Idiopathic Hypoparathyroidism, Pediatrics, *17*, 442, 1956.
Steinberg, H. and Waldron, B. R.: Idiopathic Hypoparathyroidism, Medicine, *31*, 133, 1952.

Pseudohypoparathyroidism (Seabright Bantam Syndrome)

This condition is congenital and hereditary. It is differentiated from true hypoparathyroidism by inability to respond to the presence of normal parathyroid hormone. This syndrome was first described by Albright, Burnett, Smith and Parson (1942), who reported that these patients had a tendency to be unusually thick-set and short with brachydactyly, especially in the metacarpal bones, because of early closure of the epiphyses. Mental retardation and corneal or lenticular opacities also are frequently seen. Soft tissue calcific deposits may be present, some of which can be felt on physical examination. Tetany is present, with low serum calcium and elevated serum inorganic phosphatase. The term "Seabright Bantam Syndrome" was suggested by a comparison to this breed of chickens in which the roosters present a feminine type of plumage, presumably because of an insufficient response to male sex hormone, indicating an end-organ refractory state.

Calcifications in the basal ganglia as well as elsewhere in the soft tissues have been described. The skull bones are thickened. The bony changes in the long bones sometimes are like those of an osteochondrodystrophy, with marked epiphyseal irregularities, softening and malformations which tend to return to a normal state when growth ceases. Changes in the vertebral column are not striking, consisting mainly of some demineralization of bone with accentuation of the vertical trabeculae, some irregular calcification within the bodies and interspersed dense and rarefied areas.

References

Albright, F., Burnett, C. H., Smith, P. H. and Parson, W.: Pseudo-Hypoparathyroidism—an Example of Seabright-Bantam Sundrome, Endocrinology, *30*, 922, 1942.
Bakwin, H., Gorman, W. F. and Ziegra, S. R.: Pseudohypoparathyroid Tetany, J. Pediat., *36*, 567, 1950.
Cusmano, J. V., Baker, D. H. and Finby, N.: Pseudohypoparathyroidism, Radiology, *67*, 845, 1956.
Garceau, G. J. and Miller, W. E.: Osteochondrodystrophy as a Result of or in Relation to Pseudo-Hypoparathyroidism, J. Bone & Joint Surg., *38-A*, 131, 1956.
Howat, T. W. and Ashurst, G. M.: Pseudohypoparathyroidism, J. Bone & Joint Surg., *39-B*, 39, 1957.
Lowe, C. U., Ellinger, A. J., Wright, W. S. and Stauffer, H. M.: Pseudohypoparathyroidism (the Seabright Bantam Syndrome), J. Pediat., *36*, 1, 1950.
Singleton, E. B. and Teng, C. T.: Pseudohypoparathyroidism with Bone Changes Simulating Hyperparathyroidism, Radiology, *78*, 388, 1962.
Steinbach, H. L. and Young, D. A.: The Roentgen Appearance of Pseudohypoparathyroidism (PH) and Pseudo-pseudohypoparathyroidism. Am. J. Roentgenol., *97*, 49, 1966.

Pseudo-Pseudohypoparathyroidism

There exists a small group of patients with some of the changes seen with hypoparathyroidism, but who have neither hypocalcemia nor hypophosphatemia, and consequently no tetany or convulsive symptoms. However, these patients present changes of pseudo-hypoparathyroidism in the short bones of the hands and feet, round faces, short stature and metastatic calcifications in the soft tissues. No basal ganglia calcification lenticular abnormality or abnormal dentition has been encountered in this disorder.

References

Albright, F., Forbes, A. P. and Henneman, P. H.: Pseudo-pseudohypoparathyroidism, Tr. A. Am. Physicians, *65*, 337, 1952.
McNeely, W. F., Raisz, L. G. and LeMay, M. Dyschondroplasia with Soft Tissue Calcification and Ossification, and Normal Parathyroid Function ("Pseudo-pseudohypoparathyroidism"), Am. J. Med., *21*, 649, 1956.
Wallach, S., Englert, E., Jr. and Brown, H.: The Syndrome of Pseudo-Pseudohypoparathyroidism, Arch. Int. Med., *98*, 517, 1956.

CUSHING'S SYNDROME

Cushing's syndrome is characterized by increased trunk fat, purplish stripes on the abdomen, a full moon face, hirsutism, acneiform eruptions, hypertension, cyanosis of the face, hands, neck and feet, and decreased sugar tolerance. The skin becomes thin and dry. The patient may be irritable and drowsy, with marked muscular weakness. Polydipsia, polyphagia and polyuria also appear. A mild polycythemia may be present. A low basal metabolic rate is noted in many patients, but this may be normal or even somewhat elevated. Arteriosclerosis and nephrolithiasis are common concomitants. In females amenorrhea is frequent, and in the male loss of libido and impotence is observed. This clinical picture was originally developed by Cushing (1932), who ascribed it to basophilic adenomas of the pituitary gland. Eisenhardt and Thompson (1939) called attention to the frequency with which osteoporosis was present with pituitary basophilism. Later, Cushing's syndrome was found to be due to other causes including various adrenal cortical tumors, tumors of the ovary, the thymus, the lungs, pancreas, breast, thyroid (Eastridge, Hughes and Hamman, 1965) (Sayle and co-workers, 1965), or atrophy or inhibition of the hypothalamic nuclei, particularly of the paraventricular and the supraoptic nuclei. Heinbecker (1946) reviewed experimental evidence which indicated how these four primary causes depressed the function of the neural hypophysis and affected a dominance of the eosinophilic adrenal cortical hormone complex over the basophile thyroid complex. The role of the pituitary gland in the pathogenesis of Cushing's disease is discussed by Hunter (1966).

Atrophy of lymphoid tissue with lymphocytopenia and polymorphonuclear leukocytosis is present. When the condition occurs in children, retardation of skeletal growth takes place. The urinary excretion of 17-hydroxycorticoids usually is elevated. The diabetes associated with Cushing's syndrome is usually resistant to insulin.

Similar conditions appear in patients treated over long periods with ACTH or cortisone. In a review of 189 cases from the literature and 5 cases of his own, Knowlton (1953) found that the clinical picture was variable, that the hypertension was reversible and that the suppression of gonadal function was not universal. He found x-ray evidence of spinal demineralization in 74 per cent of cases, with compression fractures in 34 per cent. Skull osteoporosis was present in 50 per cent and rib fractures in 11 per cent.

The osseous manifestations of Cushing's syndrome are principally those of osteoporosis, due to disturbed protein metabolism leading to a lack of bony matrix formation and deficient osteoblastic activity. The widespread osteoporosis affects the spine, the ribs, pelvis and skull most severely. The peripheral cortical bone of the vertebral bodies is thinned, but because of the loss of cancellous bone the margins appear relatively dense. Increase in radiolucency of affected vertebrae results from trabecular loss. The vertical trabeculae persist better than the horizontal ones, so that not infrequently the vertebrae have prominent vertical markings. Further changes are those incident to strain and weight bearing, and appear most often in the thoracic and lumbar regions. The affected vertebrae become biconvex, with bulging intervertebral discs producing exaggerated saucer-like indentations into the upper and lower surfaces of the bodies. Sometimes a sclerotic reaction appears along the margins of the bone in contact with the discs. Nuclear intrusions into the vertebrae may be quite deep, and produce only faintly sclerotic reactions in the adjacent cancellous bone. Further loss of structural strength results in bulging of the vertical walls of the vertebrae, wedging or flattening of the bodies. In some the deformity is mild, while in others the malformation is so severe that the vertebrae are discoid or deeply biconcave in configuration (Figs. 176 and 177).

The pathologic appearance of vertebrae affected by Cushing's disease was described

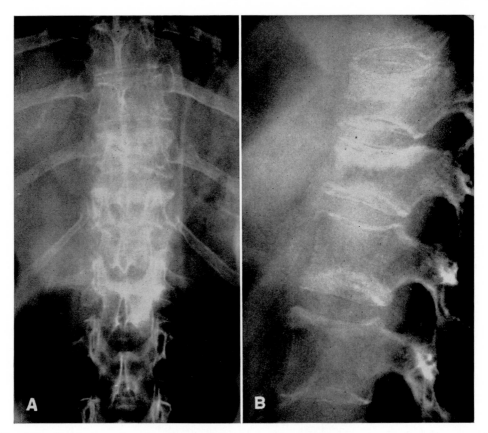

Fig. 176. Cushing's syndrome in a 46-year-old woman. The vertebrae are osteoporotic, and compressive changes with sclerotic margins are present in the superior surfaces of the twelfth thoracic and first lumbar vertebra. Similar changes are seen at the inferior aspect of the second lumbar vertebra. The intervertebral discs are bulging.

by Follis (1951) and by Sissons (1956). The principal change of osteoporosis was reflected by the diminished osteoblastic activity resulting in thin, delicate trabeculae which may be angulated and sometimes crenated. Fatty replacement of hemopoietic tissue occurred in areas where trabeculae were absent and where bony rarefaction and collapse were greatest.

As might be anticipated because of the effect of abnormal corticosteroid function, the amount of osteoid present about the trabeculae is diminished. The increased adrenal hormone inhibits protein synthesis, thereby diminishing the production of bone from osteoid. Follis noted rather thin osteoid borders about many of the thinned trabeculae in his patients. Sissons found

that the surfaces of the slender trabeculae were completely devoid of osteoid borders. Normal osteoblasts were seen, but these were reduced in number and their bone-forming activity appeared minimal. Osteoclasts were rare.

Sissons found numerous fractures of trabeculae in those vertebrae which were collapsed. He further noted that in most areas the reaction of adjacent tissues was minimal, although in one vertebra the displaced trabeculae in the collapsed area were surrounded by vascular granulation tissue and proliferating osteoblasts. Even though there was little reaction to the fractured trabeculae, they did later join into irregular masses of bone. "The structural changes in these vertebrae (see for instance Figures 2, 4, 5

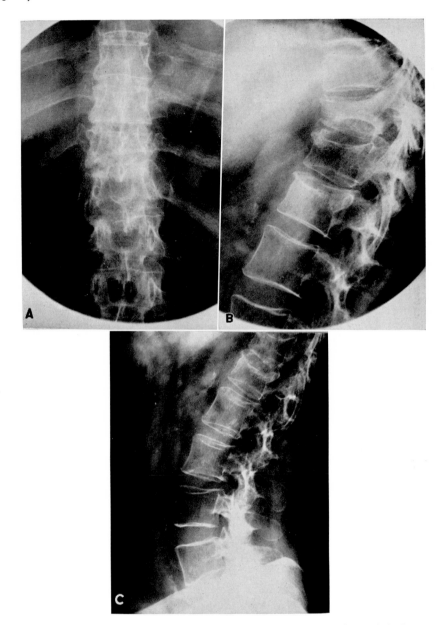

FIG. 177. Cushing's syndrome in a 37-year-old woman. Compression of the twelfth thoracic and first lumbar vertebrae, with slight sclerotic changes, together with marked osteoporosis. The lumbar vertebrae are intact, and the intervertebral discs are somewhat widened but not grossly bulging. Note the relative sclerotic appearance of the peripheries of the lumbar vertebral bodies.

and 6) indicate that 'collapse' of the osteoporotic bone structure may take place quietly and continuously, but that this process can sometimes be interrupted by a sudden and more complete compression fracture."

In the first edition of this book it was noted that occasionally osteoporotic vertebrae in patients with Cushing's disease presented compaction of the vertebral surfaces. This was attributed to compression fracture. Incidentally, an illustration of this was pub-

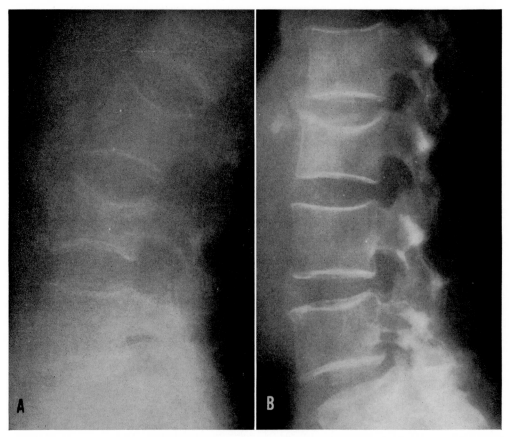

Fig. 178. *A*, Osteoporosis in a 68-year-old woman with senile osteoporosis. The anterior aspect of L3 is buckled anteriorly. The discs are widened and biconvex. Marginal bone condensation is present in the upper margin of L3 and the lower margin of L1, which also is compressed. *B*, Osteoporosis in a 74-year-old man treated with steroids for chronic myelogenous leukemia. The vertebrae are diffusely demineralized. Compression of the superior aspect of L2 with marginal bone condensation is seen.

lished by Sussman and Copleman (1942), but no specific note of its presence was made. In reviewing 16 cases of Cushing's disease from my own experience, this change was found in 3. It appears as a rather broad, band-like zone of increased density which merges rather gradually with the subjacent cancellous bone (Fig. 176).

Howland, Pugh and Sprague (1958) suggested that this compaction of the upper, and occasionally of the lower surfaces of the vertebrae may have almost specific importance in the diagnosis of Cushing's syndrome. They found it present in 29 of 69 cases, occurring only when osteoporosis was more than minimal. As a rule more than one vertebra was affected. The lower

thoracic and upper lumbar areas were involved most often, usually together with compression of the vertebrae. In a few cases this change was minimal and its recognition difficult. Post-treatment films after more than 6 months were available in 19 cases. Eight of these had marginal compressions. This remained unchanged in 2, decreased in 3 and in the remaining 3 had disappeared completely. The condensation was noted to have diminished or disappeared before any change in the osteoporosis was demonstrable radiographically.

Howland, Pugh and Sprague attributed marginal condensation to the effect of the abnormal corticosteroids on the healing of the collapsed portions of bone. A strong stimulus for osteoid formation resulted in unusually heavy callus about areas of fracture, and they attributed the heavy callus formation seen about rib and pelvic fractures in Cushing's disease to this mechanism. This does not take into account that osteoid formation and osteoblastic activity is diminished in Cushing's disease. In Sisson's article figures 4 and 5 are excellent illustrations of compacted bony trabeculae in the depressed superior surface of a lumbar vertebra which looks very much like those seen with marginal compression. It is worth recalling his observation about the minimal tissue reaction about fractured trabeculae, even though in one instance he observed newly formed bone producing thicker structures in the upper surface of a partly collapsed vertebral body (his Figure 18). Insofar as heavy callus about rib and pelvic fractures is concerned, his illustration of a rib with two fractures is illuminating (Figure 19). One of these had neither displacement nor periosteal callus, while the other was surrounded by periosteal callus.

As Howland, Pugh and Sprague point out, marginal condensation may have specific diagnostic importance in the radiologic diagnosis of Cushing's disease. On the basis of present evidence it appears that trauma is a factor in the production of this interesting phenomenon. However, the mechanism probably is equally related to deranged corticosteroid function. Similar changes appear in patients undergoing prolonged treatment with corticosteroids who do not present other manifestations of Cushing's disease (Fig. 178).

With healing of Cushing's syndrome a reversal of osteoporosis and return of the vertebrae to an approximately normal appearance has been noted in some patients still in the growth period. In others a central zone of osteoporosis persists. As normal bone is laid down at the upper and lower vertebral surfaces the demineralized area becomes sharply delineated. In some the bulging of the intervertebral discs persists, while in others it disappears. Once osteoporosis develops in the postpubertal patient it remains relatively unchanged, even when the patient recovers (Iannaccone, Gabrilove, Brahms and Soffer, 1960).

References

Brown, H. and Lane, M.: Cushing's and Malignant Carcinoid Syndromes from Ovarian Carcinoma, Arch. Int. Med., *115*, 490, 1965.

Cushing, H.: Basophile Adenomas of the Pituitary Body, Bull. Johns Hopkins Hosp., *50*. 137, 1932.

Eastridge, C. E., Hughes, F. A., Jr. and Hamman, J. L.: Cushing's Syndrome in Assocation with Carcinoma of the Respiratory Tract, Ann. Thoracic Surg., *1*, 151, 1965.

Eisenhardt, L. E. and Thompson, K. W.: Status of So-called Basophilism, Yale J. Biol. & Med., *11*, 507, 1939.

Follis, R. H., Jr.: Pathology of the Osseous Changes in Cushing's Syndrome in an Infant and in Adults, Bull. Johns Hopkins Hosp., *88*, 440, 1951.

Heinbecker, P.: Cushing's Syndrome, Ann. Surg., *124*, 252, 1946.

Howland, W. J., Jr., Pugh, D. G. and Sprague, R. G.: Roentgenologic Changes in the Skeletal System in Cushing's Syndrome, Radiology, *71*, 69, 1958.

Hundler, G. G.: Pathogenesis of Cushing's Disease, Proc. Staff Meet., Mayo Clin., *41*, 29, 1966.

Iannaccone, A., Gabrilove, J. L., Brahms, S. A. and Soffer, L. J.: Osteoporosis in Cushing's Syndrome, Ann. Int. Med., *52*, 570, 1960.

Kepler, E. J. and Keating, F. R.: Diseases of the Adrenal Glands, II. Tumors of the Adrenal Cortex, Diseases of the Adrenal Medulla and Allied Disturbances, Arch. Int. Med., *68*, 1010, 1941.

Knowlton, A. I.: Cushing's Syndrome, Bull. New York Acad. Med., *29*, 441, 1953.

O'Neal, L. W.: Pathologic Anatomy in Cushing's Syndrome, Ann. Surg., *160*, 860, 1964.

Sayle, B. A., Lang, P. A., Green, W. O., Jr., Bosworth, W. C. and Gregory, R.: Cushing's Syndrome Due to Islet Cell Carcinoma of the Pancreas, Ann. Int. Med., *63*, 58, 1965.

Silver, H. K. and Ginsburg, M. M.: Cushing's Syndrome in an Eight Year Old Girl, Am. J. Dis. Child, *100*, 405, 1960.

Sissons, H. A.: The Osteoporosis of Cushing's Syndrome, J. Bone & Joint Surg., *38-B*, 418, 1956.

Sosman, M. C.: Cushing's Disease—Pituitary Basophilism, Am. J. Roentgenol., *62*, 1, 1949.

Sussman, M. L. and Copleman, B.: The Roentgenographic Appearance of the Bones in Cushing's Syndrome, Radiology, *39*, 288, 1942.

Acromegaly

This condition is due to eosinophilic adenoma of the pituitary gland. Occasionally hyperplasia of the eosinophilic cells without adenoma formation, eosinophilic adenocarcinoma or chromophobe adenoma produces this disorder. In its fully developed form it is characterized by facial changes, notably a gross coarse thickening of the face and nose, prominence of the jaws, narrowing of the palpebral fissures, and in many cases, prognathism. The concomitant changes in the hands are a marked thickening and enlargement together with a prominent puffing of the ungual tips of the fingers. Less well known are prominent widening and beading of the distal tips of the upper ribs which has been termed "acromegalic rosary."

The accelerated growth is due to an excessive amount of growth hormone. When this occurs before puberty, gigantism results After the epiphyseal cartilages are united the process of enchondral growth continues at the costochondral junctions, so that the ribs and costal cartilages increase in size and length, contributing to the dorsal kyphosis. Similar changes take place in other areas such as the mandibular condyles. The hormonal effect is not limited to growing bone, but also influences the growth of tendons, fascia, ligaments and joint linings among other tissues.

Changes in the spinal column associated with acromegaly were described by Erdheim in 1931. He pointed out that the vertebral bodies were increased in their anteroposterior dimensions with relatively little increase in their height. This increase in width develops from the periosteum by endochondral ossification of proliferating cartilage. The newly formed bone can be identified roentgenologically by a thin line of demarcation from the vertebral body's original margins. This proliferation of bone is most marked in the anterior aspect of the bone but may occur on the lateral aspects as well. Erdheim pointed out that the new cortex is pathologically wide and that the increased transverse diameter of the vertebral bodies, which is most prominent in the lower thoracic spine may give the mistaken impression of reduced height. The additional intervertebral disc

fibro-cartilage arises from the perichondrium and is well differentiated into the various normal components including a calcified layer and the hyaline plate. The intervertebral discs retain their normal height (Fig. 179).

Acromegalic changes in the spine were reviewed by Chester and Chester (1940) who reported 8 cases of their own, 5 of which showed increase in the anteroposterior diameter of the dorsal vertebrae. Waine, Bennett and Bauer (1945) had the opportunity to study at necropsy the spine of an acromegalic patient who died of bacterial endocarditis. The dorsal vertebral bodies

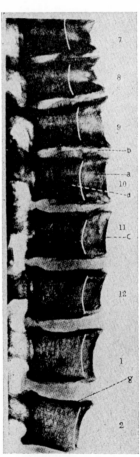

Fig. 179. Roentgenogram of half the vertebral column in case of acromegaly, originally published by Erdheim, J., Virchows Arch. f. path. Anat., *281*, 197, 1931. Note the bony overgrowth of the anterior aspects of the vertebrae. (Courtesy of Waine, H., Bennet, G. A. and Bauer, W., Am. J. Med. Sci., *209*, 671, 1945.)

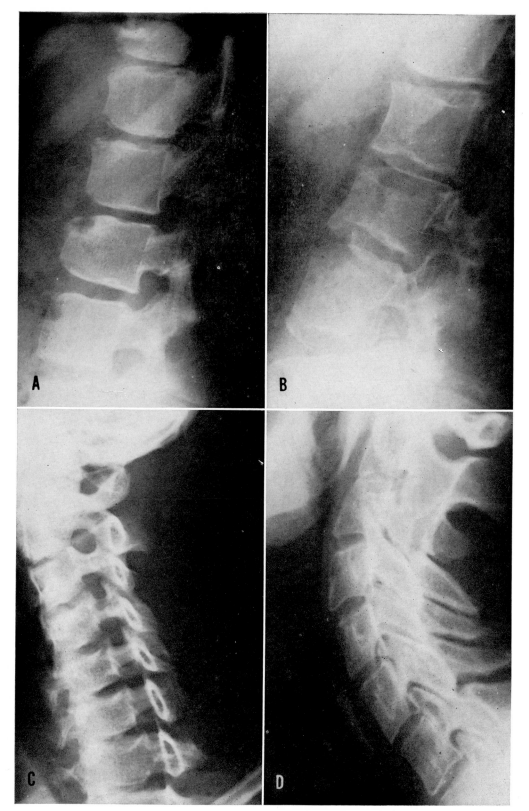

FIG. 180. A, The lumbar vertebrae of a 12-year-old girl with gigantism. Multiple nuclear intrusions are present. Some of the discs are narrowed. B, Ten years later considerable growth has occurred. The patient now is acromegalic, and practically blind. C, the cervical spine when first examined was not grossly changed. However, 10 years later, D, marked elongation of the vertebrae has taken place.

and intervertebral articulations showed massive spur formation with prominent lateral and anterior lipping of the vertebral bodies at the margins of the disc. The histologic picture resembled that of a severe degenerative bone disease. They regarded this as an overgrowth of cartilage and bone secondary to a specific hormonal stimulus.

Albright and Reifenstein (1948) were of the opinion that the bony changes in acromegaly were chiefly osteoporotic, and might best be ascribed to the hypogonadism which accompanies most of these cases. In 2 cases seen by them in an 18-year-old girl and an 18-year-old boy the spine showed only osteoporotic changes and scoliosis, with nuclear protrusions into the vertebral bodies. No bony overgrowth was present. They suggested that if this was the correct explanation, the condition should respond to estrogen therapy, and reported 2 cases in which this was accomplished. They pointed out that after closure of the epiphyses there was still possibility for restricted endochondral bone formation at certain sites, particularly the cartilaginous end plates of the vertebrae. These may again start producing endochondral bone, which together with increased periosteal bone formation accounts for the increase in the anteroposterior diameter.

Vertebral changes with acromegaly are relatively infrequent. In a review of 20 cases, Lang and Bessler (1961) found changes in the length of the vertebral bodies in 10. changes in the intervertebral disks in 12 and calcified disks in 4. Of 6 cases with lumbar spine roentgenograms, intervertebral disk changes were present in 6, with appositional growth of bone, thickening and osseous overgrowth. Change in the length of the

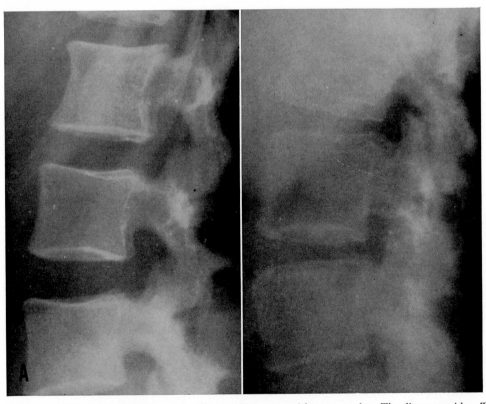

Fig. 181. *A*, The lumbar vertebrae in a 27-year-old woman with acromegaly. The discs are wide. The vertebrae are not grossly altered except for slightly increased dorsal concavities. *B*, Another female acromegalic patient with increased discal heights. A rather pronounced arthritic reaction is present in the apophyseal joints, probably unrelated to the acromegaly.

vertebral bodies, with modeling of the posterior circumference of the bodies was noted in 4.

In a review of 25 of our own cases, discernible vertebral changes were observed in 5. Some were quite subtle, others advanced. One patient was first seen at the age of 11, and was evidently far taller than she should be. She came in because of hip pain, and a slipped capital epiphysis was identified. Because of her size, a skeletal survey was made. An enlarged sella turcica was present, together with increased length of the long bones. Her lumbar vertebrae presented numerous nuclear indentations into the apposing surfaces, with a moderately increased lordotic curve and a mild right lateral scoliosis. The cervical and thoracic

vertebrae did not appear grossly changed, but a mild dorsal kyphosis was evident. She was followed over a 10-year period, and during that time evidences of acromegaly appeared. She received two courses of x-ray therapy to her pituitary gland, with apparent cessation of symptoms for a while. Operation on her pituitary finally was forced because of progressive loss of vision. Studies of her cervical spine at that time revealed a marked increase in the heights of the cervical vertebrae, and more pronounced kypho-scoliosis with healing of many of the nuclear intrusion defects (Fig. 180).

Other patients revealed increase in the height of the lumbar intervertebral discs (Fig. 181), and increased concavity in the posterior aspects of the lumbar vertebrae

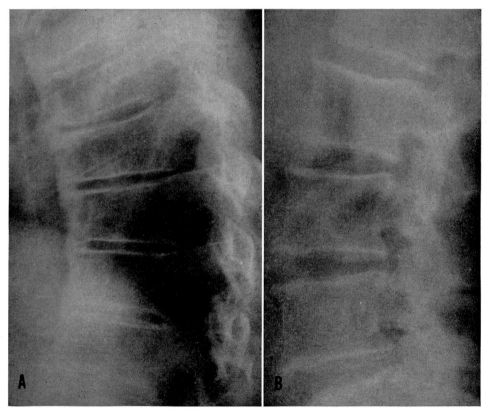

FIG. 182. *A*, The thoracic vertebrae in a 45-year-old male acromegalic known for 20 years. An increase in the anteroposterior diameter of the bodies is present, and the vertebrae are relatively flat, with slight anterior wedging. The discs are narrowed. *B*, The lumbar vertebrae are large, and there is little spondylotic reaction as compared with the heavy calcification of the anterior spinal ligament of the thoracic spine. The lumber vertebrae present indentations in their dorsal aspects. The spinous processes are unusually large.

(Fig. 182), and wedging and bony overgrowth of the anterior spinal ligament and midthoracic vertebral bodies (Fig. 182*A*). Moderate osteoporosis was fairly frequent. Prominent arthritic changes in the apophyseal joints of the lumbar vertebrae were evident in 1 patient (Fig. 182*B*). The patient who showed the most characteristic changes was the girl with gigantism who went on to acquire the characteristics of an acromegalic. The incidence of vertebral changes insofar as patterns showing all the changes noted above was infrequent, most showing one or two rather than all the structural alterations noted. This experience corresponds with that of Hamwi, Skillman and Tufts (1960), who also noted a rather scant occurrence of vertebral changes in 30 patients with acromegaly.

References

Albright, F. and Reifenstein, E. C., Jr.: *Parathyroid Glands and Metabolic Bone Disease*, Baltimore, The Williams & Wilkins Co., 1948.
Chester, W. and Chester, W. M.: Vertebral Column in Acromegaly, Am. J. Roentgenol., *44*, 552, 1940.
Erdheim, J.: Über Wirbelsäuleveranderungen bei Akromegalie, Virchow's Arch. f. path. Anat., *281*, 197, 1931.
Gilmore, J. H. and Mahan, T. K.: Acromegaly Presenting Specific Roentgenographic Changes, Radiology, *48*, 50, 1947.
Hamwi, G. J., Skillman, T. G. and Tufts, K. C., Jr.: Acromegaly, Am. J. Med., *29*, 690, 1960.
Lang, E. K. and Bessler, W. T.: The Roentgenologic Features of Acromegaly, Am. J. Roentgenol., *86*, 321, 1961.
Steinbach, H. L., Feldman, R. and Goldberg, M. B.: Acromegaly, Radiology, *72*, 535, 1959.
Waine, H., Bennett, G. A. and Bauer, W.: Joint Disease Associated with Acromegaly, Am. J. Med. Sci., *209*, 671, 1945.

Hypothyroidism

This condition is incident to diminished secretion of thyroid hormone. It may be partial, or if the gland is completely absent either as a result of destruction or surgical removal, a state of athyrosis exists. Hypothyroidism is encountered in any age group from infancy to adult life. Hypothyroidism originating in infancy or during fetal life is termed cretinism, and is recognized by thickening of the subcutaneous tissues and the characteristic facies with a dull skin, apathetic expression, enlarged and often protruding tongue, thick lips and a wide flat nose. These children also develop a protuberant abdomen with short arms and legs. Mental deficiency is common and varies from an almost complete imbecile state to the level of a moron. Growth in these children is retarded and the osseous development is considerably delayed. Bone originating in cartilage is particularly affected.

These children present evidence of dysgenesis of the epiphyses of the wrists, elbows and knees (Wilkin, 1941). Development of dentition is frequently retarded with delayed eruption of the teeth. Bony changes observed *in utero* were reported by Dorff (1934).

The radiologic changes in the spine reflect the delayed development of the skeletal structures. The gibbus deformity described below apparently may recede under thyroid treatment (Evans, 1952). The neurocentral synchondroses may have delayed union. The vertebral bodies often show some osteoporosis. Engeset, Imerslund and Blystad (1951) described fragments of irregularly ossified centers within the vertebral bodies as well as evidence of arrested longitudinal growth. In one of their cases they also reported a kyphotic angle at the first and second lumbar vertebrae similar to that noted in Hurler's disease. Swoboda (1950) reported 7 cases of infantile myxedema, all with incomplete wedging of the second lumbar vertebra producing an angular kyphosis. This was variable, and in most produces a clinical gibbus. The involved vertebral bodies had a step-like wedging anteriorly and posteriorly. Caffey (1956) mentioned a case of hypothyroidism in a boy 3 years of age in whom the maturation of the vertebrae was retarded. The first lumbar body was hypoplastic, producing a kyphotic deformity which persisted despite otherwise effective thyroid treatment. Nine years later the patient still had a marked kyphosis with spondylolisthesis and vertebral deformity. Another case of his, an untreated hypothyroid girl 8 years of age, revealed open neurocentral synchondroses together with an oval anterior notching in the vertebral bodies characteristic of the first year of life. Evans (1952), examined 13 cases of cretinism, and found minor abnormalities in 5. The other 8 all had deformities of the bodies of the twelfth dorsal or first and second lumbar vertebrae with kyphotic changes. Similarity to achondroplasia and gargoylism was pointed out.

In 1 of our patients there was a definitely increased density of the superior and inferior aspects of the various vertebrae, particularly in the dorsal region, between which a rarefied zone was present. This condition had been described by Engeset and his coworkers (1951) as a center of osteoporosis persisting after actual bone growth had become normal, indicative of the fact that the old bone remains abnormal, while new bone is laid down with normal density. A tongue formation in the twelfth thoracic and first lumbar vertebra was noted in an 8-year-old hypothyroid child who had no kyphosis (Fig. 183).

An important change associated with hypothyroidism in children is a dysgenesis in ossification centers such as the femoral head, the distal epiphyses of the femurs and the wrists, producing a stippled configuration sometimes associated with a flattening of the affected epiphyses. Under adequate thyroid treatment these changes disappear and growth proceeds normally in successful cases. This type of stippling has rarely been described in the spinal column. With healing of the hypothyroid state the signs of epiphyseal dysgenesis tend to diminish (Middlemass, 1959).

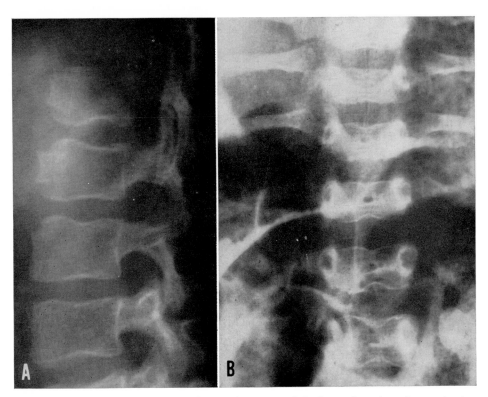

Fig. 183. A, Tongue-like deformity of the anterior aspect of the lower thoracic and upper lumbar vertebrae of an 11-year-old boy with hypothyroidism. The discs are widened and rather club-shaped. Indentations into the upper and lower surfaces of the flattened vertebrae are prominent, B, as seen in an 8-year-old cretin.

20

References

Caffey, J.: *Pediatric X-ray Diagnosis*, 5th ed., Chicago, Year Book Medical Publishers, Inc., 1967.

Dorff, G. B.: Sporadic Cretinism in One of Twins, Am. J. Dis. Child., *48*, 1316, 1934.

Evans, P. R.: Deformity of the Vertebral Bodies in Cretinism, J. Pediat., *41*, 706, 1952.

Engeset, A., Imerslund, O. and Blystad, W.: Skeletal Changes Resembling Scurvy in Infantile Hypothyreosis Before and After Thyroid Therapy, Acta radiol., *36*, 1, 1951.

Middlemass, I. B. D.: Bone Changes in Adult Cretins, Brit. J. Radiol., *32*, 685, 1959.

Reilly, W. A. and Smyth, F. S.: Cretinoid Epiphyseal Dysgenesis, J. Pediat., *11*, 786, 1937.

Swoboda, W.: Angular dorsolumbale Kyphose als unbekanntes Skeletzeichen beim kongenitalen Myxoedem, Fortschr. Röntgenstrah., *73*, 740, 1950.

VanWyk, J. J.: Hypothyroidism in Childhood, Pediatrics, *17*, 427, 1956.

Wilkins, L.: Epiphyseal Dysgenesis Associated with Hypothyroidism, Am. J. Dis. Child., *61*, 13, 1941.

Metabolic Disorders

OSTEOPOROSIS

Osteoporosis is ascribed to a disorder of tissue metabolism characterized by the failure of the osteoblasts to lay down bone matrix. Inasmuch as this is not a disease of calcium metabolism, it is associated with normal serum calcium and phosphorus levels. The most common cause appears to be the postmenopausal state caused by a deficiency in estrogen and consequent failure of adequate osteoblastic activity (Albright, Smith and Richardson, 1941). Probably next frequent is the so-called senile atrophy in which the bony structures undergo the same atrophy as other components of the body. The atrophy of disuse with diminished osteoblastic activity, the so-called idiopathic osteoporosis of unknown etiology and the osteoporosis of malnutrition with depletion of bone matrix because of insufficient protein intake are among other causes. Among the glandular causes, some of which already have been discussed, are Cushing's syndrome, the adaptation syndrome of Selye, acromegaly, gonadal disorders, and congenital osteoblastic defect as exemplified by osteogenesis imperfecta. Other conditions associated with osteoporosis infrequently include varied conditions such as pregnancy polycythemia vera, myasthenia gravis, prolonged heparin therapy, Gaucher's disease and Waldenström's macroglobulinemia. Diffuse, and often extensive demineralization of bone is noted frequently in children with leukemia, either alone or together with steroid therapy. Metastatic malignant disease with bone loss is well known. Its origin also includes disuse, hormonal alterations, hypercalcemia, and other still unknown factors. Ankylosing spondylitis also is frequently accompanied by pronounced osteoporosis which may be heightened by steroids and disuse.

Hepatogenic osteoporosis occurs when there is extensive destruction of liver parenchyma, such as results from toxic influences, biliary occlusion or external bile fistulas. Similar changes are occasionally encountered in cirrhosis or extensive liver metastases. The mechanism for this change is complex, including disturbance of calcium and fat absorption from the intestine and faulty absorption and deposition of vitamin D in the liver. Among other factors are secondary hyperparathyroidism due to lack of calcium, atrophy of the testes due to failure of the liver's inactivating functions on estrogens, and hyperplasia of the adrenal cortex due to atrophy of the testes resulting in overproduction of the adrenocortical hormone (Cocchi, 1951).

The association of hyperthyroidism with osteoporosis is ascribed to increased excretion of calcium and phosphorus in the urine and feces, the continuous negative calcium balance manifesting itself eventually as osteoporosis. Instances of juvenile hyperthyroidism with osteoporosis were described by Jacobs (1943).

Osteoporosis with ulcerative colitis was described by Ricketts, Benditt and Palmer (1945). Miyakawa and Stearns (1942) reported severe osteoporosis or osteomalacia in a 34-year-old woman who had had steatorrhea for more than 10 years.

Osteoporosis incident to the prolonged use of cortisone, hydrocortisone and corticotropin was reported by Demartini, Grokoest and Ragan (1952) and by Boland (1952). Such treatment resulted in clinical features simulating Cushing's syndrome if hyperadrenalism is produced. In the group reported by Demartini, Grokoest and Ragan 5 patients had been treated from 5 to 20 months. All were women, and 4 were in the postmenopausal age group. A predisposing factor such as prolonged bed rest, prolonged activity of the disease under treatment or postmenopausal states was present in each patient. Boland stated that 7 of his patients had spontaneous fractures. Spinal compression fractures appeared in 4, fracture of the femoral neck appeared in 2 and a pubic ramus fracture occurred in 1. Each of his patients had had long-standing rheumatoid arthritis.

The bony changes of osteoporosis of whatever cause are alike. The spongiosa and cortex are thin, and consist of normal lime-containing tissue. The trabeculae are widely separated, and red bone marrow is considerably diminished with replacement of a large portion of the marrow by fat. The trabeculae become slender, and the vertical ones stand out prominently. A meshwork of smaller horizontal trabeculae can be identified on inspection of a sliced vertebral body, but these are not identifiable on roentgenograms with the same clarity as are the vertical trabeculae (Fig. 184). This persistent vertical pattern is not a constant change, and osteoporotic vertebrae which show only diffuse demineralization of bone present radiographically with thin shell-like cortical margins and a diffuse haziness of the cancellous structures. Osteoporotic vertebrae tend towards compression fractures with little trauma, especially in those areas subject to stress. Fractures are likely to appear in the midthoracic and the upper lumbar vertebrae. Cervical vertebrae fractures in osteoporotic vertebrae are uncommon.

When osteoporosis has advanced to a certain degree, the trabeculae are no longer able to resist the weight of the body and the internal pressure of the intervertebral discs. This results in collapse of the central portion of the vertebral body producing a biconcave vertebra and expansion of the nucleus pulposus and disc in a biconvex fashion follows (Fig. 185).

Radiologic examination of the spine in early cases of osteoporosis first reveals a diffuse demineralization of the vertebral bodies, which retain their normal contours, but present a glazed appearance with sharply marked borders of increased density at the periphery. The intervertebral spaces as a rule are not disturbed. At this stage it is not uncommon for impaction fractures to occur in the anterosuperior aspect of the vertebral bodies, especially in the mid-thoracic and the thoracolumbar regions. The presence of Schmorl's nodes may be observed, but sclerosis of bone surrounding the herniated nodules of fibrocartilage is conspicuous by its absence. With further progression demineralization increases and the tensile strength of the vertebrae is lessened. This is manifested by a diffuse collapse of one or several vertebral bodies, particularly in the mid-thoracic and upper lumbar regions, together with associated widening of the intervertebral spaces. Anterior wedging of the vertebral bodies with concomitant dorsum rotundum may become prominent (Fig. 186). Combinations of diffuse flattening of the vertebral bodies together with biconvex configurations may be observed, with flattened vertical bodies more prominent in the thoracic region.

Compression fractures produce a zone of increased density just beneath the cartilaginous end plates, with reduction in the height of the vertebral body. Upward or downward displacement of an intervertebral disc can impinge into the corresponding surface of the affected vertebra. The change in density of bone involved in compaction incident to partial collapse looks much the same as that seen with Cushing's disease or iatrogenic steroid osteoporosis (Fig. 187).

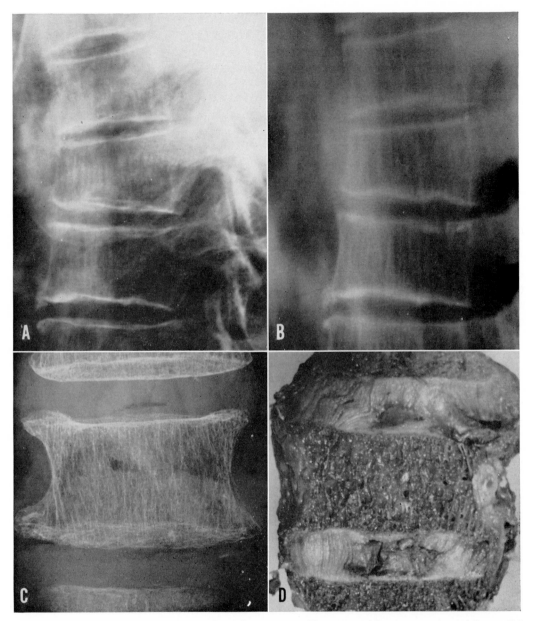

Fig. 184. *A*, The lower thoracic vertebrae in a 64-year-old woman with osteoporosis reveals parallel vertical striations and mild compressive changes. *B*, Laminagram shows these striations to better advantage. *C*, Roentgenogram of vertebral slab. The vertical markings are prominent, but horizontal strands also are present. *D*, Photograph of specimen. Note the degenerative changes in the intervertebral discs.

Involvement of the cervical spine by osteoporosis may result in demineralization of the vertebral bodies. Osteoporotic collapse of the cervical segments is uncommon. The cervical intervertebral discs likewise usually maintain normal contours unless altered by discogenic disease, which is frequent in the age group in which osteoporosis is seen most often.

The remainder of the skeleton usually shows porotic changes of lesser degree, but in advanced cases thinning of the cortices of

Fig. 185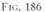

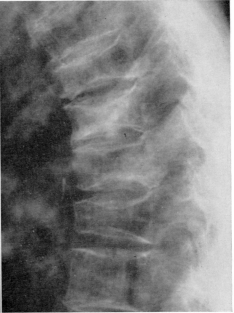

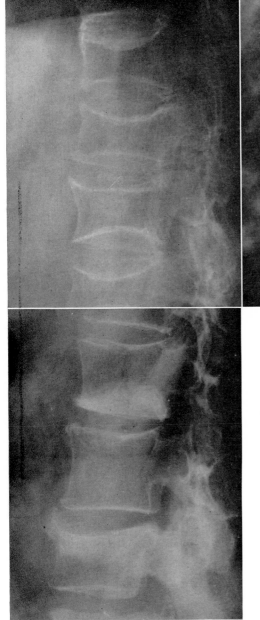

Fig. 185. Osteoporosis of the lumbar vertebrae with compressive changes and widened
discs.

Fig. 186. Midthoracic spine of a 68-year-
old woman with osteoporosis. The bodies are
narrowed and the discs expanded.

Fig. 187. Compression fracture of the
twelfth thoracic and first lumbar vertebrae in
a 65-year-old woman with osteoporosis. Note
the sclerotic changes in the inferior margin of
T11 and superior margin of L1.

Fig. 187

the long bones and widening of their medullary canals is observed fairly often. A
change associated with osteoporosis of the
postmenopausal, senile or idiopathic type, is
parietal thinness of the skull (Epstein, 1952).

The osteoporosis of the vertebral column
from the causes noted above may bear a
marked similarity to that associated with
other diseases, particularly osteomalacia,
myeloma, certain forms of hyperparathyroidism and other less common conditions mentioned before.

References

Albright, F.: Osteoporosis, Ann. Int. Med., *27*, 861, 1947.

Albright, F. and Reifenstein, E. C., Jr.: *Parathyroid Glands and Metabolic Bone Disease*, Baltimore, The Williams & Wilkins Co., 1948.

Albright, F., Smith, P. H. and Fraser, R.: Syndrome Characterized by Primary Ovarian Insufficiency and Decreased Stature, Am. J. Med. Sci., *204*, 625, 1942.

Albright, F., Smith, P. H. and Richardson, A. M.: Postmenopausal Osteoporosis, J.A.M.A., *116*, 2465, 1941.

Boland, E. W.: Clinical Use of Cortisone, Hydrocortisone, and Corticotropin, J.A.M.A., *150*, 1281, 1952.

Cocchi, U.: Hepatogenic Osteoporosis, Radiol. Clin., *20*, 362, 1951.

Demartini, F., Grokoest, A. W. and Ragan, C.: Pathological Fractures in Patients with Rheumatoid Arthritis Treated with Cortisone, J.A.M.A., *149*, 750, 1952.

Epstein, B. S.: Concurrence of Parietal Thinness with Postmenopausal, Senile or Idiopathic Osteoporosis, Radiology, *60*, 29, 1953.

Fraser, R.: The Problem of Osteoporosis, J. Bone & Joint Surg., *44-B*, 485, 1962.

Griffith, G. C., Nichos, G., Jr., Asher, J. D. and Flanagan, B.: Heparin Osteoporosis, J.A.M.A., *193*, 91, 1965.

Hanlon, D. G., Bayrd, E. D. and Kearns, T. P.: Macroglobulinemia — Report of Four Cases, J.A.M.A., *167*, 1817, 1958.

Jackson, W. P. U.: Osteoporosis of Unknown Cause in Younger People, J. Bone & Joint Surg., *40-B*, 420, 1958.

Jaffe, M. D. and Willis, P. W., III.: Multiple Fractures Associated with Long-Term Sodium Heparin Therapy, J.A.M.A., *193*, 152, 1965.

Kesson, C. M., Morris, N. and McCutcheon, A.: Generalized Osteoporosis in Old Age, Ann. Rheumat. Dis., *6*, 146, 1947.

Levin, E. J.: Congenital Biliary Atresia with Emphasis on the Skeletal Abnormalities, Radiology, *67*, 714, 1956.

Miuakawa, G. and Stearns, G.: Severe Osteoporosis (Or Osteomalacia) Associated with Long-Continued Low-Grade Steatorrhea, J. Bone & Joint Surg., *24*, 429, 1942.

Murray, R. O.: Steroids and the Skeleton, Radiology, *77*, 729, 1961.

Nicholas, J. A., Wilson, P. D. and Freiberger, R.: Pathological Fractures of the Spine, Etiology and Diagnosis, J. Bone & Joint Surg., *42-A*, 127, 1960.

Ricketts, W. E., Benditt, E. P. and Palmer, W. L.: Chronic Ulcerative Colitis with Infantilism and Carcinoma of Colon, Gastroenterology, *5*, 272, 1945.

Smith, R. W., Jr., Eyler, W. R. and Mellinger, R. C.: On the Incidence of Senile Osteoporosis, Ann. Int. Med., *52*, 773, 1960.

Snapper, I.: *Medical Clinic on Bone Diseases*, 2nd ed., New York, Interscience Publishers, 1949.

OSTEOMALACIA

This condition refers to disorders which result in the presence of abnormal amounts of osteoid in the bones because of insufficient calcification. Any condition which depletes the body's calcium stores sufficiently can cause osteomalacia. Such depletion may take place through insufficient absorption of calcium or through excessive loss. Insufficient quantities of inorganic phosphorus in the blood is another factor which militates against normal calcification of bony matrix by whatever calcium is present in the serum. The serum calcium value is within normal limits or somewhat diminished. The blood serum phosphorous level likewise may be normal or slightly lower than usual. The failure of bone to calcify properly leads to increased osteoblastic activity with a consequent elevation in the serum alkaline phosphatase content. Albright and his coworkers (1946) indicated that rickets presented all the characteristics of osteomalacia together with changes at the epiphyseal line, principally faulty calcification of the zone of provisional calcification (failure of osteoid tissue to calcify normally).

Albright and Reifenstein (1948) separated osteomalacia into four categories depending upon the degree of severity. The first group included chemical osteomalacia with normal phosphatase, the second chemical osteomalacia with high phosphatase, the third Milkman's syndrome and the fourth advanced osteomalacia. Severity depends on the relationship between serum calcium and serum phosphorus content. When minimal, the disordered deposit of calcium and osteoid tissue is not sufficient to give rise to sufficient skeletal weakness to produce a high phosphatase content because of increased osteoblastic activity. When osteoblastic activity is stimulated, and where radiologic and clinical indications of osteomalacia are lacking but still phosphatase content is elevated, there exists a group of cases in which neither pseudo-fractures nor demineralization occur. Cases with chemical osteomalacia and pseudo-fractures without obvi- ous generalized demineralization constitute the third group, of which Milkman's syndrome is probably the best example. The last classification refers to the advanced softening of bones characteristic of osteomalacia.

Osteomalacia due to simple vitamin D deficiency has not been observed in this country, but has been reported by Maxwell (1935) as occurring frequently in Northern China. Winston and Pendergrass (1954) reported a case of Milkman's disease which they attributed to simple vitamin D deficiency in an adult. Vitamin D resistant rickets and steatorrhea are other causes. The next group described by these authors is due to renal acidosis as caused by the Fanconi syndrome and renal disease of tubular insufficiency without glomerular insufficiency. A third group is idiopathic hypercalciuria and the fourth is hyperparathyroidism with osteitis fibrosa generalisata during the transitional stage following the removal of a parathyroid tumor.

There are also bizarre metabolic diseases in which osteomalacia plays a significant role. For example, Lowe (1952) mentioned marked bone loss and suggestive rachitic changes as occurring in an unusual syndrome consisting of organic acidemia, diminished renal ammonium production, hydrophthalmos and mental retardation. In one such case seen by us recently the rachitic-like disturbances responded to vigorous vitamin D therapy, but the osteomalacia, particularly of the spine, did not recede visibly. The syndrome of idiopathic hypercalciuria, caused by impaired tubular reabsorption of calcium, results in increased calcium excretion and nephrolithiasis, also includes a degree of osteomalacia among its manifestations. Evidence also has been presented to indicate that osteoporosis occurring with prolonged corticosteroid treatment may in later stages be accompanied by osteomalacia.

The radiologic features of Milkman's syndrome have received considerable attention. At first (Milkman, 1934) this was considered to be a specific disease of unknown etiology, but the work of Albright and his colleagues (1946) among others resulted in the inclusion of this syndrome with osteomalacic diseases. The condition is characterized by multiple spontaneous idiopathic symmetrical pseudo-fractures. These pseudo-fractures are actually united, the symmetrical focal bands of translucency being due to osteoid tissue. The outstanding radiologic feature consists of these translucent band-like areas. At first no deformity is present but later separation, displacement and overriding of fragments may occur. Settling of the vertebral column, formation of a heart-shaped pelvis, coxa vara, rib, ulnar and clavicular angulations are part of the picture of generalized osteomalacia. Usually no callous formation is observed. Albright and his colleagues mentioned that bone taken from a rib and vertebra of 2 patients with Milkman's disease showed characteristic changes of osteomalacia. They favored the retention of Milkman's syndrome as an entity to emphasize the fact that osteomalacia can be present without generalized decalcification, with only these united uncalcified zones. In their discussion they presented 2 cases of Milkman's syndrome associated with steatorrhea.

In a report of a 37-year-old male patient with Milkman's syndrome, Brick and Bunch (1947) stated that roentgenograms of the spine showed narrowing of the fifth and sixth dorsal vertebrae, with pseudo-fractures of the spinous processes of the fifth, sixth and seventh cervical vertebrae. There was generalized osteoporosis with pseudo-fractures of the interarticular isthmus of the third, fourth and fifth lumbar segments, of the second to fourth, the sixth, seventh, ninth, tenth and eleventh ribs, the manubrium and other bones. All in all this patient had 39 fractures. Biopsy of the tibia showed fibrosis and thinning of the cortex with unusually large Haversian canals and rarefaction of the bone.

Pseudo-fractures occur with many diseases including osteomalacia, rickets and latent rickets, renal rickets, celiac disease, chronic idiopathic steatorrhea non-tropical sprue, early and late osteogenesis imperfecta, fragilitas osseum, hyperparathyroidism, hyperthyroidism, Paget's disease, adrenal pituitary bone dystrophy, severe chronic acidosis, hyperglycemia, congenital syphilis, osteomyelitis, osteopetrosis, march fractures and bone dysplasias. The common feature to all of these is weakening of the bony framework or excessive load on the bone. Such lesions are found most often in the lower extremities, the pelvis, ribs, forearms, and wrists. In the vertebrae they may be difficult to distinguish from compression fractures. Stress fractures of the neural arches occur as well.

Albright, Burnett, Parson, Reifenstein and Roos (1946) did not entirely agree with the conclusions expressed in the preceding paragraph. They observed that the conditions listed were either rickets or osteomalacia, depending on the age of the patient, and

in the others the resemblance was purely superficial. They pointed out that in Paget's disease, polyostotic fibrous dysplasia and osteogenesis imperfecta these fractures occurred through areas of bony pathology, while in osteomalacia they occurred in bones which appear otherwise perfectly normal radiologically.

In one patient, a 27-year-old woman, osteoporosis and osteomalacia appeared soon after the delivery of a normal infant (Fig. 188). In another patient (Fig. 189) the spine roentgenograms revealed a flattening of the thoracic vertebrae and a diffuse loss of density of the lumbar vertebrae. This child had been exposed to famine. At the time these roentgenograms were made there were no clinical symptoms. Rose (1964) noted that the bones tended to bend rather than fracture, much the same as noted in this patient.

Another case observed by us was consid-

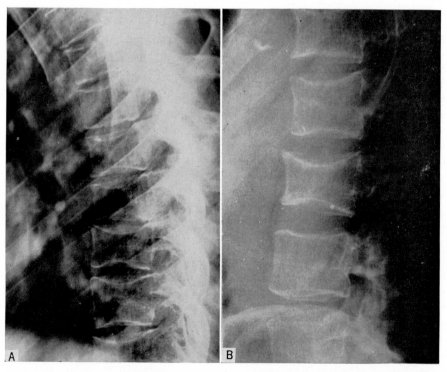

Fɪɢ. 188.   Osteoporosis and osteomalacia in a 27-year-old woman complaining of persistent back pain for a month after delivery of a normal infant. The intervertebral discs are bulging in an irregular pattern. Some of the vertebrae are less dense than others, and varying compressive changes are present.

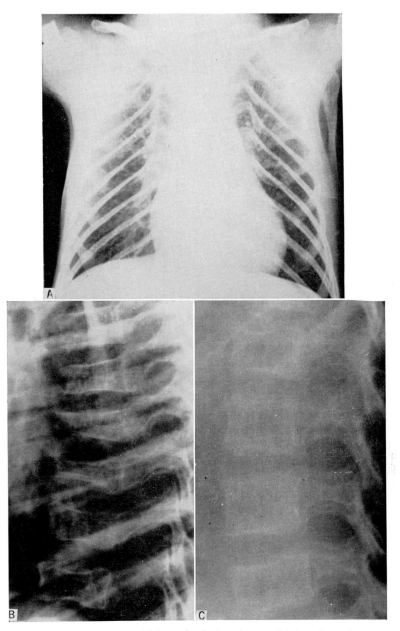

FIG. 189. Osteomalacia in an 8-year-old boy who had undergone famine about 4 years preceding this examination. The ribs are slender, and are angulated downwards beginning near the costovertebral articulations. The thoracic vertebrae are diffusely flattened, and the intervertebral discs are slightly biconvex. The lumbar vertebrae are demineralized still, but their contours are well maintained. The lumber discs are moderately bulging in appearance. The vertebral peripheries are slightly denser than their central portions.

ered as having both osteoporosis and osteo-malacia on a nutritional and biliary basis. This was a 67-year-old man who, following a subtotal gastric resection for a duodenal ulcer, was unable to accept food for a long time and developed a severe protein deficiency. A long-draining biliary fistula formed. Radiologically this was accompanied by pronounced osteoporosis resulting in practically complete demineralization of

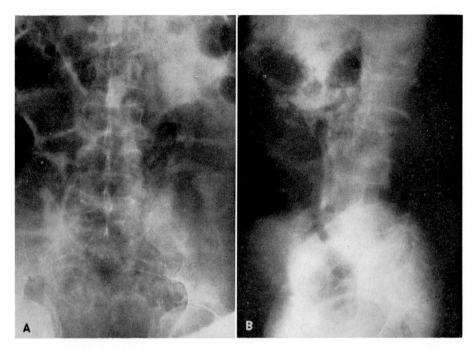

FIG. 190. Osteomalacia following subtotal gastrectomy for ulcer complicated by draining biliary fistula. Note the advanced demineralization of the vertebrae, the bulging intervertebral discs, and the inward protrusion of the femoral heads, particularly the left one.

his spine, with biconcave vertebrae and markedly enlarged and biconvex intervertebral discs (Fig. 190). This patient also developed marked decalcification of the remainder of his skeleton. The femoral heads and acetabulae protruded deeply into the true pelvis. His skull presented bilateral parietal thinness. This patient improved slowly but steadily on hormonal therapy together with an enriched diet. During this long period of recovery he fell and fractured his right hip, which was subsequently pinned with a good clinical result. Not noted at the time of the original film was a definite osteoid zone in the opposite left femoral neck. The patient complained of mild pain in the left hip, but a subsequent radiologic examination failed to disclose any evidence of fracture. About 7 months later this zone was recognized in retrospect when a current roentgenogram revealed that the left femoral neck had been fractured without known trauma, the fracture line apparently occurring through the osteoid zone. Repeated

blood chemistry studies in this patient showed the serum calcium to be between 9 and 10 mg per cent, the serum phosphatase to be between 3 and 4 mg per cent, and the serum alkaline phosphatase value to be between 10 and 15 gm per cent.

References

Albright, F., Burnett, C. H., Parson, W., Reifenstein, E. C., Jr. and Roos, A.: Osteomalacia and Late Rickets, Medicine, *25*, 399, 1946.

Albright, F. ,Butler, A. M. and Bloomberg, E.: Rickets Resistant to Vitamin D Therapy, Am. J. Dis. Child., *54*, 529, 1937.

Brick, I. B. and Bunch, R. F.: Milkman's Syndrome, New England J. Med., *237*, 359, 1947.

Camp, J. D. and McCullough, J. A. L.: Pseudofractures in Diseases Affecting the Skeletal System, Radiology, *36*, 651, 1941.

Dent, C. E.: Rickets and Osteomalacia from Renal Tubule Defects, J. Bone & Joint Surg., *34-B*, 266, 1952.

Edeiken, L. and Schneeberg, N. G.: Multiple Spontaneous Idiopathic Symmetrical Fractures, J.A.M.A., *122*, 865, 1943.

Elliot, A: Advanced Vitamin D Resistant Osteomalacia with Looser-Milkman's Syndrome, Acta med. Scandinav., *152*, 195, 1955.

Hauge, B. N.: Vitamin D Resistant Osteomalacia, Acta med. Scandinav., *153*, 271, 1956.

Juerfens, J. L., Scholz, D. A. and Wollaeger, E. E.: Severe Osteomalacia Associated with Occult Steatorrhea Due to Nontropical Sprue, Arch. Int. Med., *18*, 774, 1956.

Lowe, C. U.: Organic Acidemia, Decreased Renal Ammonium Production, Hydrophthalmos and Mental Retardation, Am. J. Dis. Child., *83*, 164, 1952.

Maxwell, J. P.: Osteomalacia and its Importance in China, Chinese Med. J., *49*, 47, 1935.

McCune, D. J., Mason, H. H. and Clarke, H. T.: Intractable Hypophosphatemic Rickets with Renal Glycosuria and Acidosis (Fanconi Syndrome), Am. J. Dis. Child., *65*, 81, 1943.

Milkman, L. A.: Multiple Spontaneous Idiopathic Symmetrical Fractures, Am. J. Roentgenol., *32*, 622, 1934.

Rose, G. A.: The Radiological Diagnosis of Osteoporosis, Osteomalacia and Hyperparathyroidism, Clin. Radiol., *15*, 75, 1964.

Segar, W. E., Iber, F. L. and Kyle, L. H.: Osteomalacia of Unknown Etiology, New England J. Med., *254*, 1011, 1956.

Winston, N. J. and Pendergrass, E. P.: Milkman's Disease (Osteomalacia), Am. J. Roentgenol., *71*, 484, 1954.

Rickets

Infantile rickets with vitamin D deficiency is associated with failure of calcification of osteoid tissue and bone development due to insufficient utilization of calcium. A reduced serum phosphorus content is present, caused by failure of absorption of phosphorus from the intestinal tract, and increased excretion of phosphorus from the intestinal and urinary tracts. The failure of osteoid calcification is characteristic of osteomalacia. The radiologic alterations in the growing bones include widened epiphyseal zones, with flaring and tuft-like configuration of the metaphyseal ends. The diffuse osteomalacia may manifest itself in the spine by a similar process. The superior and inferior surfaces of the respective vertebral bodies present a convex appearance, with the height of the vertebral bodies somewhat reduced and the intervertebral spaces proportionately widened. A mild dorsolumbar kyphosis has been observed in several cases of severe infantile rickets, an example of which is included here (Fig. 191). With proper therapy the vertebral bodies regain their height and normal osseous density.

Oppenheimer (1939) described rarefaction of the vertebrae in early stages of rapidly

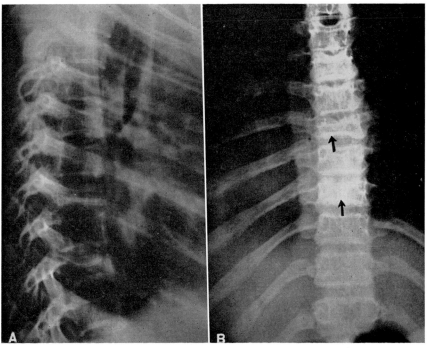

FIG. 191. Lateral and anteroposterior spine roentgenograms in rickets. The vertebral bodies are diffusely compressed (arrows) and the intervertebral discs are bulging.

progressive rickets. In less acute phases he identified globular rarefied areas arranged like clover leaves which became surrounded by calcium as the rickets healed. Broadening of the epiphyseal cartilages was not found, but compression of the vertebral bodies and expansion of the discs occurred if rarefaction was sufficiently marked.

Chronic renal insufficiency is associated with osteodystrophy, and has been mentioned in consideration of secondary hyperparathyroidism. Stunted growth sometimes follows failure of endochondral ossification at the growth zones, producing renal dwarfism in children. In adults osteosclerosis at the endplates of the vertebrae result in the "rugger-jersey" striping previously mentioned (Fig. 173). Failure of tubular reabsorption represents "vitamin D resistant rickets," associated with phosphaturia and consequent low plasma phosphorus content. These patients present skeletal deformities such as bowed legs, widened epiphyseal lines and dwarfism. Renal tubular acidosis also results in osteomalacia, with a high urinary excretion of calcium and phosphorus and nephrocalcinosis. Amino-aciduria (Fanconi syndrome) is another tubular disorder in which osteomalacia follows excessive excretion of phosphates and low blood phosphorus levels. Glycosuria is present, and other indications of tubular dysfunction include deficient resorption of water and consequent polyuria and proteinuria. In instances where cystinosis is combined with the other features of amino-aciduria the term "Lignac-Fanconi syndrome" is used. The bone lesions from this group of disorders may respond to large doses of vitamin D.

An instance of familial vitamin D resistance rickets in an adult who had been untreated was reported by Johnson and his co-workers (1966). This patient, a 28-year-old woman, developed compression of the cord secondary to bony proliferation of the neural arches, with a block at the level of the eleventh thoracic vertebra. Her father, who also had this condition, had a similar bony overgrowth without cord compression.

Dugger and Vandiver (1966) reported a 60-year-old man with vitamin D resistant rickets who had extradural compression at the twelfth thoracic vertebra due to bony proliferation of the anterior longitudinal ligament. At operation there was heavy overgrowth of bone around the articular facets, and the spinal canal was encroached upon so that the epidural space was eliminated and the dura was found adherent or closely approximated to the adjacent bone.

References

Dugger, G. S. and Vandiver, R. W.: Spinal Cord Compression Caused by Vitamin D Resistant Rickets, J. Neurosurg., *25*, 300, 1966.

Hurwitz, L. J. and Shepherd, W. H. T.: Basilar Impression and Disordered Metabolism of Bone, Brain, *89*, 223, 1966.

Johnson, C. C., Jr., Kurlander, G. J., Smith, D. M., Goodman, J. M. and Campbell, R. L.: Familial Vitamin D Resistant Rickets in Untreated Adult, Arch. Int. Med., *117*, 141, 1966.

Oppenheimer, A.: Rickets of Spinal Column, Radiol. Clin., *8*, 332, 1939.

Steinbach, H. L. and Noetzli, M.: Roentgen Appearance of the Skeleton in Osteomalacia and Rickets, Am. J. Roentgenol., *91*, 955, 1964.

HYPERVITAMINOSIS A

The bony changes associated with this condition usually appear in the long bones, with periosteal elevation nad subperiosteal calcification involving these bones as well as the clavicles and the ribs. No spine changes have been described in children. (Caffey, 1951; Bifulco, 1953).

We had the opportunity of studying intensively a patient who had been taking over 500,000 units of vitamin A daily for over 8 years. This patient, who was reported in detail by Gerber, Raab and Sobel (1954), was studied radiologically by the present author. Prominent among the findings were changes in the spine quite similar to those associated with ankylosing spondylitis. A pronounced straightening of the spine was noted together with moderate decalcification of the vertebral bodies. No change at the intervertebral spaces could be demonstrated. Of interest was the calcifica-

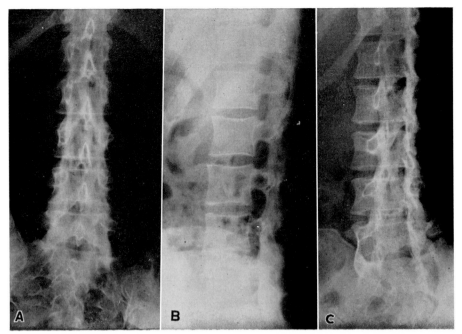

Fig. 192. Hypervitaminosis A in an adult woman. The lumbar spine is straightened, and calcification is noted aong the ligamenta flava. The articular surfaces of the lower apophyseal joints are closely apposed and roughened. The picture simulates ankylosing spondylitis.

tion along the ligamenta flava, and the intense decalcification and loss of articular surfaces of the apophyseal joints of the lumbar spine. The bony margins of the sacroiliac joints, however, retained a normal bony density (Fig. 192). Other changes noted were calcium deposits in the insertions of the various ligaments such as those at the anterior tibial spine, the insertion of the quadriceps tendon, the periphery of both hip joints, in the vicinity of the capsules of the shoulders, and at the iliolumbar ligaments.

References

Bifulco, E.: Vitamin A Intoxication, New England J. Med., *248*, 690, 1953.
Gerber, A., Raab, A. P. and Sobel, A. E.: Vitamin A Poisoning in Adults, Am. J. Med., *16*, 729, 1954.

HYPERVITAMINOSIS D

In a report by Christensen, Liebman and Sosman (1951) no vertebral involvement in cases of hypervitaminosis D was recorded.

DeWind (1961) reported the case of a 5½-year-old boy who had been subjected to an excessive intake of vitamin D over a long period of time. A pronounced degree of osteosclerosis followed. Radiographic examination of the spine disclosed dense square-appearing vertebral bodies. There was a generalized increase in bone density as well. The osseous changes were reversible, and were attributed to the effect of withdrawal of the vitamin D on the hypercalcemia. DeWind believed that the changes seen in his patient resembled somewhat that seen in severe cases of 'idiopathic hypercalcemia.'

References

Christensen, W. R., Liebman, C. and Sosman, M. C.: Skeletal and Periarticular Manifestations of Hypervitaminosis D, Am. J. Roentgenol., *65*, 27, 1951.
DeWind, L. T.: Hypervitaminosis D with Osteosclerosis, Arch. Dis. Childhood, *36*, 373, 1961.

IDIOPATHIC HYPERCALCEMIA OF INFANCY

This infrequent condition is attributed to an abnormal sensitivity in some children to vitamin D in the presence of a milk diet, resulting in excessive absorption of calcium from the gastrointestinal tract with consequent hypercalcemia, renal calcinosis, acidosis and failure to thrive.

Because of the high calcium level, marked muscular hypotonia, anorexia, vomiting, constipation and retarded growth occur. Persistent hypercalcemia results in permanent damage, with marked retardation of growth, toxic effects on the central nervous system, heart, kidneys, craniostenosis and mental retardation. Some children present a characteristic "elfin" facies, and association with cretinism has been observed. In mild cases the condition may resolve, leaving no apparent residual changes. Mental retardation and evidences of defective growth appear in more severely afflicted children, and some do not survive. Idiopathic hypercalcemia of infancy usually first appears between the ages of about 3 and 7 months. It is associated with a rise in serum calcium and urinary excretion of calcium. The blood cholesterol and urea are elevated, and a low serum alkaline phosphatase content is present. Serum phosphorus content remains normal. In most instances spontaneous cessation of idiopathic hypercalcemia takes place after about 1 year. Then normal bone is laid down, and dense bands are separated from normal bone as it is laid down at the margins of the epiphyseal cartilages. In severe cases bowing of the long bones, undertubulation, and craniostenosis with or without microcephaly may remain.

Radiographic examinations reveal extensive osteosclerosis, soft tissue calcifications and defective ossification. The osteosclerotic changes in the long bones appear at their ends, with ricket-like deformities and osteosclerotic horizontal lines. The bones appear to be rather soft, being bowed and having the epiphyseal ends invaginated into the shafts to some degree. The vertebrae partake in the osteosclerosis, their bodies particularly presenting increased density in a frame-like fashion, leaving a relatively radiolucent center. The bodies are small.

A benign form of hypercalcemia in children in known to occur, which is not as striking and is relatively self limited. The radiologic changes are minimal. It is not known whether a relationship exists between the two forms of hypercalcemia.

References

Daeschner, G. L. and Daeschner, C. W.: Severe Idiopathic Hypercalcemia of Infancy, Pediatrics, *19*, 362, 1957.

Eban, R.: Idiopathic Hypercalcaemia of Infancy, Clin. Radiol., *12*, 31, 1961.

Lowe K. G., Henderson, J. L., Park, W. W. and McGreal, D. A.: The Idiopathic Hypercalcaemic Syndromes of Infancy, Lancet, *2*, 201, 1954.

Mitchell, R. G.: The Prognosis in Idiopathic Hypercalcaemia of Infants, Arch. Dis. Childhood, *35*, 383, 1960.

Shiers, J. A., Neuhauser, E. B. D. and Bowman, J. R.: Idiopathic Hypercalcemia, Am. J. Roentgenol., *78*, 19, 1957.

Singleton, E. B.: The Radiographic Features of Severe Idiopathic Hypercalcemia of Infancy, Radiology, *68*, 721, 1957.

ALCAPTONURIA AND OCHRONOSIS

This is a rare hereditary metabolic disease in which the enzyme homogentisic acid oxidase is missing. It usually appears in adults in middle life, and affects both sexes equally. The disease is characterized by excretion of alcapton, rendering the urine dark or brown-black after exposure to the air. The chemical substance excreted is homogentisic acid, an intermediary product in the metabolism of phenylalanine, beyond which that amino-acid and tyrosin are not metabolized. A few cases have been discovered in infants because of brownish or black discoloration of the diapers. The condition is usually asymptomatic until middle age, when the patients become poorly nourished and appear chronically ill. The skin becomes a mottled yellowish or brownish color, particularly over the head, neck and torso, and to a lesser degree over the arms and legs. The ear lobes appear nodular and rigid and become a discolored greyish blue color. The nose also may acquire a bluish tint due to the deposit of homogentisic acid, and the sclerae likewise assume a slate blue or purplish appearance, with triangular brownish patches. Clubbing of the fingers occurs, and there is discoloration of the hands, the axillae and the genital regions because of pigment deposits. These people usually develop a dorsal kyphotic curve with loss of the lumbar curve. Radiologic examinations of the spine show a hypertrophic ankylosing process with osteoporosis of the vertebral bodies. The dorsal kyphosis may be prominent. Vertical or linear striations may be seen in the vertebral bodies, which may be reduced in height. Most striking is a diffuse calcification of practically all the intervertebral discs, which is considered diagnostic of this condition (Fig. 193). The intervertebral discs are markedly narrowed, and varying degrees of fusion of the vertebral bodies can be demonstrated. Dense calcification of the remaining intervertebral fibrocartilage can be identified radiologically. The cartilage as observed at necropsy is deeply pigmented, and appears black in color. Severe degeneration is prominent, so that the bony edges of the vertebrae approximate each other and ultimately fuse. Discal herniation with ochronosis is rare (McCollum and Odon, 1965). Spur formation is relatively limited.

References

Cervenansky, J., Sitaj, S. and Urbanek, T.: Alkaptonuria and Ochronosis, J. Bone & Joint Surg., *41-A*, 1169, 1959.

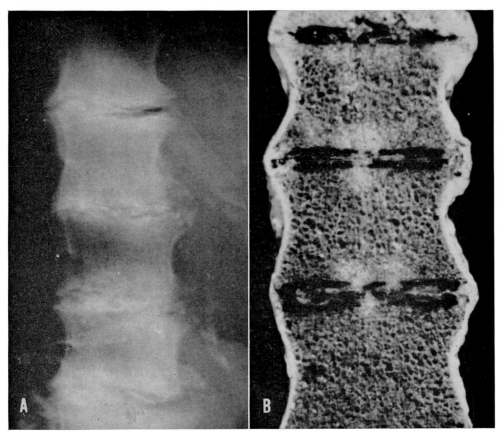

Fig. 193. *A*, Lateral lumbar spine in patient with ochronosis. The intervertebral discs are narrowed and heavy ossification rather than simple calcification is present. Considerable marginal overgrowth is present as well. *B*, Photograph of the specimen. The dense black discoloration of the discs is evident. (Courtesy of L. L. Robbins, M.D., Wittenberg, J. Gastrointestinal Bleeding and Arthropathy, J.A.M.A., *95*, 1048, 1966.)

Eisenberg, H.: Alkaptonuria, Ochronosis, Arthritis and Ruptured Intervertebral Disk, Arch. Int. Med., *86*, 79, 1950.

Harrold, A. J.: Alkaptonuric Arthritis, J. Bone & Joint Surg., *38-B*, 532, 1956.

Klaus, E., Krizek, V. and Vranesic, Z.: Die Ochronose der Wirbelsaule im Rontgenbild. Fortschr. Röntgenstr., *95*, 242, 1961.

McCollum, D. E. and Odom, G. L.: Alkaptonuria, Ochronosis and Low-Back Pain, J. Bone & Joint Surg., *47-A*, 1389, 1965.

Sacks, S.: Alkaptonuric Arthritis, J. Bone & Joint Surg., *33-B*, 407, 1951.

Smith, H. P. and Smith, H. P., Jr.: Ochronosis, Ann. Int. Med., *42*, 171, 1955.

Sutro, C. J. and Anderson, M. E.: Alkaptonuric Arthritis, Surgery, *22*, 120, 1947.

Ward, P. R. and Engelbrecht, P. J.: Alkaptonuria and Ochronosis, Clin. Radiol., *14*, 170, 1963.

Wittenberg, J.: Gastrointestinal Bleeding and Arthropathy, J.A.M.A., *195*, 1048, 1966.

PROGRESSIVE LIPODYSTROPHY

This condition is characterized by a loss of the normal fatty tissue in the upper half of the body. The adiposity of the lower trunk, pelvic regions and lower extremities becomes increased so that the lower half of the body is disproportionately bulky. The disease occurs more often in females, and may occur from childhood well into adult years. As a rule the patients are able to continue their activities, but may complain of easy fatigability. The loss of fat may be progressive. According to Ziegler (1928) the hypothetical causes are neurotrophic and endocrine disturbances, alteration of fat metabolism, race, heredity, infection and congenital defect. No one of these has been definitely identified as a single etiologic factor. The disease is neither hereditary nor familial.

No skeletal alterations have been mentioned as part of the picture of lipodystrophy. One patient, a 12-year-old boy, seen by us showed changes in the spine (Fig. 194). The anterior aspects of the middle cervical vertebrae were sharpened and angular. The thoracic vertebrae were not disturbed, but a definite convexity of the thoracolumbar junction was present.

Reference

Ziegler, L. H.: Lipodystrophies, Brain, *51*, 147, 1928.

GOUT

Gouty involvement of the vertebral column is rare. A case was described by Kersley, Mandel and Jeffrey (1950) in an 18-year-old patient with gout who was observed for 5 years. Death occurred because of sudden dislocation of the first cervical vertebra due to tophaceous softening, a condition not previously reported. Lichtenstein, Scott and Levin (1956) described a vertebral body bone section as containing heavy urate deposits within most of the intervertebral discs and extending into the contiguous bodies. In the affected joints focal chalky white or yellow tophaceous deposits were present on the articular surfaces and bone ends as well as in the deeper layers of cartilage. Hall and Selin (1960) reported urate crystal deposits in the posterior articular surfaces of the fourth and fifth lumbar vertebrae, involving the ligaments and capsules as well. The crystals did not invade the cartilage deeply, but could not be separated even by firm wiping. This patient, a 51-year-old man, had severe gout without back pain. Koskoff, Morris and Lubic (1953) reported the case of a 44-year-old man with paraplegia due to extradural deposition of sodium urate crystals in the lower thoracic spinal canal. The plain films were normal, but myelography revealed a complete block at the level of the eleventh dorsal vertebra.

Acute gouty sacro-iliac arthritis was reported by Lipson and Slocumb (1965) in a 23-year-old man who also had acute attacks of gouty arthritis of the lumbar spine. In a review of 95 gouty patients Malawista and his co-workers (1965) reported that 7 showed definite changes in the sacro-iliac joints, and equivocal changes were present in 5. These were described as sclerotic rimmed, punched out cystic lesions of varying sizes in or near the articular surfaces. Fusion of the joints without cystic changes could not be attributed with certainty to gout rather than to spondylitis. Each patient also had advanced changes in the extremities.

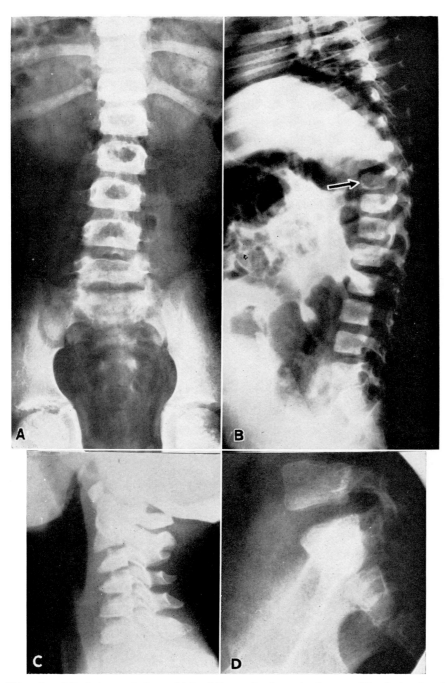

FIG. 194. *A* and *B*, Anteroposterior and lateral thoracolumbar spine in case of lipodystrophy. There is a dorsal curvature at the thoracolumbar junction. The body of the tenth dorsal vertebra at the apex of the curve is small (arrow). *C*, Same case, lateral cervical spine. Note the anterior wedging of the bodies of the third and fourth cervical vertebrae. *D*, Same case. Lumbosacral articulation. The fifth lumbar vertebral body is wider anteriorly than posteriorly, and its bony density is slightly diminished. The cancellous markings are hazy.

21

Articular chondrocalcinosis associated with attacks of acute arthritis has been described under the appellation of "pseudogout." In this condition calcium pyrophosphate crystals are deposited in the affected joints. Radiologically the changes are mainly calcification of fibrocartilaginous structures, and appear in the appendicular as well as in the spinal joints (Fig. 174). Meniscal calcifications are frequently observed, but these can appear in a wide variety of diseases. Currey and his co-workers (1966) concluded that radiologic identification of calcification of joint cartilage was not necessarily indicative of a specific condition. Patients with this change showed no definite evidence of a metabolic abnormality, and only a few had either frank gout or hyperparathyroidism. In most patients they believed that the crystal deposition was the cause of the arthropathy, either by causing local degeneration of cartilage or by entering the joint and provoking a crystal synovitis.

References

Currey, H. L. F., Key, J. J., Mason, R. M. and Swettenham, K. V.: Significance of Radiological Calcification of Joint Cartilage, Ann. Rheum. Dis., *25*, 295, 1966.

Hall, M. C. and Selin, G.: Spinal Involvement in Gout, J. Bone & Joint Surg., *42-A*, 341, 1960.

Kersley, G. D., Mandel, L. and Jeffrey, M. R.: Gout; an Unusual Case with Softening and Subluxation of the First Cervical Vertebra and Splenomegaly, Ann. Rheum. Dis., *9*, 282, 1950.

Koskoff, Y. D., Morris, L. E. and Lubic, L. G.: Paraplegia as a Complication of Gout, J.A.M.A., *152*, 37, 1953.

Lichtenstein, L. Scott, H. W. and Levin, N. H.: Pathologic Changes in Gout, Am. J. Path., *32*, 871, 1956.

Lipson, R. L. and Slocumb, C. H.: The Progressive Nature of Gout with Inadequate Therapy, Arth. & Rheum., *8*, 80, 1965.

Malawista, S. E., Seegmiller, J. E., Hathaway, B. E. and Sokoloff, L.: Sacroiliac Gout, J.A.M.A., *194*, 954, 1965.

McCary, D. J., Gatter, R. A., Brill, J. M. and Hogan, J. M.: Crystal Deposition Diseases, J.A.M.A., *193*, 129, 1965.

4

Inflammatory, Degenerative and Noxious Diseases of the Spine

ANKYLOSING SPONDYLITIS (rheumatoid spondylitis, Marie-Strümpell disease, ankylossing spondylarthritis), AND RHEUMATOID ARTHRITIS

Ankylosing spondylitis is a fairly common disease of unknown etiology which usually appears in males during the 2nd to 4th decades, and is not uncommon even later. It has a marked inflammatory component, occurs in siblings and is likely to affect the offspring of similarly afflicted parents. Mental shock, trauma and acute infectious disease sometimes precipitate its onset or aggravates its manifestations. The progress of the disease may be slow or rapid, with remissions and exacerbations. The advent of steroid therapy is a noteworthy step in the management of this disabling condition, but the prognosis remains rather gloomy insofar as progressive disability is concerned. The relief of symptoms with x-ray therapy has made a place for this modality, but the possibilities of leukemogenic effect is a deterrent to its usage.

The question whether ankylosing spondylitis and rheumatoid arthritis are the same basic disease is still unresolved. The striking resemblance of the histopathologic changes in the afflicted joints is noteworthy, as is the presence of occasional peripheral joint involvement in patients with ankylosing spondylitis and sacro-iliac and vertebral column disease in individuals whose peripheral joints are mainly involved. Ankylosing spondylitis is separated from rheumatoid arthritis on the basis of differences in the pattern of joint involvement, the difference of incidence in males and females, the absence of streptococcal and sheep red cell agglutinins in ankylosing spondylitis, the absence of subcutaneous nodules in ankylosing spondylitis and some histologic features. Gold therapy has been found more effective in rheumatoid arthritis, while x-ray therapy is more beneficial in ankylosing spondylitis. Another point is the existence of severe osteoporotic changes in the affected peripheral joints in patients with rheumatoid arthritis contrasted with its relative absence in the occasional case of ankylosing spondylitis with peripheral joint involvement. Calcification of the paraspinal ligaments is frequent in ankylosing spondylitis, but is not present with rheumatoid arthritis. Sacro-iliac joint and spinal changes are prevalent with ankylosing spondylitis, while in rheumatoid arthritis such changes are infrequent, occurring occasionally in the sacro-iliac joints and cervical spine. Nevertheless, occasional patients present peculiar combinations of changes which fit either of the rheumatoid diseases. There is much left unresolved, and while clinically a sharp differentiation usually can be made between rheumatoid arthritis and ankylosing spondylitis, certain aspects are present in both. Certain collagen diseases such as lupus erythematosus, dermatomyositis, systemic sclerosis and polyarteritis nodosa can cause confusion because of articular changes. Even determinations such as the rheumatoid serum factor (RSF) or lupus erythematosus preparations (L.E.) are not infallible. Careful consideration of clinical manifestations still helps to separate the various diseases with polyarticular manifestations.

Low back pain is one of the leading complaints of patients with ankylosing spondylitis. This sometimes is associated with changing sciatic radicular symptoms. Later the pain involves the lumbosacral and thoracolumbar areas. Initial involvement of peripheral joints sometimes confuses separation of the entities, particularly if the articular symptoms are migratory and of relatively short duration. During the active stages fever, lassitude and weight loss accompanies the stiffness of the back, and the kyphotic stance may appear rather rapidly. The period of activity may be relatively short or relentlessly progressive over a period of years, producing a fixed, rounded configuration of the thoracic spine and consequent forward thrust of the neck. Spinal involvement with rheumatoid arthritis usually is in the cervical region, and may appear in relatively young children, with ankylosis of the posterior cervical articulations. Sacroiliac involvement in rheumatoid arthritis rarely occurs, while it is frequent and early in ankylosing spondylitis. Another clinical point is that ankylosing spondylitis is rare before puberty, while rheumatoid arthritis may appear in children. Involvement of the cervical spine, and especially changes in the atlantooccipital articulation, the articulation between the dens and the anterior arch of the atlas, prominent demineralization of bone, fusion of the apophyseal joints, and pitting erosions of the spinous processes occurs both in rheumatoid arthritis and ankylosing spondylitis. With the former the thoracolumbar spine and sacro-iliac joints usually are unaffected, while with the latter changes in the entire spine are much more likely to be present.

The earliest pathologic change associated with rheumatoid disease is marked proliferation of the synovial tissues, the articular capsules and surrounding soft tissues of the joints. Vascular granulation tissue then appears over the articular cartilages. Concomitantly, a similar inflammatory process takes place in the connective tissue elements in the bone beneath the articular cartilage. The inflammation extends through the zone of temporary provisional calcification and destroys the articular cartilage nearest the bone. At the same time the articular cartilage itself is attacked. These two layers of active granulation tissue have marked potentialities for forming fibrous and bony ankylosis. This replacement of normal synovial tissue by granulation tissue, eroding cartilage and invading bone, results in marked deformities of the joints with loss of function and ankylosis.

In the early stages of the disease, increased synovial fluid of an inflammatory nature appears in the involved joints. With recession of the attack the joint effusion disappears, but in the chronic stages the hyperemia and inflamed synovial membranes become prominent. At first the synovial membrane is engorged and swollen, but retains its smoothness. Later its surfaces become granular and attached firmly to the articular cartilages as a sheet of thickened vascular fibrous tissue termed pannus. Ankylosis of the joints occurs when a pannus firmly binds two opposing surfaces, or when the surfaces meet because of ulceration through their cartilaginous boundaries leading to apposition of bony structures (Hare, 1940; Steinberg, 1942; Oppenheimer, 1945). Gibson (1957) reported that biopsies from the sacro-iliac and manubriosternal joints indicated change from fibrocartilage to fibrous tissue to chondroid and later to bone, with no truly inflammatory phase. Serial biopsies from the tips of the spinous processes showed inflammatory destruction followed by excessive bone formation. In the posterior spinal joints adhesions form rapidly after a villous synovitis, followed by chon-

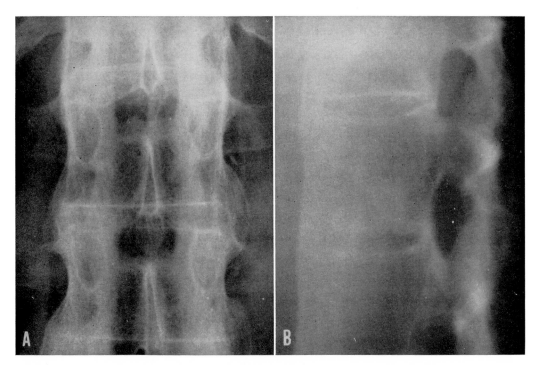

Fig. 195. *A*, Upper lumbar vertebrae of a 54-year-old man known to have ankylosing spondylitis for 35 years. The bodies are squared and the discs narrow. Paravertebral calcification in the lateral spinal ligaments. Track-like densities which outline the canal are produced by calcification in the ligaments between the apophyseal joints. *B*, the alignment of the vertebrae is straightened. The narrow discs permit contact posteriorly and anteriorly between the vertebrae. Calcification present in the anterior and posterior spinal ligaments.

droid metaplasia, ossification and ankylosis. In the intervertebral discs ossification occurs in the peripheral fibers of the annulus fibrosus and spreads from the margins of the epiphyseal rings of the body on either side to meet in the midline, producing first small spur formations and later a "bamboo spine."

The usual sites of involvement of the vertebral bodies in ankylosing spondylitis are at the upper and lower corners of contiguous vertebrae, usually at the thoracolumbar junction first, and then involving the entire thoracolumbar spine. The shaving off of these corners produces the "squared-off" appearance considered quite characteristic of ankylosing spondylitis (Fig. 195). When this process takes place relatively early in life, it may be associated with changes in the modelling of the vertebral bodies, and manifest itself by a relative increase in the height of the affected vertebral bodies. This type of change is observed occasionally in the cervical spine, and may be accompanied by fusion of the apophyseal joints and erosive changes in the spinous processes (Fig. 196). Later bony bridges (syndesmophytes) appear laterally and anteriorly on the involved vertebral bodies immediately adjacent to the discal peripheries. Consequent limitation of movement of the spine results from the changes in the apophyseal joints and the intervertebral discs. This, together with the effect of the disease process and the use of steroids can produce rather remarkable demineralization of bone (Fig. 197).

Rheumatoid disease is not entirely a disease of the articular structures, but as a disease of connective tissue in general, produces changes in the cardiovascular system, the soft tissues of the skin in the form of rheumatic nodules, and the peripheral nerves with a somewhat similar nodular change.

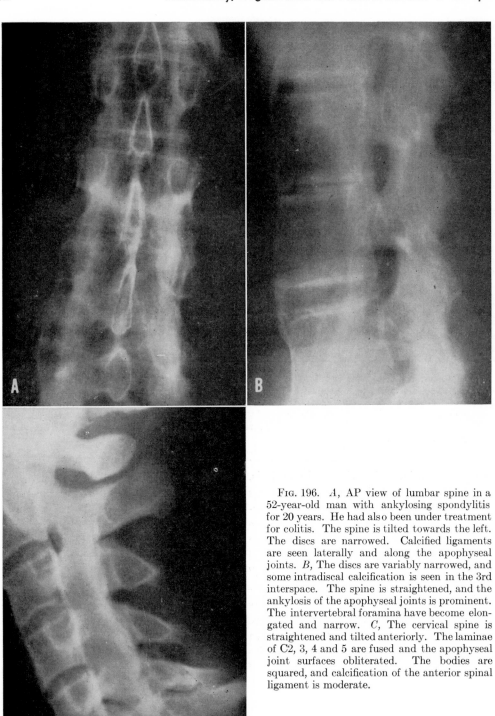

Fig. 196. *A*, AP view of lumbar spine in a 52-year-old man with ankylosing spondylitis for 20 years. He had also been under treatment for colitis. The spine is tilted towards the left. The discs are narrowed. Calcified ligaments are seen laterally and along the apophyseal joints. *B*, The discs are variably narrowed, and some intradiscal calcification is seen in the 3rd interspace. The spine is straightened, and the ankylosis of the apophyseal joints is prominent. The intervertebral foramina have become elongated and narrow. *C*, The cervical spine is straightened and tilted anteriorly. The laminae of C2, 3, 4 and 5 are fused and the apophyseal joint surfaces obliterated. The bodies are squared, and calcification of the anterior spinal ligament is moderate.

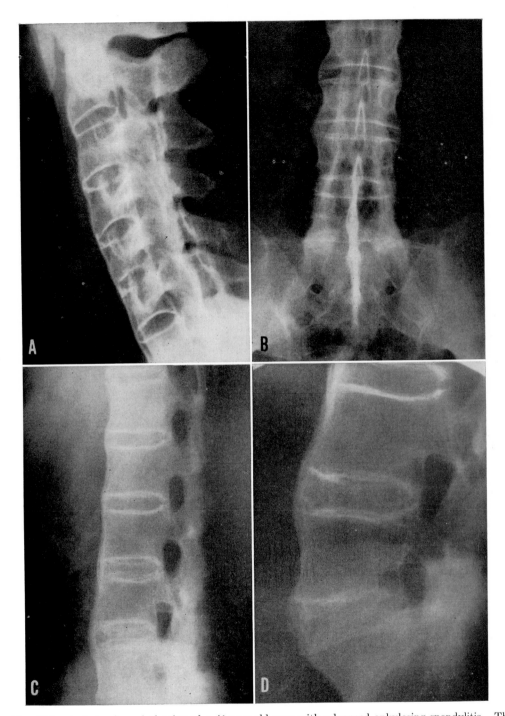

Fig. 197. *A*, Lateral cervical spine of a 41-year-old man with advanced ankylosing spondylitis. The anterior spinal ligament is heavily calcified. The apophyseal joints and their ligaments are extensively involved. The vertebral bodies are moderately demineralized, and their discs spaces are biconvex, but the edges anteriorly and posteriorly touch. *B*, The sacro-iliac joints are fused. The paraspinal ligaments are calcified. Track formation by calcification of the apophyseal joint ligaments is noted. There also is heavy calcification of the lower portion of the interspinous ligament. *C*, Marked demineralization of the lumbar vertebrae is present. The spine is straightened. *D*, Cone-down view of fourth and fifth lumbar vertebrae. The anterior spinal ligament is calcified in layers. Calcification also appears over the discal shadows, probably incident to the shadows of the paraspinal ligaments, although intradiscal calcification cannot be excluded. The posterior aspects of the inferior and superior surfaces of L4 and 5 are approximated.

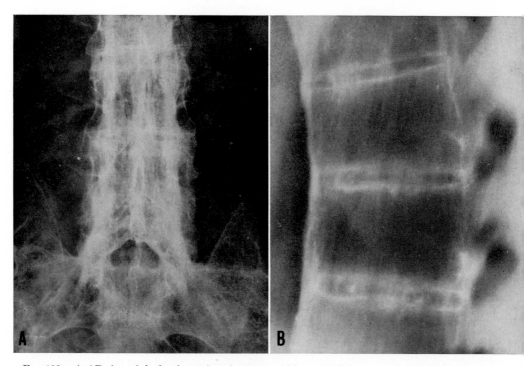

FIG. 198. *A*, AP view of the lumbar spine of a 58-year-old man with long-standing ankylosing spondylitis
Track formation is prominent and the sacro-iliac joints are fused. Diffuse demineralization of bone is
evident. *B*, Lateral laminagram of the upper lumbar vertebrae reveals narrowing of the discs, calcification
of the anterior and posterior spinal ligaments and intradiscal calcifications.

Rheumatoid arthritis produces readily
identifiable osteolytic changes in the small
articulations such as the acromioclavicular
joints, the sternoclavicular and manubrio-
sternal joints, the symphysis pubis as well as
the better known lesions in the hands,
wrists, feet and ankles. Early changes include minimal erosive and periosteal elevation patterns. Later erosion and subchondral irregularities are produced by
breakthrough of pannus, with minimal fractures through the involved bone which
finally evolve into destruction of cartilaginous boundaries and cyst-like formations.
Ankylosing spondylitis can, but is less
likely to produce similar lesions. However,
erosive changes on the plantar aspect of the
calcaneum have been seen which later are
associated with proliferation of new bone.
Similarly, peripheral joint manifestations of
ankylosing spondylitis are not uncommon in
the early stages of the disease more or less

as a transitory phenomenon. In some
patients this advances so that in addition to
the more familiar changes in the vertebral
column ankylosis and prominent trabecular
condensation develops in other joints, often
prominently in the hips. Knee, ankle,
wrist and finger involvement is infrequent,
occurring in less than 10 per cent of patients.
In these joints manifestations are likely to
be mild. The temperomandibular joints
are more likely to be affected in rheumatoid
arthritis, where erosive changes produce a
sharpening of the articular condyles and
motion becomes limited because of progressive ankylosis. However, this can also occur
with ankylosing spondylitis and scleroderma, but rarely to the same extent.

Involvement of the heart with ankylosing
spondylitis takes the form of aortic insufficiency and myocarditis with conduction
disturbances. It is of interest that many
patients with cardiac involvement present

peripheral joint changes in addition to the spinal column disorder. This form of heart disease is separated from that seen with rheumatoid arthritis in that no nodular granulomatous lesions are present and from rheumatic heart disease by the absence of other valvular changes.

According to Forestier (1939) the sacro-iliac joints are involved earliest in ankylosing spondylitis, changes having been observed by him in over 98 per cent of 153 cases. The involvement of these joints may be bilateral or unilateral. Overgaard (1945) mentioned three radiologic stages of involvement of the sacro-iliac joints. The first was scattered, slightly cloudy opacities in the para-articular bone, and slight spotted decalcifications of the subchondral osseous tissue with vague and blurred demarcation. The second consisted of bony bridges which tended to obliterate the articular spaces. The third stage was complete ankylosis. The earliest change associated with ankylosing spondylitis is a decalcification of the bone adjacent to the sacro-iliac joints, producing blurred and indistinct margins. Infrequently, advanced rheumatoid arthritis is associated with sacro-iliac changes, but not with vertebral or apophyseal joint involvement (Fig. 199).

The early radiologic spinal changes of ankylosing spondylitis are manifested in the apophyseal joints. These first present

merely a narrowing and loss of density of opposing articular facets. Later this progresses to rarefaction of bone and irregularity of the articular margins (Fig. 200). Progressively narrowed joint spaces and ankylosis eventually result. Changes in the apophyseal joints are quite difficult to interpret, particularly in the early stages of the disease. Caution is urged in evaluating minimal changes. The pathologic changes appearing in the apophyseal joints are much the same as observed in the diarthrodial joints affected by rheumatoid arthritis. The pattern of synovial villous hyperplasia, inflammatory changes, formation of pannus, erosion of articular cartilage progressing to subchondral bone and involvement of the articular ligaments and capsules with ultimate ankylosis is followed in both diseases. However, ankylosing spondylitis is primarily a disease which involves the articular structures of the spine, and thus first attacks the joint structures containing synovial membrane. It also affects the articular structures of the intervertebral discs and attacks the bone in the immediate vicinity of the discs. Bridging of the intervertebral discs follows chondroid metaplasia and enchondral calcification of the outer layers of the annulus fibrosus, terminating in bone formation and a rigid spine (Fig. 195). This involves mainly the anterior and lateral spinal ligaments. Calcification and ossification also extends along the ligamenta flava, leading to the "track" appearance considered characteristic of ankylosing spondylitis (Fig. 198). This parallel configuration follows the alignment of the destroyed apophyseal joints and the ligaments between them. Calcification of the posterior spinal ligament also can be identified, usually when there is narrowing of the intervertebral discs and approximation of the bony edges (Fig. 197). However, occasionally the intervertebral discs are relatively well maintained but mild bony proliferation along the posterior aspects of the intervertebral discs results in approximation of contiguous margins (Figs. 195, 197). Calcification can also be observed

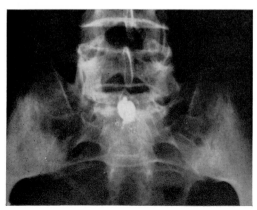

Fig. 199. Sacro-iliac joint fusion in a 48-year-old man known to have had rheumatoid arthritis for 20 years.

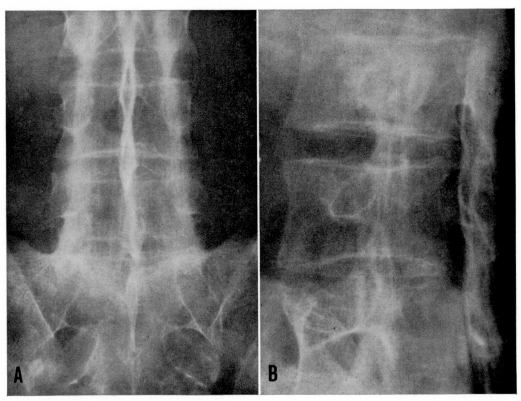

Fig. 200. *A*, Diffuse demineralization of bone and fusion of the sacro-iliac joints in a patient with ankylosing spondylitis. The apophyseal joint ligaments are mildly calcified. As seen on the oblique view, B, the surfaces of the apophyseal joints are roughened and the spaces are narrowed.

occasionally in the interspinous ligament (Fig. 197).

The appearance of the intervertebral discs in patients with ankylosing spondylitis has evoked discussion. For some time it was believed that the intervertebral discs retained their normal thickness throughout the disease. This was mentioned in 1946 by Stecher and Hauser, and in 1951 by Solovay and Gardner. Romanus and Yden (1952) described narrowing of the intervertebral discs in about one-third of their patients with ankylosing spondylitis. Pursuing this line of investigation with discography, they found that pathologic changes in the intervertebral discs were not uncommon and described the association of herniation of the nucleus pulposus with discal changes.

A review of our material disclosed that the appearance of the intervertebral discs is variable in patients with ankylosing spondylitis. In those who had the disease during the early adult years the spine became fixed in a relatively straight position, and the intervertebral discs as a rule maintained themselves fairly well (Fig. 197). In some instances the discs became rather wide, particularly in the lumbar spine. However, in the dorsal spine slight, and sometimes considerable narrowing of the intervertebral discs was noted. This change was apparent in individuals who had developed a pronounced degree of calcification and ossification of the paraspinal ligaments leading to the so-called "poker spine." In some cases the narrowing of the disc was so marked that the margins were practically in apposition one to another (Fig. 198). It was not uncommon to note areas of linear increased density at the superior and inferior margins of some of the vertebrae which had closely approximated each other. In other patients in whom the disease was less precipitous in its advance, and in whom the vertebral bodies retained a good osseous density, changes in the intervertebral discs seemed to parallel those associated with that particular age group. In individuals in early middle life, in whom a moderate dorsum rotundum had appeared, hypertrophic changes at the articular margins of the discs were not uncommon. Narrowing of the intervertebral spaces, particularly along the middle of the arc of the dorsum rotundum, was the rule rather than the exception. These changes seemed to be most pronounced in the upper two-thirds of the thoracic spine. The lower third of the thoracic spine maintained the usual height of the intervertebral discs for a longer time.

When demineralization of the vertebral bodies occurs, the intervertebral discs assume a somewhat biconvex appearance (Fig. 197). While small Schmorl's nodes are occasionally noted in the lower dorsal and upper lumbar region, their appearance in these regions, and more particularly their appearance in the remainder of the dorsal and lumbar spine, is uncommon.

As a rule, the usual lumbar lordotic curve was either straightened or shallower than normal, even though considerable dorsum rotundum had appeared. Paravertebral calcification was most intense in the vicinity of the lumbar and thoracic spine but similar changes in the cervical spine were not uncommon (Fig. 197). The appearance of the paraspinal calcification was not uniform. In several instances calcification was quite pronounced in the lumbothoracic region and absent in the upper dorsal and lower lumbar areas.

The effect of x-ray therapy on ankylosing spondylitis is beneficial but not permanently so. Favorable results have been reported by many observers, particularly in the early stages of the disease (Smyth, Freyberg, and Lampe, 1941); Hemphill and Reeves, 1945; Borak and Taylor, 1945; Baker, Conrad, Reeves and Hoyt, 1950). In some cases of a mild or moderate nature the process can be arrested or sometimes completely resolved, with improvement in the roentgenographic appearance of the involved spine. However, such progress cannot be anticipated if there has been actual destruction of cartilage and bone surfaces. The favorable effects of cortisone and corticotropin are well known and require no discussion here. However, these agents bear with them certain risks incident to their demineralizing effects. A report of pathologic fractures developing in 5 female patients with rheumatoid arthritis treated with cortisone over a long period of time was reported by Demartini, Grokoest and Ragen (1952).

An interesting complication occasionally observed in patients with advanced ankylosing spondylarthritis is reduced efficiency of the costovertebral mechanisms secondary to ankylosis of the joints between the ribs and the dorsal vertebrae. The effect of costovertebral immobility is to reduce the efficiency of the respiratory and cough mechanism, resulting in recurrent attacks of pulmonary disease (Hamilton, 1949) (Hart, Bogdanovitch and Nichol, 1950).

The clinical picture of ankylosing spondylitis has been associated with other totally unrelated conditions. Examples of these are brucellosis, which has been reported as producing changes in the sacro-iliac joints practically indistinguishable from those associated with ankylosing spondylitis (Steinberg, 1948), intestinal amebiasis (Rappaport, Rossien and Rosenblum, 1951), ulcerative colitis (Benedek and Zawadzki, 1966), ileitis (Stewart and Ansell, 1963), and that form of arthritis which not infrequently is observed in menopausal women (Greenblatt and Kupperman, 1946). Abel (1950) reported that patients with paraplegia present sacro-iliac joint changes similar to those seen with ankylosing spondylitis. Acute or chronic pelvic visceral sepsis may be responsible for destructive lesions of the sacro-iliac joints.

Destructive bone lesions with rheumatoid arthritis are occasionally encountered in the vertebrae. Of interest is the case reported by Baggenstoss, Bickel and Ward (1952) in which granulomatous nodules occurred in the body of a vertebra, producing destructive changes. X-ray examination disclosed destruction and wedging of the body of the twelfth dorsal vertebra. At necropsy there was destruction of this vertebra and a nodule in the third lumbar vertebra. These had been considered myelomatous until histologic investigation revealed bony changes including palisading of fibroblasts around a central necrotic area and destruction of adjacent bone trabeculae similar in nature to lesions present in the heart and pericardium. The necrotic focus was of a granulomatous inflammatory nature such as occurs in the viscera and subcutaneous tissues. They also mentioned 3 other cases with destruction of vertebrae without histologic confirmation. Wholey, Pugh and Bickel (1960) reported 10 cases with localized bone destruction on either side of the intervertebral disc. This was more pronounced anteriorly and was followed by spontaneous fusion and ankylosis. A certain similarity to the changes present with tuberculosis, osteomyelitis and other granulomatous lesions was observed. When fairly extensive bone destruction was present, metastatic disease had to be considered and biopsy was required sometimes to make the diagnosis. The bone destruction is less conspicuous than the other more obvious effects observed with rheumatoid arthritis. In 2 cases biopsies revealed histologic changes compatible with rheumatoid inflammation. Gibson (1957) illustrated a case of rheumatoid arthritis in an adult male patient with destruction of the intervertebral disc between the third and fourth cervical vertebrae leading to subluxation with cord pressure.

The basic difference in the pattern of vertebral destruction seen with rheumatoid arthritis as contrasted with ankylosing spondylitis was summarized by Glay and

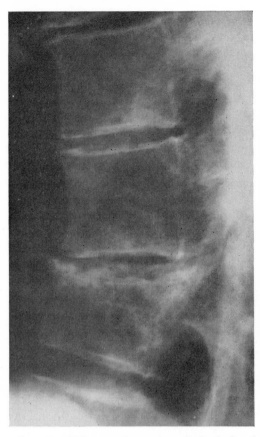

Fig. 201. The superior surface of the body of T-11 is depressed and flattened because of granulomatous involvement of bone with rheumatoid arthritis. Some sclerotic reaction is present as well.

Rona (1965). Ankylosing spondylitis is primarily a disease of the articulations, resulting in bone destruction in the immediate vicinity of the apophyseal joints and intervertebral discs. Rheumatoid arthritis affects the vertebral body, with trabecular dissolution extending to the end plates of the involved vertebrae and varying degrees of collapse (Fig. 201).

Atlantoaxial dislocation occurs with both rheumatoid arthritis and ankylosing spondylitis. Pain in the cervical region together with neurologic deficits vary with the extent of the spinal cord pressure resulting from the forward displacement of the atlas on the axis. The earliest radiologic change is a widening of the space between the anterior aspect of the dens and the posterior aspect of the anterior arch of the atlas. Normally this space measures about 2.5 mm. Sharp and Purser (1961) regard a separation of more than 3 mm as abnormal after the age of 44 years, although a gap of 4 mm may be normal in younger individuals. With more advanced displacements a lateral shift and some rotational defects occur, producing torticollis and a forward position of the head together with a flattening of the cervico-occipital curve (Fig. 202).

Atlantoaxial dislocations occur more often with rheumatoid arthritis than with ankylosing spondylitis. Inasmuch as the joint between the dens and the anterior arch of the atlas is lined with synovium, it is affected like others with the appearance of pannus, bone erosion and hyperemia. The reduction in the size of the dens and the laxity of its confining ligaments contribute to the possibility of dislocation.

Atlantoaxial dislocations are identified on

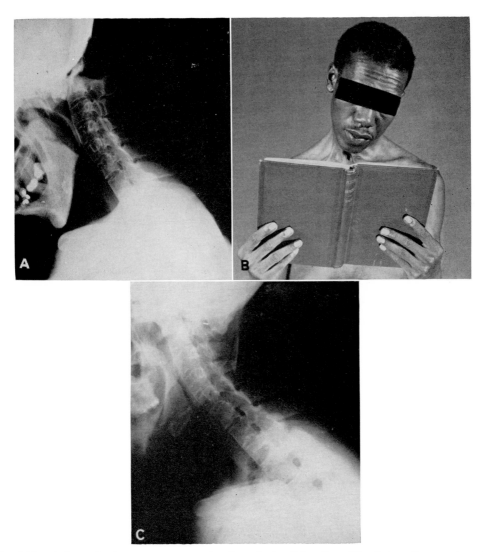

FIG. 202. *A*, Lateral spine roentgenogram showing anterior dislocation of the first on the second cervical vertebrae incidental to rheumatoid spondylitis. *B*, Note position of head of this patient. *C*, Same case, post-reduction lateral cervical spine roentgenogram. (Courtesy of Dr. M. E. Margulies, Veterans Administration Hospital, Brooklyn, N. Y.)

lateral flexion and extension studies. The characteristic change is a "V" shaped radiolucency between the two bones, the measurement at the widest part exceeding 4 mm. Cineradiographic examinations permit a permanent record of this movement, and augment rather than supplant conventional films and laminagrams which afford far better detail. The abrupt forward movement of the atlas apparent on cineradiographic studies almost give one the feeling of a "click." Not only does the arch move forward, but the position of the spinous process changes in an upwards and anterior direction, and the soft tissues anterior to the upper cervical vertebrae bulge forward as well (Figs. 203 and 204). When the change is minimal, this study may be the one which makes the diagnosis. Abnormal movement of a similar nature is seen with other conditions, such as fractures and dislocations, ununited fractures, absence of the dens, hypoplasia of the dens, and with congenital malformations such as os odontoideum.

Rheumatoid arthritis results in fusion of the neural arches of the midcervical vertebrae, which assume a slender tubular configuration. Ankylosing spondylitis also affects the cervical spine, but is more likely to be associated with ossification of the paraspinal ligaments, osteoporotic changes and sharpening of the spinous processes with some subperiosteal erosion. The apophyseal joints become fused, while the intervertebral discs retain a normal configuration or become biconvex incident to osteoporosis (Fig. 197). With exaggerated thoracic kyphosis and compensatory backward tilting of the head spondylolisthesis of the lower cervical vertebrae occasionally is observed.

Rheumatoid arthritis affects the cartilaginous end plates of the cervical vertebrae, resulting in narrowing of the disc spaces, erosive and osteoporotic changes. The spinous processes also are affected, with sharpening of their tips and subperiosteal erosions which produce small rounded lytic areas at or near their tips. In both rheumatoid arthritis and ankylosing spondylitis

rigidity of the cervical spine results in its acting as a long bone when injured, so that a transverse fracture carries with it the risk of severe cord damage (Woodruff and Dewing, 1963).

References

Abel, M. S.: Sacroiliac Joint Changes in Traumatic Paraplegics, Radiology, 55, 235, 1950.

Alpert, M. A. and Feldman, F.: The Rib Lesions of Rheumatoid Arthritis, Radiology, 82, 872, 1964.

Alpert, M. and Meyers, M.: Osteolysis of the Acromial End of the Clavicles in Rheumatoid Arthritis, Am. J. Roentgenol., 86, 251, 1961.

Baggenstoss, A. H., Bickel, W. H. and Ward, L. E.: Rheumatoid Granulomatous Nodules as Destructive Lesions of Vertebrae, J. Bone & Joint Surg., 34-A, 601, 1952.

Benedek, T. G. and Zawadzki, Z. A.: Ankylosing Spondylitis with Ulcerative Colitis and Amyloidosis, Am. J. Med., 40, 421, 1966.

Bland, J. H., Van Buskirk, F. W. V., Tampas, J. P., Brown, E. and Clayton, R.: A Study of Roentgenologic Criteria for Rheumatoid Arthritis of the Cervical Spine. Am. J. Roentgenol., 95, 949, 1965.

Borak, J. and Taylor, H. K.: Beneficial Effects of Roentgen Therapy in Advanced Cases of Rheumatoid Arthritis, Radiology, 45, 377, 1945.

Conlon, P. W., Isdale, I. C., and Rose, B. S.: Rheumatoid Arthritis of the Cervical Spine, Ann. Rheum. Dis., 25, 120, 1966.

Cruikshank, B.: Histopathology of Diarthroidal Joints in Ankylosing Spondylitis, Ann. Rheum. Dis., 10, 393, 1951.

Cruikshank, B., Macleod, J. G. and Shearer, W. S.: Subarticular Pseudocysts in Rheumatoid Arthritis. J. Fac. Radiologists, 5, 218, 1954.

Davidson, P., Baggenstoss, A. H., Slocumb, C. H. and Daugherty, G. W.: Cardiac and Aortic Lesions in Rheumatoid Spondylitis, Proc. Staff Meet., Mayo Clin., 36, 427, 1963.

DeMartini, F., Grokoest, A. W. and Ragan, C.: Pathological Fractures in Patients with Rheumatoid Arthritis Treated with Cortisone, J.A.M.A., 149, 750, 1952.

Fernandez-Herlihy, L.: The Articular Manifestations of Chronic Ulcerative Colitis. New England J. Med., 261, 259, 1959.

Forestier, J.: Sacro-iliac Changes in Early Diagnosis of Ankylosing Spondylitis, Radiology, 33, 289, 1939.

Glay, A. and Rona, G.: Nodular Rheumatoid Vertebral Lesions versus Ankylosing Spondylitis, Am. J. Roentgenol., 94, 631, 1965.

Grainger, R. G.: Procto-Colitis and Other Pelvic Infections in Relation to Ankylosing Spondylitis, J. Fac. Radiologists, 10, 40, 1959.

Greenblatt, R. E. and Kupperman, H. S.: Menopausal Arthritis, Med. Clin. North America, 30, 576, 1946.

Guest, C. M. and Jacobson, H. G.: Pelvic and Extrapelvic Osteopathy in Rheumatoid Spondylitis, Am. J. Roentgenol., *65*, 760, 1951.

Hamilton, K. A.: Pulmonary Disease Manifestations of Ankylosing Spondylarthritis, Ann. Int. Med., *31*, 216, 1949.

Hart, F. D., Bogdanovitch, A. and Nichol, W. D.: The Thorax in Ankylosing Spondylitis, Ann. Rheum. Dis., *9*, 116, 1950.

Hemphill, J. E. and Reeves, E. J.: Roentgen Irradiation in Treatment of Marie-Strümpell Disease (Ankylosing Spondylarthritis), Am. J. Roentgenol., *54*, 282, 1945.

Jones, M. D.: Cineradiographic Studies of Abnormalities of the High Cervical Spine, Arch. Surg., *94*, 206, 1967.

Lawrence, J. S., Sharp, J., Ball, J. and Bier, F.: Rheumatoid Arthritis of the Lumbar Spine, Ann. Rheum. Dis., *23*, 205, 1964.

Lemmen, L. J. and Laing, P. G.: Fracture of the Cervical Spine in Patients with Rheumatoid Arthritis, J. Neurosurg., *16*, 542, 1959.

Lynn, T. N.: Rheumatoid Spondylitis in a Prepubertal Female, J. Dis. Childhood, *91*, 282, 1945.

Margulies, M. E., Katz, I. and Rosenberg, M.: Spontaneous Dislocation of the Atlanto-Axial Joint in Rheumatoid Spondylitis, Neurology, *5*, 290, 1955.

Margulies, W.: The Occipito-Atlanto-Axial Joints in Rheumatoid Arthritis and Ankylosing Spondylitis, Am. J. Roentgenol., *86*, 223, 1961.

Martel, W. and Abell, M. R.: Fatal Atlanto-Axial Luxation in Rheumatoid Arthritis, Arth. & Rheum., *6*, 224, 1963.

Martel, W. and Duff, I. F.: Pelvo-Spondylitis in Rheumatoid Arthritis, Radiology, *77*, 744, 1961.

Martel, W. and Page, J. W.: Cervical Vertebral Erosions and Subluxations in Rheumatoid Arthritis and Ankylosing Spondylitis, Arth. & Rheum., *3*, 546, 1960.

McBride, J. A., King, M. J., Baikie, A. G., Crean, G. P. and Sircus, W.: Ankylosing Spondylitis and Chronic Inflammatory Diseases of the Intestines. Brit. Med. J., *2*, 483, 1963.

McEwen, C., Lingg, C. and Kirsner, J. B.: Arthritis Accompanying Ulcerative Colitis, Am. J. Med., *33*, 923, 1962.

O'Connell, D.: Heredity in Ankylosing Spondylitis, Ann. Int. Med., *50*, 1115, 1959.

Pratt, T. L. C.: Spontaneous Dislocation of the Atlanto-Axial Articulation Occurring in Ankylosing Spondylitis and Rheumatoid Arthritis. J. Faculty Radiologists, *10*, 40, 1959.

Rappaport, E. M., Rossien, A. X. and Rosenblum, L. A.: Arthritis Due to Intestinal Amebiasis, Ann. Int. Med., *34*, 1224, 1951.

Robinson, H. S.: Rheumatoid Arthritis-Atlanto-Axial Subluxation and its Clinical Presentation, Canadian Med. Assn. J., *94*, 470, 1966.

Romanus, R.: Pelvo-Spondylitis Ossificans in the Male (Ankylosing Spondylitis) and Genito-Urinary Infection, Acta med. scand., *145*. Suppl. 280, 1953.

Romanus, R. and Yden, J.: Diskography in Ankylosing Spondylitis, Acta radiol., *38*, 431, 1952.

Savill, D. L.: The Manubrio-Sternal Joint in Ankylosing Spondylitis, J. Bone & Joint Surg., *33-B*, 56, 1951.

Sharp, J.: Differential Diagnosis of Ankylosing Spondylitis, Brit. M. J., *1*, 975, 1957.

Sharp, J. and Purser, D. W.: Spontaneous Atlanto-Axial Dislocation in Ankylosing Spondylitis and Rheumatoid Arthritis, Ann. Rheum. Dis., *20*, 47, 1961.

Silberberg, D. H., Frohman, L. A. and Duff, I. F.: The Incidence of Leukemia and Related Diseases in Patients with Rheumatoid (Ankylosing) Spondylitis Treated with X-ray Therapy, Arth. & Rheum., *3*, 64, 1960.

Soila, P.: The Causal Relations of Rheumatoid Disintegration of Juxta-Articular Bone Trabeculae. Acta rheum. scand., *9*, 231, 1963.

Steinberg, C. L.: Brucellosis as Cause of Sacroiliac Arthritis, J.A.M.A., *138*, 15, 1948.

Travis, D. M., Cook, C. D., Julian, D. G., Cramp, S. H., Helliesen, P., Tobin, E. D., Bayles, T. B. and Nurwell, C. S.: The Lungs in Rheumatoid Spondylitis, Am. J. Med., *29*, 622, 1960.

Weed, C. L., Kulander, B. G., Mazzarella, J. A. and Decker, J. L.: Heart Block in Ankylosing Spondylitis, Arch. Int. Med., *117*, 800, 1966.

Wholey, M. H. M., Pugh, D. G. and Bickel, W. H.: Localized Destructive Lesions in Rheumatoid Spondylitis, Radiology, *74*, 54, 1960.

Woodruff, F. P. and Dewing, S. B.: Fracture of the Cervical Spine in Patients with Ankylosing Spondylitis, Radiology, *80*, 17, 1963.

JUVENILE RHEUMATOID ARTHRITIS

Juvenile rheumatoid arthritis is often referred to as Still's disease. Its pathologic manifestations are much the same as those of rheumatoid arthritis. In addition, splenomegaly, lymphadenopathy and occasionally hepatomegaly are seen fairly often. The joints most commonly affected in the polyarticular form in children are those of the hands and wrist, the feet, ankles, knees and temperomandibular joints. Accelerated epiphyseal growth causes elongated configurations of the long bones (Coss, 1946). The cervical spine is involved in about 13 per cent of the cases. The disease occurs more often in females and is seen most frequently in the 2nd to 3rd years of life. The children present a delicate, almost bird-like appearance.

In early cases of juvenile rheumatoid arthritis no radiologic changes are apparent in the spine. Later, the x-ray findings are those of spondylitis with no calcification of

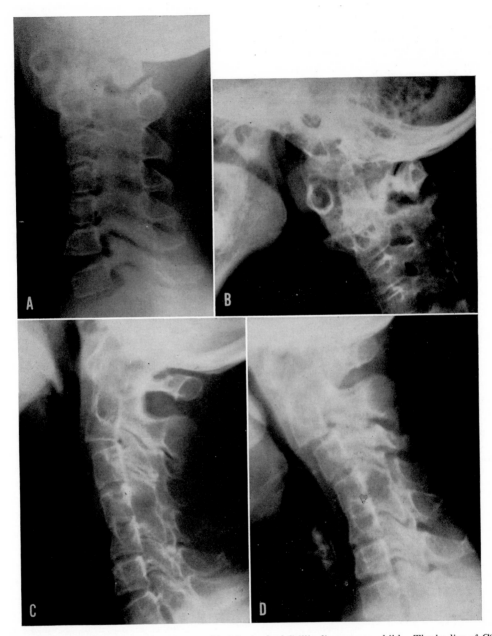

Fig. 203. *A*, Cervical spine of a 10-year-old girl who had Still's disease as a child. The bodies of C3, 4 and 5 are narrowed, and their apophyseal joints are fused. The dens is pointed, and the space between it and the anterior arch of the atlas is 4 mm. In flexion, *B*, the anterior arch moves forward. Note the change in the position of the tip, which now is higher than at rest. *C*, Lateral neck film of another patient, a 22-year-old woman who had had Still's disease as a child. The fourth and fifth vertebrae are elongated and narrowed, and their apophyseal joints are fused. There is an upward tilt of the inferior surface of C2 when the head is extended. When the head is flexed, *D*, a forward shift of C2 takes place. The dens is demineralized and appears somewhat expanded.

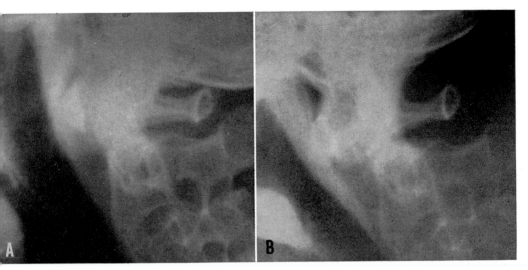

FIG. 204. *A*, Cervical spine centering on the alantoaxial articulation in a 48-year-old man with ankylosing spondylitis and neck pain. The dens is pointed. In flexion, *B*, the anterior arch moves forward, impinging on the soft tissues of the nasopharynx. The tip of the spinous process of C1 tilts upwards and forward.

the paraspinal ligaments. Some degree of decalcification of the vertebral bodies may take place early in the disease. The lumbar lordotic curve may become straightened. The intervertebral discs, according to Buckley (1943), do not become thin but may even expand. Complete ankylosis may eventually result. Saenger (1950), in a report of 4 cases in children, the oldest of which was 14 years of age, described a syndrome in which narrowing of the intervertebral discs appeared about 2 to 4 weeks after the onset of clinical symptoms. In these individuals pain was referable chiefly to the hip. Some demineralization or destruction of parts of the vertebrae appeared. Narrowing of the intervertebral spaces persisted for about 4 to 12 weeks, when sclerotic changes began to be evident in the vertebrae. During the next 2 to 8 months there was gradual widening of the intervertebral spaces with sclerosis and new bone formation in the area of destruction of the opposing bone margins. In very young children restitution to normal occurred within a year.

Later in life ankylosis of the apophyseal joints of the upper cervical vertebrae may occur. These vertebrae tend to assume a diminished anteroposterior diameter as well as height. Their intervertebral discs may narrow or disappear, resulting essentially in a small, fused upper cervical vertebral column (Fig. 203). This may to some extent simulate block vertebrae. The slender configuration of the affected segments serves to distinguish one from the other. The clinical history immediately points to the underlying rheumatoid factor. Other differences include persistence of a rudimentary intervertebral disc or other vertebral congenital malformations. Later joints affected by juvenile rheumatoid disease are prone to develop degenerative changes.

References

Barkin, R. E., Stillman, J. S. and Potter, T. A.: The Spondylitis of Juvenile Rheumatoid Arthritis, New England J. Med., *253*, 1107, 1955.

Buckley, C. W.: Spinal Arthritis in Young Subjects, Brit. Med. J., *2*, 4, 1943.

Coss, J. A., Jr.: Juvenile Rheumatoid Arthritis (Still's Disease), Med. Clin. North America, *30*, 568, 1946.

Langley, F. A.: Still's Disease, Arch. Dis. Childhood, *20*, 155, 1945.

Martel, W., Holt, J. F. and Cassidy, J. T.: Roentgenologic Manifestations of Juvenile Rheumatoid Arthritis, Am. J. Roentgenol., *88*, 400, 1962.

Saenger, E. L.: Spondylarthritis in Children, Am. J. Roentgenol., *64*, 20, 1950.

REITER'S SYNDROME

This is a disease of unknown etiology which in its complete form, consists of a triad of conjunctivitis, urethritis and arthritis. The disease is quite infrequent and has been attributed to a number of infectious origins, none of which is considered conclusive. Biopsy of synovial membrane in 1 case was reported by Bauer and Engelman (1942) as differing from the changes associated with either infectious or rheumatoid arthritis. As a rule, the joints most frequently involved are those of the elbows and wrists and, to a greater extent, the knees and ankles. Involvement of the spine and sacro-iliac joints is relatively infrequent. In the 25 cases reported by Hollander, Fogarty, Abrams and Kydd (1945), mild and nonspecific spinal involvement was encountered in only 2 cases. The characteristic roentgenographic abnormalities were those of a diffuse osteoporosis which disappeared as the condition cleared. Hollander and his co-workers studied synovial membrane removed from the right knee joint of one of their patients. In the course of removing the material it was noted that the cartilaginous surfaces of the joint were undisturbed. Their observations confirmed those of Bauer and Engelman (1942), in that an intense hyperemia and cellular reaction limited to the superficial layers of the synovium was found. They considered the disease process as distinctly different from that seen with rheumatoid arthritis. In a retrospective study of 34 cases Good (1962) found an unexpected close association with ankylosing spondylitis and clear separation from rheumatoid arthritis. Involvement of the sacro-iliac joints was noted in 13 of 27 cases with histories over 2 years in duration. Ankylosing spondylitis was diagnosed in 8 patients, and several followed a progressive course of this disease.

References

Bauer, W. W. and Engelman, E. P.: A Syndrome of Unknown Etiology Characterized by Urethritis, Conjunctivitis and Arthritis (So-Called Reiter's Disease), Tr. A. Am. Physicians, 57, 302, 1942.

Good, A. E.: Involvement of the Back in Reiter's Syndrome, Ann. Int. Med., 57, 44, 1962.
Hollander, J. L., Fogarty, C. W., Jr., Abrams, N. R. and Kydd, D. M.: Arthritis Resembling Reiter's Syndrome, J.A.M.A., 129, 593, 1945.
Mason, R. M., Murray, R. S. Oates, J. K. and Young, A. C.: A Comparative Radiological Study of Reiter's Disease, Rheumatoid Arthritis and Ankylosing Spondylitis, J. Bone & Joint Surg., 41-B, 137, 1959.
Murray, R. S., Oates, J. K. and Young, A. C.: Radiological Changes in Reiter's Syndrome and Arthritis Associated with Urethritis, J. Fac. Radiologists, 9, 37, 1958.
Reynolds, D. F. and Csonka, G. W.: Radiological Aspects of Reiter's Syndrome ("Venereal" Arthritis), J. Fac. Radiologists, 9, 44, 1958.
Weldon, W. V. and Scalettar, R.: Roentgen Changes in Reiter's Syndrome, Am J. Roentgenol., 86, 344, 1961.

WERNER'S SYNDROME

According to Thannhauser (1945) the distinguishing characteristics of this hereditary familial condition includes a premature graying of the hair and baldness, shortness of stature, scleropoikiloderma, trophic ulcers of the legs, juvenile cataracts, hypogonadism, a tendency to diabetes, osteoporosis, calcification of the blood vessels and metastatic calcification. It has been referred to as progeria of the adult. The radiologic changes, insofar as the spine were concerned, were those of an advanced spondylitis inconsistent with the patient's age. Another example of this condition was reported by Pomeranz (1948).

References

Pomerantz, M. M.: Werner's Syndrome, Radiology, 51, 521, 1948.
Thannhauser, S. J.: Werner's Syndrome (Progeria of the Adult) and Rothmund's Syndrome: Two Types of Closely Related Heredofamiliar Atrophic Dermatoses with Juvenile Cataracts and Endocrine Features, Ann. Int. Med., 23, 559, 1945.

PSORIATIC ARTHRITIS

This condition occasionally occurs coincidentally with ankylosing spondylitis or rheumatoid arthritis. It is predominantly a disease afflicting the small joints of the hands and feet, but larger joints may be involved. It has been noted that the clinical activity of the disease varies with the extent and activity of the psoriatic condition. In a case described by Jungmann and Stern (1944) fusion of certain vertebrae was observed, together with advanced changes involving the articulations of the extremities. In another case reported by Nunemaker and Hartman (1950) no spine changes were observed. Sherman (1952) described atrophic changes in the hands. In 2 cases observed by us the changes were most marked in the and wrists, with no definite alteration in the structure of the vertebral column. However, sacro-iliac joint involvement has been reported (Wright, 1961).

References

Jungmann, H. and Stern, V. S.: Joint Disease (Possible Example of Arthritis Psoriatica), Brit. J. Radiol., *17*, 383, 1944.
Nunemaker, J. C. and Hartman, S. A.: Psoriatic Arthritis, Ann. Int. Med., *33*, 1016, 1950.
Sherman, M. S.: Psoriatic Arthritis, J. Bone & Joint Surg., *34-A*, 831, 1952.
Wright, V: Psoriatic Arthritis: Comparative Radiographic Study of Rheumatoid Arthritis and Arthritis Associated with Psoriasis. Ann. Rheum. Dis., *20*, 123, 1961.

Tuberculous Spondylitis (Pott's Disease)

Tuberculous osteomyelitis of the spine in most cases results from hematogenous extension into the medullary spaces. The initial site of involvement is in the vicinity of the upper or lower vertebral cartilaginous plates, where the blood supply is most ample. Depending on the initial site of infection, a single vertebra may be affected centrally, anteriorly or epiphysially. Infection appears at times immediately beneath the anterior spinal ligament, producing a shallow excavation of the anterior aspect of the involved vertebral body. The caseating effect of tuberculosis produces a localized destruction of bone which slowly progresses. Liquefaction and abscess formation then appear. Extension of the abscess by perforation through the bone into the adjacent soft tissues is along the course of the anterior or lateral spinal ligaments. With further invasion of the adjacent soft tissues the abscesses increase in size. Those forming above the diaphragm tend to remain within the thorax or point posteriorly. Below the diaphragm tuberculous abscesses tend to enter the pelvis

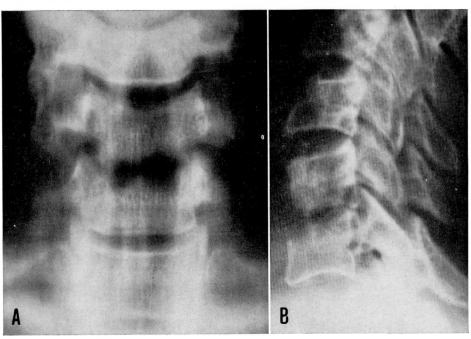

Fig. 205. *A*, AP laminagram and, *B*, lateral view of the lower cervical spine of a patient with tuberculous spondylitis. The disc between C6 and 7 is affected, and the bony margins of the adjacent vertebrae are destroyed. Soft tissue swelling in front of the involved joint is present.

along the course of the psoas muscle, pointing in the groin or the thigh. Less frequently an abscess burrows posteriorly and appears in the lumbar region.

With progressive breakdown of bone vertebral collapse takes place, accompanied by disruption of the cartilaginous plates and infection of the intervertebral discs. The initial change is a disruption of bone, usually adjacent to an intervertebral disc. This is followed by further destruction of bone, discal disintegration (Fig. 205) and ultimately, in unchecked advance, collapse of involved vertebrae with consequent spinal deformity and obliteration of intervertebral fibrocartilages. Wedging of involved vertebrae is common. The end result often is an angular kyphosis which in extreme instances reaches a 90-degree angle (Fig. 206). While extension from one vertebra to another

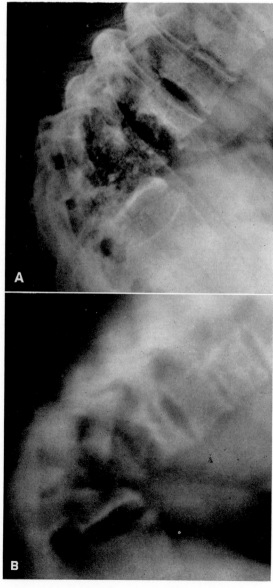

Fig. 206. *A*, Lateral thoracic spine roentgenogram showing gibbus formation with extensive tuberculous destruction. *B*, Same case, lateral body section roentgenogram.

usually is by direct continuity, involvement of multiple segments distant from one another is not uncommon.

The incidence of spinal tuberculosis was reported by Bosworth and Levine (1949) to be 3.2 per cent of a total of 12,835 tuberculous patients treated at the Sea View Hospital in New York City during the period 1940 and 1945 inclusive. This was lower than usually reported, but the lowered incidence was believed related to improved treatment. Galland (1952) pointed out that the most common cause of death, tuberculous meningitis, has been practically eliminated by modern treatment, which also has markedly reduced the incidence of tuberculosis of the spine.

Mottled, sclerotic changes in tuberculosis of the spine is more common than is generally believed (Fig. 207). Cleveland and Bosworth (1942) considered sclerotic changes in the involved bone to be a vascular phenomenon produced by loss of blood supply from thrombosis, endarteritis, occlusion or destruction of blood vessels by dissecting abscesses. Auerbach and Stemmerman (1944) pointed out that in vertebrae involved in sclerotic changes, microscopic study revealed the trabeculae to remain intact, thereby explaining the lack of collapse or other deformity. The sclerotic changes are caused by granulation tissue and caseous material filling the marrow spaces rather than by any gross increase in the density of the involved bone. Both a caseating and productive sclerotic form of tuberculosis may coexist. In their 128 cases, Auerbach and Stemmerman (1944) found that 62 per

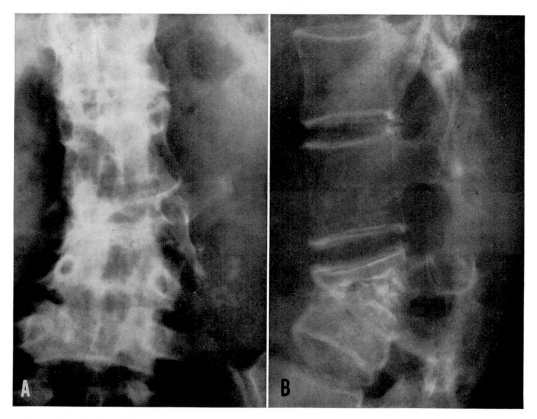

FIG. 207. *A*, AP and lateral, *B*, view of the lumbar spine of a 32-year-old man with tuberculous spondylitis treated 15 years before. The spine is angulated at L3, with a resultant gibbus formation. Note the compensatory increase in the height of L2. A calcified psoas abscess is seen on the left side. Immediately below the collapsed 3rd lumbar vertebra discal remnants with calcification are present.

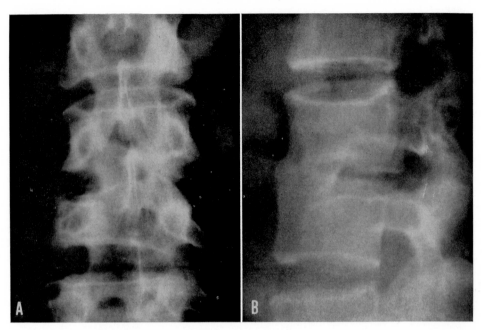

Fig. 208. *A*, AP and lateral, *B*, lumbar spine in an adult patient who had had a nephrectomy for a tuberculous kidney 10 years before. Tuberculous spondylitis was present, and has healed with bony bridging between the left lateral and anterior aspects of L3 and 4.

cent were essentially exudative in nature, 12 per cent were essentially productive and 26 per cent showed both forms of the disease.

While it is usually considered that the reparative formation of bone is more frequent in pyogenic osteomyelitis, such changes also appear with tuberculous spondylitis. Bridging of the vertebral bodies is regarded either as a reaction to irritation, with periosteal new bone formation, or ossification in ligamentous tissue rather than as evidence of healing. In some cases this is extensive enough to fuse the vertebrae as effectively as a surgical fusion (Fig. 208). Guri (1947) pointed out that in a few cases healing occurred with bony fusion of the anterior aspects of the involved vertebrae. This followed contact between two bodies resulting from destruction of the intervertebral cartilage, or by recalcification and union of the remnants of several vertebrae which had been more extensively destroyed. The amount of concurrent deformity of the spine, the shape, structure and speed of formation of these synostoses were not uniform. Pro-

tective muscle spasm may influence the final configuration of the spine.

Healing of tuberculous spondylitis is a slow process, and goes on concomitantly with the spread of the disease. There is gradual breakdown of bone, together with a reparative effort which results in the laying down of fibrous tissue and ultimately ankylosis appears. The course of tuberculosis has been markedly altered by today's therapeutic advances, so that it is uncommon in areas where such help is available to observe the usual natural history of the disease. Under adequate treatment, and in most patients who now appear with active tuberculosis, involvement of the spine is uncommon, the lesion is more or less localized and spinal deformities are avoided. In the light of previous experience, vertebral alignment alterations were common, as were psoas abscesses and other tuberculous sequelae. In some instances of tuberculosis in children which had been successfully treated in bygone days, the vertebral bodies above the involved area increased in height, thereby

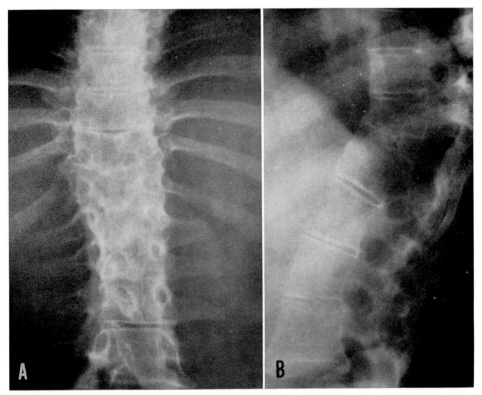

Fig. 209. *A*, AP view of the thoracolumbar spine of a 28-year-old man who had been operated upon for tuberculous spondylitis at the age of 1 year. The upper lumbar vertebrae are narrow and the transverse processes are elongated. A gibbus is present, better seen on the lateral view, *B*. The elongation and the narrowing of the upper lumbar vertebrae, and the compensatory increase in the height of the lower segments is visible. The 12th thoracic vertebra has collapsed.

compensating for the diminished size of the other segments (Fig. 207). In occasional instances of childhood tuberculosis treated with spinal fusion, impairment of blood supply resulted in diminution in the size of the affected vertebral bodies (Fig. 209).

Tuberculous spondylitis infrequently is associated with direct spread into adjacent vital areas. Instances of rupture of the aorta incident to Pott's disease were mentioned by Somerville and Wishart (1948) and by Simpson and Brobbelaar (1955).

Tuberculosis of the spine in children occurs more frequently in the thoracic region. The thoraco-lumbar area is more frequently affected in adults. Involvement of the cervical spine is less common. Paravertebral abscess formation occurs in about half the adult group, and paravertebral swelling is

an important early x-ray sign of tuberculous spondylitis. Bosworth (1945) stated that a paravertebral abscess in the thoracic region was the earliest criterion for the diagnosis of spinal tuberculosis, antedating bony or intervertebral disc changes.

Less frequent sites of involvement include the neural arches and the spinous and transverse processes. A case of isolated tuberculosis of the spinous process of the fourth lumbar vertebra was reported by Anderson, who reviewed the literature in 1940 and encountered 12 similar cases. This lesion was more frequent in adults. Involvement of a single spinous process occurred in 7 patients, and two spinous processes were affected in 5 others. The neural arch was diseased in 5 other cases. Abscess formation appeared, but no muscle spasm or deformity of the vertebral bodies was noted. Anderson stated that these lesions were less grave than those in the vertebral bodies. Judd (1940) reported a case of tuberculosis of the transverse process of the third lumbar vertebra in which the destruction of bone was accompanied by obliteration of the psoas shadow on the involved side. Operative intervention disclosed a large abscess from which 4 to 5 ounces of pus were evacuated. A sequestrum the size of an olive was found lying free in the space occupied by the transverse process. Herdner (1950) in a discussion of body section x-ray examination as applied to study of the atlas and axis mentioned 3 cases of suboccipital Pott's disease.

Tuberculosis of the sacro-iliac joints occurs in young adults, usually with tuberculosis elsewhere, the most common sites being the spine and hips. Pain, abscess formation and draining sinuses are frequently present. Pollack and Bosworth (1942) reported that sacro-iliac tuberculosis was encountered in 3.4 per cent of a thousand admissions, and described their findings in 44 cases. There were 33 males and 11 female patients varying in age between 8 and 55 years, with the peak between 21 and 25 years. In 13 cases the right sacro-iliac joint was involved, in 24 the left, and in 7 both sacro-iliac joints were diseased. Roentgenographic examination disclosed erosion, sclerosis and cavitation in 73 per cent of the cases. Sequestration could also be demonstrated. The alignment of the joint was disturbed completely in 40 cases, while 9 showed only changes in the lower half of the joint. Changes limited to the central or upper portions of the joint were seen in 1 case each. The sacrum usually showed more apparent destruction than the ilium. Isaacson and Whitehouse (1949) observed spontaneous bony ankylosis of the sacro-iliac joint in tuberculosis of this joint. The earliest fusion occurred approximately 4 months after the onset of symptoms, while the longest interval was approximately 2 years.

Intraspinal extension of tuberculosis in the form of extradural intraspinal tuberculomas is infrequent. Johnston, Ashbell and Rosomoff (1962) found a total of 9 instances of isolated extradural intraspinal tuberculomas in the current literature, noting that 200 intraspinal tuberculomas had been described in the available literature of the past 70 years. From this there were 7 reports of isolated extradural mass lesions without evidence of coexistent tuberculosis in contiguous structures, with no indications of radiologic changes in the spine or its soft tissue investments. In 2 cases myelographic block was present, at the fifth thoracic level in one and at the seventh in the other. However, extradural tuberculomas are not particularly uncommon in the presence of Pott's disease. These occur as ring-shaped lardaceous deposits which may be mistaken for meningiomas or chronic epiduritis (Arseni and Samitca, 1960). In a 25-year-old male patient recently seen by us there were signs referable to nerve root compression at the midcervical level which were unassociated with any plain film radiographic changes. Myelography disclosed an indentation into the lateral aspect of the Pantopaque column interpreted as indicative of an extradural mass. At operation it was found that a granulomatous tuberculous abscess partly covered the dura. The source of infection was a retropharyngeal tuberculous abscess.

Subdural tuberculomas occur as hard, round or ovoid masses attached to the inner aspect of the dura and imbedded in the cord as circumscribed lesions about 5 to 10 mm in diameter. They may be associated with arachnoiditis, and can be enucleated. A central area of caseation is seen, the periphery of the lesion being formed by granulation tissue. Plain film examinations in patients with subdural tuberculomas usually are not helpful, but myelographic examination will reveal evidence of partial or total block.

Intramedullary tuberculomas simulate tumors. Lin (1960) found reports of 104 such lesions in the literature, among which 16 had been removed at operation and the remaining 88 had been uncovered at necropsy. He reported the case of a 47-year-old woman who was paraplegic, incontinent and had back and radicular pain. Plain films of the spine showed some sclerotic changes in the bodies of the second and fourth lumbar vertebrae. Myelography disclosed a block at the level of the first lumbar vertebra. On opening the dura at operation there were mild adhesions between it and the cord. A gray, intrinsic mass was encountered in the lumbar enlargement, and after enucleation it measured $2.2 \times 2 \times 1.4$ cm. Its center was caseous, and acid-fast bacilli were recovered.

Tuberculous meningitis may be followed by arachnoiditis and spinal canal block, which appears early in the disease or as a late consequence. The clinical picture mimics that of a spinal cord tumor, and the diagnosis usually is made at operation if the lesion is localized.

The possibility of spinal cord compression by intraspinal intrusion of a sequestrated piece of diseased bone is rather remote, but can occur. It is of considerable interest that marked distortion of the architecture of the spine occurs with little or no evidence of cord involvement. Compression of the cord incident to direct extension from a pulmonary abscess is rare. Two such cases were reported by Norcross (1948), both involving the upper thoracic region. A unilateral tuberculous abscess with changes suggestive of a dumbbell neurofibroma was reported by Kneidel, Smith and Bishop (1950). A slight widening in the intercostal space at the level of the fifth rib was present, together with erosion of the articular tubercle and transverse process of the fifth thoracic vertebra. The vertebral body was intact, but paravertebral soft tissue swelling was noted. A complete block was found at this level. At operation caseous material was uncovered at the level of the fifth and sixth spinous processes. There was granulation tissue over the anterior and posterior dural surfaces, and a large tuberculous cavity extended to the fifth and sixth thoracic vertebral bodies.

Tuberculous involvement of the cauda equina was mentioned by Alajouanine and Thurel (1945) in a 50-year-old woman who had had low back pain with sciatica for several years. There was no evidence of a block on myelographic examination, but operation disclosed that the roots of the cauda equina on the left side were enmeshed in tuberculous fibrous tissue. In one of our patients, a 28-year-old man, scoliosis, sciatica, pain in the buttock and extreme hypersensitivity to movement of the right lower extremity appeared about a month after an injury. Plain film examination of his lumbar spine revealed an erosive process involving the superior aspect of the body of the fourth lumbar vertebra. On myelography a prominent defect and partial block were encountered at the third lumbar interspace, more marked on the right side. At operation the epidural fat was bluish-black in color, and was traversed by many large veins. On incising this membranous covering, granulomatous material containing degenerative cartilage exuded. This proved to be tuberculous in origin. Subsequently the patient developed a draining sinus into the operative wound. He was completely relieved of pain, and the bony lesion healed after conservative therapy (Fig. 210).

Infrequently tuberculosis of the spine presents with symptoms of a herniated disc without concomitant bony, dural or other manifestations. This occurred in a 67-year-old man reported by Decker, Shapiro and Porter (1959). The patient had myelographic changes indicative of a discal herniation at the fifth lumbar interspace. At operation the L5 root was tense and impinged upon by a mass that exuded purulent fluid. No primary focus could be detected.

Intraspinal block incident to gibbus formation is infrequent. The appearance of neurologic symptoms in patients with such malformations requires myelographic investigation. Paraplegia in patients with tuberculous spondylitis has been attributed to vascular impairment rather than to direct pressure, but in most cases mechanical factors are significant.

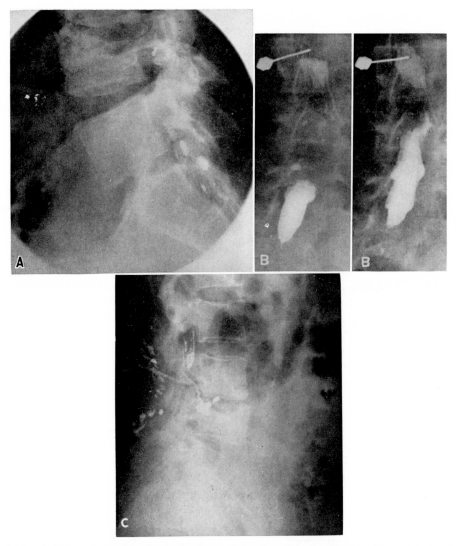

Fig. 210. *A*, Tuberculosis of the fourth lumbar vertebra in a 35-year-old man with symptoms of cauda equina compression. *B*, The first myelogram in the erect posture shows Pantopaque held up at the third lumbar interspace. Note the dentate pattern of the inferior margin of the upper Pantopaque. The next myelogram was made in the head-down position. The inferior margin of the intraspinal protrusion is delineated as corresponding with the lower aspect of the destructive process in the fourth lumbar vertebra. *C*, A draining sinus persisted 5 months after operation. This was injected with Lipiodol, and led to the posterosuperior aspect of the body of the fourth lumbar vertebra.

Trauma may be a precipitating cause of neurologic symptoms in patients with tuberculous scoliosis. In one of the cases reported by Love and Erb (1949) neurologic symptoms appeared after a fall in a hockey game. At operation the dura was found to be thickened and adherent to the arachnoid, suggesting trauma with subsequent organization.

A rare form of tuberculosis known as osteitis tuberculosa cystica, occurring as a rule in children, sometimes presents changes in the vertebrae. This condition is usually observed in the diaphyses of the long bones, is usually multiple and of metastatic origin from a primary thoracic focus. The disease is insidious, with few or no localizing signs or symptoms. The lesions consist of a circumscribed area of soft tuberculous granulation tissue and degenerated bone which tends to heal slowly. This occurs in a diffuse form with honeycomb, web-like structures or in a cystic form with destruction of the medulla and cortex. Law (1940) reported a case of the circumscribed type in a 6-year-old girl observed over a 4-year-period. The spine showed circumscribed areas of rarefaction in the third and fifth lumbar vertebrae which healed in about a year.

The radiologic changes incident to tuberculosis of the spine are slight in the early stages. The lesion rarely is diagnosed within 6 months of the onset of symptoms. The earliest alteration is a slight decalcification of the superior or inferior aspect of a vertebral body. Less frequently there may be decalcification of the central portion of the vertebra. Both changes are difficult to evaluate. Indeed, Hellstadius (1946) reported a case in which an entire vertebral body was the seat of tuberculous necrosis and the roentgenographic examination was considered to be normal. He mentioned that caseous tuberculosis may spread widely through the medullary spaces without conspicuous injury to the cortex of the bone. Consequently, little change appears on x-ray examination. The adjacent intervertebral discs are not necessarily involved even if considerable bony change has occurred. As a rule, however, the bony changes are soon accompanied by alterations in the thickness of the adjacent disc. The sharp line of definition between the bone and the intervertebral disc becomes hazy. Progressive narrowing of the disc follows extension of the infection into this area. With continued erosion partial collapse of the bodies takes place, becoming progressively more advanced as the disease further destroys bone. Extension of infection into the adjacent soft tissues is manifested by the development of paraspinal abscesses. In the cervical area soft tissue extension of tuberculous infection spreads from the anterior aspects of the vertebral bodies, pushing the trachea and esophagus forward. In the dorsal region a paraspinal unilateral or bilateral globular or fusiform bulging mass may displace the paraspinal pleural lines. It should be recalled that other diseases such as primary or metastatic tumors, osteomyelitis, or occasionally paraspinal fluid collections at times simulate this appearance.

Lumbar tuberculous osteomyelitis with extension into the psoas muscle produces a bulge on the involved side. In more advanced cases the psoas shadow may be obliterated. It is possible for healing to take place, manifested by recession of the swelling together with the appearance of calcifications within the abscess. These sometimes are faint amorphous deposits, which with progressive healing may become progressively dense.

Considerable information is obtainable by the use of body section radiography (Fig. 206). This is particularly helpful in identifying the extent of destruction of vertebrae in regions of kyphosis. Body section roentgenograms are useful in identifying areas of increased bone density, often revealing small foci of densely ossified bone within areas which are considered to be mainly destructive in nature. These bits of bone represent practically dead osseous tissue. Biopsy taken from the involved area has been advocated for diagnosis in doubtful cases.

Another change sometimes observed with tuberculosis of the vertebrae is a shallow excavation of the anterior aspect of an involved body. This represents extension of caseation under the anterior spinal ligament producing scalloped, sometimes sharply defined semicircular indentations, and may extend for three or four vertebrae above an area of kyphosis.

With the onset of healing, increased bone density appears, and sometimes spontaneous fusion of the vertebral bodies is noted. Not infrequently adjacent paraspinal abscesses develop dense, extensive calcific shadows (Fig. 207).

Spinal tuberculosis is most difficult to recognize in its early stages. Early disruption of bone, alterations in the intervertebral discs with shift of the adjacent vertebrae and paravertebral soft tissue swelling occurs more often in today's practice with osteomyelitis of pyogenic origin. Occasionally metastatic tumors and vertebral myelomas pose diagnostic problems. Interesting possibilities are encountered in those patients presenting intraspinal and intramedullary lesions. Here the diagnosis usually is made at operation. The absence of concomitant osseous changes in some of these patients heightens the complexity of this problem. Old tuberculosis encountered as incidental changes usually is easily identified. When it becomes necessary to clearly identify a bony lesion suspected to be tuberculous, one would do well to remember that the radiologic diagnosis is easily confused with osteomyelitis and that biopsy confirmation often is essential.

References

Alajouanine, T. and Thurel, R.: Fibrotic Tuberculosis of the Cauda Equina, Arch. Neurol. & Psychiat., 58, 513, 1947.

Anderson, R. L.: Isolated Tuberculosis of the Spinous Process of a Vertebra, J. Bone & Joint Surg., 22, 741, 1940.

Arseni, C. and Samitca, D. C-T.: Intraspinal Tuberculous Granuloma, Brain, 83, 285, 1960.

Auerbach, O. and Stemmerman, M. G.: Roentgen Interpretation of Pathology in Pott's Disease, Am. J. Roentgenol., 52, 57, 1944.

Bosworth, D. M.: Tuberculosis of the Spine, J. Bone & Joint Surg., 27, 491, 1945.

Bosworth, D. M. and Levine, J.: Tuberculosis of the Spine, J. Bone & Joint Surg., 31-A, 267, 1949.

Brodin, H.: Myelography with Water Soluble Contrast Medium in Lumbar and Sacrolumbar Tuberculous Spondylitis, Acta orth. scandinav., 21, 259, 1951.

Cleveland, M.: Tuberculosis of the Spine, Am. Rev. Tuberc., 41, 215, 1940.

Cleveland, M. and Bosworth, D. M.: Pathology of Tuberculosis of Spine, J. Bone & Joint Surg., 24, 527, 1942.

Decker, H. G., Shapiro, S. W. and Porter, H. R.: Epidural Tuberculous Abscess Simulating Herniated Lumbar Intervertebral Disk, Ann. Surg., 149, 294, 1959.

Guri, J. P.: Formation and Significance of Vertebral Ankylosis in Tuberculous Spines, J. Bone & Joint Surg., 29, 136, 1947.

Harris, R. I. and Coulthard, H. S.: Early Diagnosis of Pott's Disease, Ann. Surg., 114, 931, 1941.

Hellstadius, A.: Tuberculous Necrosis of Entire Vertebral Body with Negative X-ray Findings, Acta orth. Scandinav., 16, 163, 1946.

Isaacson, A. S. and Whitehouse, W. M.: Spontaneous Sacro-Iliac Obliteration in Patients with Tuberculosis, J. Bone & Joint Surg., 31-A, 306, 1949.

Jacobs, P.: Osteo-Articular Tuberculosis in Coloured Immigrants: A Radiological Study, Clin. Radiol., 15, 59, 1964.

Jakoby, R. K. and Koos, W. T.: Intradural Extramedullary Tuberculoma of the Spinal Cord, J. Neurosurg., 18, 557, 1961.

Johnston, J. D. H., Ashbell, T. S. and Rosomoff, H. L.: Isolated Intraspinal Extradural Tuberculosis, New England J. Med., 266, 703, 1962.

Key, J. A.: Pathology of Tuberculosis of Spine, J. Bone & Joint Surg., 22, 799, 1940.

Kozlowski, K.: Late Spinal Blocks After Tuberculous Meningitis, Am. J. Roentgenol., 90, 1220, 1963.

Kneidel, J. H., Smith, L. A. and Bishop, R. E.: Unilateral Tuberculous Abscess of the Thoracic Spine with Roentgen Findings of a Dumb-Bell Neurofibroma, Radiology, 54, 78, 1950.

LaFond, E. M.: An Analysis of Adult Skeletal Tuberculosis, J. Bone & Joint Surg., 40-A, 346, 1958.

Law, J. L.: Multiple Cystic Tuberculosis of Bones, Radiology, 35, 328, 1940.

Lin, T. H.: Intramedullary Tuberculoma of the Spinal Cord, J. Neurosurg., 17, 497, 1960.

Love, J. G. and Erb, H. R.: Transplantation of Spinal Cord for Paraplegia Secondary to Pott's Disease of Spinal Column, Arch. Surg., 59, 409, 1949.

Norcross, J. R.: Compression of the Spinal Cord Due to Direct Extension from a Tuberculous Pulmonary Abscess, J. Bone & Joint Surg., 30-A, 492, 1948.

Perlman, R. and Freiberg, J. A.: Bridging of Vertebral Bodies in Tuberculosis of Spine, J. Bone & Joint Surg., 25, 340, 1943.

Poppel, M. H., Lawrence, L. R., Jacobson, H. G. and Stein, J.: Skeletal Tuberculosis, Am. J. Roentgenol., 70, 936, 1953.

Rigler, L. G., Ude, W. H. and Hanson, M. B.: Paravertebral Abscess, Radiology, 15, 471, 1930.

Saenger, E. L.: Unilateral Paraspinal Abscess, Radiology, 48, 256, 1947.

Simpson, T. V. and Brobbelaar, B. G.: Rupture of the Aorta Complicating Tuberculosis of the Spine, J. Bone & Joint Surg., 37-B, 614, 1955.

Soholt, S. T.: Tuberculosis of Sacro-Iliac Joint, J. Bone & Joint Surg., 33-A, 119, 1951.

Somerville, E. W. and Wishart, J.: Pott's Disease of the Spine with Rupture of the Aorta, J. Bone & Joint Surg., 30-B, 327, 1948.

Stern, W. E. and Balch, R. E.: Surgical Aspects of Nonspecific Inflammatory and Suppurative Disease of the Vertebral Column, Am. J. Surg., 112, 314, 1966.

Strange, F. G. St.C.: The Prognosis in Sacro-Iliac Tuberculosis, Brit. J. Surg., 50, 561, 1963.

Sarcoidosis. Sarcoidosis is a systemic granulomatous disease of unknown origin. Its pulmonary manifestations are well known, as are the relatively infrequent changes in the small bones of the hands. More often the condition involves the lymph nodes, liver and spleen, the skin and the eyes. The underlying pathologic lesion is an epitheloid cell granuloma or tubercle which heals primarily by fibrosis and scarring without undergoing caseation. The systemic manifestations are referable to the extent of involvement of the various organ systems to a variable degree. Rarely do the osseous forms cause appreciable distress, except for some arthralgic pain.

Involvement of the vertebral column is uncommon. Nevertheless, cases in which lytic changes are present have been recorded. In the patient described by Rodman, Funderbuck and Myerson (1959) serial films revealed a rapid lysis which improved after spinal fusion. Wood and Bream (1959) summarized five cases, including one of their own, in which the sarcoidosis affected mainly the perivascular spaces in the meninges, the arachnoid becoming infiltrated with lymphocytes and granulomatous nodules attached to the adventitia of the small vessels. Similar perivascular infiltrations occur within the spinal cord, the destruction of nervous parenchyma being consequent thereto. The myelitis may be indistinguishable from an intramedullary tumor both radiologically and at operation. Arachnoiditis likewise may be simulated.

While it is usually accepted that the bony lesions of sarcoidosis are relatively painless, patients with severe back pain incident to vertebral lytic lesions have been reported. Extremely rapid destruction of a vertebral body in a 35-year-old woman was reported by Goobar and his co-workers (1961). Zener and his co-workers (1963) described paravertebral lower thoracic soft tissue swelling, moderate sclerosis of the ninth thoracic vertebra within which a small lytic lesion was seen and a ring-like sclerotic zone in the body of the second lumbar vertebra in a 33-year-old male patient who also had pain and local tenderness in contrast to the usual lack of symptoms in sarcoidosis of the tubular bones. In the differential diagnosis of this rare manifestation of sarcoidosis pyogenic osteomyelitis, tuberculosis, lymphoma and metastatic tumors of bone have to be considered.

References

Goobar, J. E., Gilmer, W. D., Jr., Carroll, D. S. and Clark, G. M.: Vertebral Sarcoidosis, J.A.M.A., *178*, 1162, 1961.

Jefferson, M.: Sarcoidosis of the Nervous System, Brain, *80*, 540, 1957.

Longcope, W. T. and Freiman, D. G.: A Study of Sarcoidosis Based on Combined Investigations of 160 Cases Including 30 Autopsies from Johns Hopkins Hospital and Massachusetts General Hospital, Medicine, *31*, 1, 1952.

Rodman, T., Funderbuck, E. E., Jr. and Myerson, R. M.: Sarcoidosis with Vertebral Involvement, Ann. Int. Med., *50*, 213, 1959.

Wood, E. H. and Bream, C. A.: Spinal Sarcoidosis, Radiology, *73*, 226, 1959.

Zener, J. C., Alpert, M. and Klainer, L. M.: Vertebral Sarcoidosis, Arch. Int. Med., *111*, 696, 1963.

SPONDYLOSIS (Hypertrophic osteoarthritis, osteophytosis, Bechterew's disease, spondylosis deformans)

Many names are applied to this common condition. It is commonly referred to as osteoarthritis, but the term is a misnomer because no definite inflammatory element is associated with the disease. Another name is Bechterew's disease, but Oppenheimer pointed out that the original reports were so ambiguous that Bechterew's disease has come to imply in English and French a certain type of senile kyphosis, while in the German and the Scandinavian literature Bechterew's disease is considered another name for ankylosing spondylitis. It is Oppenheimer's (1942) opinion, with which many agree, that the term Bechterew's disease be dropped, since it defines neither a clinical nor an anatomic entity. Borak (1947) preferred the term "marginal spondylosis'' if spurs were present at the edges of the vertebral bodies. The term "destructive spondylosis" was proposed if spurs coexisted with narrowing of an intervertebral disc. He further suggested that spondylosis was a factor in the development of spondylo- arthritis because of the frequency with which they occured together. Collins (1950) points out that the suffix ''sis'' or ''sos'' should not have been applied to a normal anatomic term like ''spondylo,'' which means vertebra. He suggested that the term ''osteophytosis'' would be more appro- priate, but in view of the wide acceptance of the designation ''spondylosis'' the concept be that this refers to the syndrome arising

from the effects of discal degeneration and consequent hypertrophic spurring and de- formities of the intervertebral discs and foramina.

Arthritis of the vertebral column occurs in the joints lined with synovial membrane, the apophyseal and costovertebral articulations. Inflammatory reactions in these can produce painful symptoms. Malalignment of the vertebral bodies incident to degenerative changes in the intervertebral discs also pro- duce changes in the alignment of the synovi- ally lined joints, with consequent irritation, reactive response to trauma and inflamma- tion. In the early stages little visible change occurs, but later there is thickening of the

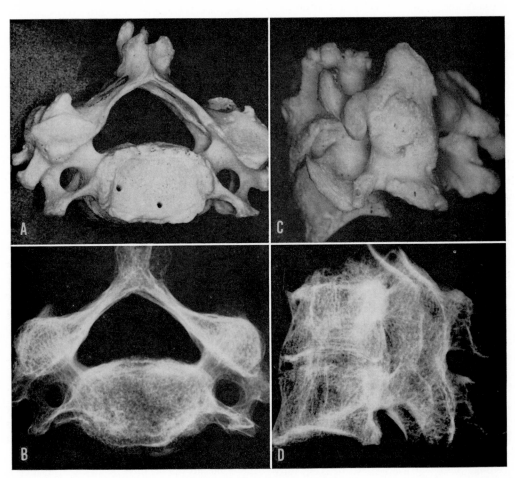

Fig. 211. *A*, Cephalad view of specimen of fused third and fourth cervical vertebrae. The spinal foramen and the foramina transversaria are not affected, and the groove for the emerging nerves are smooth and open. *B*, Roentgenogram of the specimen. *C*, Same specimen, lateral view reveals marked bony overgrowth involving the bodies and laminae. *D*, Roentgenogram of the specimen.

facets, narrowing of the joint spaces, irregularity of the articular surfaces, obliteration of the joint and ultimately ankylosis (Fig. 211). Concomitantly varying degrees of spondylosis frequently exists. The compressive effects of spondylotic ridging often is heightened by the thickening of the laminae and ligamenta flava associated with arthritis. In spinal canals with narrowing at their lateral recesses, particularly those with narrowed sagittal diameters, neurologic and nerve root symptoms out of proportion to the spondylosis or small discal protrusions are often encountered (Fig. 212).

Spondylosis is a degenerative condition which usually begins in early middle age. Most of the time it is asymptomatic unless the spondylotic deformities produce pressure on the spinal cord or nerve roots. The primary change occurs in the intervertebral discs (Horowitz, 1940). With the progressive loss of turgor and elasticity incident to advancing age there is softening and weakening of the disc margins. The softened cartilages swell outward, bulging the annulus fibrosus. These then serve as bridges over which periosteum extends with consequent formation of osteophytes. In the early stages the calcification of the bridging osteophytes is minimal, and hence largely radiotransparent. As more and more calcium is laid down and bone is formed, the spurs become prominent. Involvement of the cervical spine is frequent, and may precede

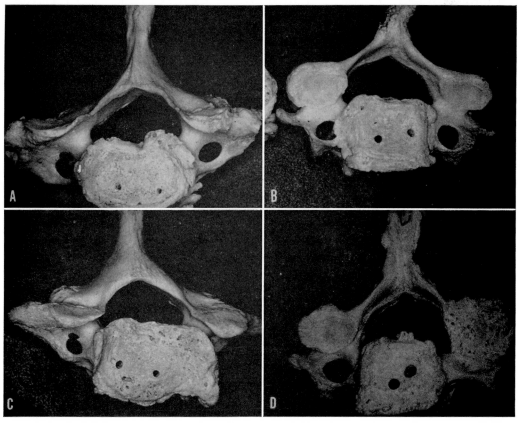

Fig. 212. A, Cephalad and caudad, B, view of a specimen of the 5th cervical vertebra with marginal osteophytosis projecting into the canal, and impinging into the intervertebral foramina at the uncovertebral junctions. C, Another specimen of a fifth cervical vertebra with prominent arthritic changes on the inferior surface of the posterior articular facet, more marked on the left side. The spurring and marginal osteophytosis impinges into the foramen for the nerve roots, and another osteophyte projects into the middle of the spinal canal.

similar spondylotic changes in the thoracic and lumbar regions. The sacro-iliac areas as a rule are not involved except for some spur formation inferiorly. The spondylotic ridges may extend around the periphery of the intervertebral joints, and protrude into the spinal canal and the intervertebral foramina (Fig. 212). Narrowing of one or more intervertebral discs develops together with changes in the normal curvature of the spine. The dorsal spine may become rounded, the usual lumbosacral lordotic curve straightens and the spine tilts to one side or the other.

As a rule the development of posterior discal spurs is less extensive than on the periphery. Keyes and Compere (1932) showed experimentally that fibrillation of the cartilage plate as a result of chronic trauma led to dehydration and escape of disc material. This resulted ultimately in loss of the disc's semi-fluid consistency and cushioning effect. As the disc became thinner, the daily trauma of living was borne in greater part by the fibrocartilaginous annulus fibrosus. Strain was placed on the vertebral bodies with consequent sclerosis, lipping and spur formation. The preponderance of anterior and lateral osteophyte formation was explained by the shift in the axis of motion posteriorly to the articular facets when the disc lost its normal configuration. An added stress forward and laterally was produced when the patient bent. This lipping and spurring also occurred in the true arthrodial joints of the articular facets with consequent bony overgrowth.

Osteophytosis usually begins to appear during the third decade, and by the time the average person is over 40 some degree of marginal osteophytosis is common. The location of osteophytes varies, most tending to develop in the concave portions of the spine and in areas subject to strain. A wide range of calcification along the lateral and anterior aspects of the vertebral column is observed, from rather delicate bone bridges to deposits over a centimeter thick. It is sometimes stated that osteophytosis on the left side of the thoracic spine is inhibited by the pulsations of the aorta (Culver and Pirson, 1960), but this is not always so (Fig. 213). While osteophytes usually are asymptomatic, they can produce symptoms when large enough to press on the trachea, the esophagus and adjacent soft tissues. In the cervical spine pressure on the vertebral artery can be of sufficient intensity to produce vertebro-basilar insufficiency. Strategically situated spurs producing pressure on nerve roots passing through the intervertebral foramina can set up inflammatory reactions and produce a clinical picture which cannot be distinguished from discal herniation (Fig. 214).

Excessive bending and strain, as may be seen in laborers or others engaged in occupations requiring considerable and prolonged muscular effort, is accompanied by the appearance of large paravertebral ligamentous calcifications. These appear mainly at the bending points, particularly in the thoracolumbar region. It is not unusual, however, to find almost the entire spine so affected. The ligamentous calcifications can exceed 1.5 cm in thickness, and sometimes can be seen separated by a radiolucent thin line from the vertebral borders. Increase in the dorsal convexity of the spine can be prominent, and the intervertebral discs become narrowed. The small joints may be affected to a lesser extent. It is of interest that extensive changes such as these often appear with little in the way of symptoms (Fig. 213).

With the more prominent changes in the dorsal convexity of the spine seen with kyphosis senilis, there is usually close approximation of the anterior aspects of the thoracic vertebral margins together with calcification of the paraspinal ligaments. This usually is quite mild. Fusion of the anterior lips of the apposing thoracic vertebrae occurs fairly frequently. An almost characteristic stance, with the neck thrust forward and downwards so that it appears almost horizontal, is often present. With this there may be some forward slipping of the fifth or sixth cervical

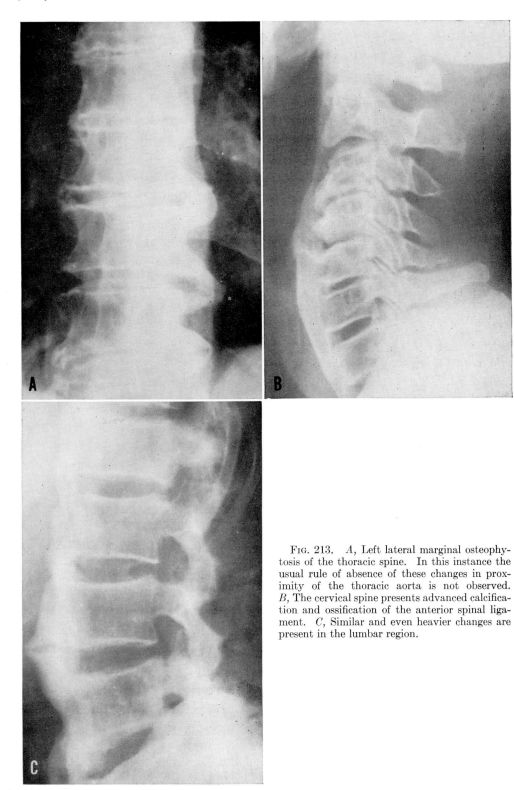

Fig. 213. *A*, Left lateral marginal osteophytosis of the thoracic spine. In this instance the usual rule of absence of these changes in proximity of the thoracic aorta is not observed. *B*, The cervical spine presents advanced calcification and ossification of the anterior spinal ligament. *C*, Similar and even heavier changes are present in the lumbar region.

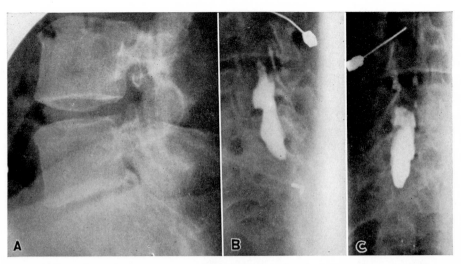

Fig. 214. *A*, Lateral conedown roentgenogram of lumbosacral articulation. A spur is seen protruding dorsally from the posteroinferior aspect of the fifth lumbar vertebra. The lumbosacral interspace is narrowed. *B* and *C*, Right and left oblique myelograms showing indentation of the Pantopaque column. At operation the defect was found to be due to a heavy spur corresponding to that seen in *A*.

vertebrae. Emphysema and various cardio-pulmonary disturbances often are associated with kyphosis dorsalis senilis.

Mention has been made in various reports (Gunsel, 1952; Kertzner and Madden, 1950; Borak, 1947) that large anteriorly placed cervical spurs may be associated with dysphagia. Indentations against the esophagus are often seen, particularly if the spurs project over half a centimeter anteriorly. However, this should not be accepted as a cause for dysphagia unless every other possibility has been excluded (Fig. 215). The role of spondylotic spur formation in the production of other conditions simulating organic disease is part of the picture of radicular and spinal cord compression. Mention should be made of the simulation of anginal pain incident to hypertrophic spondylotic changes in the cervico-thoracic spine and of occipital headache incident to spondylosis of the upper cervical spine.

Occasionally calcification is identified in the posterior spinal ligament. In the few cases I have seen there were no concomitant clinical manifestations. Recently Onji and his coworkers (1967) reported cervical myelopathy with posterior paravertebral

ossification in the cervical spine in 18 patients. The calcification was most prominent in the posterior longitudinal ligament from C1 to C6. Myelographic examination revealed a narrow spinal canal, particularly at C3 and C4, corresponding to the bulk of the calcified ligament.

The neurologic picture associated with spondylosis deformans is usually referable to the area in which pathologic alterations have produced pressure upon the spinal cord or upon the nerve roots. If an inflammatory reaction is present, symptoms may be produced without specific nerve or spinal cord pressure. It is difficult to generalize on the correlation with pain, and one has to conclude that while considerable deformity is known to occur without pain in some, others may have considerable pain with similar or lesser deformities.

Cervical spondylosis can produce a wide range of clinical manifestations. Unless recognized in time, many patients with remedial lesions are consigned to the category of degenerative spinal cord disease and some of these certainly could have been helped. The diagnosis of amyotrophic lateral sclerosis, multiple sclerosis, progressive lateral

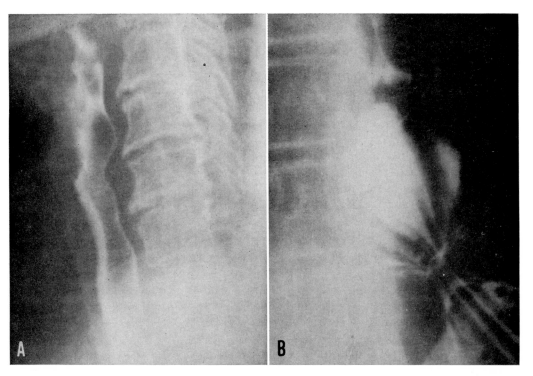

FIG. 215. *A*, This 67-year-old woman's dysphagia was attributed to the anterior cervical spurs, but on further investigation, *B*, it was found that she had a large hiatal hernia with peptic esophagitis.

sclerosis as well as spinal cord tumor or less clearly defined degenerative or vascular disease requires careful consideration and investigation for the possibility that the symptoms may be part of a compressive disorder which can be relieved surgically. The possibility that an obscure disease such as porphyuria exists should also be excluded.

Radiographic examination of the cervical spine begins with adequate plain film roentgenograms. The demonstration of prominent paravertebral calcifications in itself usually is not of fundamental importance. The changes which must be clearly defined by the radiologist include the alignment of the vertebrae, the configuration of the intervertebral discs, the presence of spurring extending posteriorly and laterally so as to impinge against the spinal canal and the intervertebral foramina, and especially an estimation of the sagittal diameter of the spinal canal. The most important of these is the last one, because diminution of the cervical spinal canal space is a fundamental change which influences any others which may cause cord or nerve root compression. The sagittal diameter of the cervical spinal canal can be determined from true lateral roentgenograms, preferably made with a 6-foot target-film distance. The measurement is taken from the middorsal aspect of the respective vertebral bodies to their corresponding points at the roof of the canal. This point is at the white line formed by the base of the spinous process. With this, observation should be made of a similar measurement taken from the dorsal aspect of the intervertebral discs, especially if visible calcific spurs are seen. Measurements have been reported for each vertebral level and have been discussed before (pages 54, 74). A sagittal diameter of 15 mm or less is regarded by us as significant. Sagittal depths 13 mm or under are considered important, especially in the presence of symptoms which suggest radicular or spinal cord disease. Stenosis of the cervical spinal canal relatively limited to the levels of the fifth, sixth and seventh vertebrae is particularly significant because of the frequency with which spondylotic changes occur there.

No specific relationship exists between the changes identified on plain film examinations of the cervical spine and the symptoms of radicular and cord compression. It is likely that advanced bone changes will appear without complaints, and equally possible that minimal radiographic alterations coexist with severe symptoms. While useful information is obtained, particularly as to the presence of uncovertebral spurring, similar projections into the anterior aspect of the canal, and possible stenosis of the cervical spinal canal, the presence of symptoms should be the guide to further exploration. A negative examination in the presence of a clinical picture indicative of radiculopathy and myelopathy is misleading if one does not go on with myelography. The possibility of cord compression by osteophytes which are not visible on plain film roentgenograms and the dynamic effects of movement, such as infolding of a hypertrophied yellow ligament against the dorsal aspect of the cord, cannot be identified without help from myelography. In a narrow canal, a relatively small cartilaginous spur and a thickened yellow ligament can effectively pinch the spinal cord. This is exaggerated during forced extension of the head. Such a sequence of events can sometimes be clearly demonstrated on lateral cinemyelographic examinations (Fig. 79).

Myelography is most important in the evaluation of the cervical spinal canal. I prefer positive contrast examination with the use of an adequate amount of Pantopaque to fill the entire cervical subarachnoid space. Usually this requires about 15 to 18 ml of contrast material. As mentioned before, cineradiographic recording of the passage of the Pantopaque through the spinal canal is made in every case. With cervical myelography observations are made in the frontal, oblique and lateral positions,

and cross-table films are obtained as required with the head in the neutral, flexed and extended positions. I do not place the patient on his back in most cases, because with adequate filling of the cervical canal one can get the required information as to the configuration of its dorsal aspect. Studies are made with the patient in the supine position if there is need to fill the fourth ventricle and the sylvian aqueduct. Otherwise, it is entirely possible to fill the region of the foramen magnum and the posterior cranial fossa with the patient in the prone and oblique positions. Control of the contrast material is best accomplished with the aid of image intensification fluoroscopy and television monitoring.

There are some advocates of air myelography for the investigation of the cervical spinal canal. The advantage offered is the superior visualization of the spinal cord. Wilson, Weidner and Hanafee (1966) found this helpful in determining the presence of cord atrophy, which, they felt, was a contraindication to surgery. However, I still regard positive contrast examinations as preferable because of the ease of the examination and the fact that the entire subarachnoid space can be studied actively during motion cineradiography.

One of the important details in cervical myelography is the observation of the entrance of Pantopaque into the upper thoracic and lower cervical regions. Here, a temporary holdup in the passage of Pantopaque into the lower cervical canal and a backup of contrast material into the thoracic canal can be a significant observation (Fig. 216). The flow of Pantopaque in the cervical canal should be recorded cineradiographically because it is practically impossible to remember accurately just what one sees fluoroscopically. Usually the Pantopaque passes into the lateral gutters on either side of the canal, and spills over anteriorly from one side to the other. Holdup of such passage can be momentary, and still be significant. The effects of flexion and extension of the head also provides helpful information, particu-

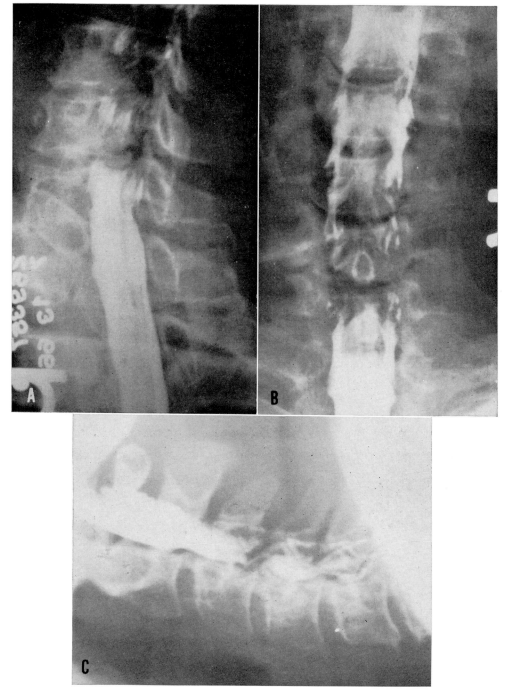

Fɪɢ. 216. *A,* A 53-year-old man with shoulder and arm weakness and muscular atrophy. A hold-up in the passage of Pantopaque is seen at C7 when the head is moderately extended. A small amount passes craniad. *B,* After the head was flexed and the patient placed prone, the cervical canal is well filled. Multiple ridge defects are present at C5, 6 and 7 interspaces. The spinal cord is flattened and widened. *C,* Cross-table view reveals multiple spondylotic spurs with retention in the upper spinal canal. At operation discal ridge together with herniation found at C3 interspace. Ridges present at C4, 5, 6 and 7, the last one being the largest. This patient was incapacitated before operation, and had been diagnosed as having a demyelinating disease. The plain film identification of a narrow cervical spinal canal led to myelography as the first step in further investigation.

larly as to the indentations produced by
infolding of the ligamenta flava and the
changes in the configurations of the Pantopaque column caused by anterior filling defects. Evaluation of lateral defects in the
column are more accurate when cineradiographic recordings supplement the spot
films usually available.

In the presence of cervical spondylotic
changes affecting the spinal canal, one may
encounter myelographic alterations varying
from a complete block to more subtle
changes suggesting the presence of indentations produced by spurs intruding into the
anterior and anterolateral aspects of the
canal. It is important to consider the fact
that the deformities themselves are not necessarily the most important factors in the
production of symptoms. Indeed, in many
instances the cervical spinal canal filled
during a routine myelography disclosed
rather prominent filling defects which were
of no clinical importance, much the same as
occurs in the lumbar spinal canal. For a myelographic defect to assume diagnostic significance one must keep in mind the association
of symptoms, the architecture of the canal in-

sofar as available space for the spinal cord
and nerve roots is concerned, and the fact
that the clinical picture in the same patient
can vary from day to day.

Cervical spondylosis appears in many
forms. With a single small spur strategically
situated so that it compresses a nerve root,
the clinical picture is one that suggests a
herniated cervical disc. The plain film examination may be within normal limits,
and myelographic examination discloses
only a lateral defect in the Pantopaque
column. In such instances a differential
diagnosis between a hypertrophic spur or a
discal herniation is not clearly possible. One
might justifiably regard the condition as
two aspects of the same pathologic process
(Fig. 217).

In other patients, a whole series of spurs
along the floor of the cervical spinal canal
can appear. This results in the so-called
"wash-board configuration" of the floor of
the spinal canal, manifested myelographically by multiple radiolucent defects at the
various levels (Fig. 218). Each one may
cause some degree of obstruction, and observation of Pantopaque passing from one side

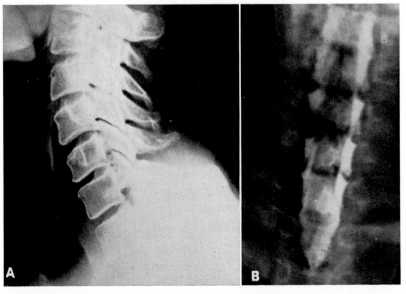

Fig. 217. A, Lateral cervical spine roentgenogram. The vertebral bodies are well formed and aligned.
B, Cervical myelogram. A semicircular defect is present on the left side at the sixth cervical interspace.
At operation this was found to be due to a dense cartilaginous spur. The clinical picture was that of a
lateral herniated disc.

of the canal to the other as it fills the cervical subarachnoid space is best made cineradiographically. In these patients defects also appear at the lateral margins of the affected interspaces (Fig. 219). The extent of the lesions also vary, some being prominent and others less so in the same patient. In some patients such ridges may involve the fourth, fifth and sixth interspaces. Relief can best be obtained by adequate release of the compressive forces by laminectomy and facetectomy for relief of cord and nerve root compression (Epstein and co-workers, 1963, 1965). Others prefer anterior cervical diskectomy and fusion (Rosomoff and Rossman, 1966), but for the present our

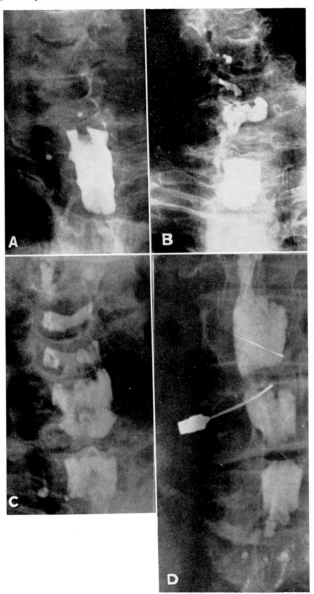

Fig. 218. *A, B* and *C,* Successive spot films made during cervical myelography. At the time A was exposed there was a temporary delay at the seventh cervical interspace. A few seconds later a small amount passed above this region (*B*), and within a minute a "wash-board" ribbed effect was present, *C.* This patient had symptoms of cervical spinal cord compression. *D,* Same case. The patient had no symptoms referable to the lumbar spine, but radiologically presented the same type of "washboard" deformity.

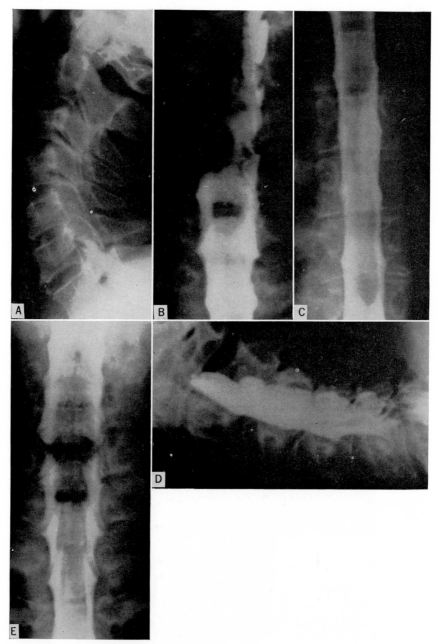

Fig. 219. A 58-year-old woman with weakness of both arms and progressive spastic gait and weakness of both legs for about 4 years. *A*, Lateral roentgenogram of cervical spine shows only mild hypertrophic spondylotic changes. *B*, Myelography showed a partial block at the level of the fifth cervical interspace, with the Pantopaque flowing to the right of the spinal canal. *C*, Film of thoracic canal showing the Pantopaque backing up in this region. *D*, Transcervical view with head in moderate extension. A large indentation is present at C6 in the anterior aspect of the column. Note the upward displacement of that nerve root, as well as the flattening of the cord. At operation a large ridge was present. The laminae of C6 were unusually dense and thickened, contributing to the compression of the cord. *E*, After the cervical canal was filled, a ridge defect becomes evident at the fifth interspace. The spinal cord is widened.

group prefers not to use the anterior approach and do not regard cervical fusion as the operation of choice. Our results with multiple laminectomies indicate that as a rule no significant loss of function of the neck follows this procedure.

The influence of thickening of the ligamenta flava and of the neural arches on compressive syndromes of the spinal cord and nerve roots is important. This is especially so when there is developmental narrowing of the cervical spinal canal together with spondylosis and arthritic changes in the apophyseal joints. Demonstration of the effects of neural arch changes on the Pantopaque column is best made on lateral and cross-table myelograms, and requires adequate filling of the cervical spinal canal.

The pulsatile activity in the cervical spinal canal is prominent. Changes in the movement of the Pantopaque column, however, are rather difficult to evaluate except when one can demonstrate an active pulsation above a lesion and diminished movement below it.

Observation of the caudad flow when the patient is returned to the erect position sometimes provides important information

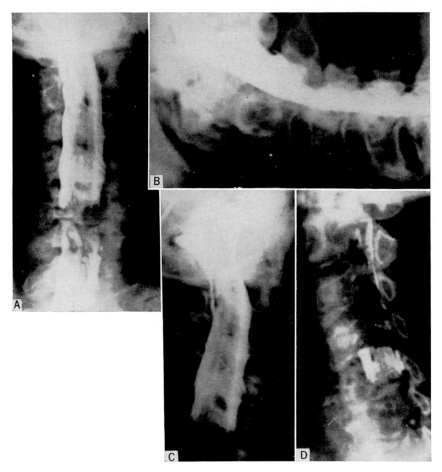

Fig. 220. A 48-year-old woman with intense pain in the right arm, weakness and paresthesias, and weakness of both lower extremities. *A*, The flow of Pantopaque in the cervical canal was held up at the interspace between the fifth and sixth segments. A transverse defect, wider on the right side, is present. *B*, Transcervical view with canal filled. Note the dorsal indentations at the fourth, fifth and sixth interspaces. *C*, With the patient placed erect, a marked delay is noted in the downward passage of the Pantopaque at the sixth interspace. The oil below the column has passed rapidly down the spinal canal. *D*, Film made about 3 minutes after *C*. Some Pantopaque is still held up above the ridge. Verified at operation.

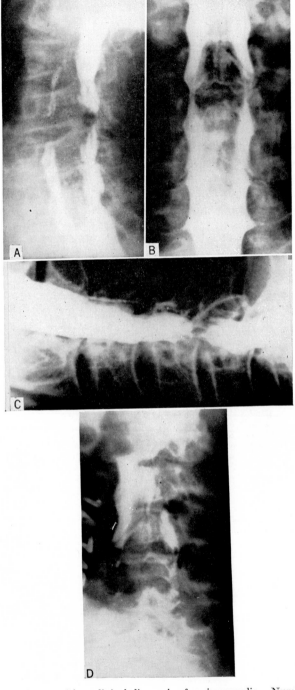

Fig. 221. A 60-year-old man with a clinical diagnosis of syringomyelia. Numbness and burning both hands and feet, weakness of both arms and legs, broad based gait. Temperature, touch and vibratory sense intact. *A*, A delay in the passage of Pantopaque at the fourth interspace was noted. *B*, The column then became spread, producing a spindle-shaped defect which at first glance was believed to be suggestive of an intramedullary tumor. *C*, Transcervical study shows compression of cord from below as well as from above, leading to the diagnosis of a large ridge defect associated with thickening of the neural arch and ligamentum flavum. *D*, When the patient was placed erect, the Pantopaque below the defect passed rapidly down the spinal canal, but that above was held up, and presented a widened configuration simulating that of a tumor. At operation a large ridge was found at the C4–5 interspace.

(Fig. 220). A definite holdup in the presence of multiple ridge defects may indicate the uppermost significant lesion. Retention of Pantopaque in the upper cervical spinal canal occasionally causes some difficulty in the adequate removal of the contrast material. In these instances flexion and extension of the head and neck, and particularly coughing and straining during these movements, is helpful in mobilizing the droplets. Even with these maneuvers, at times droplets remain in the lateral margins of the cervical canal, particularly if the arachnoidal extensions are prominent. It is of interest that Holt and Yates (1966) found cystic arach-

noidal diverticula which excavated the posterior root ganglia in 36 out of 120 cervical spines removed at necropsy from elderly patients. Their observation of the significance of apophyseal joint arthritis in the presence of cervical spondylosis also is helpful in putting together the anatomic picture of these conditions.

In the presence of multiple ridges the extent of compression of the cord may involve several levels, producing a flattening of the cord which is seen on frontal myelograms as a spreading and thinning of the lateral margins of the Pantopaque column. Indeed, this sometimes cannot be distin-

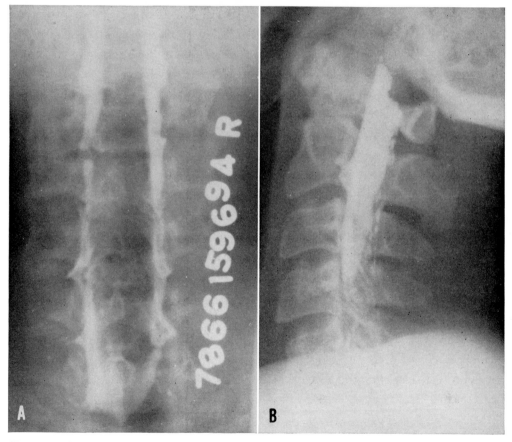

Fig. 222. *A*, A 51-year-old woman with numbness of both hands and unsteady gait for 3 months. The patient was at work when she became quadriplegic within an hour. Atrophy of both shoulder girdles was present, and the tendon reflexes were increased. Clinical diagnosis was possible spinal cord tumor. Myelography revealed a symmetrical, elongated widening of the cord from C4 to C7, with some prominence of the axillary pouches and thin lateral margins of the Pantopaque column. On placing the patient erect, *B*, a delay in the descent was observed, but there was a peculiar flattening of the column at C4. The spinal canal is narrow. At operation large ridges were present at C5 and 6, and the neural arches were heavy, resulting in a marked pinching of the cord.

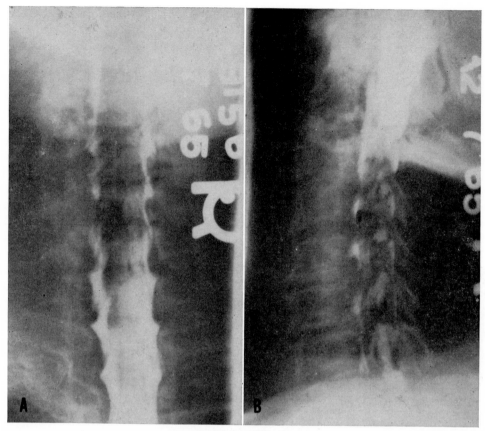

Fig. 223. *A*, A 58-year-old man with weakness of both arms, gradual in onset, with muscle atrophy and paresthesias of the upper extremities. The patient no longer could care for himself. CSF proteins 94 mg per cent. On manometrics, partial block when head placed in extension. Plain films showed narrow canal with spondylosis. Myelography revealed a wide cord, multiple ridge defects with delay in descent when patient was placed erect, *B*.

guished from an intramedullary tumor if one were to rely on anteroposterior films alone (Figs. 221 and 222). Even with oblique and lateral myelograms there may be difficulty in differential diagnosis because the configuration of the Pantopaque column in these projections do not always reflect either the indentations of spurs or the bulging of a spinal cord tumor. It might be helpful to note the sagittal diameter of the canal and the type of dorsal indentation into the contrast column, keeping in mind that a narrow canal is more likely to be one affected by spondylotic changes. In these patients the cord practically fills the canal, with very little Pantopaque present below and above it (Fig. 223).

The coexistence of herniated discs and spondylotic spurs and neural arch malformations is not rare (Fig. 216). It is difficult to distinguish these lesions one from another, especially in patients with multiple defects such as occur with middle and lower cervical spondylotic lesions. Both laterally situated spurs and herniated discs cause defects in the vicinity of the axillary pouches. Midline discal herniations and spurs similarly produce defects in the center of the Pantopaque column. It is possible in the same patient to have one of these caused by a herniated disc and another by a spondylotic spur, or there may be a situation in which a large bulbous protrusion from an articular facet projects deeply into the spinal canal and causes enough compression to seriously impair cord function (Fig. 224).

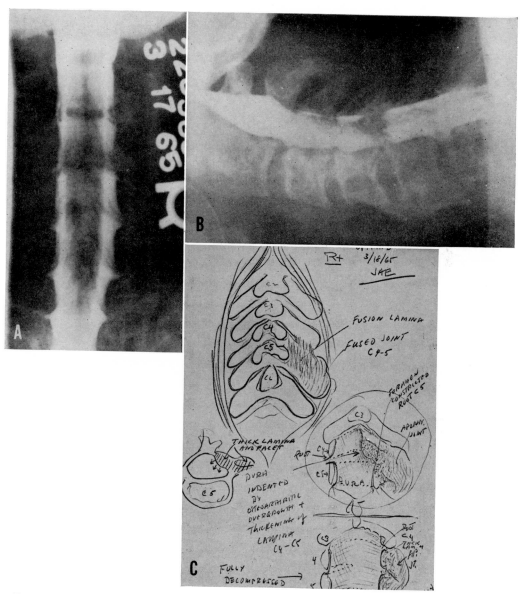

Fig. 224. A, An 81-year-old man with a falling gait for 4 months, with no pain but symptoms of lateral column disease. Ridge defect at C4, with local widening of the cord and identation into the right axillary pouch. B, On transcervical examination a large indentation is seen into the superior aspect of the cord, and a smaller spur is present anteriorly. At operation, C, there was fusion of the right laminae of C4 and 5, both being heavy with osteophytic overgrowth. This caused extradural compression and was corrected by laminectomy and foraminotomy.

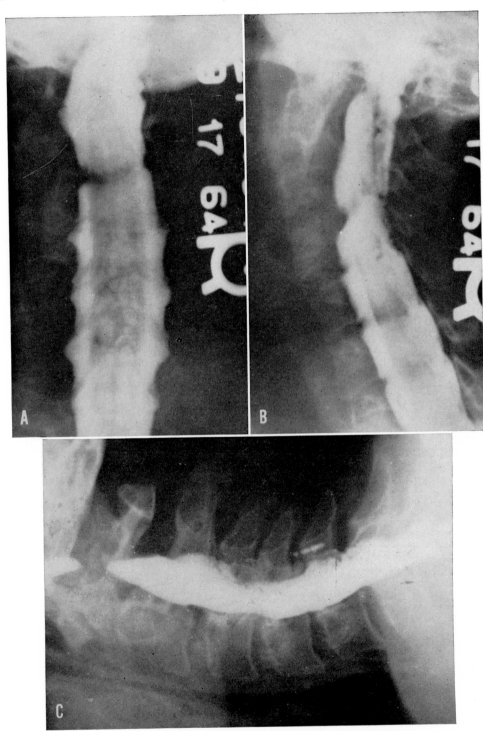

FIG. 225. *A*, A 49-year-old man with pain and limited motion of left arm and shoulder for about 5 months, with numbness and weakness. Unsteady gait for about a year attributed to labyrnthitis. Myelogram reveals an indentation on the left side of the C3 interspace. On oblique views, *B*, the defect persists. On transcervical studies, *C*, an indentation into the dorsal aspect of the canal is seen at C3, 4 and 5. At operation the C3 root was surrounded by coarse, vascular adhesions. The root was freed from its attachment to a prominent spur directly beneath it, and the spur was removed. This was followed by a satisfactory recovery.

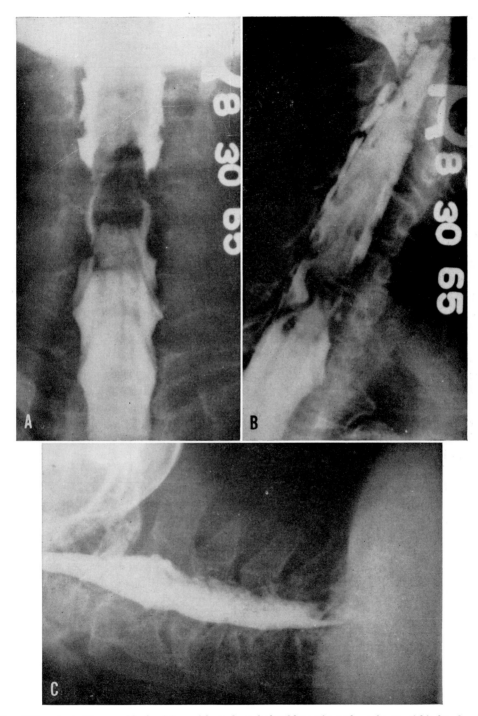

Fig. 226. *A*, A 49-year-old physician with neck and shoulder pain and weakness of his hands which became incapacitating. Symptoms had been present intermittently for about 9 years, and had made it impossible to work. Myelography revealed a large filling defect centrally at C5 and 6 interspaces, with holdup of both craniad and cephalad passage of Pantopaque. Large tortuous dilated veins were present, *B*. On transcervical examination compression from thickened laminae was observed at the involved interspaces, *C*. At operation laminectomy and foraminotomy at the C5 and 6 interspaces revealed marked encroachment on the canal both dorsally and ventrally by huge spurs which were removed. At C6 on the left side there was also a discal herniation which was corrected.

Clinically significant cervical spondylotic lesions appear mainly in the lower cervical spine. Involvement of the fifth and sixth cervical interspaces is observed most often. However, spondylotic changes involving the third, fourth and seventh cervical interspaces also occur. Most often these are part of a more generalized picture in that multiple cervical segments are involved. Occasionally, however, an isolated spondylotic spur defect is identified above or below the more commonly affected fifth and sixth interspaces (Fig. 225). As with other lesions causing spinal cord compression and obstruction in the canal, discal and spondylotic lesions are accompanied by dilatation of the veins, both in the epidural and subarachnoid spaces (Fig. 226). These contribute to the obstructive process.

Spondylotic change in the thoracic spine is frequent, and usually affects the anterior and lateral aspects of the vertebral bodies. Rarely are there any alterations in the configuration of the spinal foramina which compress the cord and nerve roots. Discal degeneration with herniation occurs, but usually is unassociated with alterations in the sagittal diameter of the spinal canal or with spondylotic spurs which intrude into the lumen sufficiently to compromise the cord. In examination of anatomic preparations of dried spinal columns it was rare to encounter a prominent intrusion into the spinal canal in the thoracic region even though the cervical and lumbar vertebrae of the same specimen presented marked spondyloarthritic changes with stenosis of the canal in these regions.

The size and configuration of the lumbar spinal canal and intervertebral foramina are important in the production of symptoms referable to the conus, the cauda equina and the emerging nerve roots. The available space may be the decisive element in the complex of herniated disc, spondylotic spurring, stenosis of the spinal canal and neurologic disturbances. The sagittal diameter of the lower lumbar spinal canal is more difficult to evaluate than the corresponding measurement in the cervical region. A fairly accurate estimation of depth can be obtained by measurement of the intervertebral foramina as seen on true lateral lumbar spine roentgenograms. The vertical dimension of the fifth lumbar vertebra is not as readily measured as those above.

Normally the lumbar vertebrae present a fairly constant structural pattern. The vertebral foramina of the first and second segments are rounded, much like those of the lowermost thoracic vertebrae. The vertical dimension is equal to or slightly greater than the interpedicular measurement. The lower three lumbar vertebrae present a more variable pattern, and a wide range in the configurations of the spinal foramina is encountered (Fig. 227). There is a relationship between the sagittal diameter of the spinal canal and narrowing of the lateral recesses. This diminishes the space available for the cauda equina and particularly for the emerging nerve roots as they pass through the intervertebral foramina. It is not possible to obtain direct radiographic evidence of narrowing of the lateral recesses, but the correlation is accurate enough to permit the assumption that a patient with a stenosed spinal canal will also have constriction of the lateral recesses. Under this circumstance a small discal herniation or a strategically

Fig. 227. *A,* Sagittal measurements of the spinal foramina can be made on these five selected specimens of the lumbar vertebrae. Note the variations in the configuration of the spinal foramina varying from very wide to very narrow. *B,* Lateral roentgenogram in a patient with a narrow lumbar canal compared with one in which the foramina are wide. (From Epstein, B. S., Epstein, J. A. and Lavine, L.: The Effect of Anatomic Variations in the Lumbar Vertebrae and Spinal Canal on Cauda Equina and Nerve Root Syndromes, Am. J. Roentgenol., *91,* 1055, 1964.)

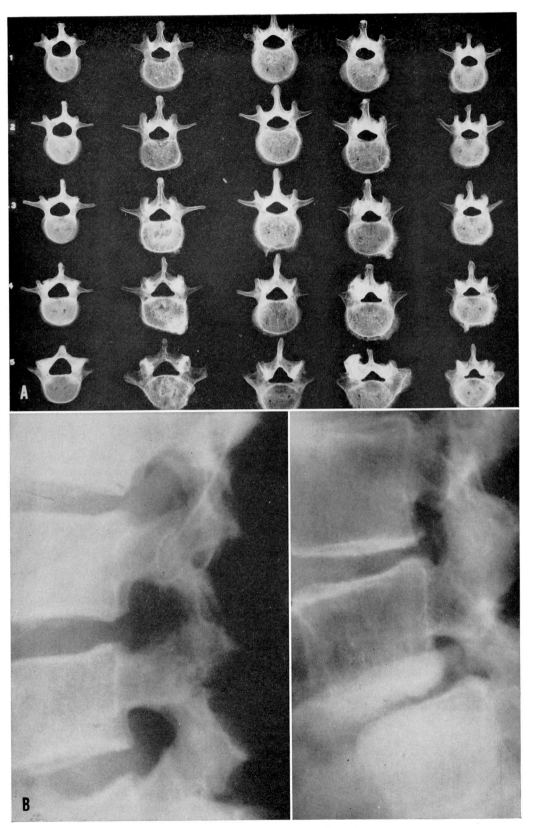

Fig. 227. (*Legend on opposite page.*)

placed spondylotic spur is capable of producing marked compressive changes on an emerging nerve root. The normal measurement is about 1.5 cm in the lower lumbar region, and slightly greater above (Epstein, Epstein and Lavine, 1964).

In considering the available space in the lumbar spinal canal, account must be taken of several other factors, including thickening of the neural arches, spondylotic ridges and spurs along the posterior vertebral margins and the articular facets, thickening of the ligamenta flava and spondylolisthesis. Congenital variations in the neural arches, especially in the lumbosacral region, also influences the available space. Changes in posture, straining and coughing also alter the room available for the cauda equina because of engorgement of the epidural venous plexuses. This can often be demonstrated by having the patient strain during myelography. The Pantopaque column is seen to narrow and its upper level moves cephalad, sometimes for a considerable distance (Figs. 70 and 72).

Spondylotic spurs appear in diverse forms. In some, particularly younger individuals, the spur is localized to a single area, and may be unidentifiable on plain film roentgenograms because of insufficient calcification (Fig. 228). Localized spurs which are sufficiently calcified can be seen (Fig. 214), but may require myelographic investigation to evaluate them more accurately. We have found many instances in which filling defects produced by spurs could not be differen-

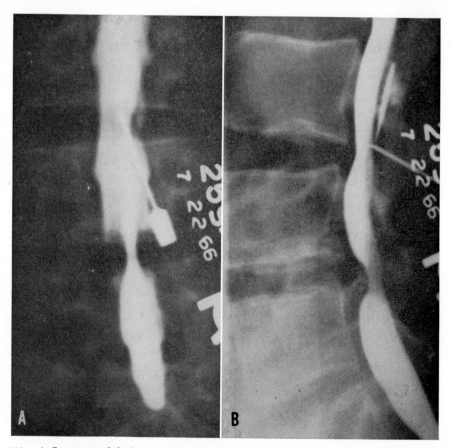

Fig. 228. *A*, Large spondylotic spur intruding into the fourth lumbar interspace in a 16-year-old boy with a narrow canal. Bilateral defects are seen in the AP view, but in the lateral view, *B*, it is evident that the intrusion is from the floor of the canal, leaving only a small dorsal channel for passage of fluid. A bit of Pantopaque has entered the subdural space above the needle tip.

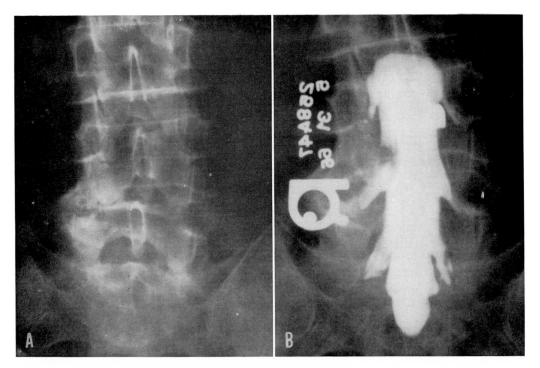

Fig. 229. *A*, A 48-year-old man diagnosed as having a demyelinating disease. The fourth lumbar interspace is narrowed, and spondylotic spurring is present on the right margin which intrudes into the Pantopaque column, *B*. This was considered of no clinical importance.

tiated form those produced by herniated discs. The presence of both discal degeneration, some herniation and bony spur formation in one involved area is not rare.

The clinical picture associated with spondylotic ridges and spurs depends on the extent of the compression on the cauda equina and the emerging nerve roots and concomitant inflammatory reactions, which vary considerably from time to time. In wide canals prominent defects often are asymptomatic (Fig. 229). Pain, often with a changing pattern of midback and radicular involvement, is a common complaint. With severe compression of the cauda equina the initial symptoms occasionally simulate peripheral vascular disease. Intermittent claudication, aggravated by exertion, has been attributed to ischemia of the cauda equina. This may be consequent to other obstructive lesions, as, for example, large midline herniated discs. It is important to note that similar complaints result from

compressive changes produced by spondylosis and neural arch thickening, and that relief can be obtained by means of adequate surgical decompression (Verbiest, 1954) (Spanos and Andrew, 1966) (Foffe, Appleby and Arjona, 1966). Radicular pain often is intense, and may be bilateral. Sensory changes also appear, and absence of the ankle jerk and depression of the patellar reflex is frequent. Sphincteric disturbances, however, are infrequent.

Myelographic examination is required for accurate evaluation of the effects of spondyloarthritis. However, the extent of the defects do not necessarily indicate the clinical severity of the condition, especially in patients who have wide spinal canals. These pose perplexing problems when multiple defects are present, some obviously unrelated to the patient's complaints and others of considerable significance being less apparent. The plain film roentgenograms provide a lead as to the size of the spinal canal.

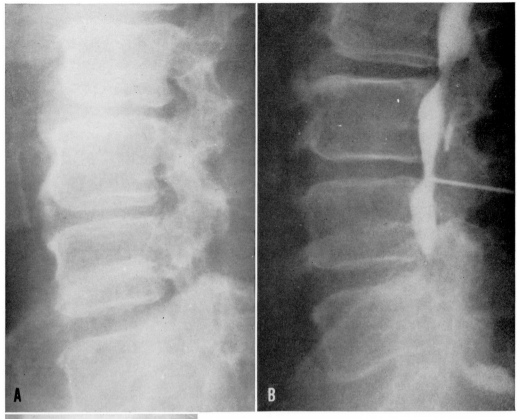

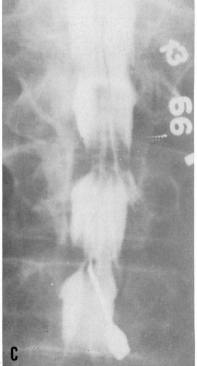

Fig. 230. *A*, Lateral roentgenogram of the lumbar spine of a 68-year-old man with bilateral claudication and leg pain. The spinal canal is narrow. Difficulty was encountered in performing lumbar puncture, *B*, and a tap at L3 showed a slow drip of fluid. After injecting 3 ml of Pantopaque, the canal is seen to be narrow, with a tapered, almost complete block at L4 disc. Multiple ridges are present, *C*, and the fila of the cauda equina are thickened. Both femoral pulses were adequate. Operation was refused.

Another indication of a narrow canal appears when lumbar puncture is attempted and difficulty in getting a good flow of cerebrospinal fluid follows a proper tap. In these patients instillation of a few drops of Pantopaque under image intensification control with the patient semi-erect can be helpful (Fig. 230).

Ridge defects in the lumbar spinal canal appear mainly anteriorly, and may be more prominent on one side than the other. Together with this there frequently are indentations into the dorsal aspect of the dural sac caused by thickening of the ligamenta flava and of the neural arches. The flow of Pantopaque often is impeded by these intrusions. In some instances only a thin ventrally placed channel is left for the flow of cerebrospinal fluid. Multiple defects are common, with Pantopaque accumulating in the hollows of the dorsal aspects of the vertebral bodies. In some a partial or complete block results in a tapered thin configuration of the caudal aspect of the Pantopaque column (Figs. 230, 232 and 233). Pantopaque may flow past this area, but it may be several hours before the caudal sac is visualized. Drainage of Pantopaque under these circumstances is difficult. It is interesting, nevertheless, to see how often most of the Pantopaque can be syphoned off. If this does not work, it is advisable to perform another lumbar puncture, selecting the widest interspace for the second attempt.

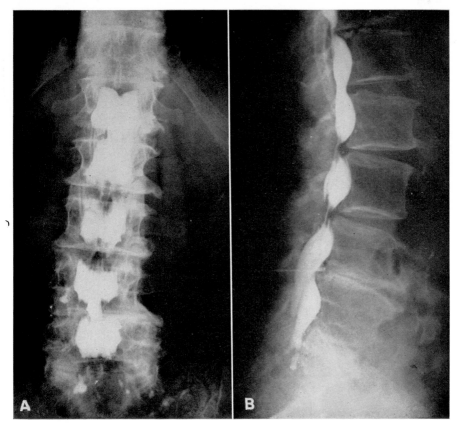

FIG. 231. Anteroposterior and lateral myelograms of a 59-year-old man completely incapacitated because of pain and weakness of both lower extremities. Large ridge defects are present at each lumbar level. Note the narrow configuration of the Pantopaque column at each discal space produced by the bulging at the disc as well as pronounced thickening of the neural arches and ligamenta flava. Considerable relief after multiple laminectomies.

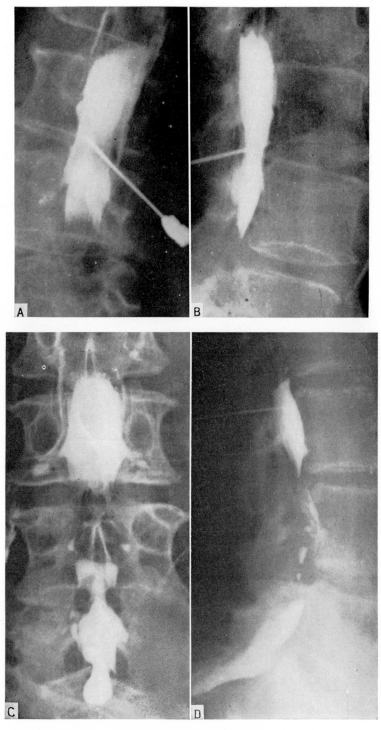

Fig. 232. Pronounced narrowing of the lumbar canal, with a tapered partial block at L3. Markedly thickened neural arches and ligamenta flava together with large ridges at L3 and 4 were found (courtesy of M. Elkin, M.D., Albert Einstein College of Medicine). *C* and *D*, Another patient with a tapered block at L3 caused by a combination of thickened neural arch, heavy ligamenta flava, spondylotic ridges and a small discal herniation.

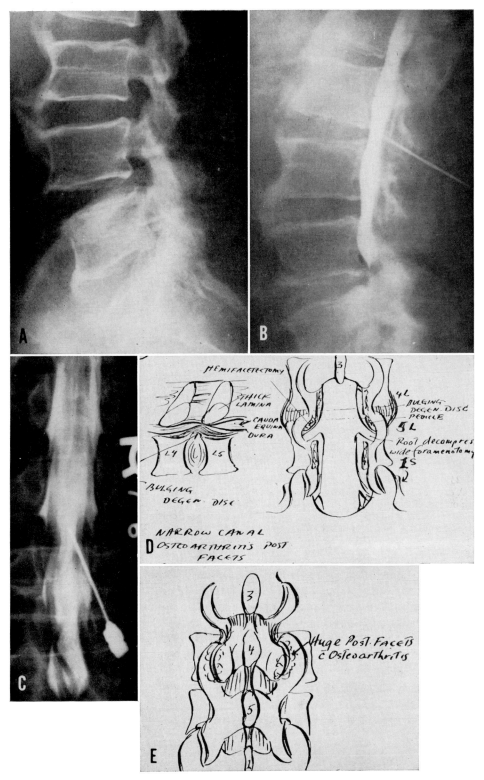

Fig. 233. *A*, A 68-year-old man with long-standing low back pain, weakness of both lower extremities with numbness and pain. Plain film examination revealed a narrow lower lumbar spinal canal. Myelography disclosed a tapered block at L4, *B*, and thickening of the roots of the cauda equina, *C*. A dilated vein is seen in the left side of the canal at the upper level of L4. At operation the articular facets at L4 and 5 were highly hypertrophied and overgrown with bone. A bulging degenerated disc contributed to the block, *D*. He was discharged free from symptoms.

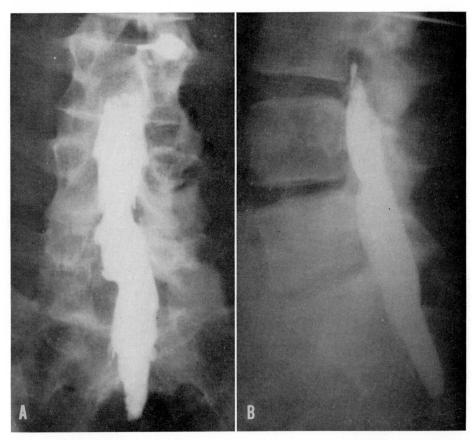

Fig. 234. *A*, Combined spondylotic and herniated disc defects in the lower lumbar spine of a 38-year-old man. A deep indentation is present on the right side of the fifth lumbar interspace, and a shallow defect is present on the left side of the fourth interspace. On lateral views, *B*, an indentation anteriorly is seen at L4. At operation a combined disc herniation and spondylotic spur was present at L5, while the 4th interspace was not explored because it did not fit the clinical pattern of right-sided pain. Good recovery followed operation.

Cinemyelographic studies supplement fluoroscopic and spot film examinations in the same way as in the cervical spinal canal. Instillation of Pantopaque under image intensification control has proven particularly helpful in avoiding extravasation. Nevertheless, some leakage may take place during the examination even after an atraumatic spinal puncture has been accomplished. This is more likely to occur when the lumbar canal is narrow, and usually is of no consequence (Fig. 228).

The coexistence of herniated discs and spondylotic spurs is not uncommon. They may appear together in the same patient, both at the involved single discal level or at multiple levels. When multiple lesions are present, especially in patients with stenosed lumbar canals, adequate laminectomy and foramenotomy are required if relief is to be obtained (Fig. 234).

Thickening of the neural arches alone occasionally results in significant stenosis of the lumbar spinal canal. This is more likely to compromise the cauda equina and the emerging lumbar nerve roots in patients with congenitally narrowed spinal canals, and makes the presence of a minor discal protrusion that much more significant. Frontal myelograms in these patients reveal a waist-like defect, and lateral films disclose the indentation into the dorsal aspect of the dural sac (Fig. 235). Only a single vertebra may be involved, but more often two or three adjacent neural arches are involved (Figs. 230, 231, 233, and 235).

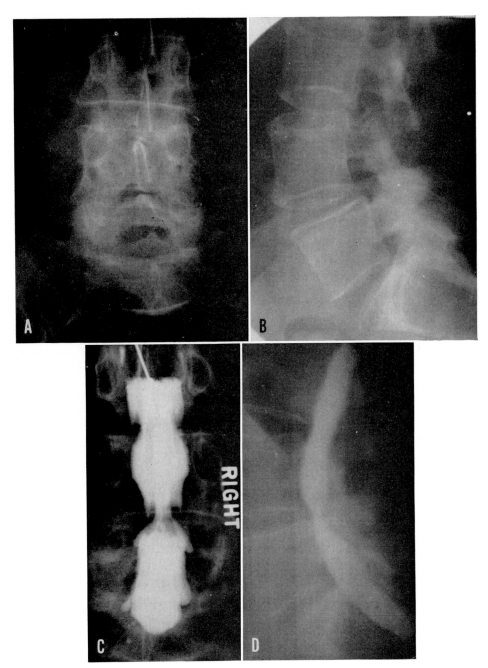

Fig. 235. *A*, AP lumbar spine of a 57-year-old woman with radicular pain in both lower limbs. The 4th lumbar interspace is narrowed, and the left apophyseal joint is coronally placed while the right is oblique. Arthritic changes are present in the apophyseal joints, *B*. On myelographic examination a waist-like defect is present at L4, *C*. On lateral examination there is a deep indentation into the dorsal aspect of the column at L4, *D*. At operation this was found to be due to marked thickening of the laminae and the ligamenta flava which sharply pinched the nerve roots and the cauda equina at this site.

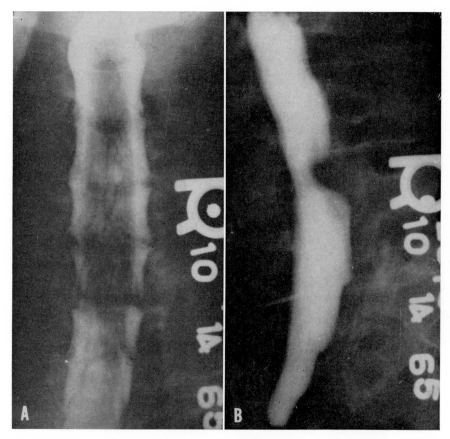

Fig. 236. *A*, A 61-year-old man with numbness, weakness and diminished sensation of the right hand and paresis of the hand muscles. Large ridges are present at the fifth, sixth and seventh cervical interspaces. *B*, A large filling defect is present at the L4 level on the right side. This was asymptomatic. Symptoms were relieved by cervical laminectomy and foramenotomy, which disclosed multiple ridges.

Spondylotic narrowing of both the cervical and lumbar spinal canal occasionally occurs (Fig. 236). With symptoms referable to both the arms and legs, together with evidence of cervical myelopathy, the first attack usually is made in the cervical region. After a suitable interval, if symptoms referable to the lumbar area persist, further surgical correction is made.

References

Allen, K.: Neuropathies Caused by Bony Spurs in the Cervical Spine with Special Reference to Surgical Treatment, J. Neurol., Neurosurg. & Psychiat., *15*, 20, 1952.

Bakay, L. and Leslie, E. V.: Surgical Treatment of Vertebral Artery Insufficiency Caused by Cervical Spondylosis, J. Neurosurg., *23*, 596, 1965.

Bick, E. M.: Vertebral Osteophytosis, Pathologic Basis of Its Roentgenology, Am. J. Roentgenol., *73*, 979, 1955.

Borak, J.: Spondylosis and Spondylarthritis, Ann. Int. Med., *26*, 427, 1947.

Bradshaw, P.: Some Aspects of Cervical Spondylosis, Quart. J. Med., *26*, 177, 1957.

Brain, R.: Some Aspects of the Neurology of the Cervical Spine, J. Fac. Radiologists, *8*, 74, 1956.

Brain, W. R., Northfield, D. and Wilkinson, M.: The Neurological Manifestations of Cervical Spondylosis, Brain, *75*, 187, 1952.

Brain, R. and Wilkinson, M.: The Association of Cervical Spondylosis and Disseminated Sclerosis, Brain, *80*, 456, 1957.

Breig, A., Turnbull, I. and Hassler, O.: Effect of Mechanical Stresses on the Spinal Cord in Cervical Spondylosis, J. Neurosurg., *25*, 45, 1966.

Brish, A., Lerner, M. A. and Braham, J.: Intermittent Claudication from Compression of Cauda Equina by a Narrowed Spinal Canal, J. Neurosurg., *21*, 207, 1964.

Cave, A. J. E., Griffiths, J. D. and Whitely, M. M.: Osteo-Arthritis of the Luschka Joints, Lancet 1, 176, 1955.

Clarke, E. and Robinson, P. K.: Cervical Myelopathy: A Complication of Cervical Spondylosis, Brain, 79, 483, 1956.

Collins, D. H.: *The Pathology of Articular and Spinal Diseases*, Baltimore, The Williams & Wilkins Co., 1950.

Crandall, P. H. and Batzdorf, U.: Cervical Spondylotic Myelopathy, J. Neurosurg., 25, 57, 1966.

Crandall, P. H. and Hanafee, W. M.: Cervical Spondylotic Myelopathy Studies by Air Myelography, Am. J. Roentgenol., 92, 1260, 1964.

Culver, G. J. and Pirson, H. S.: Preventive Effect of Aortic Pulsations on Osteophyte Formation in the Thoracic Spine, Am. J. Roentgenol., 84, 937, 1960.

Davis, D. and Ritvo, M.: Osteoarthritis of the Cervicodorsal Spine (Radiculitis) Simulating Coronary Artery Disease, New England J. Med., 238, 857, 1948.

Epstein, B. S. and Epstein, J. A.: Osteoarthritis and Spondylosis of the Spine, Rheumatism, 13, 82, 1957.

Epstein, B. S., Epstein, J. A. and Lavine, L.: The Effect of Anatomic Variations in the Lumbar Vertebrae and Spinal Canal on Cauda Equina and Nerve Root Syndromes, Am. J. Roentgenol., 91, 1055, 1964.

Epstein, J. A.: Diagnosis and Treatment of Painful Neurological Disorders Caused by Spondylosis of the Lumbar Spine, J. Neurosurg., 17, 991, 1960.

Epstein, J. A. and Davidoff, L. M.: Chronic Hypertrophic Spondylosis of the Cervical Spine with Compression of the Spinal Cord and Nerve Roots, Surg., Gynec. & Obst., 93, 27, 1951.

————: Recognition and Management of Spinal Cord and Nerve Root Compression Caused by Osteophytes, Bull. Rheum. Dis., 3, 29, 1953.

Epstein, J. A. and Epstein, B. S.: Neurological and Radiological Manifestations Associated with Spondylosis of the Cervical and Lumbar Spine, Bull. New York Acad. Med., 35, 370, 1959.

Epstein, J. A., Epstein, B. S. and Lavine, L.: Nerve Root Compression Associated with Narrowing of the Lumbar Spinal Canal, J. Neurol., Neurosurg. & Psychiat., 25, 165, 1962.

————: Cervical Spondylotic Myelopathy. The Syndrome of the Narrow Canal Treated by Laminectomy, Foramenotomy and the Removal of Osteophytes, Arch. Neurol., 8, 307, 1963.

Epstein, J. A., Lavine, L., Aronson, H. A. and Epstein, B. S.: Cervical Spondylotic Radiculopathy. The Syndrome of Foraminal Constriction Treated by Foramenotomy and Removal of Osteophytes, Clinical Orthopaedics, 40, 113, 1965.

Forestier, J. and Rotès-Querol, J.: Senile Ankylosing Hyperostosis of the Spine, Ann. Rheum. Dis., 9, 231, 1950.

Friedenberg, Z. B. and Miller, W. T.: Degenerative Disc Disease of the Cervical Spine. A Comparative Study of Asymptomatic and Symptomatic Patients, J. Bone & Joint Surg., 45-A, 1171, 1963.

Friedmann, E.: Narrowing of the Spinal Canal Due to Thickened Lamina. A Cause of Low-back Pain and Sciatica, Clin. Orthopedics, 21, 190, 1961.

Günsel, E.: Röntgenbefunde bei "Globus hystericus," Med. Klin., 47, 1250, 1952.

Gunther, L. and Kerr. W. J.: Radicular Syndromes in Hypertrophic Osteoarthritis of Spine, Arch. Int. Med., 43, 212, 1929.

Hadley, L. A.: Anatomicoradiographic Studies of the Spine, New York State J. Med., 39, 969, 1939.

————: The Covertebral Articulations and Cervical Foramen Encroachment, J. Bone & Joint Surg., 39-A, 910, 1957.

————: Tortuosity and Deflection of the Vertebral Artery, Am. J. Roentgenol., 80, 306, 1958.

————: Anatomico-roentgenographic Studies of the Posterior Spinal Articulations, Am. J. Roentgenol., 86, 270, 1961.

Hanraets, P. R. M. J.: *The Degenerative Back*, Amsterdam, Elsevier Publishing Co., 1959.

Hardin, C. A., Williamson, W. P. and Steegman, A. T.: Vertebral Artery Insufficiency Produced by Cervical Osteoarthritic Spurs, Neurology, 10, 855, 1960.

Hartsock, C. L.: Headache Due to Arthritis of the Cervical Spine, Med. Clin. North America, 24, 329, 1940.

Heck, C. V.: Hoarseness and Painful Deglutition Due to Massive Cervical Exostoses, Surg., Gynec. & Obst., 102, 657, 1956.

Highman, J. H.: Complete Myelographic Block in Lumbar Degenerative Disease, Clin. Radiol., 16, 106, 1965.

Hinck, V. C., Clark, W. H., Jr. and Hopkins, C. E.: Normal Interpediculate Distances (Minimum and Maximum) in Children and Adults, Am. J. Roentgenol., 97, 141, 1966.

Holt, S. and Yates, P. O.: Cervical Nerve Root "Cysts," Brain, 87, 481, 1964.

————: Cervical Spondylosis and Nerve Root Lesions, J. Bone & Joint Surg., 48-B, 407, 1966.

Horwitz, M. T.: Degenerative Lesions in Cervical Portion of Spine, Arch. Int. Med., 65, 1178, 1940.

Hussar, A. E. and Guller, E. J.: Correlation of Pain and the Roentgenographic Findings of Spondylosis of the Cervical and Lumbar Spine, Am. J. Med. Sci., 232, 518, 1956.

Hutchinson, E. C. and Yates, P. O.: The Cervical Portion of the Vertebral Artery, Brain, 79, 319, 1956.

Joffe, R., Appleby, A. and Arjona, V.: "Intermittent Ischaemia" of the Cauda Equina Due to Stenosis of the Lumbar Canal, J. Neurol., Neurosurg. & Psychiat., 29, 315, 1966.

Josey, A. I.: Headache Associated with Pathological Changes in the Cervical Region, J.A.M.A., 140, 944, 1949.

————: Importance of Cervical Spine to the Internist, Ann. Int. Med., 35, 375, 1951.

Kertzner, B. and Madden, W. A.: Dysphagia Caused by Exostoses of the Cervical Spine, Gastroenterology, 16, 589, 1950.

Kovacs, A.: Subluxation and Deformation of the Cervical Apophyseal Joints, Acta radiol., 43, 1, 1955.

Nathan, H.: Osteophytes of the Vertebral Column, J. Bone & Joint Surg., *44-A*, 243, 1962.

Nugent, C. R.: Clinicopathologic Correlations in Cervical Spondylosis, Neurology, *8*, 273, 1959.

Onji, Y., Akiyama, H., Shimomura, Y., Ono, K., Hukuda, S. and Mizuno, S.: Posterior Paravertebral Ossification Causing Cervical Myelopathy, J. Bone & Joint Surg., *49-A*, 1314, 1967.

Oppenheimer, A.: The Apophyseal Intervertebral Articulations, Roentgenologically Considered, Radiology, *30*, 724, 1938.

————: Calcification and Ossification of Vertebral Ligaments (Spondylitis Ossificans Ligamentosa), Radiology, *38*, 160, 1942.

Pallis, C., Jones, A. M. and Spillane, J. D.: Cervical Spondylosis, Brain, *77*, 274, 1954.

Patterson, H. A. and Byerly, G.: Esophageal Obstruction Due to Lesions of the Cervical Spine, Ann. Surg., *147*, 863, 1958.

Payne, E. E. and Spillane, J. D.: The Cervical Spine: An Anatomico-Pathological Study of 70 Specimens with Particular Reference to the Problem of Cervical Spondylosis, Brain, *80*, 571, 1957.

Penning, L.: Some Aspects of Plain Radiography of the Cervical Spine in Chronic Myelopathy, Neurology, *12*, 513, 1962.

Roth, M.: Vertebro-medullary Interrelations as Observed on Gas Myelography, Acta radiol., *4*, 569, 1966.

Ryan, G. M. S. and Cope, S.: Cervical Vertigo, Lancet, *2*, 1355, 1955.

Sarpyener, M. A.: Congenital Stricture of the Spinal Canal, J. Bone & Joint Surg., *27*, 70, 1945.

————: Spina Bifida Aperta and Congenital Stricture of the Spinal Canal, J. Bone & Joint Surg., *29*, 817, 1947.

Schnitker, M. T. and Curtzwiler, F. C.: Hypertrophic Osteosclerosis (Bony Spur) of the Lumbar Spine Producing the Syndrome of Protruded Intervertebral Disc with Sciatic Pain, J. Neurosurg., *14*, 121, 1957.

Schorr, S., Fränkel, M. and Adler, E.: Right Unilateral Thoracic Spondylosis, J. Fac. Radiologists, *8*, 59, 1956.

Scoville, W. B.: Cervical Spondylosis Treated by Bilateral Facetectomy and Laminectomy, J. Neurosurg., *18*, 423, 1961.

Sheehan, S., Bauer, R. B. and Meyer, J. S.: Vertebral Artery Compression in Cervical Spondylosis Neurology, *10*, 968, 1960.

Smith, C. F., Pugh, D. G. and Polley, H. F.: Pathologic Vertebral Ligamentous Calcification: an Aging Process, Am. J. Roentgenol., *74*, 1049, 1955.

Smith, J. R. and Kountz, W. B.: Deformities of Thoracic Spine as Cause of Anginoid Pain, Ann. Int. Med., *17*, 604, 1942.

Stoltmann, H. F. and Blackwood, W.: The Role of the Ligamenta Flava in the Pathogenesis of Myelopathy in Cervical Spondylosis, Brain, *87*, 45, 1974.

Stoops, W. L. and King, R. B.: Chronic Myelopathy Associated with Cervical Spondylosis, J.A.M.A., *192*, 281, 1965.

Taylor, A. R.: Mechanism and Treatment of Spinal-Cord Disorders Associated with Cervical Spondylosis, Lancet, *1*, 717, 1953.

Teng, P.: Spondylosis of the Cervical Spine with Compression of the Spinal Cord and Nerve Roots, J. Bone & Joint Surg., *42-A*, 392, 1960.

Teng, P. and Papatheodorou, C.: Combined Cervical and Lumbar Spondylosis, Arch. Neurol., *10*, 298, 1964.

Verbiest, H. A.: A Radicular Syndrome from Developmental Narrowing of the Lumbar Canal, J. Bone & Joint Surg., *36-B*, 230, 1954.

————: Further Experiences on the Pathological Influence of a Developmental Narrowness of the Bony Lumbar Vertebral Canal, J. Bone & Joint Surg., *37-A*, 576, 1955.

Virtama, P. and Kivalo, E.: Impressions on the Vertebral Artery by Deformations of the Unco-Vertebral Joints. Post-Mortem Angiographic Studies, Acta radiol., *48*, 410, 1957.

Wilson, G., Weidner, W. and Hanafee, W.: Comparison of Gas and Positive Contrast in Evaluation of Cervical Spondylosis, Am. J. Roentgenol., *97*, 648, 1966.

Wilson, J. C., Jr.: Degenerative Arthritis of Lumbar Intervertebral Joints, Am. J. Surg., *100*, 313, 1960.

Yden, S. and Romanus, R.: Destructive and Ossifying Spondylitic Changes in Rheumatoid Arthritis, Acta orthop. Scandinav., *22*, 88, 1952.

HYPERTROPHIC OSTEOARTHROPATHY

Osteoarthropathy occurs as a concomitant of various cardiac and pulmonary diseases, especially chronic inflammatory diseases such as bronchiectasis and tuberculosis. It has also been observed with pulmonary tumors, liver and blood diseases and chronic intestinal conditions such as colitis. Clinically it may simulate rheumatoid arthritis (Temple and Jaspen, 1948). As a rule the condition is manifested mostly in the tubular bones and in the small bones of the hands. The predominant change is a roughening and thickening of the periosteum with consequent proliferation of the cortex. Involvement of the spine in hypertrophic osteoarthropathy is uncommon. In an extensive report of this condition Mendlowitz (1942) mentioned that the vertebrae were rarely involved.

Camp and Scanlan (1948) reported on several cases of a condition they termed chronic idiopathic hypertrophic osteoarthropathy. They defined this as a lesion occurring predominantly in males at the age of puberty or adolescence, and characterized by an osteoarthropathic syndrome of clubbing of the digits, enlargements of bones of the joints and thickening of the skin of the face in the absence of any primary disease. The disease manifests itself by thickening of subperiosteal bone following approximately the same distribution as noted in pulmonary hypertrophic osteoarthropathy. In their discussion they stated that the vertebrae were rarely involved.

References

Camp, J. D. and Scanlon, R. L.: Chronic Idiopathic Hypertrophic Osteo-Arthropathy, Radiology, 50, 581, 1948.
Keats, T. E. and Bagnall, W. S.: Chronic Idiopathic Osteoarthropathy, Radiology, 62, 841, 1954.
Mendlowitz, M.: Clubbing and Hypertrophic Osteoarthropathy, Medicine, 41, 269, 1942.
Temple, H. L. and Jaspin, G.: Hypertrophic Osteo-Arthropathy, Am. J. Roentgenol., 60, 232, 1948.

Interspinal Osteoarthrosis ("Kissing Spine")

An increase in the usual lordotic curve of the lumbar spine may produce approximation and contact of the tips of the spinous processes. This results in trauma and injury to the interspinous tissues and painful arthritic changes may follow. Other causes include Paget's disease, when the mass of the spinous processes are increased, or atrophy of the vertebral bodies and the intervertebral discs which results in approximation of the tips of the spinous processes. The condition may also be due to congenitally high spinous processes and low vertebral bodies or both anomalies together. It has been observed as part of the picture of spondylosis deformans. The lesion occurs most often in elderly patients. It is characterized by a chronic and sometimes severe pain, which may be aggravated by rotational movements or bending forward or backward. Radiologically, the tips of the involved spinous processes can be seen in contact with each other, with bony sclerosis and overgrowth of the opposing edges.

References

Franck, S.: Surgical Treatment of Interspinal Osteoarthrosis ("Kissing Spine"), Acta orth. Scandinav., 14, 127, 1943.
Rissanen, P. M.: "Kissing Spine" Syndrome in the Light of Autopsy Findings. Acta Orthop. Scand., 32, 132, 1962.

Osteomyelitis

While pyogenic infection of the vertebral column is relatively uncommon, it occasionally presents a perplexing problem in diagnosis. The usual cause is a staphylococcic metastasis from a distant focus of infection. However, numerous other organisms produce osteomyelitis of the spine. The association of vertebral osteomyelitis with genitourinary infections, postpartum and other uterine infections and after operations on the pelvic organs or the genitourinary tract has been attributed to spread of infection by way of the open system of veins along the vertebral column. The nutrient arteries of the vertebrae offer another and perhaps easier avenue of infection. Serial radiographic examinations are important in following the progress of the disease because of the lag between clinical and radiologic manifestations. Body section radiography is important in evaluating small lesions. In patients with meningeal irritation or spinal canal obstruction myelography is essential, particularly in the presence of advancing neurologic symptoms.

In pyogenic osteomyelitis of the spine complaints can be classified as predominantly cervical, thoracic, or abdominal and as involving the central nervous system, depending upon the extent of bony involvement, and its relationship to the segmental nerves, pleura, and abdomen. The onset may be insidious or acute, and the progression of the infection varies considerably. Slowly progressive spinal osteomyelitis is easily confused with tuberculosis. Associated with bone infection are fever, leukocytosis, muscle spasm and signs of meningeal irritation when the infection extends into the spinal canal. With osteomyelitis of the lumbar spine the pain may be referred to the hip and leg, with pain, contractures, and limitation of motion. The vertebral body is involved most often but infection of the neural arches or the spinous and transverse processes alone has been reported. The lumbar spine is the most commonly affected region, the dorsal spine is less commonly involved, and the cervical spine and coccyx present the lowest incidence of osteomyelitis.

The radiologic evidences of osteomyelitis of the vertebral column usually lag as much as 4 to 8 weeks behind the pathologic changes. If adequate treatment is instituted, and the response satisfactory, no radiologic spine changes may develop. In the early stages of the disease involvement of bone is limited to a small focus of rarefaction, usually in the superior or inferior aspects of the involved vertebral body close to the cartilaginous plate. Radiologic examination then may disclose nothing of significance, or a faintly

decalcified focus. An early sign is slight narrowing of the intervertebral disc in the suspected area. When the disease has progressed so that there is appreciable destruction of bone, the rarefied area becomes more apparent (Fig. 237). Collapse of the vertebral body occurs when the bone is sufficiently weakened. Involvement of the intervertebral disc occurs frequently by direct extension through the cartilaginous plate. Adjacent to the intervertebral plate granular destruction of the bone takes place. When the infection has extended completely through the intervertebral disc to the supra- or infrajacent vertebral body, a roughly demarcated and rather ragged appearance of the opposing bone surfaces appears (Fig. 238).

The disc itself is narrowed either by herniation into the vertebral spongiosa or by spread of infection into the disc. Osteomyelitis of the spine is frequently accompanied by rather rapid bony regeneration. Spur

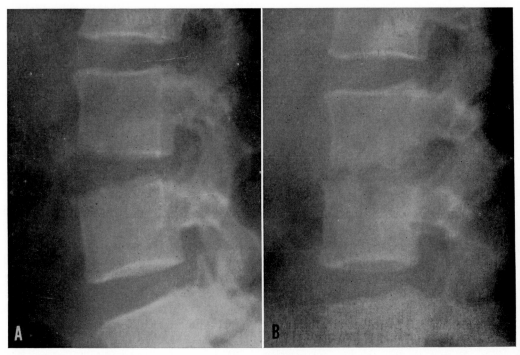

Fig. 237. *A*, A 47-year-old woman with early osteomyelitis of the lumbar spine manifested by erosions along the bony margins of the anterior aspect of the third lumbar interspace. *B*, Four months later the disc is practically obliterated and the osseous changes have advanced. The patient was seen before the days of antibiotic therapy. She recovered under conservative treatment. An abscess formed in the left buttock, and Staphylococcus aureus was isolated from the purulent discharge.

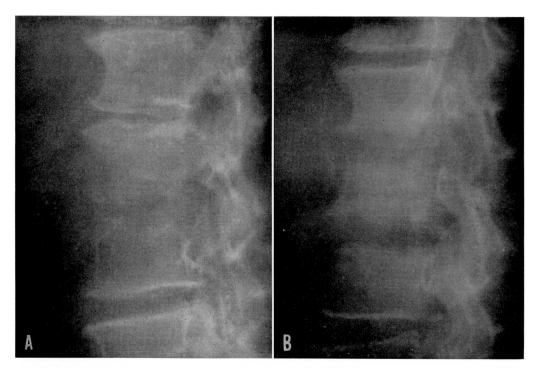

Fig. 238. *A*, A 66-year-old diabetic woman who fell 1 month before admission. Fever and low back pain with tenderness of the midlumbar spine appeared about a week thereafter. A gross erosion is seen in the third and fourth lumbar vertebrae, and that intervertebral disc is narrowed. Four months later, *B*, the lesion has progressed so that L3 has become narrowed, while the disc actually is widened. The diagnosis was verified by biopsy and a positive culture for Staphylococcus aureus.

formations may appear at the same time as destructive changes (Fig. 239). The appearance of proliferating bone may be encountered within 4 to 6 weeks after the disease becomes apparent radiologically. The end result is a complete fusion of opposing vertebral bodies (Fig. 240). Extension of the calcification outside of the confines of the vertebral bodies is infrequent, but occasionally lime salts are deposited in abscesses adjacent to infected vertebrae. The tendency for osteomyelitis to heal with bone proliferation is considered useful in distinguishing osteomyelitis from tuberculosis of the spine.

Several noteworthy complications can appear. Extension of infection from the cervical vertebrae into the soft tissues of the neck may result in marked widening of the retrotracheal space, with pressure against the trachea and constriction of the esoph-

agus. The usual lordotic curve of the cervical vertebrae is straightened, particularly when there is collapse of the anterior aspect of the involved vertebae. An instance of osteomyelitis of the dens was reported by Frank (1944) in a 43-year-old man with a finger infection followed by cellutitis and bacteremia. X-ray examination of the neck at first was negative. Osteoporosis of the odontoid was noted within 3 weeks, followed by pathologic fracture through its base. Necropsy showed acute osteomyelitis of the odontoid process. Another such case was reported by Leach, Goldstein and Younger (1967) with meningeal irritation. Osteomyelitis of the transverse processes of the mid-cervical vertebrae was described by Finch (1947) in a baby 3 weeks old. This child was first seen with an abscess at the tip of a finger. When reexamined 3 weeks later, paralysis involving

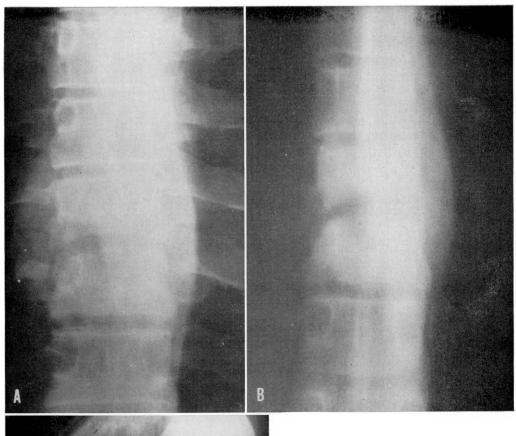

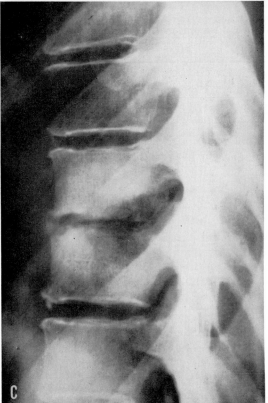

Fig. 239. *A,* AP film of the thoracic spine of a 49-year-old diabetic woman with back pain for 5 weeks. Paravertebral swelling is present. The 8th thoracic interspace is narrowed and its bony margins are irregular. *B,* Laminagram reveals bony destruction on both sides of the interspace. On lateral examination, *C,* the narrowed disc and irregular bony edges are apparent. Some sclerotic reparative effort is present. Diagnosis of osteomyelitis verified by biopsy and positive culture for Staphylococcus aureus.

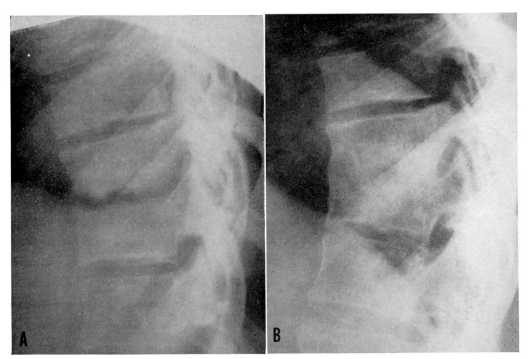

Fig. 240. *A*, Osteomyelitis of the 10th and 11th thoracic vertebrae in a 49-year-old man with fever and back pain. The disc is narrowed and erosions are present in its bony margins. Seven months later, *B*, healing has taken place by bony union after spine fusion had been done.

both arms, shoulders and hands was present. A lump which became large and fluctuant appeared in the midline of the back of the neck. Thick green pus was aspirated, from which Staphylococcus aureus was cultured. Healing took place by fusion of the involved vertebral bodies and their neural arches.

Osteomyelitis of the thoracolumbar spine may invade the adjacent soft tissues and sometimes enters the thoracic cavity, perforating into a bronchus and manifesting itself by purulent expectoration. Such a case was described by Johnson and James (1945) in a 34-year-old patient with suppurative osteomyelitis of the spine due to typhoid fever 22 years before admission. In this case a paravertebral abscess formed which perforated into the lung. Brill and Silberman (1938) described a case of pyogenic osteomyelitis of the spine with mediastinal abscess and spinal cord compression.

Extension of osteomyelitis into the soft tissues adjacent to the thoraco-lumbar verte-

brae and psoas abscess formation is not infrequent (Fig. 239). Sinus formation may occur with extension of the infection to more remote areas, sometimes emerging to the skin. In such case injection of the fistulous tract with positive contrast material may help identify the source of the infection. We have observed several cases in which osteomyelitis of a lumbar vertebra was limited to a transverse process, and radiologically presented only a small area of rarefaction. The contrast injection in these people disclosed large sinus tracts with purulent collections deep in the tissues adjacent to the spine, and extending a considerable distance from the original small infected area (Fig. 241). Shehadi (1939) reported a case of osteomyelitis involving the inferior articular process of the second lumbar vertebra, in which serial roentgenograms over an 8-year period revealed a gradual bisappearance of this structure. Cure was spontaneous.

25

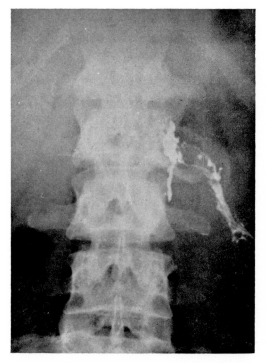

FIG. 241. Lipiodol injection of sinus tract leading to the primary osteomyelitic focus in the left transverse process of the second lumbar vertebra.

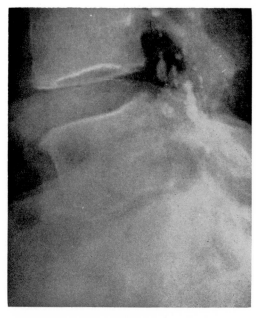

FIG. 242. Lateral roentgenogram of lumbosacral spine. Osteomyelitis destroying the anteroinferior aspect of the fifth lumbar vertebra following operation for herniated disc.

Osteomyelitis of the neural arches is not as frequent as involvement of the vertebral bodies. It may be associated with extension of the infection into the epidural space, producing spinal cord irritation and compression. In such cases myelography constitutes an important part of the examination.

Instances of infection of vertebral bodies after trauma are infrequent. Such a case was reported by Atstatt (1939) in which chills and fevers followed fracture of the second lumbar vertebra due to a fall. This patient developed a secondary hematogenous osteomyelitis secondary to a streptococcus infection, as disclosed by necropsy.

The role of lumbar puncture in the development of osteomyelitis of the spine has been recognized (Redo, 1953). Roentgenograms reveal narrowing of the involved intervertebral disc, followed by sclerosis or rarefaction and destruction of the involved vertebral bodies.

Osteomyelitis of the lumbar spine following operation for herniated disc is a complication which occurs occasionally. In 4 such cases in our experience surgery had been preceded by myelography. The infection first manifested itself in the anterior aspect of the involved vertebral bodies, and infection appeared clinically about 2 weeks after the operation had been done. In 2 of these cases a slow but satisfactory response followed antibiotic therapy. In the other the response was not as satisfactory, and the infection took a long time before healing by sclerosis took place (Fig. 242).

Osteomyelitis of the sacrum and sacroiliac joints may be directly introduced, follow infections in the adjacent soft tissues or be of metastatic origin. The infection may involve the body of the sacrum, with destruction of its midportion and formation of sinus tracts to its immediate vicinity or extending as far distally as the hip region. With healing, the lytic areas gradually fill in and eventually become densely sclerotic (Fig. 243). The process may be indolent and last a long time, resulting in destruction and deformity of the sacrum and later pronounced sclerosis.

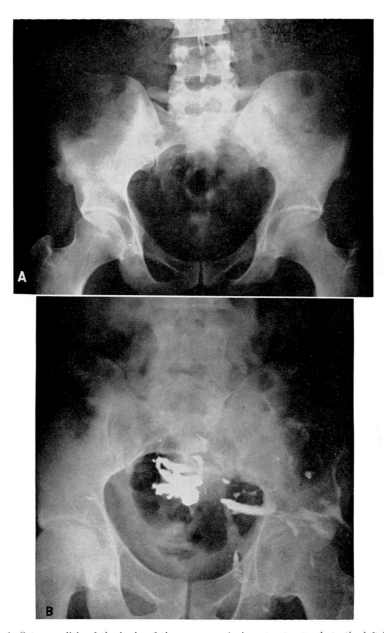

FIG. 243. *A*, Osteomyelitis of the body of the sacrum. A sinus tract extends to the left hip region. A rarefied destructive focus is present in the sacrum, overshadowed by gas in the bowel. *B*, Same case, lipiodol injection of the sinus tract. The contrast medium collects in the hollow of the sacrum.

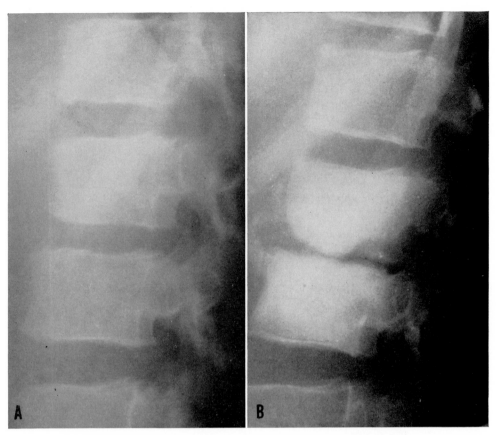

Fig. 244. *A*, Osteomyelitis of L1 and 2 in a 16-year-old boy first seen with upper abdominal girdle pain, weakness of both legs and 20 pound weight loss. Minimal changes are present in the bone adjacent to the anterior aspect of the L1 disc. Positive culture from biopsy. *B*, Six months later healing occurred with marked sclerosis of the bodies of L1 and 2 and bony bridging along the anterior and lateral aspects of these vertebrae. The disc had narrowed markedly.

Rarely, healed osteomyelitis presents as a densely sclerotic vertebra, simulating a so-called "ivory vertebra." We have had but one verified example of this unusual variation in a 16-year-old boy who responded to treatment by prolonged rest and antibiotic medication. The density of the vertebra did not alter perceptibly over a period of observation of about a year after symptoms disappeared (Fig. 244).

A benign form of osteitis appears in the spine in children (Bremner and Neligan, 1953; Pritchard and Thompson, 1960; Jamison and co-workers, 1961). This appears with symptoms of a systemic infection, followed by back pain and stiffness with gradual progression of symptoms for about 6 weeks. After that symptoms recede and usually recovery takes place. The clinical course often is mild, and the specific etiologic agent cannot be identified. The radiologic changes include gradual narrowing of the intervertebral disc, followed by areas of destruction of the contiguous margins of the adjacent vertebral bodies. Healing occurs spontaneously, and is associated with sclerosis of the involved vertebral margins and some restoration of the disc. It is still unknown whether this is a separate disease or a variant of the better known infectious spondylitis caused by bacterial infection.

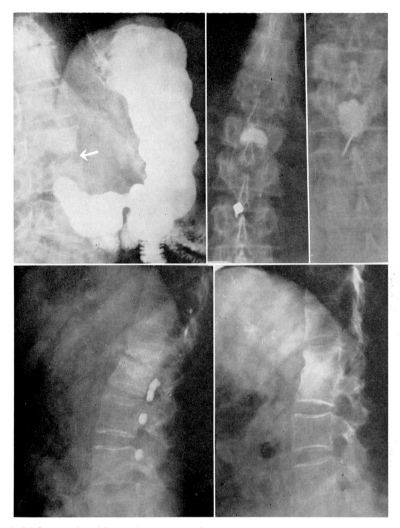

FIG. 245. *A*, Right anterior oblique view of stomach. A destructive process is present at the first lumbar interspace, with involvement of the opposing bone surfaces. This was an incidental observation in a patient in whom the clinical diagnosis was perforating duodenal ulcer. *B*, Myelogram outlining the superior and inferior aspects of the intraspinal protrusion. *C*, Lateral spine roentgenogram made 6 weeks later, 5 weeks after operation when an inflammatory granulation was found impressing into the spinal canal. Some effort at bony repair is apparent. *D*, Seven months after identification of the lesion verified as osteomyelitis. Complete healing after antibiotic and chemotherapeutic treatment.

The onset of symptoms of cord compression and nerve root deficits indicates the need for myelographic investigation. These symptoms, or bizarre abdominal pain, can appear at any stage of infection, and sometimes precede visible bony changes in the involved vertebrae. More often, however, there is concomitant osseous involvement (Fig. 245). Sometimes it is difficult to distinguish such bone destruction from that incident to vertebral metastases, tuberculosis, granulomatous osteomyelitis incident to other organisms such as brucellosis, cryptococcosis and fungal infections. If evidences of an intraspinal block are obtained, surgical relief is required. At this time the etiologic agent responsible for the disease usually can be identified.

References

Adlerman, E. J. and Duff, J.: Osteomyelitis of Cervical Vertebrae as a Complication of Urinary Tract Disease, J.A.M.A., *148*, 283, 1952.

Billington, R. W.: Spondylitis Following Cerebrospinal Meningitis, J.A.M.A., *86*, 683, 1924.

Bremner, A. E. and Neligan, G. A.: Benign Form of Acute Osteitis of Spine in Young Children, Brit. M. J., *1*, 856, 1953.

Brill, N. Q. and Silberman, D. E.: Pyogenic Osteomyelitis of the Spine, Mediastinal Abscess and Compression of the Spinal Cord, J.A.M.A., *110*, 2001, 1938.

Campbell, J. A. and Silver, R. A.: Roentgen Manifestations of Epidural Granulomas, Am. J. Roentgenol., *72*, 229, 1954.

De Feo, E.: Osteomyelitis of Spine Following Prostatic Surgery, Radiology, *62*, 396, 1954.

Donahue, C. D.: Osteitis of the Spine, J. Urol., *61*, 405, 1949.

Downing, F. H.: Collapse of Intervertebral Disc Following Spinal Puncture, U. S. Naval Bull., *43*, 666, 1944.

Finch, P. G.: Staphylococcic Osteomyelitis of the Spine in a Baby Aged Three Weeks, Lancet, *2*, 134, 1947.

Findlay, L. and Kemp, F. H.: Osteomyelitis of the Spine Following Lumbar Puncture, Arch. Dis. Childhood, *18*, 102, 1943.

Frank, T. J. F.: Osteomyelitis of the Odontoid Process of the Axis (Dens of the Epistopheus), M. J. Australia, *1*, 198, 1944.

Giaccai, L. and Idriss, H.: Osteomyelitis Due to Salmonella infection, J. Pediat., *41*, 73, 1952.

Gilmour, W. N.: Acute Haematogenous Osteomyelitis, J. Bone & Joint Surg., *44-B*, 841, 1962.

Greenspan, R. H. and Feinberg, S. B.: Salmonella Bacteremia, Radiology, *68*, 861, 1957.

Guri, J. P.: Pyogenic Osteomyelitis of Spine, J. Bone & Joint Surg., *28*, 29, 1946.

Hall, J. E. and Silverstein, E. A.: Acute Hematogenous Osteomyelitis, Pediatrics, *31*, 1033, 1963.

Henson, S. W. and Coventry, M. B.: Osteomyelitis of the Vertebrae as the Result of Infection of the Urinary Tract, Surg., Gynec. & Obst., *102*, 207, 1956.

Hurwitz, A. and Albertson, H. A.: Cervical Osteomyelitis and Urinary Tract Infection Caused by Escherichae Coli, New England J. Med., *243*, 562, 1950.

Jamison, R. C., Heimlich, E. M., Miethke, J. C. and O'Loughlin, B. J.: Nonspecific Spondylitis of Infants and Children, Radiology, *77*, 355, 1961.

Johnson, E. K. and James, A.: Suppurative Typhoid Spine Perforating into the Bronchus, Am. J. Surg., *68*, 103, 1945.

Kulowski, J.: Pyogenic Osteomyelitis of Spine, J. Bone & Joint Surg., *18*, 343, 1936.

Lame, E. L.: Vertebral Osteomyelitis Following Operation on the Urinary Tract or Sigmoid, Am. J. Roentgenol., *75*, 938, 1956.

Leach, R. E., Goldstein, H. and Younger, D.: Osteomyelitis of the Odontoid Process, J. Bone & Joint Surg., *49-A*, 369, 1967.

Leigh, T. F., Kelly, R. P. and Weens, H. S.: Spinal Osteomyelitis Associated with Urinary Tract Infection, Radiology, *65*, 334, 1955.

Liming, R. W. and Youngs, F. J.: Metastatic Vertebral Osteomyelitis Following Prostatic Surgery, Radiology, *67*, 92, 1956.

Martin, P.: Pyogenic Osteomyelitis of Spine, Brit. Med. J., *2*, 688, 1946.

Pease, C. N.: Injuries to Vertebrae and Intervertebral Disks Following Lumbar Puncture, Am. J. Dis. Child., *49*, 849, 1935.

Pritchard, A. E. and Thomson, W. A. L.: Acute Pyogenic Infections of the Spine in Children, J. Bone & Joint Surg., *42-B*, 86, 1960.

Schein, A. J.: Bacillus Pyocyaneus Osteomyelitis of Spine, Arch. Surg., *41*, 740, 1940.

Selig, S.: Bacillus Proteus Osteomyelitis of Spine, J. Bone & Joint Surg., *16*, 189, 1934.

Shehadi, W. H.: Primary Pyogenic Osteomyelitis of Articular Process of Vertebrae, J. Bone & Joint Surg., *21*, 969, 1939.

Sherman, M. and Schneider, G. T.: Vertebral Osteomyelitis Complicating Postabortal and Postpartum Infection, Southern M. J., *48*, 338, 1955.

Smith, D. AeF.: Benign Form of Osteomyelitis of Spine, J.A.M.A., *101*, 335, 1933.

Solomon, H. A. and Bachman, A. L.: Pyogenic Osteomyelitis of Thoracic Spine Presenting as Primary Pulmonary Disease, Am. J. Roentgenol., *49*, 219, 1943.

Stenstrom, R.: Spondylitis Caused by Salmonella Typhimurium, Acta radiol., *49*, 355, 1958.

Stern, W. E. and Balch, R. E.: Surgical Aspects of Nonspecific Inflammatory and Suppurative Disease of the Vertebral Column, Am. J. Surg., *112*, 314, 1966.

Stern, W. E. and Crandall, P. H.: Inflammatory Intervertebral Disc Disease as a Complication of the Operative Treatment of Lumbar Herniations, J. Neurosurg., *16*, 261, 1959.

Stone, D. B. and Bonfiglio, M.: Pyogenic Vertebral Osteomyelitis, Arch. Int. Med., *112*, 491, 1963.

Sullivan, C. R., Bickel, W. H. and Svien, H. J.: Infections of Vertebral Interspaces after Operations on Intervertebral Disks, J.A.M.A., *166*, 1973, 1958.

Wear, J. E., Baylin, G. J. and Martin, T. L.: Pyogenic Osteomyelitis of Spine, Am. J. Roentgenol., *67*, 90, 1952.

Wiley, A. M. and Trueta, J.: The Vascular Anatomy of the Spine and its Relationship to Pyogenic Osteomyelitis, J. Bone & Joint Surg., *41-B*, 796, 1959.

Typhoid Osteomyelitis

Typhoid osteomyelitis may develop long after the infection supposedly has been cured. Spota and Bardeci (1950) reported a 44-year-old woman with osteomyelitis of the upper dorsal spine 20 years after typhoid infection. The neural arch was involved to a greater extent than the body, and paraplegia developed because of subarachnoid block due to extradural pressure from a typhoid abscess. Steingraber (1947) mentioned that typhoid spondylitis may appear during the convalescent period, approximately 4 weeks after the disappearance of symptoms. It has been shown that patients with sickle cell anemia are prone to develop bone infarcts which subsequently become infected with salmonella organisms. Similarly, patients with salmonella bone or joint infections are often found to have sickle cell anemia of the SS type (Walker, 1963).

The basic pathologic change is bone destruction caused by infected embolic infarcts. The intervertebral disc is secondarily affected by rupture of the focus through the cartilage, much the same as in pyogenic osteomyelitis (Keith and Keith, 1926). Healing with osteosclerosis and bone bridging may take more than a year to complete.

References

Keith, D. Y. and Keith, J. P.: Typhoid Osteitis and Periostitis, J.A.M.A., *87*, 2145, 1926.
Miller, G. A. H., Ridley, M. and Medd, W. E.: Typhoid Osteomyelitis of the Spine. Brit. Med. J., *1*, 1068, 1963.
Spota, B. B. and Bardeci, C. A.: Espondilitis Tifica con Compresion Medular Dorsal, Prensa med. argent., *37*, 3035, 1950.
Steingraber, M.: Über Spondylitis Typhosa, Zentralbl. f. Chirurg., *72*, 762, 1947.
Walker, G. F.: Typhoid Spine in a Nigerian with Sickle Haemoglobin, J. Bone & Joint Surg., *45-B*, 683, 1963.

Brucella Spondylitis

Involvement of the spine with undulant fever is frequent, occurring in from 10 to 65 per cent of patients. Males are affected more frequently. The disease affects the vertebral bodies, the neural arches, and extends into the intervertebral discs and the adjacent ligaments. Further progression into the spinal canal, with involvement of the meninges and the adjacent nerve roots takes place. Bony changes involve multiple and sometimes separated vertebrae (Purriel,

Risso and Espasandin, 1943). Di Rienzo (1943, 1950) reported that an early sign was lack of definition of the bone structures, with some attempt at bone regeneration which appears in the more chronic forms, and sometimes is quite marked. Extensive bony overgrowth may be concomitant with newly formed destructive areas. In young people the destruction of the vertebral bodies and the intervertebral discs may be extensive. At the end stages of the disease the appearance is that of a chronic destructive spondylitis. Calcification of the anterior spinal ligament is fairly common, that of the posterior spinal ligament is rare.

Aguilar and Elvidge (1961) called attention to the early appearance of a step-like erosion in the margin of the vertebral body opposing an involved disc. Thinning of the disc and faint osteophytic bridging appear soon thereafter, followed by areas of rarefaction of the corners and the vertebral bodies. Conspicuous hypertrophic bridging may then appear, simulating hypertrophic spondylosis, with heavy beaks of bone bridging the borders of the interspaces involved, indistinguishable in chronic cases from degenerative spondylosis. They point out that brucellar spondylitis is usually limited to one level, more often in the lumbar region than in the thoracic or cervical levels.

Zammit (1958) observed cord compression in 8 of 62 cases. This occurred with bone involvement as a rule, but there was one instance where there were no signs of bone change but myelography revealed a block at the level of the third lumbar vertebra due to an epidural abscess. Zammit found that the fourth lumbar vertebra was the one most commonly involved. Of his 62 cases, 5 occurred in the cervical spine, 16 in the thoracic spine, combined thoracic and lumbar involvement was present in 4, and lumbar involvement was present in 7.

The diagnosis is best established by identification of the causative organism. The radiologic changes are not necessarily characteristic, and difficulty in diagnosis between brucellar spondylitis and other infectious diseases such as tuberculosis, osteomyelitis, granulomatous conditions such as actinomycosis, coccidiomycosis, or hydatid disease are best resolved clinically. Little trouble should be encountered in identifying osteomyelitic disease from such conditions as Scheuermann's disease and hypertrophic spondylosis.

References

Aguilar, J. A. and Elvidge, A. R.: Intervertebra Disc Disease Caused by Brucella Organism, J. Neurosurg., *18*, 27, 1961.
Bishop, W. A., Jr.: Vertebral Lesions in Undulant Fever, J. Bone & Joint Surg., *21*, 665, 1939.
Di Rienzo, S.: La Espondilitis Brucelosica, Radiologia, *6*, 171, 1943.
————: Brucellar Spondylitis, Rev. argent. noteam, cien. med., *1*, 737, 1944.
————: Die brucellos Spondylitis, Fortschr. Röentgenstrah., *73*, 333, 1950.
Kelly, P. J., Martin, W. J., Schinger, A. and Weed, L. A.: Brucellosis of Bones and Joints, J.A.M.A., *174*, 347, 1960.
Purriel, P., Risso, R. and Espasandin, J.: Localizacion de la Brucelosis en la Columna Vertebra, Radiologia, *6*, 243, 1943.
Spink, W. W.: Pathogenesis of Human Brucellosis, Ann. Int. Med., *29*, 238, 1948.
Zammit, F.: Undulant Fever Spondylitis, Brit. J. Radiol., *31*, 683, 1958.

Syphilis of the Spine

Congenital syphilis follows infection of the fetus through the placental circulation. Destructive changes take place, particularly in the growing ends of the extremities, with granulation tissue replacing bone. Periosteal elevation, osteoporosis and nonspecific band-like zones of radiolucency appear. Osseous changes in the vertebrae with congenital syphilis are rare. McLean (1931) reported zones of increased and diminished density in the superior and inferior aspects of involved vertebrae, with no visible bone destruction. He considered these to correspond with the transverse bands present in the long bones. Péhu and Boucomont (1933) reported a 15-month-old infant with syphilitic spondylitis involving the twelfth thoracic and first and second lumbar vertebrae. A gibbus was present, but no paravertebral swelling was seen. Tissue removed from this region was described as being consistent with but not pathognomonic of syphilitic spondylitis.

Vertebral syphilis in later life follows periosteal and osseous spirochetal invasion, producing osteoperiostitis of the involved vertebrae, with granulomatous extension into the adjacent soft tissues. Occlusion of blood vessels by syphilitic arteritis causes bone destruction. The irregular foci of destruction and reconstruction of bone are usually more marked in the anterior portions of the involved vertebrae. The intervertebral discs are quite resistant, but with extensive involvement become narrowed or almost completely destroyed.

The cervical vertebrae are involved most often with syphilitic spondylitis. Three such cases were reported by Sgalitzer (1941), with intense pain and destructive lesions involving particularly the ventral aspects of the involved bodies. The thoracic spine is not affected as often as either the cervical or the lumbar vertebrae.

The radiologic appearance of syphilis of the spinal column varies greatly. When only a single vertebra is involved, the diagnosis may be difficult, the only evidence being a destructive process in the anterior aspect of the vertebral body. When reparative changes take place, the presence of overgrowth of bone into the paravertebral soft tissues offers some help. With more extensive involvement the concomitant destruction and production of bone and the overflow of reparative bone into the adjacent soft tissues is more easily recognized. The intervertebral spaces may be visible even though extensive destruction occurs adjacent to them, while close by irregular deposits of ossification are prominent. Bridging between the involved vertebrae may be quite extensive, and the calcification may involve the paraspinal ligaments (Fig. 246).

In our experience are 5 cases of syphilitic spondylitis in adults. Two had extensive destruction of the midcervical vertebrae, with marked distortion of the vertebral

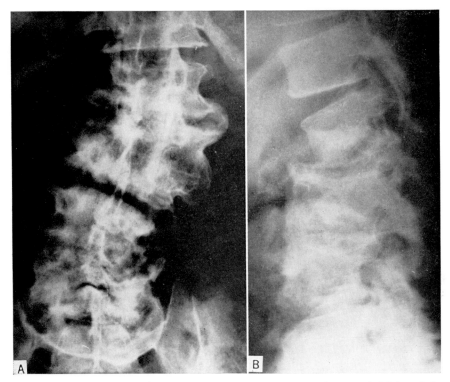

FIG. 246. Syphilitic osteitis with heavy bony repair, large osteophytes and shifting of the vertebral bodies.

bodies and destroyed intervertebral discs. In both the cervical spine remained almost vertical in alignment, probably because healing after treatment had rendered the midcervical spine a practically solid, irregular column of bone. The other cases involved the second, third and fourth lumbar vertebrae. The involved bodies were dense and sclerotic. The intervertebral spaces were narrowed and irregular, but still could be identified. Heavy solid perivertebral calcification with large spurs was present.

The occurrence of gummas within the spinal canal is rare. Such a case was reported by Ray (1940) in a 41-year-old male who presented a clinical syndrome consistent with the diagnosis of a tumor of the cauda equina. At operation the nerve roots were slightly swollen and loosely stuck together by what appeared to be a low-grade inflammatory process. A yellowish-white tumor mass about 2 cm in its widest diameter was enountered. The tumor appeared to rise in one of the main roots on the left side, and was slightly adherent to the dura. Because of the general inflammatory appearance of the region, a syphiloma or tuberculoma was suspected. The diagnosis of syphilis was confirmed by biopsy. The patient did well on anti-syphilitic treatment.

References

Abernethy, C.: Syphilitic Spondylitis, Brit. Med. J., *1*, 1112, 1931.

Freedman, E. and Meschan, I.: Syphilitic Spondylitis, Am. J. Roentgenol., *49*, 756, 1943.

Gill, A. W. and Frazier, A. D.: Syphilitic Spondylitis, Brit. Med. J., *2*, 606, 1933.

McLean, S., III: Correlation of the Roentgenologic Picture with the Gross and Microscopic Examination of Pathologic Material in Congenital Osseous Syphilis, Am. J. Dis. Child., *41*, 607, 1931.

Péhu, M. and Boucomont, J.: Mal de Pott Syphilitique, Rev. Franç. d. Pediat., *9*, 664, 1933.

Ray, B. S.: Gumma Simulating Tumor of Cauda Equina, J.A.M.A., *114*, 401, 1940.

Sgalitzer, M.: Vertebral Syphilis, Radiology, *37*, 75, 1941.

NEUROPATHIC JOINTS (Charcot's Arthropathy)

Included in this group are changes in the spine usually secondary to central nervous system syphilis, and appear rarely with diabetes, cauda equina tumors, spina bifida, traumatic paraplegia, transverse myelitis, and hematomyelia (Holland, 1952). The primary pathologic process is degeneration and partial disappearance of the articular cartilages, which are invaded by fibrous connective tissue from an inflammatory pannus. The zone of preliminary calcification becomes exposed by stripping away of the cartilage, beneath which further cartilage proliferates and becomes converted into subchondral bone. This accounts for the sclerotic eburnated bone seen at the base of large defects in the articular cartilages. A generalized atrophy of the trabeculae of cancellous bone is often seen. As a result of this combined degeneration of cartilage and proliferation of subchondral bone, osteophytes develop either as free bone fragments or as amorphous, dense, scattered conglomerates which appear to grow in a purposeless fashion. Such bony proliferation in the spine occurs first in the regions of the articular margins, resembling hypertrophic spondylosis. Associated with this are areas of degeneration of bone resulting in radiolucent foci within malformed vertebral bodies. The appearance of bone atrophy and degeneration, together with the extensive deposition of proliferating bone both adjacent to the vertebral column and some distance from it is fairly characteristic of the Charcot joint. These changes are accompanied by calcification in the adjacent soft tissues.

The usual site is the lumbar spine. Occasionally the thoracic vertebrae or a single vertebra is involved. The differential diagnosis between neuropathic osteoarthropathy and syphilitic osteoperiostitis of the spine on purely radiologic grounds may be difficult. The more frequent involvement of the cervical spine with syphilitic spondylitis, and the purposeless diffuse proliferation of bony growth into the soft tissues seen with Charcot's disease is of some help. Incidentally, the blood and cerebrospinal fluid specific serological reactions may be normal in about half the cases.

The cause for neuropathic disturbances in the joints is commonly ascribed to trauma, combined with analgesia and consequent loss of warning pain. In an analysis of 134 cases, with a total of 214 Charcot joints, Steindler, Williams and Puig-Guri (1942) noted that in only 57 was there a definite picture of tabes. Delano (1946) noted that the explanation of all neuropathic arthropathies was ascribed to a common origin of trophic disturbance. He regarded this as inadequate to explain the lavish and purposeless production of new bone around the involved joints, which to him suggested that a profound disturbance of regional nutrition was taking place. He describes a patient paralyzed from the waist down for 15 years following a fracture of the first lumbar vertebra. Radiographic examination showed extensive irregular bony overgrowth and osteosclerosis, consistent with joint neuropathy.

The occurrence of other neuropathic joints in association with Charcot's diseaes of the spine is well known. Goodman (1949) described such a case in a 64-year-old white male with tabetic neurosyphilis in which the elbows, knees and hands were involved as well as the lumbar spine. Neuropathic joints associated with syringomyelia are reported most often in the arms, but sometimes involve the legs (Skall-Jensen, 1952). Involvement of the spine, if it occurs at all, is most unusual. Congenital indifference to pain is associated with neuropathic joints, but no instances of vertebral involvement have been reported (Murray, 1957; Siegelmann, Heimann and Manin, 1966).

The association of diabetes with neuropathic joints has come into prominence. Knuttson (1951) reported 4 cases involving the joints of the legs and feet, but no involvement of the spine was mentioned. Four additional cases with osseous destruction of the feet were reported by Beidelman and

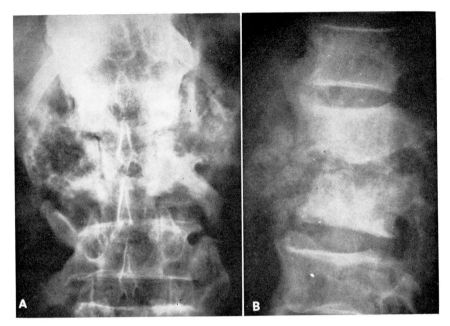

FIG. 247. Charcot's disease of the upper lumbar vertebrae, with prominent bone destruction, large amorphous calcific deposits adjacent to the involved first lumbar interspace.

Duncan (1952). No spinal involvement was noted by these authors. Zucker and Marder (1952) presented a case of Charcot spine due to diabetic neuropathy in a patient with severe pseudotabes. They believed this to be the first case of Charcot spine reported as a result of diabetic neuropathy. Extensive destruction and disorganization of the second, third and fourth lumbar vertebrae were present, together with considerable bone production within the area of the destroyed vertebrae.

We observed a male patient 45 years old with Charcot's disease of the spine (Fig. 247) who presented dissolution of the superior half of the body of the second lumbar vertebra, so that the intervertebral space between the first and second lumbar vertebrae appeared widened. Large, heavy, dense bony bridges between the vertebrae apparently were strong enough to keep them apart. Large amorphous calcific deposits were spread in the adjacent soft tissues for more than 3.5 cm on both sides and anteriorly. The anterior aspect of the first lumbar vertebra inferiorly and the second lumbar verte-bra superiorly were partially destroyed, and a slight gibbus formation was present. This patient suddenly became paraplegic, and myelography revealed a block at the level of the first lumbar vertebra. At operation this was found to be due to compression of the spinal canal by granulomatous tissue from the involved bony walls.

References

Beetham, W. P., Jr., Kaye, R. L. and Polley, H. F.: Charcot's Joints, Ann. Int. Med., 58, 1002, 1963.
Beidelman, B. and Duncan, G. G.: Charcot Joints and Infectious-Vascular Lesions of Bones in Diabetes Mellitus, Am. J. Med., 12, 43, 1952.
Delano, P. J.: Pathogenesis of Charcot's Joint, Am. J. Roentgenol., 56, 189, 1946.
Goodman, R. D.: Multiple Charcot Joints, Am. J. Roentgenol., 62, 531, 1949.
Hodges, P. C., Phemister, D. B. and Brunschwig, A.: Charcot's Neuropathic Lesion of the Spine, New York, Thomas Nelson & Sons, 1941.
Holland, H. W.: Charcot's Arthropathy of Spine, Brit. J. Radiol., 25, 267, 1952.
Katz, I., Rabinowitz, J. G. and Dziadiw, R.: Early Changes in Charcot's Disease, Am. J. Roentgenol., 86, 965, 1961.
Knuttson, F.: Diabetic Arthropathy, Acta radiol., 36, 114, 1951.
Murray, R. O.: Congenital Indifference to Pain, Brit. J. Radiol., 30, 2, 1957.

Siegelman, S. S., Heimann, W. G. and Manin, M. C.:
    Congenital Indifference to Pain, Am. J. Roent-
    genol., *97*, 242, 1966.
Skall-Jensen, J.: Osteoarthropathy in Syringomy-
    elia, Acta radiol., *38*, 382, 1952.
Thomas, D. F.: Vertebral Osteoarthropathy or
    Charcot's Disease of the Spine, J. Bone & Joint
    Surg., *34-B*, 248, 1952.
Zucker, G. and Marder, M. J.: Charcot Spine Due
    to Diabetic Neuropathy, Am. J. Med., *12*, 118,
    1952.

Fungus, Protozoan and Parasitic Infestations

Actinomycosis follows infection with fungi of the actinomyces group, the most frequent being actinomyces bovis. Other members of the genus may also be pathogenic, and the clinical manifestations are identical. The portal of entry is usually the mouth, the organisms resting in carious teeth, pyorrhetic gums or the tonsils. They assume pathogenicity upon entrance into the subcutaneous tissues after local trauma or other disease processes. The characteristic granulomatous lesions produce local swellings in the jaws, the so-called "lumpy jaw." Abscess formation is accompanied later by sinus tracts discharging to the skin, and from this pus may be cultured the causative fungus, or the characteristic sulfur granules may be identified as yellowish-gray granular masses.

Actinomycosis can then spread to other regions, particularly the chest and the gastrointestinal tract. Vertebral involvement may follow extension of the granulomas to the paravertebral soft tissues. Less often infected emboli rest in the medulla of a vertebra and set up an intraosseous granuloma. When the outside tissues are infected, extension to the periosteum and the cortex results in destruction of bone. A reparative effort is mainfested by the appearance of bone sclerosis which may be quite intense at the margins of the infected bone (Fig. 248).

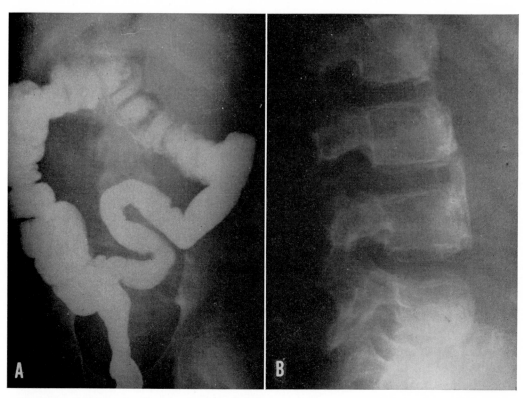

FIG. 248. *A*, Perirectal actinomycosis with tubulation and straightening of the distal colon and depression of the splenic flexure by an enlarged spleen. The spine, *B*, presents a heavy bone bridge connecting the anterior aspects of L3 and 4. Erosive changes are present at the anterior margin of L2. Diagnosis of actinomycosis of the bowel and spine confirmed at necropsy. (Courtesy of P. Steinhorn, M.D., New Hyde Park, N. Y.)

With extension of the disease numerous channel-like areas of destruction permeate the vertebra producing an appearance variously described as "soap-bubble," "honeycomb" or "lattice-like." This may involve all or any part of the vertebra including the spinous and transverse processes. Infection extends to the adjacent ribs, visceral cavities or the skin with multiple sinus tracts. As a rule, multiple vertebrae are diseased, but it is not uncommon in this relatively rare condition to observe involvement of a single vertebra, usually depending on the point of origin of the infection. The intervertebral discs as a rule are spared, and collapse of involved vertebrae even when extensively diseased is uncommon, although occasional instances of angular deformities are known (Lubert, 1944).

The symptoms of vertebral actinomycosis are inconstant and varied. Pain, tenderness, limitation of motion and nerve root pain are all dependent on the location of the disease and its spread to adjacent soft tissues. Prior to the advent of chemotherapeutic and antibiotic agents the prognosis was poor, but this has now changed for the better (Brett, 1951; Cope, 1951).

Involvement of the spinal canal with actinomycosis is rare. A case with meningeal involvement and compression of the spinal cord was reported by Lamartine de Assis and Mignone (1946) in a 52-year-old male with cutaneous and thoracic spine lesions. Necropsy disclosed purulent exudate in the tissues around the spinal column, and there was extensive thickening of the dura with spots of inflammatory exudate. The cord was intact.

Blastomycosis (American blastomycosis; Gilchrist's disease) is caused by infection with the fungus Blastomyces dermatitidis. The portal of entry is the skin, upon which small papulo-pustules form. These gradually enlarge, become crusted over and form irregular, patchy papillomatous tumors which expand peripherally and heal centrally with a flat scar. This local form of blastomycosis is relatively benign. When systemic dissemination occurs, there may be involvement of the lungs, the internal organs and the bones. Occasionally the primary focus is in the lungs, and the lesion can be mistaken for tuberculosis or bronchogenic carcinoma.

Meyer and Gall (1935) mentioned 12 cases of blastomycosis of the spinal column in a review of mycotic diseases of the spine. In a review of 63 cases collected from the literature by Jones and Martin (1941), 25 instances of vertebral involvement were noted, and paravertebral abscesses were observed in 14. Colonna and Gucker (1944) observed that the bony manifestations of blastomycosis suggested an ordinary osteomyelitis and presented no characteristic features. Baylin and Wear (1953) indicated that spinal blastomycosis might simulate tuberculosis.

Involvement of the spinal canal is rare. Craig, Dockerty and Harrington (1940) reported a case of an intravertebral and intrathoracic blastomycoma which simulated a dumbbell tumor. Another case with spinal cord involvement was reported by Greenwood and Voris (1950), with erosion of the pedicles of the sixth and seventh dorsal vertebrae and foci of destruction in the body of the eighth dorsal vertebra.

Coccidiomycosis ("valley fever") is caused by infection with the fungus Oidium coccidioides (Coccidioides immitis). The portal of entry in most cases is the pulmonary tract, and the initial lesions resemble tuberculosis, with a clinical picture resembling an upper respiratory infection. Recovery from the primary infection usually takes place within a few weeks, leaving the patient hypersensitive to the organism. Re-infection endogenously or through the skin may introduce the secondary or granulomatous phase, and the disease enters a prolonged period of exacerbation and remission during which time metastatic involvement of the skeleton as well as the visceral organs may occur. The disease appears more often in males, and only a small proportion of infected patients develop the granulomatous phase. According to Benninghoven and Miller (1942) the lesion may exist in the spine as a single central focus, but most often multiple marginal vertebral changes take place because of extension to the bone from paravertebral abscesses. Miller and Birsner (1949) stated that in their series of 17 cases there was no bone involvement caused by extension from soft tissue abscesses or granulomas. The spine was involved in 6, and most frequently the lumbar vertebrae were involved. The lesion was predominantly lytic, with no involvement of the intervertebral discs. Some sclerosis was present, and they noted calcification in the paravertebral soft tissues. Denenholtz and Cheney (1944) reported that in a case observed by them $8\frac{1}{2}$ months after the onset of the disease there was destruction of the intervertebral disc between the tenth and eleventh thoracic vertebrae as well as osseous erosion. They suggested that differential diagnosis from tuberculosis might be quite difficult.

Adhesive meningitis incident to coccidiomycosis was reviewed by Newton and Cohen (1963). This was most frequent in the basal meninges, leading to obstructive hydrocephalus. However, involvement of the spinal meninges also occurred, and in 2 cases produced extensive distortion and block of the Pantopaque column. This might be confused with adhesive arachnoiditis from other causes, and had to be differentiated from other lesions such as vascular malformations, extensive ependymomas or other diffuse neoplasms. A case of quadriplegia caused by involvement of the cervical spine with coccidioides immitis was reported by Jackson, Kent and Clare (1964). In this 22-year-old-male patient there was complete destruction of the body of the fifth cervical vertebra, and involvement of the posterior portion of the body of the sixth, with a fracture through the pedicle of C6.

Torulosis (Cryptococcosis; European blastomycosis) is a fungus infection due to the Torula histolytica (Cryptococcus hominis). The portal of entry is believed to be the upper respiratory tract, from which there follow disseminated discrete lesions. In a summary of 10 cases from the literature, including 1 of their own, Carton and Mount (1951) reported a case in which a cauda equina tumor was simulated. Spinal tap disclosed cloudy fluid, with a total protein of 4200 mg per cent. The plain spine roentgenograms were normal. Laminectomy revealed a solid, firm, tenacious gray-white mass occupying the spinal canal from the upper portion of the first lumbar vertebra to the upper portion of the fourth lumbar vertebra. The arachnoid was thickened. When this was opened, 2 to 3 ml of purulent fluid exuded, from which the Cryptococcus neoformans was recovered. Ley, Jacas and Oliveras (1951) recorded a case of torula granuloma of the cervical spinal cord in which the plain films showed widening of the spinal canal and erosion of the pedicles. This occurred in an 8-year-old child with quadriparesis. The true nature of the disease was not known until histologic study showed the characteristic torula organisms. The lesion seen at operation was an extensive granuloma simulating a spinal cord tumor.

Bone involvement in cryptococcosis was discussed by Collins (1950) who mentioned that in over 200 reported cases 17 examples of bone involvement were encountered. In his first case a destructive lesion was present in the upper three lumbar vertebrae, with cortical erosion and no osteoblastic reaction in the soft tissues. Abscess formation in the adjacent lumbar musculature was noted. In his second case, abscesses were present in the cervical, lumbar and sacral regions with areas of bone destruction in the pedicle of of the fourth lumbar vertebra. A cryptococcic granuloma of the thoracic spinal cord was reported by Skultety (1961) in a 60-year-old male patient. The lesion was intramedullary, and there was involvement of the cord and its membranes by the granulomatous mass. At the first examination myelography was considered normal, but a review disclosed some stringy deformity of the Pantopaque column at the level of the sixth thoracic vertebra which raised the question as to a vascular anomaly. Skultety noted that only 8 cases of actual involvement of the cord or cauda equina with a granulomatous mass lesion of cryptococcic origin had been found, but that other examples of cryptococcic meningitis with perivascular infiltration or myelitis have been observed.

It is not possible to distinguish one fungus infection from another radiologically.

Toxoplasmosis

This is a disease caused by toxoplasma, a protozoan organism of uncertain status, usually classed with the sporozoa. This protozoan may infect many tissues, the central nervous system being often involved. It was first described as causing encephalomyelitis in infants, giving rise to a syndrome of hydrocephalus accompanied by convulsive seizures, enlargement of the head and increased intracranial pressure. Radiographic examination of the skull often shows calcifications in the cerebral hemispheres. Dyke, Wolf, Cowen, Paige and Caffey (1942) mentioned that in the vertebral column the provisional zones of calcification in the superior and inferior margins of the vertebral bodies were exaggerated into heavy white borders. Internal to the heavy white lines were parallel linear zones of decreased density similar to the deep transverse zones of the ends of the shafts of the long bones. These authors considered the lesions as probably not specific for toxoplasmosis since they had been observed in several other infectious and nutritional disturbances.

References

Baylin, A. J. and Wear, J. M.: Blastomycosis and Actinomycosis of the Spine, Am. J. Roentgenol., 69, 395, 1953.

Benninghoven, C. D. and Miller, E. R.: Coccidioidal Infection of Bone, Radiology, 38, 663, 1942.

Brett, M. S.: Advanced Actinomycosis of the Spine Treated with Penicillin and Streptomycin, J. Bone & Joint Surg., 33-B, 205, 1951.

Carton, C. A. and Mount, L. A.: Neurosurgical Aspects of Cryptococcosis, J. Neurosurg., 8, 143, 1951.

Collins, V. P.: Bone Involvement with Cryptococcosis (Torulosis), Am. J. Roentgenol., 63, 102, 1950.

Colonna, P. C. and Gucker, T., 3rd.: Blastomycosis of Skeletal System, J. Bone & Joint Surg., 26, 322, 1944.

Conaty, J. P., Biddle, M. and McKeever, F. M.: Osseous Coccidioidal Granuloma, J. Bone & Joint Surg., 41-A, 1109, 1959.

Cope, V. Z.: Actinomycosis of Bone, J. Bone & Joint Surg., 33-B, 215, 1951.

Craig, W. McK., Dockerty, M. B. and Harrington, S. W.: Intravertebral and Intrathoracic Blastomycoma Simulating a Dumbbell Tumor, South. Surg., 9, 750, 1940.

Denenholz, E. J. and Chency, G.: Chronic Coccidiomycosis, Arch. Int. Med., 74, 311, 1944.

Dyke, C. G., Wolf, A., Cowen, D., Paige, B. H. and Caffey, J.: Toxoplasmic Encephalomyelitis, Am. J. Roentgenol., 47, 830, 1942.

Gosling, H. R. and Gilmer, W. S.: Skeletal Cryptococcosis (Torulosis), J. Bone & Joint Surg., 38-A, 660, 1956.

Greenwood, R. C. and Voris, H. C.: Systemic Blastomycosis with Spinal Cord Involvement, J. Neurosurg., 7, 450, 1950.

Jackson, F. E., Kent, D. and Clare, F.: Quadriplegia Caused by Involvement of Cervical Spine with Coccidioides Immitis, J. Neurosurg., 21, 512, 1964.

Jones, R. R. Jr. and Martin, D. S.: Blastomycosis of Bone, Surgery, 10, 931, 1941.

LaMartine de Assis and Mignone: Actinomycosis of the Thoracic Vertebrae with Pachymeningitis and Compression of the Cord, Arq. di Neuropsychiat., 4, 21, 1946.

Ley, A., Jacas, R. and Oliveras, C.: Torula Granuloma of Cervical Spinal Cord, J. Neurosurg., 8, 327, 1951.

Lubert, M.: Actinomycosis of the Vertebrae, Am. J. Roentgenol., 51, 669, 1944.

Mazet, R., Jr.: Skeletal Lesions in Coccidioidomycosis, Arch. Surg., 70, 497, 1955.

Meyer, M. and Gall. M. B.: Mycosis of Vertebral Column, J. Bone & Joint Surg., 17, 857, 1935.

Miller, D. and Birsner, J. W.: Coccidioidal Granuloma of Bone, Am. J. Roentgenol., 62, 229, 1949.

Neuhauser, E. B. D. and Tucker, A.: Roentgen Changes Produced by Diffuse Torulosis in Newborn, Am. J. Roentgenol., 59, 805, 1948.

Newton, T. H. and Cohen, N. H.: Coccidioidal Meningitis, Acta radiol., 1, 886, 1963.

Skultety, F. M.: Cryptococcic Granuloma of the Dorsal Spinal Cord, Neurology, 11, 1066, 1961.

Toone, E. C., Jr. and Kelly, J.: Joint and Bone Disease Due to Mycotic Infection, Am J. Med. Sci., 231, 263, 1956.

Young, W. B.: Actinomycosis with Involvement of the Vertebral Column, Clinical Radiol., 11, 175, 1960.

Parasitic Infestations of the Spine

Echinococcosis (Hydatid disease) results from ingestion of the ova of echinococcus granulosus. Infestation is usually incurred during childhood from contact with dogs or cats. Unless there is involvement of the brain or the orbit, symptoms do not develop until later in life when the slowly growing tumors make themselves apparent. Involvement of the spine with hydatid disease has been described by many authors. Bellini (1946) reported that bone involvement occurred in approximately 1 per cent of cases. The six-hooked embryo reaches the bone by way of the arterial circulation, and establishes itself in highly vascularized areas such as the epiphyseal ends of long bones or the spongy bone of the vertebral bodies. Vertebral hydatosis shows no tendency to formation of cyst-like spaces, and for that reason the height of the vertebrae usually is not changed and the intervertebral cartilages remain undisturbed. Often calcification or replacement of the lamina by newly formed bone takes place. The contiguous ribs may be involved. Viterbo (1948) reported the occurrence of a large osteolytic bone defect in the right half of the body of the first lumbar vertebra, with no evidence of deformity or gibbus formation and normal intervertebral discs in a 32-year-old woman. Following immobilization, repair occurred, and re-examination showed in addition a paravertebral mass containing calcification and sclerosis.

Schlanger and Schlanger (1948) mentioned that echinococcosis infestation of the spine is relatively frequent. Although the x-ray signs are insignificant at the beginning of the disease, clinically it may produce alarming symptoms originated by extention and infiltration of the meninges by the cysts. Spinal blocks may occur early in the disease and are demonstrated by myelographic examination. They mentioned that the initial stage may present a partially destructive area in a transverse process far below the area of myelographic block, together with small clear bubble-like areas of radiolucency of the adjacent vertebral bodies. If the disease continues, destruction increases and the bubble-like character of the bone lesion disappears, being replaced by a destructive process.

Spontaneous or operative fistulas appear and obscure the bone picture. A widening of the interpedicular spaces in a case of hydatid disease of the twelfth thoracic vertebra was described by Oosthuizen and Fainsinger (1949). In their case myelography disclosed a local block. They noted a hollowing out of the posterior surface of the involved vertebral body and observed that the findings could not be distinguished from those produced by any other expanding lesion in a similar situation.

In 4 of the 5 cases reported by Woodland (1949) there were symptoms of spinal cord pressure. The original site of the hydatid infection was the upper lumbar spine in 3 and the midthoracic spine in 2. No pathognomonic radiographic signs could be observed, but Woodland (1949) suggested that the absence of periosteal reaction, minimal vertebral collapse and intervertebral disc narrowing, slight sclerotic reaction with areas of destruction and involvement of contiguous ribs might be of some diagnostic aid. Rocca, Frano and Alayza (1950) reported a case of primary echinococcosis of the body of the sixth thoracic vertebra with cord compression and recovery after operation.

The differential diagnosis of hydatid disease of the spine, particularly in the presence of central nervous system derangements, is difficult. Included in consideration must be tuberculosis, malignant disease, neurofibroma, hemangioma and large perineurial sacral cysts. Myelography is important in determining the extent of encroachment into the spinal canal, and surgical relief may become necessary.

Schistosomiasis (Bilharziasis) is caused by any of three blook flukes. These produce vesical or urinary symptoms (Schistosoma hematobium), or intestinal manifestations (Mansoni or Japonicum). The disease is due to contact with water contaminated with cercariae discharged by infested snails. The primary infection occurs through the skin with distribution by way of the blood. Infection of the vertebral column by this disease is rare, but a case was mentioned by

Gama and Marques de Sa (1945) in a 42-year-old male who had pain in the back and paraplegia. A myelographic examination showed partial block at the level of the sixth dorsal vertebra and complete block at the level of the twelfth dorsal vertebra. At operation an intramedullary granuloma containing eggs of Schistosoma mansoni was found. Schistosomiasis also produces a granulomatous tumor, myelitis or cauda equina radiculitis. The absence of evidence of urinary or bowel schistosomiasis and a normal myelogram does not necessarily exclude the lesion (Bird, 1964).

Cysticercosis follows ingestion of raw or partially cooked pork infected with Cysticercus cellulosa. Infection also occurs through ingestion of contaminated water or food, particularly uncooked vegetables. The clinical aspects and diagnosis of spinal cysticercosis was described by Bartschi-Rochaix and de la Cuadra (1946), who reported that the symptoms simulated intracranial or spinal disorders. A primary meningeal intracranial reaction was associated with a severe and widespread spinal arachnoiditis. The diagnosis of spinal arachnoiditis was made by the characteristic findings on spinal tap and myelography. Cysticercosis also manifests itself by single or multiple cyst-like masses in the spinal subarachnoid space, with a clinical picture of cord compression. Myelography reveals intradural extramedullary filling defects which are more or less spherical in shape. A positive cysticercosis reaction in the cerebrospinal fluid makes the diagnosis. These cysts also produce a complete block at times (Cabieses, Vallenas and Landa, 1959; Santin and Vargas, 1966).

References

Bärtshci-Rochaix, W. and de la Cuadra, J.: Spinal Cysticercosis, Helvetica medica acta, *13*, 192, 1946.
Bellini, M. A.: Osteohydatidosis, Radiology, *47*, 569, 1946.
Bird, A. V.: Acute Spinal Schistosomiasis, Neurology, *14*, 647, 1964.
Cabieses, F., Vallenas, M. and Landa, R.: Cysticercosis of the Spinal Cord. J. Neurosurg., *16*, 337, 1959.

Murray, R. O. and Haddad, F.: Hydatid Disease of the Spine, J. Bone & Joint Surg., *41-B*, 499, 1959.
Osthuizen, S. F. and Fainsinger, M. H.: Hydatid Disease, Radiology, *53*, 248, 1949.
Robinson, R. G.: Hydatid Disease of the Spine and its Neurological Complications, Brit. J. Surg., *47*, 301, 1959.
Rocca, E. D., Franco, J. and Alayza, F.: Hidatosis Vertebra, Rev. Neurospsyquiat., *13*, 643, 1950.
Santin, G. and Vargas, S.: Roentgen Study of Cysticercosis of Central Nervous System, Radiology, *86*, 520, 1966.
Schlanger, P. M. and Schlanger, H.: Hydatid Disease, Am. J. Roentgenol., *60*, 331, 1948.
Viterbo, F.: Contributo Radiologico alla Conoscenza della Disti da Echinocco Vertebrale, Radiol. med., *34*, 75, 1948.
Woodland, L. J.: Hydatid Disease of Vertebrae, M. J. Australia, *2*, 904, 1949.

"IVORY VERTEBRAE"

This condition is one in which a distinctive radiologic appearance may be associated with various etiologic factors, all quite different. The usual roentgenographic picture is a vertebra with a dense, white appearance in contrast to the normal or possibly osteoporotic appearance of the remainder of the vertebral column. Such changes have been associated with Hodgkin's disease, Paget's disease (Fig. 249), myelomas, osteosclerotic metastases, particularly from carcinomas of the prostate, and occasionally from the breast. Barsony and Schulhof (1930) believe the sclerotic changes might be a reaction to a low grade infectious process. We have recently had a 16-year-old male patient who had a classically dense, ivory vertebrae following a staphylococcic infection verified by culture of bone obtained at biopsy (Fig. 244).

References

Bársony, T. and Schulhof, O.: Der Elfenbeinwirbel, Fortschr. Röntgenstrah., *42*, 597, 1930.
Engels, E. P., Smith, R. C. and Kravitz, S.: Bone Sclerosis in Multiple Myeloma, Radiology, *75*, 242, 1960.
Golding, F. C.: The Radiological Diagnosis of the Reticuloses, Brit. J. Radiol., *24*, 478, 1951.
Húlten, O.: Ein Fall von "Elfenbeinwirbel" bei Lymphogranulomatose, Acta radiol., *8*, 245, 1927.
Ochsner, H. C. and Moser, R. H.: Ivory Vertebra, Am. J. Roentgenol., *29*, 635, 1938.

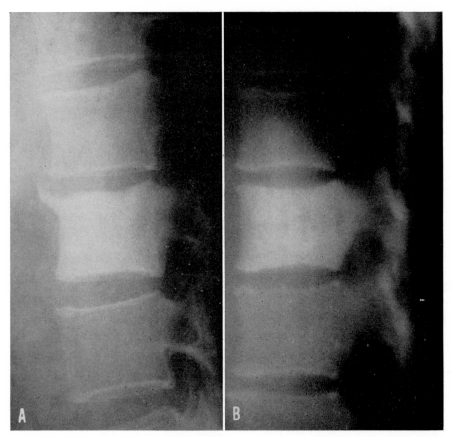

Fig. 249. *A*, Ivory vertebra due to Paget's disease. *B*, Ivory vertebra due to metastasis from carcinoma of the breast.

CALCIFIED MEDULLARY DEFECTS

These were described by Ferguson (1947) as solitary rounded areas made up of irregular nodules of amorphous calcification, in or near the metaphyseal regions of the long bones, frequently in the center of the medullary cavity. They are 1 to 2 cm in diameter, and as a rule, are solitary lesions which are sharply demarcated from the adjacent reticular bone. Ferguson believed that the lesion represented degenerated islands of cartilage which had become calcified. In a review of 6,000 roentgenograms, 120 calcified islands were found, most often in the femoral condyles, the iliac wings, the proximal portions of the tibia and head of the humerus. Their etiology is not established, but 27 per cent of the lesions were found in patients suffering

from blood vessel abnormalities. The possibility of bone infarction was strongly considered by him.

We have encountered 11 cases of sclerotic bone islands within the vertebral bodies. Two of these are illustrated here (Figs. 250 and 251). These irregular, slightly lobulated dense sclerotic foci measured up to 3.5 cm in their widest diameter. As a rule, they were sharply delimited from the adjacent cancellous bone, and did not distort the outlines of the vertebral body. The lesions were solitary and were encountered as incidental findings. They were not associated with any specific symptoms. Ackermann and Schwarz (1958) were able to demonstrate the benign sclerotic nature of this condition on biopsy material.

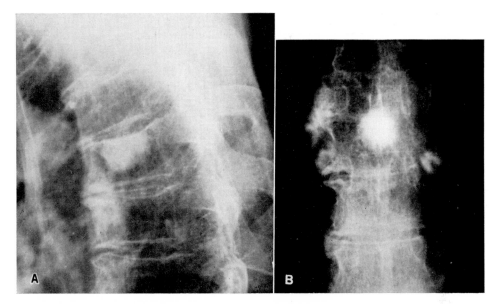

FIG. 250. Localized enostosis in the body of the seventh thoracic vertebra.
Incidental finding made during course of chest examination.

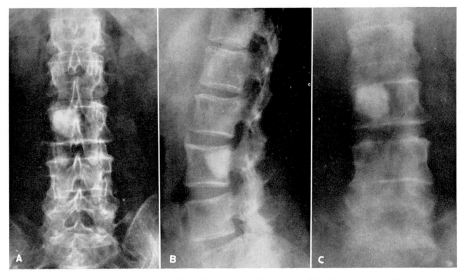

FIG. 251. Calcified medullary defect in body of the third lumbar vertebra.
Anteroposterior, lateral and anteroposterior body section roentgenograms.

References

Ackermann, W. and Schwarz, G. S.: Non-Neoplastic
Sclerosis in Vertebral Bodies, Cancer, *11*, 703, 1958.
Ferguson, G. H.: Roentgen Diagnosis of the Ex-
tremities and Spine. *Annals of Roentgenology*,
17, 2nd ed., New York, Paul B. Hoeber, Inc., 1949.
Steel, H. H.: Calcified Islands in Medullary Bone,
J. Bone & Joint Surg., *32-A*, 405, 1950.

CAISSON DISEASE

Caisson disease is due to an accumulation
of nitrogen gas in the blood vessels within
the bones, with resultant aseptic necrosis.
The common sites for involvement are the
heads of the femur or humerus. The

necrotic lesions may break down and be invaded by, or eventually replaced by, new bone or fibrous tissue. Medullary calcifications in the diaphyseal ends of the long bones and secondary hypertrophic arthritis appear as the disease proceeds to healing (Phemister, 1940). Rendich and Harrington (1940) encountered no spinal involvement in 4 cases. Coley and Moore (1940) suggested that the reason the vertebrae escape in this condition is the high proportion of red as compared to fatty marrow. They pointed out that the tissues with the poorest blood supply in relationship to nitrogen content are the bone marrow and the spinal cord. Those tissues with high nitrogen content are enclosed in bone, thus preventing free diffusion of nitrogen into contiguous tissues. This makes them dependent upon a comparatively poor blood supply for absorption and elimination. Consequently nitrogen elimination from these tissues is retarded when bubbles are present in the blood.

References

Coley, B. L. and Moore, M., Jr.: Caisson Disease, Ann. Surg., *111*, 1065, 1940.
McCallum, R. I., Walder, D. N., *et al.*: Bone Lesions in Compressed Air Workers, J. Bone & Joint Surg., *48-B*, 207, 1966.
Phemister, D. B.: Changes in Bones and Joints Resulting from Interruption of Circulation, Arch. Surg., *41*, 436, 1940.
Rendich, R. A. and Harrington, L. A.: Caisson Disease of Bone, Radiology, *35*, 439, 1940.

Osteitis Condensans Ilii

Although not a disease of the vertebral column, its close association with the sacroiliac region makes inclusion desirable. This benign, self-limited condition occurs mostly in females of the childbearing age, and may be associated with recurrent attacks of low-back pain. Roentgenographic examination reveals a condensation of bone in one or both iliac bones adjacent to the sacro-iliac joints. Gillespie and Lloyd-Roberts (1953) encountered this condition in 2.2 per cent of 760 lumbosacral spines, and noted sacral as well

as iliac bone involvement. In 1 case with histologic verification they found that the bone was harder than normal and bled less readily. The bone tissue showed no qualitative abnormality, but was gradually thickened by deposition of lamellar bone of normal structure. The ligaments and cartilage were normal. These writers postulate a vascular deficiency as a cause, with resultant sclerosis. Rendich and Shapiro (1936) reported 1 case in which a fusion of the sacro-iliac joint was done and a biopsy of the involved bone was obtained. This presented condensation of osseous tissue with obliteration of the evident former lacunae. There appeared to be no osteolytic or osteoplastic change in the bone.

References

Gillespie, H. W. and Lloyd-Roberts, G.: Osteitis Condensans, Brit. J. Radiol., *26*, 16, 1953.
Hare, H. F. and Haggart, G. E.: Osteitis Condensans Ilii, J.A.M.A., *128*, 723, 1945.
Isley, J. R. and Baylin, G. J.: Prognosis in Osteitis Condensans Ilii, Radiology, *72*, 234, 1959.
Knuttson, F.: Changes in the Sacro-Iliac Joints in Morbus Bechterew and Osteitis Condensans, Acta radiol., *33*, 557, 1950.
Rendich, R. A. and Shapiro, A. V.: Osteitis Condensans Ilii, J. Bone & Joint Surg., *18*, 899, 1936.
Shipp, F. L. and Haggart, G. E.: Management of Osteitis Condensans Ilii, J. Bone & Joint Surg., *32-A*, 841, 1950.
Sicard, J. A., Gally, L. and Haguenau, J.: Osteitis Condensantes, a Etiologie Inconnue, J. de Radiol. et d'Electrol., *10*, 503, 1926.

Paget's Disease (Osteitis Deformans)

This disease was originally named osteitis deformans by Sir James Paget in 1877, because he believed that it represented a mild, progressive inflammatory lesion of bone of an unusual nature. It is generally conceded today that the origin of Paget's disease is unknown. The histologic appearance of the affected bone was described by Schmorl (1931, 1932), who stressed the so-called mosaic structures consisting of many irregular islands of newly-formed bone cemented together by heavily staining lines, indicating rapid absorption and still more extensive and hasty reformation of bone. These rapid sequences of bone resorption and regeneration eventually lead to secondary medullary fibrosis. The pathologic appearance of involved vertebrae is quite variable. The cancellous tissue becomes thickened and whitish, compressing the marrow cavity. Progression of the disease is accompanied by softening of the bone and progressive deformity. The initial phases occur in small isolated foci consisting of thickened trabeculae. Productive changes follow the initial softening and the end result may, in isolated cases, be a so-called "ivory vertebra" (Fig. 249) in which the entire body assumes a dense, white appearance as seen radiologically. This appearance is not in accord with the actual density of the bone, which may be relatively soft, compressible and entirely unlike ivory in its consistency. Paget's disease occurs in a monosteitic form, or more often as a diffuse disease. Usually the lumbar spine and sacrum are in-

volved to the greatest extent, the dorsal spine next in frequency, and the cervical spine is infrequently involved.

Compression of the spinal cord in Paget's disease was reported by Wyllie (1923) in 4 cases. Colclough (1949) was able to collect a total of 27 cases up to 1948, and added 2 of his own. Nineteen had been operated upon with varying degrees of return of function. The point of exact block can be discovered by myelography. A case of Paget's disease in which compression of the spinal cord was caused by hypertrophied laminal arches of the first, second, and third thoracic vertebrae was reported by Teng, Gross, and Newman (1951). An unusual case of Paget's disease affecting the first and second cervical vertebrae with spinal cord compression was described by Whalley (1946) in a 66-year-old man in whom there was a spontaneous forward dislocation of the head on the cervical spine. Roentgenograms showed massive new bone formation, fusion

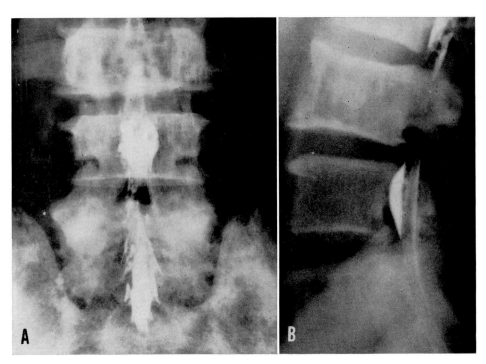

Fig. 252. A, A 56-year-old man with severe leg pain and difficulty in walking. Spinal tap accomplished with difficulty at L4 interspace. After instillation of 1.5 ml of Pantopaque under image intensification control the opaque medium gathers in the hollows of L2 and 4. The canal is markedly narrowed. Extensive Paget's disease, B, is seen. It was not possible to remove the Pantopaque.

of the vertebrae, kyphosis, and dislocation of the head, with narrowing of the spinal canal. At necropsy there was encroachment of the bony overgrowth on the spinal canal and its contents. Dickson, Camp and Ghormley (1945) mentioned that in their series there was evidence of compression of the cord following pathologic fracture of the vertebrae in 6 cases. Laminectomy had been performed 4 times on 1 patient in a period of 5 years.

Myelographic block was encountered in 3 cases reported by Latimer, Webster and Gurdjian (1953). Other instances of cord compression have been reported by Schreiber and Richardson (1963), Hartman and Dohn (1966) and Klenerman (1966). Difficulty in obtaining a free flow of cerebrospinal fluid from a spinal tap is frequently encountered when the canal is narrowed by hypertrophic changes in the vertebral bodies and the neural arches, and is accentuated when bulging discs are also present (Fig. 252). The need for surgical relief sometimes is acute. Extradural block produced by bony overgrowth above the level of the cauda equina may produce gradual symptoms easily mistaken for a degenerative disease of the spinal cord (Fig. 253).

Malignant degeneration of Paget's disease is well known. Its occurrence is mainly in the long bones and pelvis, occasionally in the skull, and infrequently in the spine. Campbell and Whitfield (1943) reported that in a search of the literature they found but 3 cases of sarcoma of the vertebrae. Involvement of other bones was present, so that it was difficult to determine the primary lesion. Their search revealed an incidence of osteogenic sarcoma of various bones in Paget's disease of from 7.5 to 14 per cent. In 3 cases reported by them compression of the spinal cord and cauda equina was associated with severe pain and neurologic changes. Summey and Pressly (1946) collected 76 cases of sarcomatous degeneration of Paget's disease of bone from the literature, of which 9 were in the vertebral column, almost always in conjunction with changes elsewhere

in the skeleton. Paget's sarcoma is highly malignant, may be multicentric in origin and is frequent in situations where the original disease is relatively infrequent, as in the humerus. In bones commonly affected, such as the pelvis or vertebrae, sarcomatous degeneration is relatively uncommon.

The radiologic diagnosis of Paget's disease is often made incident to other examinations in which the vertebral column happens to be visualized. In many the disease is entirely unsuspected. The earlier stages may be manifested by a slight diffuse increase in the density of an involved vertebra which in some instances presents vertically parallel thickened trabecular markings (Fig. 254). These may occupy the entire vertebral body or in some instances are limited to a relatively small portion of the vertebra. The change at times simulates the vertical striations present with vertebral hemangiomas. The changes are most frequently seen in the vertebral body but sometimes occur in the neural arch as well. Involvement of the spinous and transverse processes is relatively uncommon, but sometimes is extensive (Fig. 255). In other instances the disease manifests itself by the presence of small, somewhat circular shadows of increased density within the vertebral body. As a rule, these are multiple and in early stages are unaccompanied by any changes in the configuration of the vertebrae. As the disease advances there is flattening of the involved vertebra, sometimes with bulging of its borders. A diffuse increase in the density of the vertebral body approximating the cotton wool appearance usually associated with Paget's disease in the flat bones appears. Mention has already been made of the monosteitic form of Paget's disease involving a single vertebra. Our experience has been that this is relatively uncommon. Frequently both the thoracic and the lumbar spine are involved at the same time. In the more advanced forms of the disease the vertebrae assume flattened elongated appearance (Fig. 256). In these instances involvement of the neural arches

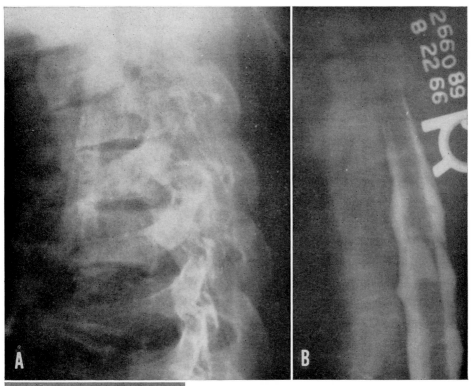

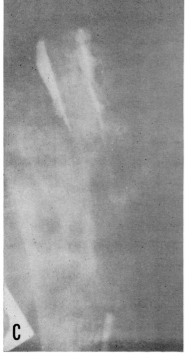

FIG. 253. *A*, A 53-year-old woman with known Paget's disease for 20 years. Progressive weakness and paresthesia of the lower extremities had been present for about 10 months. Lately there was also fecal incontinence and diminished pain sensation at the T5 level. Clinical diagnosis was degenerative cord disease. Lateral thoracic spine reveals Paget's disease. Myelography, *B* and *C*, after instillation of 8 ml of Pantopaque reveals a cephalad block at T5. A small amount passed the block, and on caudad flow disclosed the upper level of the block. The cord above the block is swollen. At operation an extradural block at T3, 4 and 5 was relieved by laminectomy.

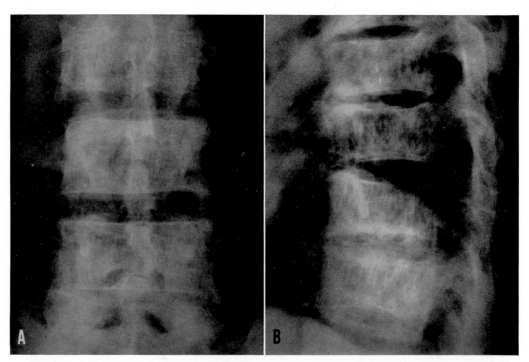

FIG. 254.   *A*, Extensive Paget's disease in which the bone is altered by vertical parallel thickened trabeculae. *B*, Some flattening of the vertebral bodies is present.

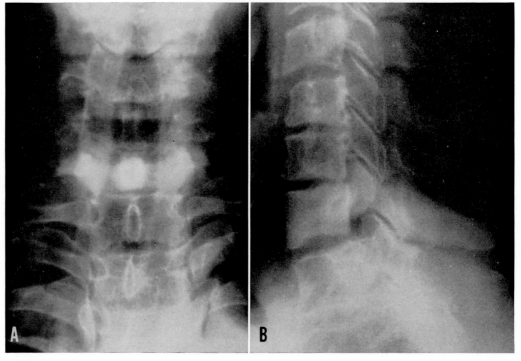

FIG. 255.   *A*, Extensive bone sclerosis due to Paget's disease of C7, involving the neural arch, *B*, and spinous process as well as the body.

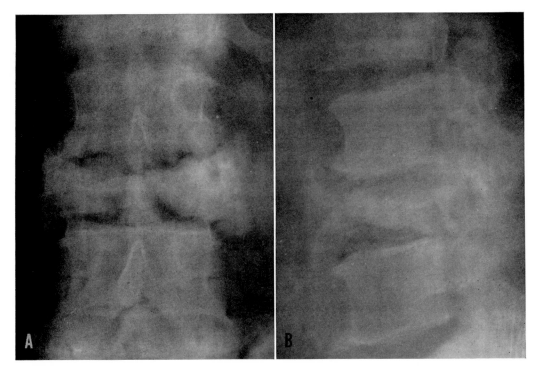

FIG. 256. *A*, Advanced Paget's disease with spreading and compression of L2. Vacuum phenomenon is noted in the adjacent discs. *B*, Lateral projection reveals anterior bulge of the vertebral body.

is frequent. Deformity of the intervertebral discs is no more common in patients with Paget's disease than is observed in the similar age groups. However, a loss of density of a vertebral body with encroachment of the intervertebral fibrocartilage into the involved vertebra with a consequent loss of the height of that vertebral body is seen occasionally. In 1 of our cases the intervertebral space between the fourth and fifth lumbar vertebrae practically disappeared into the degenerated softened inferior aspect of the fourth lumbar vertebra.

Snapper (1951) mentioned that in patients over 40 years of age, with hypertrophic changes in the spine, Paget's disease may start in the osteophytic proliferations and then gradually spread to the vertebral bodies.

One sometimes encounters difficulty in evaluating the status of a patient suspected of Paget's disease from the spinal roentgenograms alone. Investigation of the other bones, and particularly of the pelvis and skull, may prove helpful in differential diagnosis from prostatic carcinoma or other metastases.

References

Campbell, E. and Whitfield, R. D.: Osteogenic Sarcoma of Vertebrae Secondary to Paget's Disease, New York State J. Med., *43*, 931, 1943.

Caughey, J. E., Gwynne, J. F. and Jefferson, N. R.: Dystrophia Myotonica Associated with Familial Paget's Disease (Osteitis Deformans) with Sarcomata, J. Bone & Joint Surg., *39-B*, 316, 1957.

Colclough, J. A.: Compression of Spinal Cord by Osteitis Deformans, Surgery, *25*, 760, 1949.

Dickson, D. D., Camp, J. D. and Ghormley, R. K.: Osteitis Deformans, Radiology, *44*, 449, 1945.

Hartman, J. T. and Dohn, D. F.: Paget's Disease of the Spine with Cord or Nerve Root Compression, J. Bone & Joint Surg., *48-A*, 1079, 1966.

Janetos, G. P.: Paget's Disease in the Cervical Spine, Am. J. Roentgenol., *97*, 655, 1966.

Klenerman, L.: Cauda Equina and Spinal Cord Compression in Paget's Disease, J. Bone & Joint Surg., *48-B*, 365, 1966.

Lake, M.: Paget's Disease (Osteitis Deformans), J. Bone & Joint Surg., *33-B*, 323, 1951.

Latimer, F. R., Webster, J. E. and Gurdjian, E. S.: Osteitis Deformans with Spinal Cord Compression, J. Neurosurg., *10*, 583, 1953.

Porretta, C. A., Dahlin, D. C. and Janes, J. M.: Sarcoma in Paget's Disease of Bone, J. Bone & Joint Surg., *39-A*, 1314, 1957.

Russel, D. S.: Malignant Osteoclastoma and the Association of Malignant Osteoclastoma with Paget's Osteitis Deformans, J. Bone & Joint Surg., *31-B*, 281, 1949.

Schmorl, G.: Uber Ostitis Deformans Paget, Virchow's Arch. path. Anat., *283*, 694, 1932.

Schreiber, M. H. and Richardson, G. A.: Paget's Disease Confined to One Lumbar Vertebra, Am. J. Roentgenol., *90*, 1271, 1963.

Teng, P., Gross, S. W. and Newman, C. M.: Compression of Spinal Cord by Csteitis Deformans (Paget's Disease), Giant Cell Tumor and Polyostotic Fibrous Dysplasia (Albright's Syndrome) of Vertebrae, J. Neurosurg., *8*, 482, 1951.

Wiberg, G.: Paget's Disease (Osteitis Deformans) with Symptoms of Compression of the Cord Treated Surgically, Rev. Assoc. Med. Argent., *62*, 740, 1948.

Wyllie, W. G.: Occurrence in Osteitis Deformans of Lesions of Central Nervous System, Brain, *46*, 337, 1923.

Radiation Effects

The effect of intensive x-ray irradiation on the vertebral column has been known for a long time (Desjardins, 1930; Warren, 1943). Smithers, Clarkson and Strong (1943) reported radiation myelitis in a patient who received a depth dose of 5800 r in 39 days for carcinoma of the esophagus. The lesion developed 15 months later, presenting a Brown-Séquard syndrome considered to be due to intramedullary gliosis. Radiation myelitis of the brain stem was reported by Boden (1948) as occurring in 5 fatal and 5 nonfatal cases in a series of 161 patients who had received x-ray therapy for malignant tumors of the nose, mouth, larynx or cervical lymph nodes, the myelitis appearing in the cervical spinal cord. A long time interval occurred between the appearance of symptoms and the cessation of treatment. Initial symptoms were numbness and tingling of the hands and feet, precipitated by flexion or extension of the neck, and often associated with shoulder or neck pain. In a few cases the symptoms were transient, disappearing in from 3 to 9 months. In others parasthesias were followed by weakness or spastic paralysis of one or more extremities, and later bowel or

bladder dysfunction. In the fatal cases there was intercostal paralysis and death from bronchopneumonia or urinary tract infection. Greenfield and Stark (1948) reported on post-irradiation neuropathy in 3 cases where neurologic disability followed intensive million-volt x-ray therapy to the retroperitoneal region. In each case a flaccid paralysis appeared, and the chief site of injury was believed to be the anterior horn cells in the lumbosacral segments of the cord. No histologic material was available. These authors calculated the doses to be from 5000 to 6000 r, delivered to the retroperitoneal areas for nodes from primary testicular tumors. The x-ray examination and myelograms of these patients were all within normal limits. Seven cases of fatal damage to the brainstem after x-ray therapy for malignant tumors of the middle ear, pharynx or parotid gland were reported by Boden (1950) who concluded that the limit of tolerance of the central nervous system was from 3500 to 4500 r, depending on the size of the field used. The x rays affected primarily the blood vessels rather than the neurones, and the eventual neurologic lesions resulted from impaired circulation. Radiologic examination in these people showed no evidence of bone change.

The latent period for the appearance of radiation damage to the brain and spinal cord varies from about 4 months to over 7 years. Rapid progress corresponds to the presence of an acute necrotizing myelitis associated with a fibrinoid degeneration of blood vessels and a mild glial response. With more protracted damage there is cystic degeneration and gliosis of the grey matter, demyelinization and gliosis of white matter and sclerosis and hyalinization of the blood vessels (Malamud and co-workers, 1954). Transient radiation myelopathy also can be encountered (Jones, 1964), starting with symptoms referred to as the "barber's chair sign," with abnormal sensation of an electric discharge down the spine and limbs on flexing the neck. Neck flexion is regarded as the trigger mechanism for this phenomenon, which also is referred to as Lhermitte's sign. Jones considered hypertension as an important factor in the incidence of radiation myelopathy. Other factors include not only the radiation dose, but also the shape of the spinal canal, which again brings into focus the importance of the relative space available in the canal for the cord. In his cases of transient myelopathy there were no histologic changes. Dynes and Smedal (1960) found the average interval between completion of treatment and the development of myelitis was over 23 months. Paresthesias, sensory changes and evidences of long tract involvement was transitory in some patients. However, with more extensive damage the final result may be paraplegia or quadriplegia. With supervoltage treatment it has been estimated that doses beyond the 5,000 rad range were more likely to be followed by a radiation reaction.

Radiographic evidence of destruction of bone following x-ray therapy was reported by Spitz and Higginbotham (1951) in a 46-year-old man who developed an osteogenic sarcoma following irradiation for testicular seminoma. Roentgenograms of this patient showed destruction of the laminae of the third, fourth and fifth lumbar vertebrae with calcific flecks in the soft tissues, and distinct bulging of the right psoas shadow. Extraskeletal osteogenic sarcoma arising in irradiated tissue was also reported by Auerbach, Friedman, Weiss and Amory (1951) in a case of testicular tumor following intensive treatment. Necropsy revealed postradiation effects and a huge osteogenic sarcoma of the right lumbar muscles, with invasion of adjacent vertebrae and ribs, and lung and lymphatic metastases. Four years had intervened between x-ray therapy and the clinical onset of the malignant disease. The roentgenograms showed a calcific mass in the soft tissues, not connected with bone or skin.

Retardation of bone growth, with deformity of muscular bony architecture, atrophy, and scarring of the skin and fibrosis of subcutaneous tissues were reported by Murphy and Berens (1952) as a late sequela

following heavy irradiation in children. These authors commented that changes usually cannot be avoided if a clinical cure is to be attained. In a detailed report on the irradiation effects of roentgen therapy on the growing spine Neuhauser, Wittenborg, Berman and Cohen (1952) described 45 patients who had had x-ray therapy over the spine, together with post-mortem examinations of 11. These authors suggested, as a preliminary guide, that dosages under 1000 tissue roentgens usually fails to produce a gross permanent defect in a growing child, irrespective of the age at which treatment is given. Children over 2 years of age may tolerate between 1000 and 2000 r delivered to the spine, with only minor growth disturbances, but dosages in excess of 2000 r, irrespective of age, will probably produce growth disturbances. In their series these were associated with gross abnormality in the contour of the vertebrae. Scoliosis was rarely produced if the spine was uniformly irradiated. The significant changes in the eleven post-mortem examinations were non-specific growth retardation and irregularity of ossification of the epiphyseal cartilage. These changes may lead to an irregular advance of the line of ossification, but no alterations of osseous contour were described. Benign cartilaginous exostoses of the types seen in multiple and familial form appear to arise with greater frequency in bones where epiphyses had been irradiated than in the normal population. Their findings were much the same as those described by Arkin and Simon (1950) in their experimental study of the production of scoliosis by irradiation in which vertebral epiphyseal growth was suppressed by irradiating the vertebral bodies asymmetrically. Whitehouse and Lampi (1953) followed 4 patients who had been treated for renal tumors in infancy and childhood for 10 years, and described vertebral damage which they associated with dosage factors.

Rubin and his co-workers (1962) followed patients treated for Wilms' tumor and neuroblastoma for periods of from 4 to

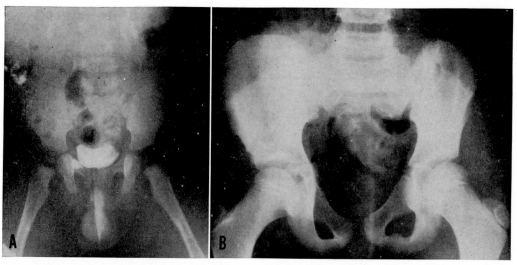

FIG. 257. *A*, Roentgenogram of the pelvis of a 9-month-old boy with a retroperitoneal neuroblasotma. The left ureter is displaced. *B*, Six years later after operation and x-ray therapy over the left hemipelvis, shielding the hip and pubic areas, hypoplasia of the left iliac bone is present. The spine was not included in the field, and remains straight. Radiation tissue dose was 1200 r.

23 years, with tumor doses ranging from 3 to 4 thousand r in 3 to 4 weeks. Three types of change in contour were observed. These included horizontal transverse lines of increased density parallel to the epiphyseal plates, producing an "os within os" contour, irregularity or scalloping of vertebral plates associated with loss in axial height and changes in the growth pattern of the bone. In some gross contour abnormalities with flat, small or beaked vertebrae such as seen in osteochondrodystrophy or achondroplasia were noted. Other changes noted included reduction in the size of the spinal canal with interpedicular spaces below normal. This was observed more often in the lumbar region and was regarded as incident to cessation of cartilaginous growth. Measurable scoliosis was produced. They cautioned against treating over the iliac crest because this might produce severe hypoplasia and underdevelopment of the sacrum (Fig. 257).

The effects of ingestion of radium were described by Stevens (1942) in a 36-year-old man who in 1926 was described as having Hodgkin's disease and as a heroic measure had been given injections of radium chloride intravenously. Radiation necrosis of the jaw, with sequestration of bone containing radium, followed. Destructive changes appeared in the dorsal vertebrae before the mandibular destruction became apparent.

The histology of irradiation sarcoma does not differ from spontaneous ostoegenic sarcoma. The tumors are essentially of the pleomorphic spindle cell variety. In many giant cells are prominent, and cartilaginous and myxomatous changes are not uncommon (Jones, 1953).

References

Arkin, A. M. and Simon, N.: Radiation Scoliosis, J. Bone & Joint Surg., *32-A*, 396, 1950.

Auerbach, O., Friedman, M., Weiss, L. and Amory, H. I.: Extraskeletal Osteogenic Sarcoma Arising in Irradiated Tissue, Cancer, *4*, 1095, 1951.

Boden, G.: Radiation Myelitis of the Cervical Spinal Cord, Brit. J. Radiol., *21*, 464, 1948.

————: Radiation Myelitis of Brain-Stem, J. Fac. Radiologists, *2*, 79, 1950.

Dejardins, A. U.: Osteogenic Tumor: Growth Injury of Bone and Muscular Atrophy Following Therapeutic Irradiation, Radiology, *14*, 206, 1930.

Dynes, J. B. and Smedal, M. I.: Radiation Myelitis, Am. J. Roentgenol., *83*, 78, 1960.

Greenfield, M. M. and Stark, F. M.: Post-Irradiation Neuropathy, Am. J. Roentgenol., *60*, 617, 1948.

Itabashi, H. H., Bebin, J. and De Jong, R. N.: Postirradiation Cervical Myelopathy, Neurology, 7, 844, 1957.

Jones, A.: Irradiation Sarcoma, Brit. J. Radiol., 26, 273, 1953.

————: Transient Radiation Myelopathy (with Reference to Lhermitte's Sign of Electrical Paresthesia, Brit. J. Radiol., 37, 727, 1964.

Looney, W. B.: Late Skeletal Roentgenographic, Histopathological, Autoradiographic and Radiochemical Findings Following Radium Deposition, Am. J. Roentgenol., 75, 559, 1956.

Looney, W. B., Hasterlick, R. J., Brues, A. M. and Skirmont, E. A.: Clinical Investigation of the Chronic Effects of Radium Salts Administered Therapeutically (1915–1931), Am. J. Roentgenol., 73, 1006, 1955.

Malamud, N., Boldrey, E. B., Welch, W. K. and Fadell, E. J.: Necrosis of Brain and Spinal Cord Following X-Ray Therapy, J. Neurosurg., 11, 353, 1954.

Murphy, W. T. and Berens, D. L.: Late Sequelae Following Cancericidal Irradiation in Children, Radiology, 59, 35, 1952.

Neuhauser, E. B. D., Wittenborg, M. H., Berman, C. Z. and Cohen, J.: Irradiation Effects of Roentgen Therapy on Growing Spine, Radiology, 59, 637, 1952.

Rubin, P., Duthie, R. B. and Young, L. W.: The Significance of Scoliosis in Postirradiated Wilm's Tumor and Neuroblastoma, Radiology, 79, 539, 1962.

Smithers, D. W., Clarkson, J. R. and Strong, J. A.: Roentgen Treatment of Cancer of Esophagus, Am. J. Roentgenol., 49, 606, 1943.

Spitz, S. and Higginbotham, N. L.: Osteogenic Sarcoma Following Prophylactic Roentgen-Ray Therapy, Cancer, 4, 1107, 1951.

Stevens, R. H.: Radium Poisoning, Radiology, 39, 39, 1942.

Ward H. W. C.: Disordered Vertebral Growth Following Irradiation, Brit. J. Radiol., 38, 459, 1965.

Warren, S.: Effects of Radiation on Normal Tissues. IX. Effects on Nervous System, Arch. Path., 35, 127, 1943.

Whitehouse, W. M. and Lampe, I.: Osseous Damage in Irradiation of Renal Tumors in Infancy and Childhood, Am. J. Roentgenol., 70, 721, 1953.

Fluoride poisoning occurs in individuals who have been in contact with various forms of fluorides, such as cryolite miners as described by Moller and Gudjonsson (1932), who reported widespread osteophitic formations at the attachments of ligaments, tendons and periosteum together with widespread osteosclerosis. Cryolite is the double fluoride of sodium and aluminum, containing as much as 54 per cent of fluorine. Bone changes in chronic fluorine intoxication were reported by Bishop (1936) in a laborer who for 18 years had been exposed to the dust of fertilizer made by crushing a phosphate rock which had a high fluorine content. Sclerosis of the entire skeleton except the skull was noted, with marked increase in density of the bones, together with vertebral osteophytes and calcifications of the attachments of some of the ligaments. In a chemical analysis of the bone in Bishop's case, Wolff and Kerr (1938) found an increase in fluorine content up to 20 times that of normal. The fluorine content was highest in the vertebrae and in the long bones, and had been deposited as calcium or magnesium fluoride. Wilkie (1940) reported 2 cases of fluorine osteosclerosis which occurred secondary to exposure to hydrofluoric acid fumes over a long period of time.

A much more common form of exposure is that secondary to the consumption of drinking water of high fluorine or fluoride content, such as may occur in North Africa, India or Argentina. The literature on this was cited by Greenwood (1940), who reported fluoride osteosclerosis in such patients. The effect of drinking contaminated water was graphically described by Kilborn, Outerbridge and Lei (1950). This happened in a Chinese village in which the inhabitants drank water contaminated by fluorine, and consequently developed fluorosis. Pigs, which shared the human water supply, were also affected, but other animals which used pond water containing no fluorine escaped. These authors described the skeleton of an affected male who died at the age of 37 and whose skeleton was available for study 1 year later. All the bones were markedly thickened, porous, rough and brittle. There was complete ossification of the intervertebral discs with fusion of the vertebrae making the spine one long rigid bone. Chemical study showed about 20 times the normal fluorine content for many of the bones, with an even higher ratio for the teeth. Roentgenograms showed increase density, thickened trabeculae and narrowing of the marrow cavities.

In a report on the roentgenographic
changes and urinary fluoride excretion
among workmen engaged in the manufacture
of inorganic fluorides Largent, Bovart and
Heyroth (1951) mentioned that 22 cases had
been reported in the American literature, including 6 in their paper. There appeared to
be a correlation between the level of fluoride
excretion in the urine and the presence or
absence of changes in the bone density.
These authors concurred with other observers in that the increased density of bone
is particularly prominent in the vertebral
column, but they noted that in their cases
little or no hypertrophic changes existed.
This observation was in accord with that
made by Linsman and McMurray (1943)
who had also reported a case of fluoride
osteosclerosis from drinking water in which
necropsy showed no evidence of osteophyte
formation.

Calenoff (1962) reported eburnation of
vertebrae which otherwise were normal in
size and shape in a 52-year-old man who had
been taking 4 to 5 drops of a solution of 1 part
of hydrofluoric acid and 2 parts of water for
about 9 years because he believed it would
help his teeth. Calcification of the paraspinal ligaments, particularly the ligamenta
flava, the intertransverse and the interspinous ligaments were reported as conspicuous changes in endemic fluorosis by
Singh and his co-workers (1962). A large
number of osteophytes were observed in
various muscle attachments. Slow and
gradual cord and nerve root compression
with a picture like that seen with cervical
spondylosis also occurs with endemic fluorosis
probably caused by a combination of factors
including thickening of ligaments, exostoses
and displacement of the cord resulting in
cord compression (Singh and Jolly, 1961).

In a study of the lumbar vertebrae in 1015
patients over age 45 Bernstein and co-
workers (1966) noted that the incidence of
osteoporosis was lower in a high fluoride
intake area. Evidence of osteoporosis, reduced bone density and collapsed vertebrae

was higher in a low fluoride area, especially
in women. Visible calcification of the abdominal aorta was higher in the low fluoride
intake area, especially in men. They concluded that fluoride consumption might be
important in the prevention of osteoporosis,
and play some part in preventing calcification of the aorta.

References

Bernstein, D. S., Sadowsky, N., Hegsted, D. M.,
  Guri, C. D. and Stare, F. J.: Prevalence of Osteo-
  porosis in High- and Low-fluoride Areas in North
  Dakota, J.A.M.A., *198*, 499, 1966.
Bishop, P. A.: Bone Changes in Chronic Fluorine
  Intoxication, Am. J. Roentgenol., *35*, 577, 1936.
Calenoff, L.: Osteosclerosis from Intentional In-
  gestion of Hydrofluoric Acid, Am. J. Roentgenol.,
  87, 1112, 1962.
Greenwood, D. A.: Fluoride Intoxication, Physiol.
  Rev., *20*, 582, 1940.
Kilborn, L. G., Outerbridge, T. S. and Lei, H-P.:
  Fluorosis, Canad. M.A.J., *62*, 135, 1950.
Largent, E. J., Bovard, P. G. and Heyroth, F. F.:
  Roentgenographic Changes and Urinary Fluoride
  Excretion Among Workmen Engaged in the
  Manufacture of Inorganic Fluorides, Am. J.
  Roentgenol., *65*, 42, 1951.
Linsman, J. F. and McMurray, C. A.: Fluoride
  Osteosclerosis from Drinking Water, Radiology,
  40, 474, 1943.
Moller, P. F. and Gudjonsson, S. V.: Massive
  Fluorosis of Bones and Ligaments, Acta radiol., *13*,
  269, 1932.
Singh, A., Dass, R., Hayreh, S. S. and Jolly, S. S.:
  Skeletal Changes in Endemic Fluorosis, J. Bone
  & Joint Surg., *44-B*, 802, 1962.
Singh, A. and Jolly, S. S.: Endemic Fluorosis,
  Quart. J. Med., *30*, 357, 1961.
Stevenson, C. A. and Watson, A. R.: Fluoride
  Osteosclerosis, Am. J. Roentgenol., *78*, 13, 1957.
Waldbott, G. L.: Incipient Fluorine Intoxication
  from Drinking Water, Acta med. Scandinav., *106*,
  157, 1956.
Wilkie, J.: Fluorine Osteosclerosis, Brit, H.
  Radiol., *13*, 213, 1940.

Lead Poisoning

The lead line associated with ingestion of
lead in growing children is well known.
However, such changes do not as a rule appear in the vertebrae, and in a review of
10 cases of lead poisoning in our series the
roentgenograms of the spine were normal
even when the epiphyseal lines of the long
bones showed dense lead lines.

5

Neoplasms of the Vertebral Column

NEOPLASTIC METASTATIC DISEASE

The most frequent of spinal tumors are metastatic neoplasms. Involvement usually occurs by extension through the blood stream, either the systemic circulation or through the venous vertebral plexus. Invasion of tumor into regional lymph nodes is believed to occur by embolization through the lymphatics to the affected glands. The question as to whether lymphatic drainage is an acceptable route for metastases to the vertebral column is discussed by Willis (1952). According to him lymphatics have not been demonstrated in the bone marrow, and cancerous permeation of the lymphatics in the deep fascia, periosteum and soft tissues adjacent to affected bones is rarely present. As a result of his work and a review of the literature, Willis concluded that the association of lymph node metastatic deposits and metastases to adjacent bones was purely coincidental, and that the hypothesis of lymphatic entry of neoplastic metastases into bone should be abandoned. Direct extension of malignant neoplasms into the vertebral column is relatively infrequent. The periosteum and cartilage maintain an effectual barrier against such penetration. When this barrier is disrupted, however, neoplastic invasion of bone through the destroyed periosteum may occur.

Metastatic invasion of the vertebral bodies by the hematogenous route involves the red marrow first. The tumor cells encroach into the spaces surrounding the bony trabeculae, and later extend towards and destroy the cortex. As a rule, the periosteum of the vertebral bodies confine the tumor so long as it remains intact. If, however, there is periosteal destruction by local pressure, the tumors extend beyond their confines and bulge into the adjacent tissues in much the same way as a paravertebral inflammatory or granulomatous process. Such neoplastic extension is less prominent than observed either with tuberculosis or pyogenic infections, but can be quite pronounced (Fig. 258), and can precede visible bony changes.

Metastases frequently are designated as being either osteoplastic or osteoclastic, the former with increased bony density, while the latter connotes osseous destruction and demineralization. Both may coexist not only in the same patient, but also in the same vertebra (Fig. 259). The demineralization of bone with osteoclastic metastases is due to the fact that the tumor crowds out the calcium-bearing stroma. In more advanced cases, with obliteration of the vascular supply because of the packing of carcinomatous cells, necrosis of bone may occur with replacement of the neoplasm by degenerated, devitalized bone and metastatic tissue. Increased bone formation with osteoplastic metastases has not been entirely explained. Willis regarded this as a reaction of bone to diffusable products from the tumor cells. He pointed out that various tumors possessed different intrinsic properties. For example, the highly osteoplastic nature of bone metastases from carcinoma of the prostate may be associated with a

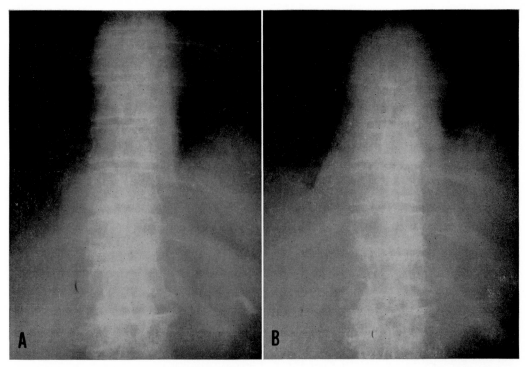

Fig. 258.   *A*, Metastatic lesion of the tenth thoracic vertebra from a kidney carcinoma.   Considerable paravertebral soft tissue swelling is present, but the bone involvement at this time is minimal.   *B*, Four months later the soft tissue swelling has increased and definite bone destruction is present.

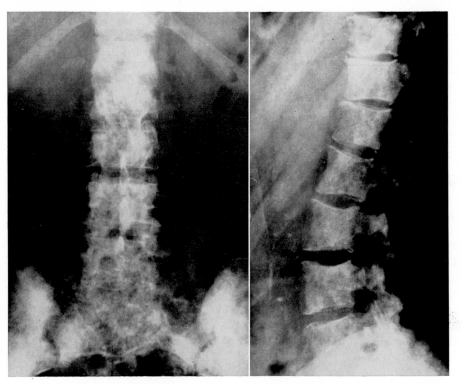

Fig. 259.   Anteroposterior and lateral roentgenograms of the lumbosacral spine showing mixed lytic and osteoblastic metastases from carcinoma of the breast.

substance which causes rapid proliferation of bone. The high serum acid phosphatase content indicates that the substance possibly is of enzymatic character. The association of osteoplastic metastases with slow-growing tumors such as scirrhous carcinomas of the breast, or prostatic carcinomas, and the association of osteoclastic metastases with tumors of an anaplastic nature or with tumors deficient in stroma, such as thyroid or renal carcinomas, is of interest. This rule, however, is not inviolable. It is not rare to find prostatic metastases in bone in which the lytic element is prominent, or sclerotic metastases with the more rapidly advancing tumors such as those of the breast or kidney.

The usual symptom of spinal metastases is pain. However, it is well known that extensive skeletal metastases may exist without symptoms referable to the involved vertebrae. This occurs when the vertebral body maintains its configuration, and when there is no extension of the tumor to cause pressure on or invade the periosteum (Fig. 260). Pain is due mainly to pressure on the richly innervated periosteum and on nerve roots and the spinal cord. The clinical picture sometimes suggests a herniated disc if a single nerve root in the lumbar or cervical spinal canal is impinged upon (Fig. 261). Extension of a neoplasm higher in the spinal canal may be associated with a syndrome of compression of the spinal cord. An interesting observation was made in several patients with severe pain in the vicinity of a vertebra in which marked destruction was evident radiologically, but in whom the vertebral body had retained its normal height. With collapse of the vertebra, and

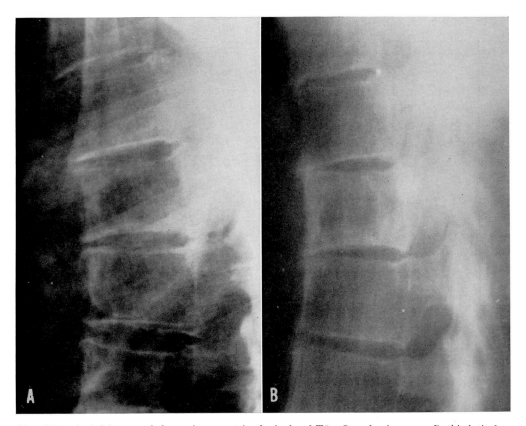

Fig. 260. *A*, A faint rounded area is present in the body of T5. On a laminagram, *B*, this lytic focus surrounded by slight osteosclerosis is clearly recognized as a metastatic lesion. The primary was a breast carcinoma.

27

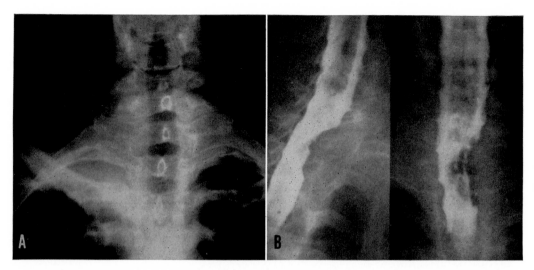

Fig. 261. *A*, A 57-year-old woman with pain in the neck radiating to her right arm. Clinical diagnosis was possible herniated cervical disc. AP study of the cervical spine reveals an opacity in the right apex, with no visible bone destruction. *B*, Myelographic examination reveals a prominent indentation into the right side of the lower cervical and upper thoracic epidural space. This was found to be due to intrusion through the intervertebral foramina from a Pancoast tumor of the right pulmonary apex.

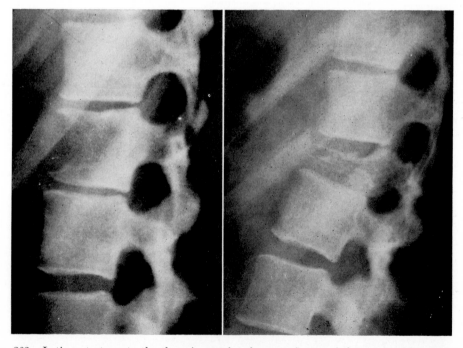

Fig. 262. Lytic metastases to the thoracic vertebra from carcinoma of the cervix with midback pain. Within 4 months the vertebra collapsed so that a vertebra plana resulted, with narrowing of the intervertebral foramina between the twelfth thoracic and first lumbar vertebra. The intervertebral discs were undisturbed.

probably with lessening of tension on the periosteum, pain became less marked and in some actually disappeared (Fig. 262). The intervertebral discs resist invasion by metastatic tumor. Destruction and fragmentation occur, however, when the support of the underlying bone is lost, so that the disc fragments and then is invaded by tumor. If the collapse of a subjacent vertebra is uniform, the disc above and below can remain intact (Fig. 262).

The common sites of origin of tumors which metastasize to the vertebral column are the breast, prostate, thyroid, kidney and lung. Less commonly tumors of the ovary, the uterus, the testes, the pancreas, biliary and the gastrointestinal tracts involve the spine. Melanomas frequently metastasize to the vertebrae. Other tumors are those of the bladder, the salivary glands, the lips, and various bone and soft tissue sarcomas. Of considerable importance is the occurrence of spinal metastases in patients with lym-

phomas and leukemia. Another group of interest includes neoplasms of the brain which extend into the spinal canal by way of the cerebrospinal fluid circulation. These will be discussed later.

The radiologic identification of metastatic tumors in the vertebral column depends upon the identification of bone destruction or production. Frequently fairly large metastatic deposits exist with no visible disturbance in the contour or bony density of the affected vertebral segments. Snure and Maner (1937) pointed out that cortical bone accounted for most of the detail of the bony structures depicted on roentgenograms, while the spongiosa accounted for the general bony density. Destructive changes in the marrow spaces, usually the first to be involved, easily go undetected until sufficient destruction of bone occurs to present itself on the roentgenograms as a shadow of decreased density sometimes visible on one projection only (Fig. 263). Their findings were borne out

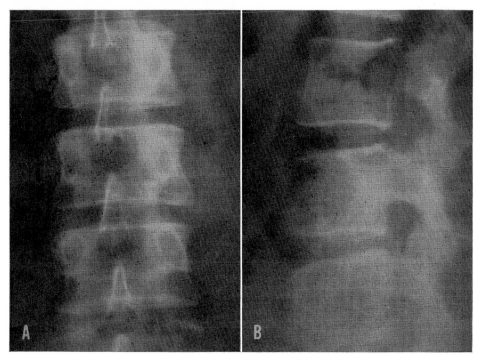

Fig. 263. *A*, AP view of the lumbar spine in a 43-year-old woman with a breast carcinoma taken as part of a skeletal survey. No bony destruction is visible, but on the lateral film, *B*, gross destruction of the anterior aspect of L3 is evident.

by Ardran (1951), who described experiments in which a 3-mm hole drilled vertically through the center of a vertebral body was seen only on a lateral roentgenogram and could not be identified on frontal films, where it was obscured by the spinous process. This hole was then filled with water and roentgenograms under the same conditions showed that the loss of bone could no longer be identified. Ardran then enlarged the hole by stages to approximately 14 mm in diameter and roentgenologic studies showed that when filled with water the defect was only slightly visible as a porosed area. He concluded that an area of destruction of bone over 1 cm in diameter in the center of a vertebral body may exist without definite x-ray evidence of its presence. Further experiments were performed in which slices of bone were removed from the anterior aspect of a vertebral body parallel to the anterior spinal ligament in which over 1 cm of bone had to be removed before the deficiency became apparent on the anteroposterior view.

An early roentgenologic sign of metastatic disease is slight, somewhat spotty decalcification of a vertebral body, often associated with a slight change in its contour. Similarly, there may be early loss of cortical markings in a pedicle, transverse or spinous process or lamina (Fig. 264). By the time this occurs the metastasis usually is quite large and of sufficient extent to have disrupted the spongiosa sufficiently to permit some collapse of bone. Usually this is associated with some extension to the cortex from the inner aspect of the vertebral body, weakening the buttressing effect of the solid bone. Nevertheless, the thing to watch for is slight decrease of density associated with the minimal changes in the configuration of a vertebral body, transverse process or neural arch or pedicle. This may be so slight as to involve only a centimeter or so, and sometimes may be seen only on one projection, either frontal or lateral, depending upon the location of the destroyed bit of bone. Less frequently, particularly where

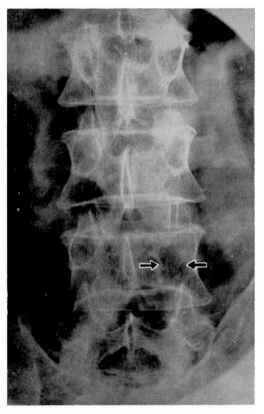

FIG. 264. Lytic metastasis to the left pedicle of the fourth lumbar vertebra extending to the inferior articular process (arrows) from a carcinoma of the kidney.

there is an osteosclerotic reaction such as occurs with carcinoma of the prostate, the initial indication of a metastatic deposit may be a small somewhat circular, usually poorly defined area of increased density only a few millimeters in diameter. In occasional cases, particularly in metastases from breast tumors, areas of radiolucency coexist with small spotty areas of increased bony density. Occasionally sclerotic changes in an involved vertebrae are so extensive that they produce the appearance of so-called "ivory vertebrae" (Fig. 249B), especially when limited to a single segment.

With progression of metastatic involvement and increasing weakness of the vertebral body, distortion follows either as a diffuse flattening or, not infrequently, the destroyed region involves part of the anterior aspect of a vertebra. It is not uncommon to observe a vertebra in which one lateral half is diminished considerably in height, and the zone of distinction between the destroyed area and the uninvolved bone is fairly sharply demarcated. The use of laminagraphy has helped considerably in the demonstration of small or obscure lesions both of an osteolytic and osteoplastic nature (Fig. 260).

Vertebral metastases frequently are multiple. The extent of metastases to the individual vertebrae is variable, and no constant pattern of involvement can be described for any specific type of neoplastic deposit, keeping in mind the tendency for certain tumors to produce more or less characteristic patterns, such as the sclerotic deposits from prostatic cancer.

Metastases to the neural arches, the pedicles and the transverse and spinous processes are quite common (Fig. 265). Neoplastic deposits in the pedicles and laminae are of particular importance because of their close relationship to the spinal canal and the probability of pressure against the spinal cord or nerve roots by direct extension. Stereoroentgenograms of the spine are helpful in studying the configuration of the pedicles. The initial change may be nothing more than decalcification of a single pedicle,

with no bony reaction, and is easily overlooked (Fig. 264). In more advanced cases a destructive process may extend into the lamina. Involvement of the transverse processes usually can be easily identified because these areas are not covered by adjacent bone. Destructive changes in the spinous processes are sometimes identified on the anteroposterior view by the absence of the shadow of the spinous process across the vertebral body. However, it is better to obtain lateral soft tissue studies, coning down on the suspected area.

The role of intraspinal metastatic deposits as a cause of pain and neurologic symptoms is well recognized. As a rule, these deposits are associated with involvement of the adjacent vertebral body or neural arch, and produce epidural cord compression and spinal canal block (Fig. 266). Occasionally one encounters an epidural deposit without bone destruction. In others, the osseous involvement may be minimal, and situated at quite a distance from the intraspinal metastasis. When such deposits are situated low in the spinal canal, the clinical picture may simulate a herniated disc (Fig. 267). This occurred in 9 of 11 cases described by Epstein (1952). In 4 of these, the plain roentgenograms made before myelography were considered to be normal, while in

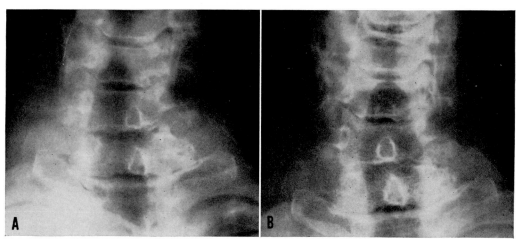

FIG. 265. *A*, A 56-year-old man with a known lymphoma for 16 months had severe pain in the supraclavicular fossa with radiation down the left arm. A lytic lesion is present in the left transverse process of C7. After x-ray therapy, *B*, pain cleared and the lesion recalcified.

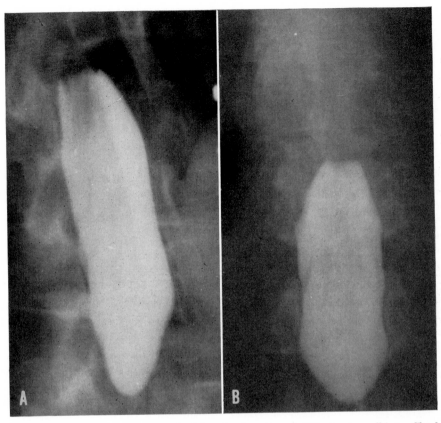

Fig. 266. *A*, A 48-year-old woman with diffuse back pain and difficulty in walking. She had been operated upon 2 years before for a neurofibrosarcoma of the pelvis. Plain film roentgenograms revealed destruction of the right pedicle of T11. On myelographic examination a complete extradural block is revealed, with slight displacement of the cord from right to left as seen on a slightly oblique view. On the direct frontal view, *B*, both sides are enveloped in tumor. A dentate appearance of the cephalad end of the column is present (*A*).

2 others there was discussion as to whether a slight decrease in the density of the fifth lumbar or first sacral segment indicated metastatic involvement. In 4 cases a faint lytic lesion of the fifth lumbar or first sacral vertebra had been overlooked, only to be identified on myelograms and a later review of the preceding films. In 1 the metastatic nature of a faint decalcification of the body of the fifth lumbar vertebra in its postero-superior aspect was confirmed by the co-existence of ischial metastases. Myelographic examination of this group showed a fairly characteristic defect, consisting of a deviation and tapering of the caudal sac contralateral to the side of the major tumor deposit. In these cases the caudal sac as-sumed the appearance of an inverted in-clined cone of varying height deviated away from the lesion, while the ipsilateral axillary pouch was blunted or obliterated. The axillary pouch on the opposite side was either pressed against the Pantopaque column, or was unidentifiable. This defect was noted in 7 cases, but in the others the deformity could not be definitely differenti-ated from that of a herniated disc. At operation the deposits of malignant tissue were irregular, nodular in shape and varied in thickness from a few millimeters to over 1.5 cm. The nerve roots were deflected by the metastases, and in 2 cases encrustations of tumor tissue about the involved nerve roots were noted. No invasion of the dura itself

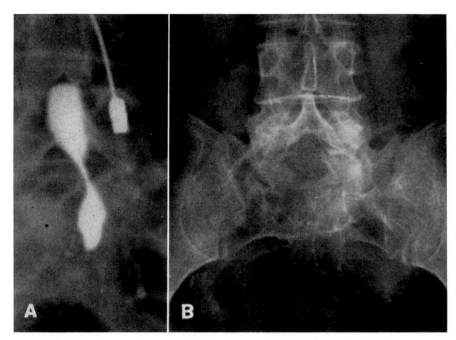

Fig. 267. Epidural metastasis from "benign" metastasizing thyroid deforming the thecal sac. The clinical diagnosis had been a herniated disc. The thyroid gland was not enlarged, and plain spine films were normal. At operation the bone appeared normal. Relief of symptoms followed operation and x-ray therapy. Four years later, *B*, pain recurred and osseous metastases were found in the right side of the sacrum extending towards the midline.

was identified. In 9 cases invasion of bone a short distance from the epidural metastases was found at operation but no visible connections were noted between the osseous malignancies and the epidural deposits. More extensive deposits may envelop the distal end of the cauda equina producing complete block or a pencil point deformity of the caudal sac (Fig. 268).

Metastatic deposits high in the lumbar or in the cervicodorsal spinal canal may be associated with symptoms of spinal cord compression. In such instances destruction of bone points towards the involved area. However, myelographic examination in some of these individuals will show that the extradural block is somewhat distant from the visible bony destruction. At operation extension of neoplastic tissue into the spinal canal can be seen to account for this discrepancy. In our patients with metastases to the upper lumbar, thoracic or cervical spinal canal the usual change was partial or a

complete extradural arrest of the passage of Pantopaque. In some instances the column was deviated contralaterally, passing above the block through a thin lateral channel. In the great majority adjacent bony destruction was present but in several the bone appeared to be intact both radiologically and at operation. However, since only the neural arches and the spinal canal surfaces were investigated one can make no statement as to what was going on in the vertebral body, even though the roentgenograms were normal. Intraspinal block also occurs without actual epidural extension of tumor, but from direct compression of collapsed bone as well (Fig. 270).

Intraspinal metastatic deposits occasionally occur with lymphomas. Smith and Stenstrom (1948) noted this in 11 of 308 cases of Hodgkin's disease. Symptoms of spinal cord block were present in 3 cases. I have observed 10 similar cases. One patient, a 17-year-old boy with a verified

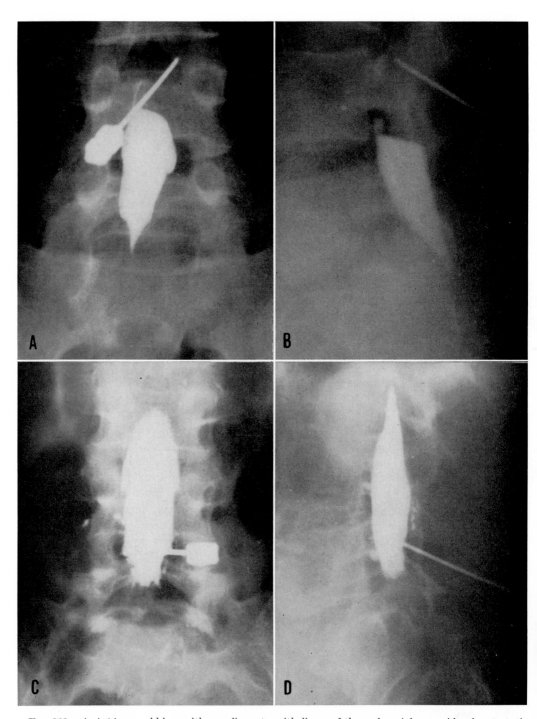

Fig. 268. *A*, A 14-year-old boy with a malignant perithelioma of the scalp. A large epidural metastatic deposit is present in the lower lumbar spinal canal with no bone involvement visible. Relief of symptoms followed x-ray therapy. *B*, The caudal sac is compressed into a pointed structure which is displaced dorsad. *C* and *D*, Another patient, a 9-year-old boy with epidural metastases from a neuroblastoma. The caudal sac is blunted and sharply terminated at the L4 interspace.

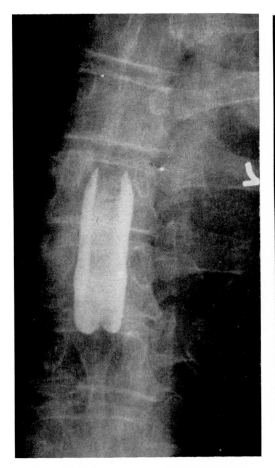

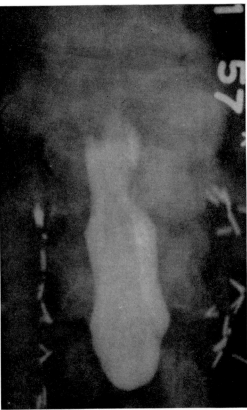

Fig. 269. Intraspinal epidural metastasis, mid-thoracic region, from a carcinoma of the breast. The plain film roentgenograms were normal, and no osseous destruction was observed at operation.

Fig. 270. *A*, A 63-year-old woman with metastases from a breast carcinoma and a complete block at T11. At operation there were no epidural deposits. The obstruction was caused by compression from a tumefied vertebra and neural arch.

lymphoblastoma, converted into an acute lymphatic leukemia. Late in the disease he developed symptoms of spinal cord compression at about the level of the tenth thoracic vertebra. Myelographic examination disclosed a complete extradural block at this site, and laminectomy revealed a cuff of tumorous tissue extending cephalad for about 5 cm. On histologic examination this tissue was found to be composed of leukemic cells. The patient did well after operation and postoperative x-ray therapy. He expired about 5 months later, and necropsy disclosed extensive metastases from his lymphoblastoma. Apparently the leukemic transformation had receded back to the original condition. No evidence of recurrence of the spinal canal lesion was found. At operation the bits of bone removed for laminectomy disclosed deposits of leukemic cells, while the necropsy report indicated the existence of bony involvement with lymphoblastoma. In 2 other individuals with known lymphomas a preoperative diagnosis of spinal canal block by lymphomatous tissue was made because of spinal cord compression. At operation, one of these patients was found to have an ependymoblastoma, and the other had a metastasis from an unsuspected carcinoma of the lung. The obvious moral is that one cannot assume with certainty the histologic nature of a lesion because of a coexistent neoplasm elsewhere.

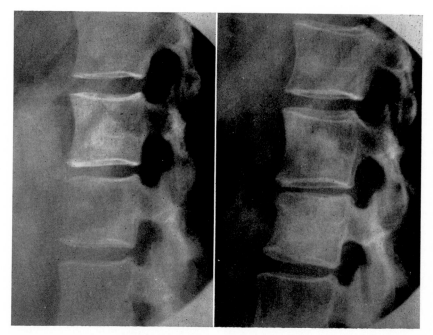

FIG. 271.   Lytic metastases from carcinoma of the breast to the second lumbar vertebra.
Restoration of bone after x-ray therapy.

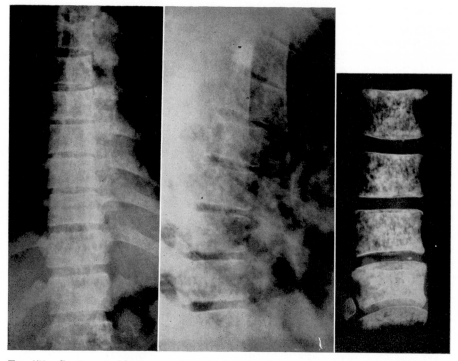

FIG. 272.   Spotty osteoblastic metastases to the spine from an unsuspected carcinoma of the
stomach, with verification at necropsy.

The effectiveness of x-ray therapy in restoring bone in lytic metastases of the vertebral column is well known and requires no further comment here (Fig. 271). Mention must be made of the great usefulness of hormonal therapy in producing recalcification of vertebral bodies.

Special mention is made of skeletal metastases from gastrointestinal malignancies. With these a form of osteosclerosis occurs within the medullary canals of the long bones as well as of the vertebral bodies, producing diffuse and spotty areas of increased density. This may be associated with secondary anemia. Four cases observed by us had numerous small nodular shadows of increased density within the vertebral bodies as well as in the medullary canals of the long bones (Fig. 272). Rarely generalized osteosclerosis appears secondary to metastatic medulloblastoma, usually from the cerebellum (Black and Keats, 1964).

The help obtainable from vertebral column scans in the diagnosis of bone metastases is considerable (Fig. 101). It should be recalled, however, that positive scans also appear with Paget's disease, osteomyelitis and other processes with active reformation of bone.

References

Ardran, G. M.: Bone Destruction Not Demonstrable by Radiography, Brit. J. Radiol., *24*, 107, 1951.

Auerbach, O. and Trubowitz, S.: Primary Carinoma of Liver with Extensive Skeletal Metastases and Panmyelophthisis, Cancer, *3*, 837, 1950.

Barron, K. O., Hirano, A., Araki, S. and Terry, R. D.: Experiences with Metastatic Neoplasms Involving the Spinal Cord, Neurology, *9*, 91, 1959.

Bertin, E. J.: Metastasis to Bone as the First Symptom of Cancer of the Gastrointestinal Tract, Am. J. Roentgenol., *51*, 614, 1944.

Black, S. P. W. and Keats, T. E.: Generalized Osteosclerosis Secondary to Metastatic Medulloblastoma of the Cerebellum, Radiology, *82*, 395, 1964.

Blumer, H., Aronoff, A., Chartier, J. and Shapiro, L.: Carcinoma of the Stomach with Myelosclerosis: Presentation of a Case and Review of the Literature, Canadian M.A.J., *84*, 1254, 1961.

Campbell, J. A. and Silver, R. A.: Roentgen Manifestations of Epidural Granulomas of the Spine, with a Report of Ten Cases, Am. J. Roentgenol., *72*, 229, 1954.

Cohen, D. M., Dahlin, D. C. and MacCarty, C. S.: Apparently Solitary Tumors of the Vertebral Column, Proc. Staff Meet., Mayo Clin., *39*, 509, 1964.

Cole, J. O. Y.: Bone Metastases in Advanced Breast Cancer: Radiological Appearances Following Hypophysectomy, Clinical Radiol., *16*, 295, 1965.

Deucher, W. G.: Roentgen Therapy for Metastatic Neoplasms, Am. J. Roentgenol., *50*, 197, 1943.

Ehrlich, J. C. and Kaneko, M.: Metastasizing "Adenoma" of the Thyroid Gland. A Brief Reconsideration, with Report of Two Cases, J. Mt. Sinai Hosp., *24*, 804, 1957.

Epstein, B. S.: Myelographic Diagnosis of Epidural Metastases in Lumbosacral Spinal Canal, Am. J. Roentgenol., *68*, 730, 1952.

Feiring, E. H. and Hubbard, J. H., Jr.: Spinal Cord Compression Resulting from Intradural Carcinoma. Report of Two Cases, J. Neurosurg., *23*, 635, 1965.

Freid, J. R.: Skeletal and Pulmonary Metastases from Cancer of the Kidney, Prostate and Bladder, Am. J. Roentgenol., *55*, 153, 1946.

Freid, J. R. and Goldberg, H.: Treatment of Metastases from Cancer of the Breast; with a Section on Hormonal Therapy of Breast Cancer, Julian B. Herrman, Am. J. Roentgenol., *63*, 312, 1950.

Gyepes, M. T. and D'Angio, G. J.: Extracranial Metastases from Central Nervous System Tumors in Children and Adolescents, Radiology, *87*, 55, 1966.

Heiser, S. and Swyer, A. J.: Myelography in Spinal Metastases, Radiology, *62*, 695, 1954.

Jarvis, L. J.: Involvement of the Sacrum by Recurrent Carcinoma of the Rectum, Am. J. Roentgenol., *84*, 339, 1960.

Lafferty, J. O. and Pendergrass, E. P.: Carcinoma of Testicle with Metastasis to Bone, Am. J. Roentgenol., *63*, 95, 1950.

Lenz, M. and Greid, J. R.: Metastases to Skeleton, Brain and Spinal Cord from Cancer of Breast, and Effect of Radio-Therapy, Ann. Surg., *93*, 278, 1931.

Marshall, S., Tavel, F. R. and Schulte, J. W.: Spinal Cord Compression Secondary to Metastatic Carcinoma of the Prostate Treated by Decompressive Laminectomy, J. Urology, *88*, 667, 1962.

Milch, R. A. and Changus, G. W.: Response of Bone Tumor Invasion, Cancer, *9*, 340, 1956.

Norman, A. and Kambolis, C. P.: Tumors of the Spine and Their Relationship to the Intervertebral Disk, Am. J. Roentgenol., *92*, 1271, 1964.

Odell, R. T. and Key, J. A.: Lumbar Disk Syndrome Caused by Malignant Tumors of Bone, J.A.M.A., *157*, 213, 1955.

Outerbridge, R. E.: Malignant Adenoma of Thyroid with Secondary Metastases to Bone, with Discussion of So-Called "Benign Metastasizing Goiter," Ann. Surg., *125*, 282, 1947.

Pendergrass, E. P. and Selman, J.: Dysgerminoma of Ovary with Widespread Metastases, Radiology, *46*, 377, 1946.

Russo, P. E.: Malignant Melanoma in Infancy, Radiology, *48*, 15, 1947.

Scott, M. G.: Carcinoma of Pancreas with Direct Involvement of Spine, Stomach and Colon, Brit. J. Radiol., *25*, 671, 1952.

Sherman, R. S. and Ivker, M.: The Roentgen Appearance of Thyroid Metastases to Bone, Am. J. Roentgenol., *63*, 196, 1950.

Simon, F. and Moon, A. C.: Pitfalls in the Diagnosis of Pancoast Tumor, Radiology, *82*, 235, 1964.

Smith, M. J. and Stenstrom, K. W.: Compression of Spinal Cord Caused by Hodgkin's Disease, Radiology, *51*, 77, 1948.

Snure, H. D. and Maner, G. D.: Metastatic Malignancy in Bone, Radiology, *28*, 172, 1937.

Stein, J. J.: Metastasis to Bone from Carcinoma of Gastrointestinal Tract, Radiology, *35*, 486, 1940.

Toomey, F. B. and Felson, B.: Osteoblastic Bone Metastases in Gastrointestinal and Bronchial Carcinoids, Am. J. Roentgenol., *83*, 709, 1960.

Tyler, A. F.: Epithelioma of Lip Metastatic to the Vertebra, Am. J. Roentgenol., *48*, 76, 1942.

Wagoner, G. W., Hunt, A. D., Jr. and Pendergrass, E. P.: Relative Importance of Cortex and Spongiosa in Production of Roentgenogram of Normal Vertebral Body, Am. J. Roentgenol., *53*, 40, 1945.

Willis, R. A.: *The Spread of Tumours in the Human Body*, London, Butterworth & Co., Ltd., 1952.

Wolf, A.: Tumors of Spinal Cord, Nerve Roots, and Membranes, in *Surgical Diseases of the Spinal Cord, Membranes and Nerve Roots*, C. A. Elsberg, New York, Paul B. Hoeber, Inc., 1941.

Woll, E. and Vickery, A. L.: Primary Fibrosarcoma of Heart with a Vertebral Metastasis, Arch. Path., *43*, 244, 1947.

Plasma-cell Myeloma (Multiple myeloma)

Myelomas are fairly common tumors which arise from plasma cells in the bone marrow. Subdivision into groups on the basis of cytologic variations is now regarded as unsound, and the variations in the size and appearance of the pathologic cells reflect stages in the maturation of these abnormal cells rather than specific cellular origins. The myeloma cell is regarded by some as a derivative of the reticulum cell, and multiple myeloma has been included with the leukemias and lymphomas by some observers. Occasionally numerous plasma cells are encountered in the peripheral blood, referred to as plasma-cell leukemia in such infrequent appearances. The disease affects the red bone marrow at first, and may exist without clinical manifestations for a considerable time. Later the liver, spleen, kidneys, lymph nodes and the lungs also become involved. The bones most often observed with myelomatous changes are the spine, the ribs, the pelvis, the skull and the long bones approximately in the order named. The rate of progression of the disease is variable, and in some the condition remains static for a long time. In others a relentless, painful and rapid course is encountered.

Discussion as to whether myeloma may exist as a solitary lesion has not clearly resolved this problem. Cutler, Buschke and Cantril (1936) referred to a type in which the lesion was first solitary and then became generalized, and another in which the lesion was relatively benign and remained localized. Raven and Willis (1949) found what they regarded as 18 acceptable cases of solitary plasmacytomas of the spine. This occurred more often in males. Two forms were described, one with marked destruction of bone in a well demarcated and sharply defined location, and the other a cystic and trabeculated expansion of bone. Paul and Pohle (1940) regarded solitary bone myeloma as an unusual but not rare disease. In a review of 45 cases they observed two forms, one simulating giant cell tumor and the other an osteolytic lesion seen more frequently in the spine and usually limited to a single vertebra. Gootnick (1945) also found solitary myelomas most often in the spine in his study of 61 cases. Wright (1961) reviewed a small group of patients who survived from 16 to 35 years after radical surgery for solitary plasmacytoma.

While it is possible that solitary myelomas appear once in a while, the generalized form of the disease is in such predominance that it would appear reasonable to regard them as manifestations of the same condition. Toth and Wintermantel (1943) reported a case originating in the pubic bone with later generalized spread, and commented that the seemingly solitary myeloma was not a specific condition. Aegerter and Robbins (1947) and Bayrd and Heck (1947) believed all myelomas to be multiple even though a single bone might be involved initially and for a long time. White and Tillinghast (1950)

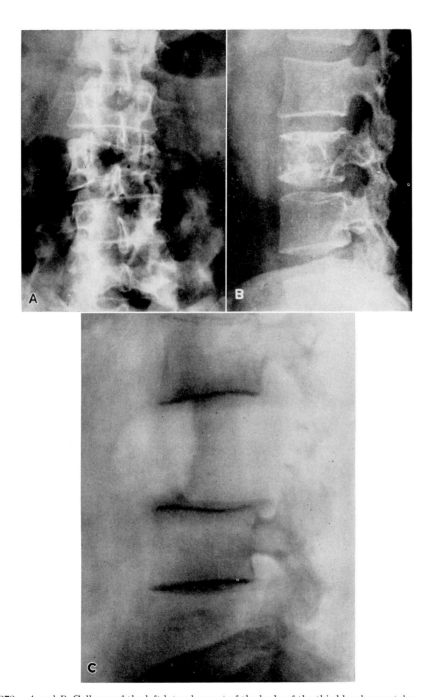

FIG. 273. *A* and *B*, Collapse of the left lateral aspect of the body of the third lumbar vertebra. The reticular appearance as seen on the lateral view suggested the diagnosis of "giant cell tumor." *C*, Same case. Lateral lumbar spine roentgenogram made 16 months later. There has been complete disappearance of the third lumbar vertebra. The fifth lumbar vertebra is practically gone, only a thin sliver of bone remaining visible. Diagnosis of multiple myeloma confirmed at necropsy.

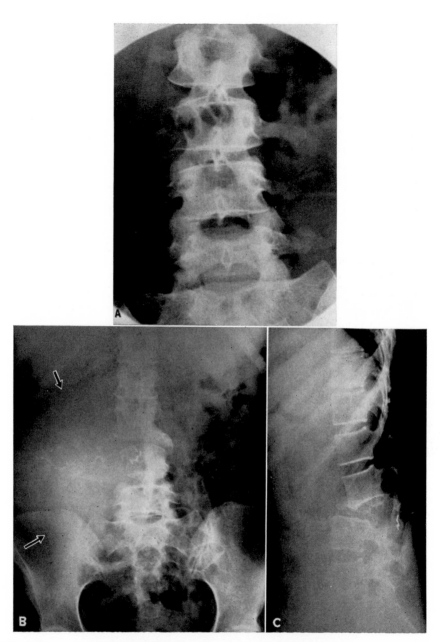

Fig. 274. *A*, Expansion of the right lateral aspect of the body of the third lumbar vertebra, believed to be due to a benign bone tumor. *B*, Same case, 2 years later. The diagnosis of myeloma had been established at operation done to relieve spinal canal block. A large paravertebral soft tissue mass practically filling the right side of the abdomen had appeared. Within this (arrows) was a reticular formation of new bone. *C*, Same case, lateral lumbar spine roentgenogram showing collapse of the third lumbar vertebra anteriorly. The posterior aspect is markedly involved as well, but remains higher.

also believed the solitary myeloma to be rare and might be only an early manifestation. Dalgaard and Dalgaard (1952) reported 3 lesions which at first occurred in the vertebral bodies but terminally presented involvement of other bones and organs. In several instances we have followed patients who were regarded as having isolated vertebral myelomas, who underwent prolonged courses but at necropsy revealed evidence of multiple involvement (Figs. 273 and 274). It is of interest that in both these patients the intial diagnosis had been giant cell tumor involving a single vertebra, and that in one the diagnosis had been considered as verified by biopsy.

The usual clinical picture observed with multiple myeloma is one in which pain predominates. Initial complaints often are referred to the back or the chest, and may be mild until exaggerated by a pathologic fracture. Occasionally complaints are caused by extension of tumor into adjacent soft tissues, producing neuritic, pleural or abdominal pain. Progressive weakness and anemia are common. Later stages are accompanied by visceral disturbances involving the gastrointestinal tract, the urinary system and the central nervous system. Cord involvement results from tumor perforation of the vertebrae and impingement on the spinal cord or the cauda equina and the peripheral nerves emerging from the intervertebral foramina. More often myelomatous destruction of the vertebrae, including the pedicles and neural arches, are responsible for the initial complaints. With collapse of bone there may be intrusion into the canal with or without concomitant tumorous intrusion producing extradural pressure. The dura is resistant to invasion by tumor, and instances of intradural extension of myeloma are rare (Fig. 275). Occasionally a peripheral neuritis of unknown pathogenesis occurs with multiple myeloma. Abnormal bleeding occasionally is incident to hemopoietic depression. Renal failure may follow deposition of abnormal proteins in the tubules, leading to uremia and death. The kidneys also may be affected by deposition of uric acid, part of the process of hyperuricemia due to increased purine metabolism incident to the formation and breakdown of tumor cell nucleic acids. Nephrocalcinosis incident to hypercalcemia also occurs, as does metastatic calcification in other organs. Indeed, secondary hyperparathyroidism may develop in response to the chronic renal insufficiency, leading to considerable difficulty in differential diagnosis.

Diagnosis is greatly facilitated by the demonstration of plasma cells in the bone marrow and hyperproteinemia with reversal of the albumin-globulin ratio. Electrophoretic study of the blood protein is important, keeping in mind the fact that a wide variety of abnormal proteins may be present in patients with multiple myeloma, and that similar changes also are encountered in other conditions such as Hodgkin's disease, lupus erythematosus, cirrhosis of the liver, lymphatic leukemia and carcinomatosis. The presence of cryoglobulins in the blood, a form of serum protein which precipitates on exposure to cold and redissolves at body temperature, also may indicate the presence of multiple myeloma as well as of other conditions.

Amyloidosis occurs in from 6 to 10 per cent of patients with muliple myeloma. This is associated with excessive formation of abnormal globulin. Para-amyloid, regarded as an abnormal protein product of malignant plasma cells, also precipitates in various locations as well as in plasmacytomas themselves. Deposits of amyloid or para-amyloid may be responsible for symptoms referable to the gastrointestinal tract, the liver, spleen and lungs, and the heart. Deposition in the spinal canal may produce extradural compression, and can occur in the absence of contiguous myelomatous involvement of adjacent vertebrae.

Hypercalcemia occurs in about half the patients, but no change in phosphate or alkaline phosphatase levels appear. The peripheral blood smear usually is normal, except in the unusual instance of a plasma-

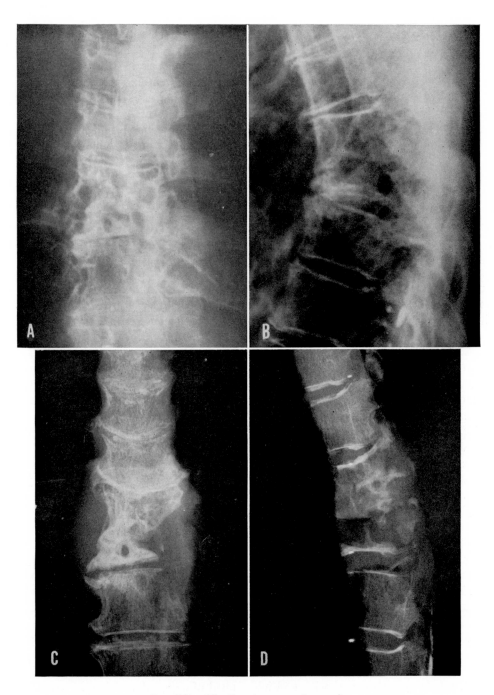

FIG. 275.   (*Continued on opposite page.*)

cell leukemic state. The presence of Bence-Jones proteinuria has been estimated to occur in from 10 to 85 per cent of patients. Geschickter and Copeland (1949) commented that the reported incidence of such proteinuria would be greater if proper laboratory tests for its existence were made routinely.

The radiologic manifestations of myeloma include mainly the punched-out, sharply demarcated rarefied areas seen especially in the skull, the pelvis, the ribs and long bones. Expanding lesions producing multiloculated ballooned-out areas with pronounced thinning of the cortex and numerous traversing string-like bands of bone appear in the various bones. Perforation of the cortex is associated with escape and proliferation of myeloma in the adjacent tissues, sometimes with invasion of the brain and parenchymatous organs. In some instances myelomas cannot be distinguished from metastatic

malignancy without the help of other examinations, particularly bone marrow and electrophoretic studies. Skeletal surveys are important because extensive lesions may be present in other bones, particularly the skull, without concomitant symptoms. When difficulty is encountered in evaluating a diffuse loss of bone in the spine, the identification of the characteristic punched-out lesions in the skull can be decisive. However, even here there may be some trouble because occasionally metastatic disease, especially from the breast and lungs, is known to produce quite similar changes.

The radiologic manifestations of vertebral involvement with myeloma are varied. The common change is one of bone loss presenting a picture not unlike that seen with osteoporosis. This may be observed in early instances with little loss of the configuration of the involved vertebrae, but more often some irregularity or deformity of the verte-

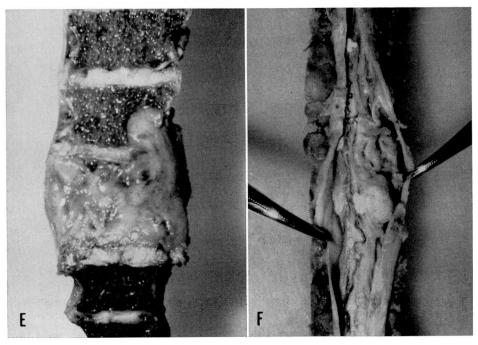

Fig. 275. *A*, AP roentgenogram of the thoracic spine in a 71-year-old woman with multiple myeloma. The 5th thoracic vertebra is collapsed, and there is extensive myelomatous infiltration in the adjacent soft tissues, *B*. A gibbus formation is present. *C* and *D*, Roentgenograms of the excised specimen. *E*, Photograph of the specimen showing extension of myeloma through the intervertebral disc. *E*, On opening the dura it was found that myeloma had invaded and perforated the dura and impinged against the thoracic spinal cord and the adjacent nerve roots.

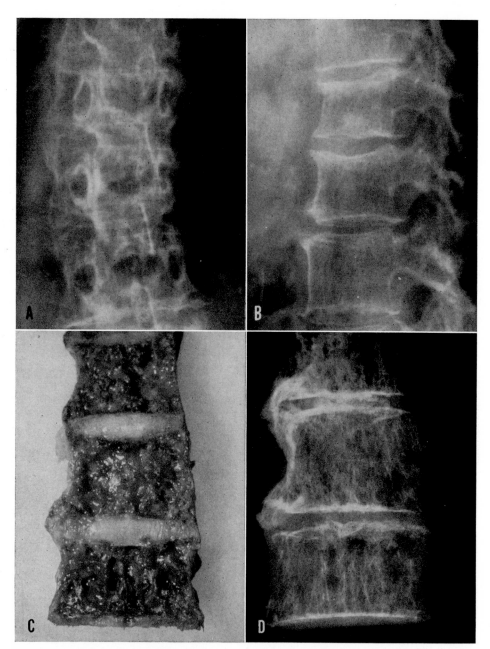

FIG. 276. *A*, A 60-year-old woman with pain in the midback and ribs. Marked demineralization of bone is present. On the lateral view, *B*, some vertical striation of bone is seen. *C*, Photograph of specimen shows that the bone has been replaced by a gelatinous material which bulges from the bone surface. *D*, Roentgenogram of the specimen reveals loculation and destruction of cancellous and cortical bone by myeloma.

bral margins appears as the integrity of the cortical bone is impaired by the myelomatous destruction with little or no concomitant repair. The intervertebral discs maintain their integrity, and a widened biconvex appearance of these structures reflects the retained turgescence of the disc and the softening of the adjacent bone. Compression fractures are commonly present, with wedging of the vertebrae or in some instances, flattening of the more involved segments (Fig. 276). On close inspection of the vertebrae loss of cortical bone is apparent, and faint irregularly distributed elongated areas of trabecular destruction can be made out. With loss of the integrity of the subchondral bone changes also appear in the intervertebral disc (Fig. 277). Softening of the vertebral body leads to a wrinkled configuration of their margins (Fig. 278). In advanced cases the vertebrae become markedly demineralized, their trabeculae destroyed and cortex grossly thinned out. This may in-

volve the pedicles, the neural arches and the transverse and spinous processes as well. Collapse of both the vertebral bodies and the intervertebral discs, with extension of myelomatous tissue into contiguous vertebrae and adjacent soft tissues, results in gross distortion of the involved segments and widening of the paravertebral soft tissues (Fig. 275). In some the involved vertebrae are grossly flattened, in others a gibbus formation appears. The patient and his friends may actually notice diminution in height as well as gross postural change over a short period of time.

In rare instances the first manifestation of a vertebral or a sacral myeloma may be localized as a rarefied, relatively small lesion (Fig. 274A) which can be confused with other tumors. Later observation and demonstration of myeloma cells on biopsy is required to clarify these problem cases. Another uncommon manifestation of myeloma is one in which there is a grossly lytic

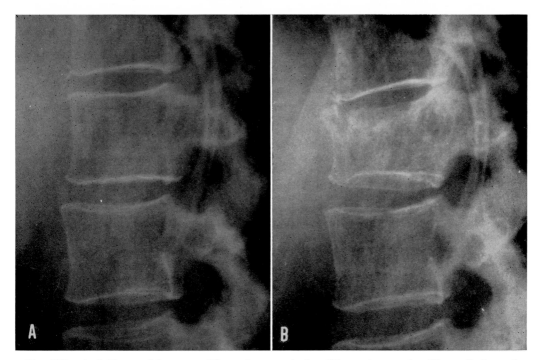

FIG. 277. A, A 60-year-old woman with myeloma producing diffuse osteoporosis. The cortical margins are thin. Vertical striations persist, but there are poorly defined, irregular radiolucencies indicative of bone destruction. B, Five months later the body of L1 has collapsed partly and the upper surface is broken through and fragmented.

lesion without evidence of deformity of the adjacent structures (Fig. 273). Rarely one may observe a myeloma which apparently involves the sacrum, or only a pedicle and neural arch, with relatively little destruction of the vertebral body (Fig. 279). Intradural extramedullary tumors without adjacent bone lesions also are infrequent (Sod and Wiener, 1959), and are identified only after operation.

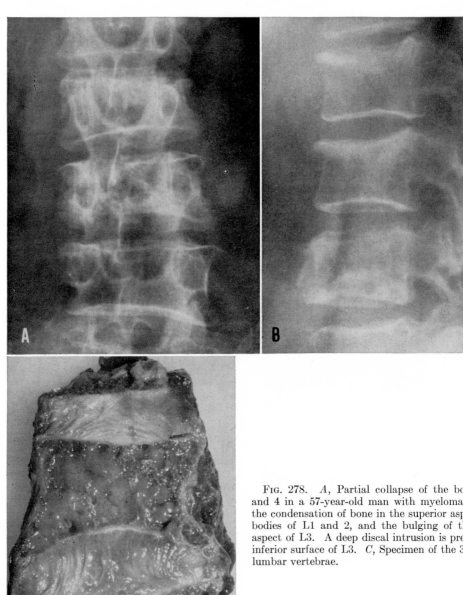

Fig. 278. *A*, Partial collapse of the bodies of L3 and 4 in a 57-year-old man with myeloma. *B*, Note the condensation of bone in the superior aspects of the bodies of L1 and 2, and the bulging of the anterior aspect of L3. A deep discal intrusion is present in the inferior surface of L3. *C*, Specimen of the 3rd and 4th lumbar vertebrae.

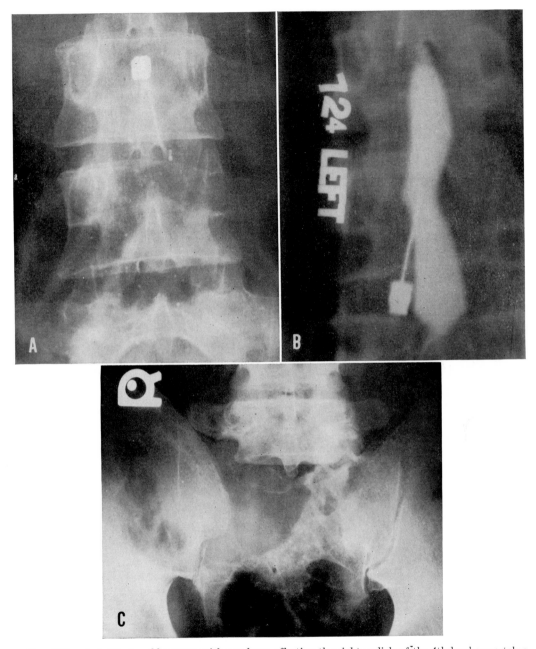

Fig. 279. *A*, A 62-year-old woman with myeloma affecting the right pedicle of the 4th lumbar vertebra and the adjacent lamina. The clinical picture was that of a herniated disc. *B*, Myelography reveals a lateral indentation into the Pantopaque column at this site. *C*, Another 60-year-old patient with a clinical picture suggesting discal herniation. A large lytic lesion involves the upper right sacrum and iliac bone, proved to be a myeloma.

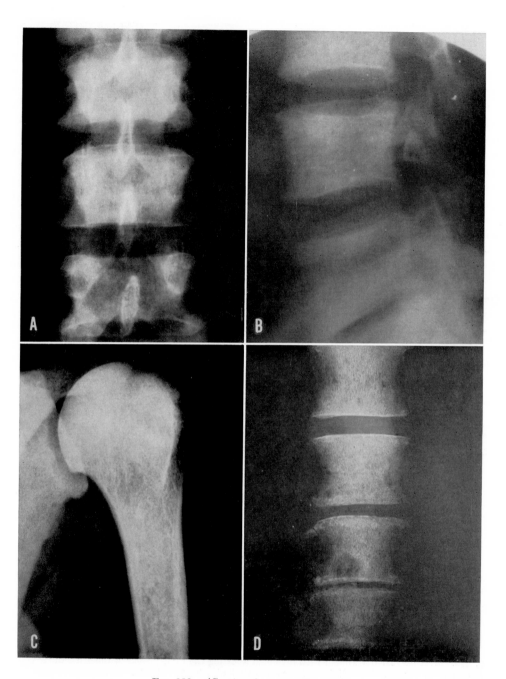

Fig. 280.   (*Continued on opposite page.*)

Bone sclerosis as the predominating change in multiple myeloma is infrequent. Langley, Sabean and Sorger (1966) found 18 reports in the literature, and added an additional 5. In my series of 85 cases there were 3 (Fig. 280). The most apparent change is one which is readily confused with myelosclerosis, with diffusely disposed intramedullary sclerotic changes. These may overshadow the usual lytic lesions to such an extent that they are unidentifiable, but their presence sometimes can be brought out on radiographic examination of bone slabs. Increase in the density of cortical bone also occurs, as does combined lytic and sclerotic lesions (Fig. 280).

Symptoms referable to the spinal cord or the cauda equina follow either intrusion of myelomatous tissue into the spinal canal or the intervertebral foramina. Collapse of a vertebral body also causes extradural compression, and may be unassociated with actual tumorous invasion of the canal. In most instances there will be adequate radiographic evidence of bone destruction. However, in some there are no visible osseous defects and yet at operation tumorous changes are apparent (Fig. 281). In others myelomatous tissue exuding from adjacent bone may wrap itself around the cord for one or more segments. Occasionally a deposit of myeloma occurs without adjacent tumor in bone. Blockage of the spinal canal from para-amyloid deposits also occur.

Myelographic examination discloses either a partial or complete block. When the lesion is low in the canal, the defect can simulate that due to a herniated disc (Fig. 279), particularly if close to an intervertebral disc. Spinal canal block is observed more often in the thoracic and cervical canal. Here the defect indicates the presence of an extradural lesion. In occasional cases there is but slight evidence of bone destruction. In 2 of 12 cases seen by us the only defect visible was a single destroyed pedicle, but

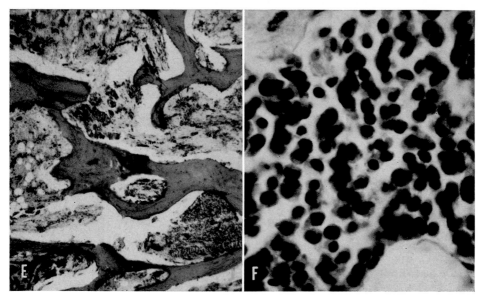

Fig. 280. *A*, AP and lateral, *B*, films of the lumbar spine of a 68-year-old woman who had been treated for myelofibrosis of 2 years. She had secondary anemia. Bone marrow aspiration revealed myeloma. A skeletal survey disclosed a diffuse pattern of sclerosis. Before death plasma cells in large quantities were found in the peripheral blood. *C*, The left upper humerus reveals osteosclerotic changes characteristic of those present in other bones. *D*, At necropsy the vertebrae were hard, but numerous small areas of rarefaction containing mucinous material were found. These proved to be myelomatous deposits. *E*, Low power and, *F*, high power photomicrographs reveal cellular marrow containing plasma cells in nests, sheaths and as single cells.

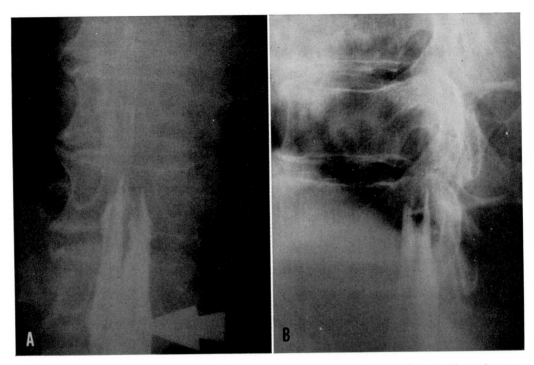

Fig. 281. *A*, Extradural block in the lower thoracic spinal canal in a 65-year-old man with myeloma extending from the right pedicle. No bone defects visible on the roentgenograms. The pattern of extradural compression is visible on the lateral examination *B*, as well.

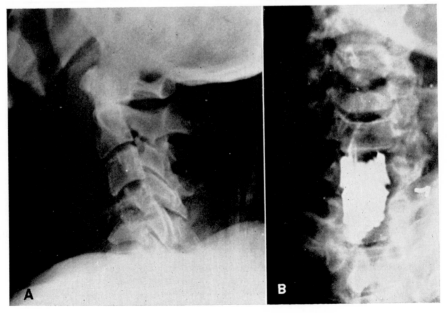

Fig. 282. *A*, Myelomatous destruction of the fourth and fifth cervical vertebrae.
B, Same case, with complete block demonstrated myelographically.

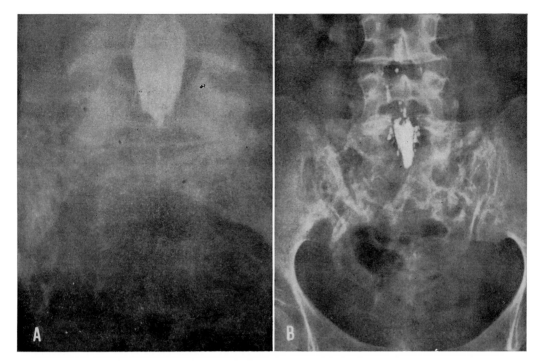

FIG. 283. *A*, A 55-year-old woman considered to have a herniated disc. There is a tapered complete block at L5. Extensive reticular destruction of the right upper sacrum is present. This proved to be a plasma cell myeloma. After x-ray therapy, *B*, sclerosis replaced the tumor and the caudal sac now is relatively normal. This film was made 2 years after conclusion of treatment.

at operation the cord was encased by myeloma. The cuff-like myelomatous deposit can be irregular, so that the cord itself is displaced more to one side than the other, much the same as in other extradural tumors. The most common myelographic defect is a complete extradural block associated with visible bone involvement (Fig. 282).

X-ray therapy sometimes is useful in controlling pain. In some patients who respond favorably considerable sclerosis of bone is observed (Fig. 283).

In differential diagnosis the conditions to be considered include osteoporosis, hyperparathyroidism, metastatic tumor of diverse origin, Cushing's disease and occasionally leukemia and lymphomas. The combination of lytic, sometimes bubble-like bone lesions, characteristic cells in the bone marrow and the demonstration of abnormal proteins on electrophoresis are helpful in identifying myelomas.

References

Aegerter, E. and Robbins, R.: Myeloma of Bone, Am. J. Med. Sci., *213*, 282, 1947.

Bayrd, E. D. and Heck, J. F.: Multiple Myeloma, J.A.M.A., *133*, 147, 1947.

Briggs, G. W.: Amyloidosis, Ann. Int. Med., *55*, 943, 1961.

Carson, C. P., Ackerman, L. V. and Maltby, J. D.: Plasma Cell Myeloma, Am. J. Clin. Path., *25*, 849, 1955.

Christopherson, W. M. and Miller, A. J.: A Re-Evaluation of Solitary Plasma-Cell Myeloma of Bone, Cancer, *3*, 240, 1950.

Clarke, E.: Spinal Cord Involvement in Multiple Myelomatosis, Brain, *79*, 332, 1956.

Cutler, M., Buschke, F. and Cantril, S. T.: Course of Single Myeloma of Bone, Surg., Gynec. & Obst., *62*, 918, 1936.

Dalgaard, E. B. and Dalgaard, J. B.: Solitary Plasmocytoma with Terminal Dissemination, Acta radiol., *37*, 231, 1952.

Engles, E. P., Smith, R. C. and Krantz, S.: Bone Sclerosis in Multiple Myeloma, Radiology, *75*, 242, 1960.

Evison, G. and Evans, K. T.: Bone Sclerosis in Multiple Myeloma, Brit. J. Radiol., *40*, 81, 1967.

Geschichter, C. F. and Copeland, M. M.: *Tumors of Bone*, 3rd Ed., Philadelphia, J. B. Lippincott Co., 1949.

Gootnick, L. T.: Solitary Myeloma, Radiology, *45*, 385, 1945.

Hallen, J. and Rudin, R.: Pericollagenous Amyloidosis. Acta med. scandinav., *179*, 483, 1966.

Kurnick, N. B. and Yohalem, S. B.: Peripheral Neuritis Complicating Multiple Myeloma, Arch. Neurol. & Psychiat., *59*, 378, 1948.

Kyle, R. A. and Bayrd, E. D.: "Primary" Systemic Amyloidosis and Myeloma, Arch. Int. Med., *107*, 344, 1961.

Langley, G. R., Sabean, H. B. and Sorger, K.: Sclerotic Lesions of Bone in Myeloma, Canadian M. A. J., *94*, 940, 1966.

Leonard, B. J.: The Pathology of Myelomatosis, Clin. Radiol., *12*, 20, 1961.

Lichtenstein, L. and Jaffe, H. L.: Multiple Myeloma, Arch. Path., *44*, 207, 1947.

Lumb, G. and Prossor, T. M.: Plasma Cell Tumors, J. Bone & Joint Surg., *30-B*, 124, 1948.

McKissock, W., Bloom, W. H. and Chynn, K. Y.: Spinal Cord Compression Caused by Plasma-Cell Tumors, J. Neurosurg., *18*, 68, 1961.

Odelberg-Johnson, O.: Osteosclerotic Changes in Myelomatosis, Acta radiol., *52*, 139, 1959.

Paul, L. W. and Pohle, E. A.: Solitary Myeloma of Bone, Radiology, *35*, 651, 1940.

Raven, R. W. and Willis, R. A.: Solitary Plasmocytoma of Spine, J. Bone & Joint Surg., *31-B*, 369, 1949.

Sharnoff, J. G., Belsky, H. and Melton, J.: Plasma Cell Leukemia or Multiple Myeloma with Osteosclerosis, Am. J. Med., *17*, 582, 1954.

Snyder, L. J. and Cohen, C.: Multiple Myeloma with Spinal Cord Compression as Initial Finding, Ann. Int. Med., *26*, 1169, 1948.

Sod, L. M. and Wiener, L. M.: Intradural Extramedullary Plasmacytoma, J. Neurosurg., *16*, 107, 1959.

Toth, B. J. and Wintermantel, J. A.: Apparently Solitary Myeloma with Subsequent Generalization, Radiology, *41*, 472, 1943.

White, S. and Tillinghast, A. J.: Multiple Myeloma, Am. J. Roentgenol., *63*, 851, 1950.

Wright, C. J. E.: Long Survival in Solitary Plasmacytoma of Bone, J. Bone & Joint Surg., *43-B*, 767, 1961.

Yentis, I.: The So-Called Solitary Plasmacytoma of Bone, J. Fac. Radiologists, *6*, 132, 1956.

————: Radiological Aspects of Myelomatosis, Clin. Radiol., *12*, 1, 1961.

Spinal Lymphomas

Included in this group are Hodgkin's disease, lymphosarcoma, giant follicular lymphoma and reticulum cell sarcoma. Histologic variations usually permit identification of individual tumors. Reed-Sternberg cells are associated with Hodgkin's disease. Lymphosarcomas are associated with disappearance of lymphoid germinal centers, filling of sinusoids with lymphoid cells and varying patterns of infiltration with lymphoblasts and lymphocytes. Abnormal cells may enter the peripheral blood late in the disease, presenting a picture of lymphocytic leukemia. Giant follicular lymphoma later may become malignant and appears then as lymphosarcoma. Reticulum cell sarcomas are characterized by abundant reticulum surrounding groups of tumor cells. There is evidence that these subdivisions are not absolute, and that the entire group represents a series of interrelated tumors arising from the lymphoid and reticuloendothelial system. A relationship with leukemia also has been postulated.

Lymphomas spread by direct extension from involved lymph nodes or by way of the vascular and lymphatic channels. The frequency of bone involvement has been variously estimated as from 20 to 70 per cent, depending on whether the examinations were conducted radiologically or at necropsy. If small bone lesions are sought, the incidence approaches the higher figure. The vertebral column is involved most often. Reticulum cell sarcomas are of interest in that such tumors sometimes originate in the spine (Coley, Higgenbotham and Groesbeck, 1950; MacCormack, Ivins, Dahlen and Johnson, 1952).

Involvement of the spinal cord and the cauda equina usually occurs because of extradural pressure. Tumorous invasion of the cauda equina and of individual nerve roots also has been noted (Hunt, Poser and Williamson, 1960; Van Allen and Rahme, 1962). Primary epidural lymphomas occasionally are encountered (Bucy and Jerva, 1962), or there may be extension of tumor from adjacent lymph nodes through intervertebral foramina (Verda, 1944; Smith and Stenstrom, 1948). The clinical picture associated with intraspinal lymphomas is related to the site of compression, the extent of the lesion, and the degree of involvement of the cauda equina and nerve roots. As a rule the symptoms are much the same as seen with other epidural tumors. Primary epidural spinal lymphomas have a tendency to appear in younger patients. Cord compression may be the first clinical evidence of a lymphoma, and may require laminectomy for immediate relief of pressure. The use of x-ray therapy and chemotherapy in the management of lymphomas is well known.

The radiologic picture of lymphomas of the spine is varied. A single vertebra may be invaded, but often several are involved as part of general osseous extension. Vertebral metastases usually are lytic, with diffuse demineralization of bone and persistent trabecular strands of increased density. With this type of metastatic invasion extensive involvement of a number of vertebrae can exist with relatively little change seen on x-ray examination (Fig. 284). The yellowish tumor tissue has a rubbery consistency, so that the configuration of the involved vertebrae is retained. In some instances a sclerotic reaction occurs, resulting in an "ivory vertebra," a relatively infrequent but sometimes striking manifestation of vertebral lymphoma (Hulten, 1927; Dresser and Spencer, 1936) (Fig. 285). Another infrequent change is the gross collapse of a vertebral body with maintenance of the intervertebral discs above and below (Fig. 286). More often compressive changes appear in an irregular fashion, and the destruction of bone is much the same as seen with other metastases. Occasionally some sclerosis is evident along the compressed margins of an involved vertebra, simulating that seen with Cushing's disease or in patients with compressive vertebral fractures incident to steroid therapy or osteoporosis.

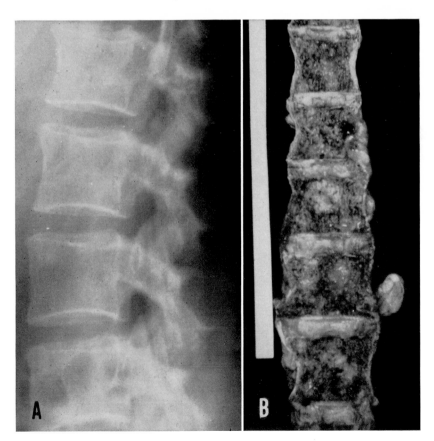

Fig. 284. *A*, Lower thoracic and upper lumbar vertebrae in a 38-year-old woman with Hodgkin's disease. There were no symptoms referable to the spine. The plain film roentgenograms were considered to be within normal limits. At necropsy, *B*, 3 weeks later extensive involvement of cancellous bone was found.

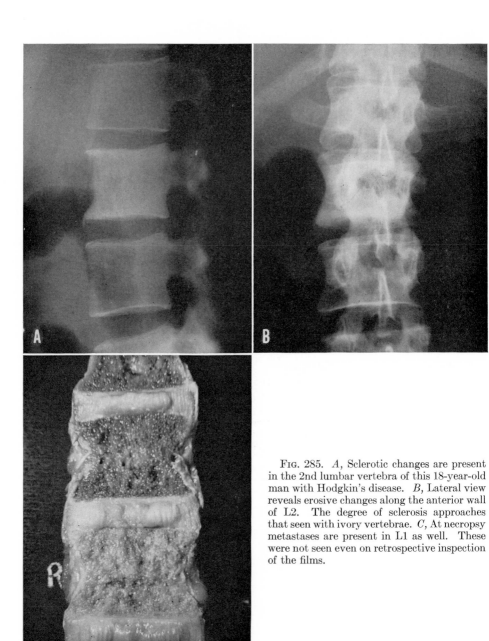

Fig. 285. *A*, Sclerotic changes are present in the 2nd lumbar vertebra of this 18-year-old man with Hodgkin's disease. *B*, Lateral view reveals erosive changes along the anterior wall of L2. The degree of sclerosis approaches that seen with ivory vertebrae. *C*, At necropsy metastases are present in L1 as well. These were not seen even on retrospective inspection of the films.

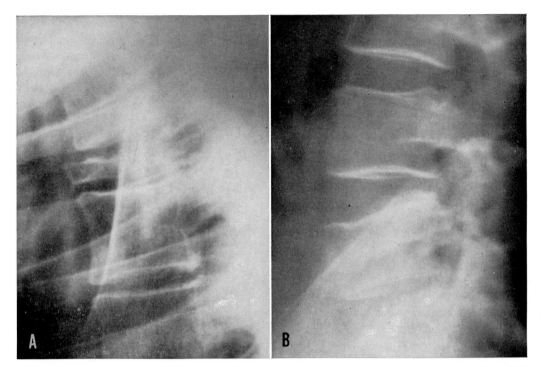

FIG. 286.   *A*, A 54-year-old man with Hodgkin's disease for more than 13 years. Vertebra plana of T4 found on spine survey because of diffuse pain. *B*, The body of L5 also is involved, with partial collapse of its upper surface.

The intervertebral discs, particularly in young people, retain their elasticity and produce deep indentations into the adjacent vertebral surfaces. However, if there is softening beneath the disc, the bone may give way and the interspace may become widened locally (Fig. 286). With more advanced softening of a vertebral body, bulging of the lateral margins occurs, so that the affected segment presents a slight convexity on its lateral or anterior aspect. Another infrequent change is the appearance of a reticular bony network, more likely to involve the transverse processes and the adjacent ribs, although the vertebral body or the sacrum may be altered (Fig. 287). Erosive changes along the anterior aspect of a vertebral body is regarded as more or less characteristic of lymphomatous invasion (Figs. 286 and 288) (Mosely, 1962).

Paravertebral swelling in lymphomas occurs incident to the appearance of lymph nodes in the adjacent soft tissues (Fig. 289), a condition which can be identified by lymphangiography. Penetration of the cortex of a diseased vertebra also can result in paravertebral swelling indistinguishable from lesion producing a similar change such as metastatic disease from other tumors, granulomas or infections.

The diagnosis of lymphomatous invasion of the spine usually is made when the patient is known to have the disease. The ivory vertebra of Paget's disease or other tumorous invasion rarely causes difficulty, and the appearance of vertebra plana also must be regarded in the light of the accompanying primary disease inasmuch as similar changes appear with myeloma or other tumors. Usually the vertebra plana of eosinophilic granuloma appears in younger patients. Quite often one is astounded by the extent of lymphomatous invasion of the spine present at necropsy and the relatively minor radiologic changes apparent before death. However, detailed radiologic investigations,

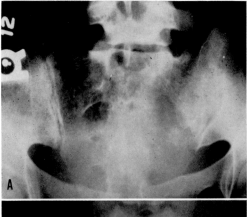

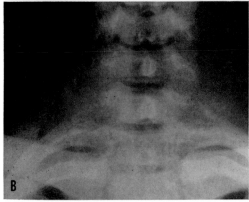

FIG. 287. *A*, A 20-year-old woman with lymphosarcoma manifested by reticular destruction of the
upper sacrum. *B*, Another patient, a 28-year-old
man who also had a reticular type of bone destruction in the cervicothoracic region.

including body section roentgenograms,
usually indicate the presence of disease even
in the absence of gross bony changes. In
such instances strontium scans of the spine
offer considerable help.

Involvement of the spinal cord and the
cauda equina usually is incident to compressive changes and extradural invasion of the
canal either from adjacent bone or from
adjacent tumorous nodes extending into the
intervertebral foramina. Diagnosis is facilitated by myelography. It is important to
suspect all evidences of medullary or cauda
equina compression as secondary to invasion
of the canal even if the plain roentgenograms
are entirely normal. Myelography should
be considered for evaluation of intraspinal
extension. Usually there is evidence of

extradural block (Figs. 290 and 291), most
often in the thoracic spinal canal. However,
localized intrusions can simulate discal herniations as well. Another uncommon form of
lymphomatous involvement is envelopment
of the roots of the cauda equina by tumor
tissue. This produces a picture of diffuse
radiculopathy and can be identified, sometimes with difficulty, by identification of
swollen nerve roots. Localized invasion of
a single nerve root also has been reported
(Hunt, Poser and Williamson, 1960).

References

Bucy, P. C. and Jerva, M. J.: Primary Epidural
    Spinal Lymphosarcoma, J. Neurosurg., *19*, 142,
    1962.
Cockshott, W. P. and Evans, K. T.: Childhood
    Paraplegia in Lymphosarcoma (Burkitt's Tumour),
    Brit. J. Radiol., *36*, 914, 1963.
Coles, W. C. and Schulz, M. D.: Bone Involve-
    ment in Malignant Lymphoma, Radiology, *50*,
    458, 1948.
Coley, B. L., Higinbotham, N. L. and Groesbeck,
    H. P.: Primary Reticulum-Cell Sarcoma of Bone,
    Radiology, *55*, 641, 1950.
Dennis, J. M.: The Solitary Dense Vertebral Body,
    Radiology, *77*, 618, 1961.
Dresser, R. and Spencer, J.: Hodgkin's Disease and
    Allied Conditions of Bone, Am. J. Roentgenol.,
    36, 809, 1936.
Edwards, J. E.: Primary Reticulum Cell Sarcoma
    of Spine, Am. J. Path., *16*, 835, 1940.
Húlten, O.: Ein Fall von "Elfenbeinwirbel" bei
    Lymphogranulomatose, Acta radiol., *8*, 245, 1927.
Hunt, T. R., Poser, C. M. and Williamson, W. P.:
    Lymphoma of Spinal Nerve Root, J. Neurosurg.,
    17, 342, 1960.
Ibbot, J. W. and Whitelaw, D. M.: The Relation
    Between Lymphosarcoma and Leukemia, Cana-
    dian M. A. J., *94*, 517, 1966.
MacCormack, J. L., Ivins, J. C., Dahlin, D. C. and
    Johnson, E. W., Jr.: Primary Reticulum Cell
    Sarcoma of Bone, Cancer, *5*, 1182, 1952.
Mosely, J. E.: Patterns of Bone Change in the
    Malignant Lymphomas, J. Mt. Sinai Hosp., *29*,
    463, 1962.
Murphy, W. T. and Bilge, N. C.: Compression of
    the Spinal Cord in Patients with Malignant
    Lymphoma, Radiology, *82*, 495, 1964.
Musshoff, K., Busch, M. and Kaminski, H.:
    Lymphogranulomatose (Morbus Hodgkin) mit
    Knochenbefall, Fortschr. Röntgenstrahl., *101*,
    117, 1964.
Oberfield, R. A.: Coexistence of Chronic Lymphatic
    Leukemia and Hodgkin's Disease, J.A.M.A., *195*,
    177, 1966.
Smith, M. J. and Stenstrom, K. W.: Compression
    of Spinal Cord Caused by Hodgkin's Disease,
    Radiology, *51*, 77, 1948.

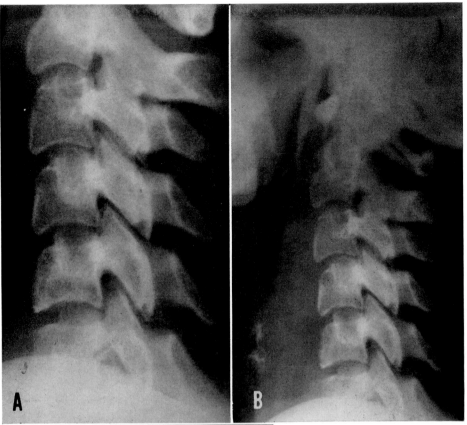

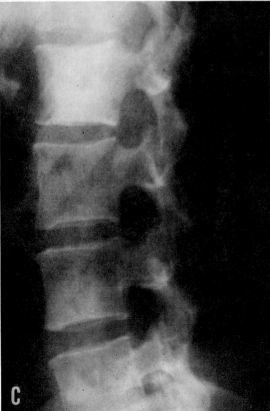

Fig. 288. *A,* A 24-year-old woman in the terminal stage of Hodgkin's disease. Erosive changes are present along the anterior aspect of the body of C5, which also bulges forward. *B,* Soft tissue swelling is present in the prevertebral area. *C,* Sclerotic changes also involve the body of T12. There were no symptoms attributable to these lesions, which were confirmed at necropsy.

433

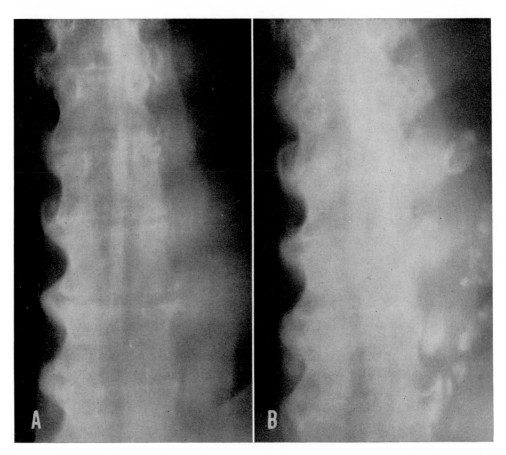

Fig. 289.   *A*, Laminagram of the lower thoracic spine in a 45-year-old man with Hodgkin's disease reveals soft tissue swelling to the left, just above the diaphragm.   *B*, Lymphangiogram discloses the lymphoid nature of the lesion, which did not affect bone insofar as could be determined radiologically.

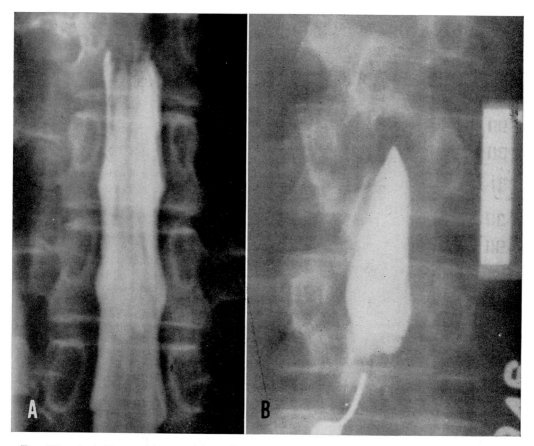

Fig. 290. *A,* A 61-year-old man with weakness of both legs progressing quickly to paraplegia. Plain film examination of the spine was normal. Myelography revealed a complete block at T10. The Pantopaque column terminates in a brush-like configuration. *B,* Another patient with Hodgkin's disease, a 50-year-old woman, also with no changes on plain spine films, but a tapered extradural block at L2.

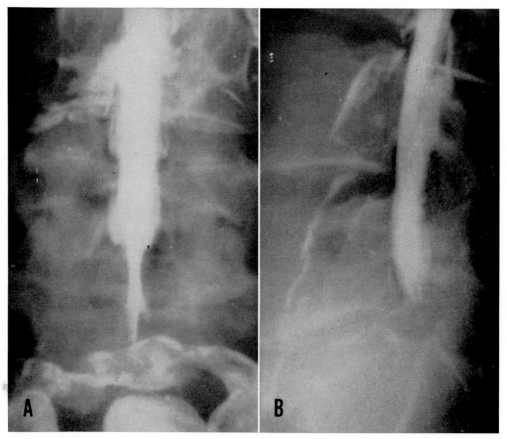

F<small>IG</small>. 291. *A*, Epidural metastases involving the caudal sac in a 32-year-old man with Hodgkin's disease.
Relief of pain followed x-ray therapy. There was no visible bony involvement.

Van Allen, M. W. and Rahme, E. S.: Lymphosar-
comatous Infiltration of the Cauda Equina, Arch.
Neurol., *7*, 476, 1962.
Verda, D. J.: Malignant Lymphoma of Spinal
Epidural Space, Surg. Clin. North America, *24*,
1228, 1944.
Viets, H. R. and Hunter, F. T.: Lymphoblastom-
atous Involvement of the Nervous System.
Arch. Neurol. & Psychiat., *29*, 1246, 1933.
Wilson, T. W. and Pugh, D. G.: Primary Reticu-
lum-Cell Sarcoma of Bone, Radiology, *65*, 343,
1955.
Witten, R. M., Fayos, J. V. and Lampe, I.: The
Dorsal Paraspinal Mass in Hodgkin's Disease,
Am. J. Roentgenol., *94*, 947, 1965.

E<small>NDOTHELIOMA</small> <small>OF</small> B<small>ONE</small> (Ewing's Sarcoma)

Ewing (1940) described this neoplasm as
an endothelial myeloma arising from the
vascular endothelium in the bone marrow.
Today it is generally accepted that the
tumor more likely is derived from the mesenchymal connective tissue framework of the
marrow. The basic cell type as described by
Ewing was a small polyhedral cell with well-
defined margins and a small hyperchromatic
nucleus. Jaffe (1945) attributed this to the
effects of degeneration, and described cells
with poorly delimited boundaries containing
fairly large round or ovoid nuclei. The histologic differential diagnosis may be difficult, these cells being quite similar to those
seen in skeletal metastases from neuro-
blastomas, reticulum cell sarcomas, lymphomas, multiple myelomas and other round
cell tumors. Ewing's tumor arises most
often in the long bones or the pelvis, and is
mainly destructive, extending along the
marrow cavity with little bony reaction. It

occurs in young people and clinically simulates an infectious or granulomatous lesion with fever, leukocytosis and local pain. In differential diagnosis the possibilities include tuberculous or pyogenic osteomyelitis, eosinophilic granuloma and osteogenic sarcoma among the others mentioned above. While the tumor is radiosensitive, the prognosis is dismal. Few patients survive for 5 years. The tumor metastasizes widely, affecting the viscera, lungs and skeletal systems. When the vertebrae are involved the marrow spaces become extensively infiltrated, with areas of necrosis and perforations of the tumor under the paraspinal ligaments and into the epidural space.

The radiologic aspects of spinal involvement with Ewing's tumor are varied. Swenson (1943) reported a case in which destruction and wedging of the ninth thoracic vertebra had been interpreted as tuberculosis of the spine, and a spinal fusion had been done. A paraspinal soft tissue mass was present. In a review of 37 cases Hamilton (1940) mentioned 2 with spinal involvement. One was a 17-year-old female with Ewing's tumor of the first and second lumbar vertebrae with slight kyphosis, tenderness and partial paraplegia, treated with laminectomy followed by x-ray therapy. This patient was living $7\frac{1}{2}$ years later (Case No. 35). His second case (No. 27) occurred in a 9-month-old infant and involved the sacrum, the tumor being of a lytic nature. Death occurred 15 months after admission. A case of Ewing's tumor simulating osteomyelitis in a 2-year-old infant was reported by Swenson and Teplick (1945). Extensive metastases involving almost every bone in the body, including marked decalcification of the spine, was noted within 2 months after admission. A finding of interest in this case was marked arterial calcification in the upper and lower extremities. These authors speculated that the rapid bone destruction produced hypercalcemia with subsequent metastatic calcification of the vessel walls.

A series of 91 histologically proven cases, of which the end-result after 5 or more years of observation was known in 73 cases, was reported by Coley, Higinbotham and Bowden (1948). Only 3 survived 5 years or

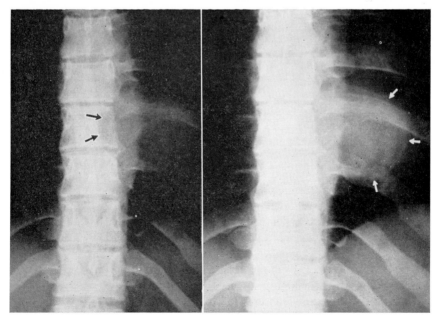

Fig. 292. *A*, Ewing's tumor of the seventh thoracic vertebra. The left pedicle and the adjacent portion of the vertebral body are destroyed (arrows). *B*, Same case, soft tissue roentgenogram. Note the large paravertebral soft tissue mass extending to the left (arrows).

more regardless of treatment. Neurological complications were frequent and disturbing. In 14 cases studied at necropsy, vertebral metastases were encountered in 4, and in 74 cases vertebral metastases were suspected on clinical grounds in 21. In 3 cases pathologic fractures of the vertebrae were observed. In 3 the site of the primary lesion was in the sacrum, and none was noted primarily in the spine.

In our material there were 2 verified cases of spinal Ewing's tumor. In the first (Fig. 292), a 10-year-old boy, the eighth thoracic vertebra had a lytic lesion involving the left lateral aspect of the body. Adjacent thereto was a large soft tissue swelling. The diagnosis was verified by biopsy. Girdle pain at the level of the seventh rib had been present intermittently for about a year but became rapidly progressive a few days before admission. Other neurologic signs included increased reflexes in the lower extremities, loss of bladder control and progressive weakness which progressed to a complete paraplegia at admission. At laminectomy tumor tissue extended into the left side of the spinal canal epidurally from the sixth to the eighth thoracic vertebra, deviating the cord towards the right.

The second case was a 23-year-old woman who had pain in the back following a fall, with numbness in the left buttock and pain radiating to the left posterior thigh. This patient had had a swelling over the right second metatarsal bone for 13 years. Myelography disclosed displacement of the Pantopaque column from right to left at the fifth lumbar vertebra. The caudal sac assumed a sharp tapered appearance, associated with epidural metastases. At laminectomy a tense reddish mass deflected the cord from the fourth lumbar vertebra downward towards the right. This mass was extradural and encapsulated. Biopsy showed this tumor to be an endothelial myeloma. X-ray examination of the hand showed a destructive lesion of the shaft of the second metatarsal bone consistent with the diagnosis of a Ewing's tumor. This patient did

quite well for about 3 years following operation with x-ray therapy both to the spine and to the hand, with regeneration of the bone of the hand. The plain roentgenograms of the spine before myelography were normal and reinspection of the films after operation failed to disclose any evidence of bony destruction.

References

Barden, R. P.: The Similarity of Clinical and Roentgen Findings in Children with Ewing's Sarcoma (Endothelial Myeloma) and Sympathetic Neuroblastoma, Am. J. Roentgenol., 50, 575, 1943.

Coley, B. L., Higinbotham, N. L. and Bowden, L.: Endothelioma of Bone, Ann. Surg., 128, 533, 1948.

Ewing, J. E.: Neoplastic Diseases, 4th Ed., Philadelphia, W. B. Saunders Co., 1940.

Hamilton, J. F.: Ewing's Sarcoma, Arch. Surg., 41, 29. 1940.

Jaffe, H. L.: The Problem of Ewing Sarcoma of Bone, Bull. Hosp. Joint Diseases, 6, 82, 1945.

Lichtenstein, L. and Jaffe, H. L.: Ewing's Sarcoma of Bone, Am. J. Path., 23, 43, 1947.

Lumb, G. and Mackenzie, D. H.: Round-Cell Tumours of Bone, Brit. J. Surg., 43, 380, 1956.

McCormack, L. J., Dockerty, M. B. and Ghormley, R. K.: Ewing's Sarcoma, Cancer, 5, 85, 1952.

Neely, J. M. and Rogers, F. T.: Roentgenological and Pathological Considerations of Ewing's Tumor of Bone, Am. J. Roentgenol., 43, 204, 1940.

Stout, A. P.: A Discussion of the Pathology and Histogenesis of Ewing's Tumor of Bone Marrow, Am. J. Roentgenol., 50, 334, 1943.

Swenson, P. C. and Teplick, J. G.: Ewing's Sarcoma, Radiology, 45, 594, 1945.

Wang, C. C. and Schulz, M. D.: Ewing's Sarcoma: A Study of Fifty Cases Treated at the Massachusetts General Hospital, 1930–1952 Inclusive, New England J. Med., 248, 571, 1953.

SARCOMAS OF THE VERTEBRAL COLUMN

Osteogenic sarcoma arises from the primitive bone-forming mesenchyme. The proliferating connective tissue is often anaplastic, and produces both tumor osteoid and bone tissue. Occasionally the proliferating connective tissue develops cartilage which rapidly undergoes further differentiation into bone. Osteogenic sarcomas appear more often in males in adolescent and early adult life. However, cases are encountered in adults, some with malignant degeneration of Paget's disease. Previous irradiation also

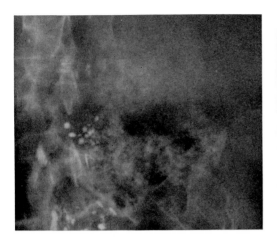

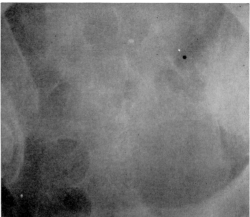

Fig. 293. Sclerosing osteogenic sarcoma probably originating from a transverse process.

Fig. 294. Osteolytic variety of osteogenic sarcoma involving the left hemisacrum of a 57-year-old woman with sciatic pain.

may be a causative factor. While the usual sites of origin are in the long bones, particularly in the vicinity of the knee and shoulder, such tumors also arise in the pelvis or spine. It is believed that osteogenic sarcomas first appear in the cancellous bone, and gradually erode through the cortex, perforating the periosteum and expanding into the adjacent soft tissues. It is during this stage that the destruction of bone and elevation of the periosteum may be demonstrated.

In some the bone forming tendency of the tumor is manifested by calcifications in the tumor (Fig. 293). As the tumor expands into the adjacent soft tissues foci of bone formation can be demonstrated in the periphery of the tumor as well as in its center. Extension through articular cartilage is rare. The histologic pattern of osteogenic sarcoma is variable. The diagnosis is based on the presence of a frankly sarcomatous stroma and the direct formation of tumor osteoid and bone.

In addition to the bone forming of osteogenic sarcoma one occasionally encounters such a tumor which is predominantly lytic (Fig. 294). These tumors are characterized by the coexistence of necrotic softening and hemorrhage with little or no evidence of tumor osteoid or pathologic bone formation. Roentgenologically they are difficult to identify, and the lytic sarcomatous nature of the disease requires histologic examination for identification.

The occurrence of osteogenic sarcoma in the vertebral column is infrequent. Geschickter and Copeland (1949) identified 187 cases of sclerosing osteogenic sarcoma from a total of 750 osteogenic sarcomas. The favorite site of origin was in the metaphyses of the long bones adjacent to the epiphyseal lines. They mentioned that only a few isolated cases occurred in the ribs, vertebrae, and the pelvis. In reviewing their Table 17, 1 case of sclerosing osteogenic sarcoma of the sacrum is noted in the 109 cases listed. In Table 18, also headed as osteogenic sclerosing sarcoma, 1 case involving the second and third lumbar vertebrae was noted out of a total of 78 cases. Under a heading of osteogenic osteolytic sarcoma 1 case involving the vertebrae is listed out of a total of 62. Listed in Table 22, also headed as osteogenic osteolytic sarcoma, no examples of vertebral tumors were encountered in 88 cases.

In my experience 3 cases of osteogenic sarcoma of the osteolytic variety were observed. In one the fourth lumbar vertebra was involved, and the radiographic picture was that of a slightly flattened, decalcified vertebra with slightly bulging edges. The

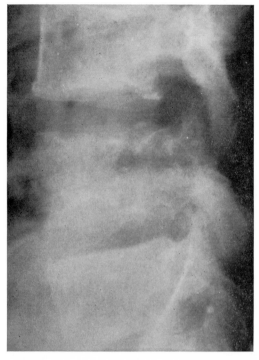

FIG. 295. A 47-year-old man who developed low back pain and sciatica after trauma, diagnosed as a herniated disc. Osteogenic sarcoma of L4 was found, with considerable destruction of bone in the dorsal aspect of the body of the vertebra and the pedicles.

intervertebral discs were normal, and its appearance suggested a lytic metastasis (Fig. 295). The true nature of the tumor was discovered at necropsy. The second was in an 18-month-old infant. The third case involved the fifth thoracic vertebra and its nature was discovered at laminectomy for spinal cord compression.

Fibrosarcoma. Lichtenstein (1952) described fibrosarcoma of bone as a primary malignant fibroblastic tumor which does not form osteoid or bone, either locally or in its metastases. This tumor usually originates in cancellous bone, and manifests itself by outward growth, perforating the cortex and extending into the adjacent tissues (Fig. 296). Occasionally fibrosarcomas arise from the periosteum, and extend directly through the cortex. Stout (1948) considered these relatively benign growths of the fibroblasts,

and presented an example of a fibrosarcoma of the periosteum of the coccyx which pressed forward to indent the rectum. This tumor did not recur 16 years after resection.

In my series there are 5 cases of fibrosarcomas of the spine. These occurred in young and middle-aged adults, and involved the fourth lumbar vertebra in one case, the fifth lumbar vertebra in another (Fig. 297) and the upper portion of the sacrum in the remaining three (Fig. 298). The lesion was characterized by a faint diffuse lytic process with a mild sclerotic reaction within the tumor. In 3 cases myelographic examination was done because the clinical picture simulated that of a herniated disc. The distal end of the Pantopaque-filled thecal sac was tapered and deviated contralaterally. At operation the change was found to be due to epidural extension of the tumor tissue from the bone malignancy (Fig. 297). In 2 of these cases the roentgenograms made before myelography had been considered within normal limits and the lesion was identified only after the operative findings were known.

Chondrosarcoma. This is a malignant tumor of mature cartilage which not infrequently appears as a degenerative lesion in benign enchondromas, or less often, as malignant degeneration of the cartilaginous cap of an osteochondroma. Chondrosarcomas were classified by Lichtenstein and Jaffe (1943) as central, originating within bone, while those which appeared as malignant degeneration of the cartilaginous cap of an osteochondroma were referred to as peripheral chondrosarcomas. These tumors usually occur in adults between 30 and 50 years of age. The most common sites for this tumor are the long bones, the pelvis and the ribs, but they have been reported in the spine as well.

In our experience we have an instance in which a chondroma arising from the lamina of the seventh dorsal vertebra underwent malignant degeneration, eroded into its body and extended into the adjacent soft tissues (Fig. 299). The presenting symptoms were

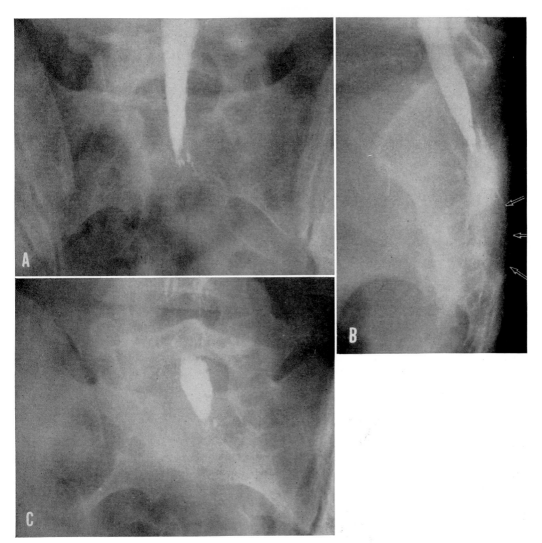

Fig. 296.   *A*, A 47-year-old man with a clinical diagnosis of left herniated lower lumbar disc.   AP myelo-gram reveals a tapered caudal sac shifted slightly to the left.   There is a faint lytic process involving the upper right sacrum.   *B*, The dorsal plate of the sacrum is destroyed (arrows).   At operation a fibrosarcoma of the sacrum was found.   *C*, After x-ray therapy the lesion filled in and the caudal sac distended.

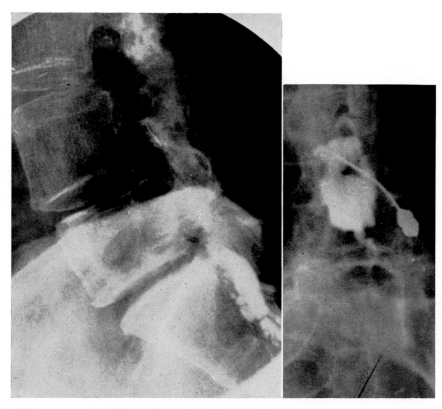

Fig. 297. Fibrosarcoma of the fifth lumbar vertebra with destruction of the posterior aspect of the vertebral body. Complete block is present at the fourth lumbar interspace.

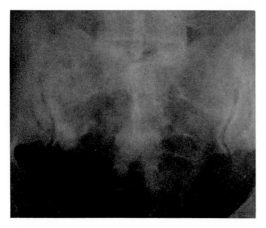

Fig. 298. Fibrosarcoma of the upper right sacrum in a 58-year-old woman with right sciatic pain for 2 months. A sclerotic reaction is present in the tumor.

slowly progressive, starting with pain in the back and terminating with paraplegia. This patient, a 27-year-old male, was afflicted with hereditary multiple exostoses and undoubtedly one of these lesions was the source for the osteochondrosarcoma which caused his death. Another patient succumbed to a similar lesion involving the upper lumbar vertebrae (Fig. 300). The development of chondrosarcoma on the lesions of Ollier's disease has also been described.

Chondrosarcomas of bone are relatively slow growing tumors which metastasize late. They tend to be locally invasive for a long time before penetrating bone and extending into the adjacent tissues or metastasizing distally. This occurred in another of our cases in which the sacrum and coccyx were affected (Fig. 301).

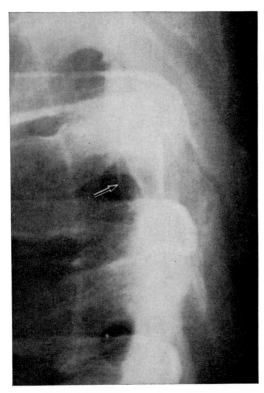

FIG. 299. Osteochondrosarcoma originating in the base of the spinous process of T7, extending into the spinal canal causing extradural compression. Note the curvilinear thin calcific line indenting into the canal (arrow). The patient was a 59-year-old man who had girdle pain at that level.

An unusual case of a chondrosarcoma extending into the abdominal venous trunks from the lower spine was described by Ernst (1900). In a review of 40 chondrosarcomas of bone O'Neil and Ackerman (1952) described 2 cases involving the spine, one arising from the spinous process and lamina of the second cervical vertebra, and the other from the body of the sixth dorsal vertebra.

Angiosarcomas are malignant tumors of blood vessels which are better designated as hemangio-endotheliomas. The usual site of occurrence is at the proximal ends of the long bones, particularly the femurs and humeri, the hands, feet, pelvis, and rarely the vertebrae. The tumor is predominantly a destructive one which gives rise to a wide expansion of the bone, and presents a rather

characteristic appearance which has been described as "soap bubbles."

The neoplasm is formed by blood vessels, and is characterized by an interwoven network of anastomosing vascular channels. The increased circulation in the tumor may give rise to an audible bruit, and sometimes a pulsation within the tumor can be detected on physical examination.

The incidence of hemangio-endotheliomas in the spine must be infrequent. I have not found any specific reference to this tumor as involving the vertebrae except for mention by Brailsford who included the vertebrae among the sites of origin.

Mesenchymal chondrosarcomas occur in a single bone, and after a long interval, appear in other bones. Visceral spread occurs terminally. The tumor is believed to be derived from cartilage-forming mesenchyme, and probably is multicentric in origin. Lichtenstein and Bernstein (1959) reported such a tumor in a 26-year-old man with paraplegia from extradural cord compression at the fourth and fifth thoracic vertebrae. One of our patients was a 48-year-old man who presented with symptoms of cord compression. His spine roentgenograms were normal, but myelography revealed a block at the fourth thoracic level. He did well after decompression, and the diagnosis was osteochondroblastoma. Three years later he returned with similar symptoms. Roentgenograms of his spine disclosed a lytic lesion on the left side of the third thoracic vertebra with extension into the adjacent soft tissues. An extradural block was again demonstrated, and at operation it was found wrapped in tumor tissue. This now was diagnosed as mesenchymal chondrosarcoma (Fig. 302). Since then he has had two local recurrences, both requiring decompressive operations 1 and 3 years later. Dahlin and Henderson (1962) reported 10 such tumors in various locations, all in adults. These tumors metastasized to unusual locations, sometimes after a remarkable delay.

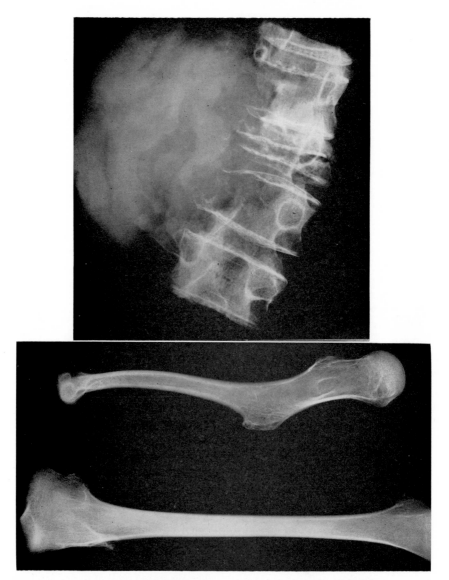

Fig. 300.   Roentgenogram of necropsy specimen of sarcoma destroying second, third and fourth lumbar vertebrae.   Note the large paravertebral soft tissue extension.   The long bone specimens show multiple hereditary exostoses.   It was believed that the spine sarcoma originated from one of these even though no other exostoses could be found in the vertebrae.

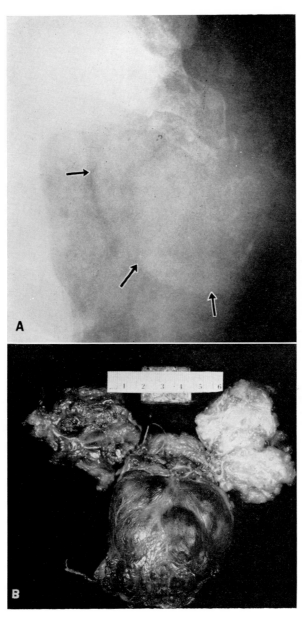

FIG. 301. *A*, Osteochondrosarcoma of the sacrum with destruction of its distal half. A large soft tissue mass is seen (arrows). *B*, Same case, Operative specimen.

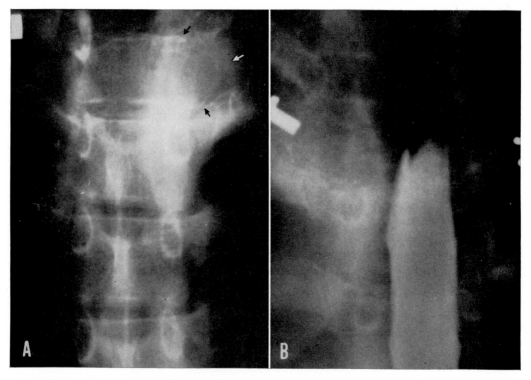

Fig. 302. *A*, A lytic lesion involves the left side of the body of T4. When this 38-year-old man was first seen his spine was normal, but myelography revealed a complete block in the upper thoracic canal after a 3-week period of numbness of both legs and a sensory level at T-4. At operation the dura was compressed by intraspinal extension of an "osteochondroblastoma." The present study 3 years later reveals destruction of the left side of T3, with extension of tumor into the adjacent soft tissues (arrows). *B*, Myelography reveals a complete block. At operation the cord was wrapped in tumor, which proved to be a mesenchymal chondrosarcoma. (From Epstein, B. S.: Spinal Canal Mass Lesions, Radiol. Clin. North America, *4*, 185, 1966.)

References

Aronstram, E. M., Ludden, T. E. and Matuska, W. H.: Chondrosarcoma of the Thoracic Spine, J. Thoracic Surg., *31*, 725, 1956.

Brailsford, J. F.: *Radiology of Bones and Joints*, 5th Ed., Baltimore, The Williams & Wilkins Co., 1953.

Carter, J. H., Dickinson, R. and Needy, C.: Angiosarcoma of Bone, Ann. Surg., *144*, 107, 1956.

Coventry, M. B. and Dahlin, D. C.: Osteogenic Sarcoma, J. Bone & Joint Surg., *39-A*, 741, 1957.

Dahlin, D. C. and Coventry, M. B.: Osteogenic Sarcoma, J. Bone & Joint Surg., *49-A*, 101, 1967.

Dahlin, D. C. and Henderson, E. C.: Mesenchymal Chondrosarcoma, Cancer, *15*, 410, 1962.

Ernst, P.: Ungewöhnliche Verbreitung einer Knorpelgeschwulst in der Blutbahn, Beitr. z. path. Anat. u. z. allg. Path., *28*, 255, 1900.

Geschickter, C. F. and Copeland, M. M.: *Tumors of Bone*, 3rd Ed., Philadelphia, J. B. Lippincott Co., 1949.

Gokay, H. and Bucy, P. C.: Osteochondroma of the Lumbar Spine, J. Neurosurg., *12*, 72, 1955.

Jaffe, H. L.: *Tumors and Tumorous Conditions of the Bones and Joints*, Lea & Febiger, Philadelphia, 1958.

Lichtenstein, L.: *Bone Tumors*, 3rd Ed., St. Louis, The C. V. Mosby Co., 1965.

Lichtenstein, L. and Jaffe, H. L.: Chondrosarcoma of Bone, Am. J. Path., *19*, 553, 1943.

Lichtenstein, L. and Bernstein, D.: Unusual Benign and Malignant Chondroid Tumors of Bone, Cancer, *12*, 1142, 1959.

O'Neil, L. W. and Ackerman, L. V.: Chondrosarcoma of Bone, Cancer, *5*, 551, 1952.

Stout, A. P.: Fibrosarcoma, Cancer, *1*, 30, 1948.

Chordomas

These infrequent, slowly growing malignant tumors originate from remnants of the notochord and occur mostly at the cephalic and caudal ends of the vertebral column. Horowitz (1941) showed that the topographic distribution of heterotopic chordal vestiges correspond closely to the sites of chordomas. Schmorl (1928) demonstrated spinal chordal remnants in 9 adult cadavers in dissection of over 3000 human vertebral columns. In 6 these were placed posteriorly in the vertebral bodies; in 2 centrally, and in 1 instance laterally. While these tumors occur predominantly in the region of the clivus Blumenbachii and the sacrococcygeal region, they also are found in the cervical, thoracic and lumbar spine. They never originate in the intervertebral discs.

In a study of 59 cases by Dahlin and MacCarty (1952) 15 chordomas were found in the vincinity of the clivus Blumenbachii, and 32 in the sacrum. Of the remainder, 9 occurred in the cervical region, 2 in the fourth lumbar vertebra and 1 in the eleventh thoracic vertebra. Wood and Himadi (1950) in a report of 16 cases, encountered 7 in the clivus, 1 in the nasopharynx, 5 in the vertebrae, and 3 in the sacrococcygeal region. A review of the literature by Faust, Gilmore and Mudgett (1944) disclosed 252 cases. Of these 92 were cranial, including the spheno-occipital and nasopharyngeal regions, 34 were vertebral in location and 122 were caudal or sacrococcygeal in location. Four were mentioned as occurring in the other regions. Littman (1953) summarized the literature on sacrococcygeal chordoma and gathered 168 cases in patients varying in age from infancy to over 80 years.

Chordomas are usually round or lobulated masses of soft gelatinous tissue containing areas of cystic degeneration, necrosis, hemorrhage and sometimes calcification. In their early stages the growths usually are circumscribed, but as they grow penetration of the capsule occurs and the tumor invades adjacent bony structures and soft tissues. This is particularly apparent in sacral chordomas, where large presacral and infra-sacrococcygeal soft tissue masses appear (Fig. 303). In the cervical area, these tumors may project into the retropharyngeal region sufficiently to manifest themselves by dysphagia or other symptoms of a retropharyngeal mass. Chordomas arising from the odontoid process have also been encountered. Tumors occurring in the vertebral column in areas other than the proximal and distal ends usually arise within a vertebral body. The illustrations of chordomas entering the posterior and anterior cranial fossae published by Adson, Kernohan and Woltman (1935) are of considerable interest.

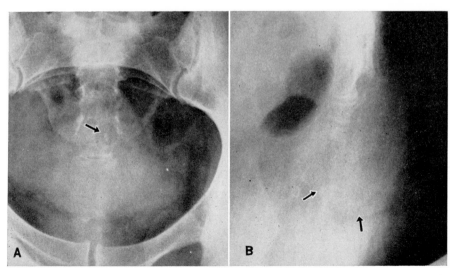

Fig. 303. *A*, Sacrococcygeal chordoma, with destruction of coccyx with a central locule to the left of the midline in the lower sacrum (arrow). A soft tissue mass is seen just below the coccyx. *B*, Same case. Note the bony destruction and the adjacent soft tissue tumor (arrows).

Chordomas present microscopic changes which simulate the embryonic notochord, being composed of large polyhedral cells with small nuclei and vacuolated cytoplasm distended with glycogen and mucin-like material. The cells are arranged in cords, separated by a fine trabeculated stroma of connective tissue.

In an early stage, when chordoma has not destroyed its bony confines or protruded into an area in which altered function might bring the patient to the physician, the tumor may be symptomless. Once growth starts the clinical picture depends on the area invaded and the extent of the tumor. Sometimes chordomas reach a considerable size. In the case reported by Faust, Gilmore and Mudgett (1944) a sacrococcygeal chordoma extended into the lower quadrant of the abdomen. In our experience 3 sacral chordomas reached a diameter of more than 15 cm.

Chordomas originating in the spine may first manifest themselves because of pressure on the spinal cord or nerve roots. In those tumors originating low in the lumbar spine, a clinical picture suggestive of a herniated disc may be encountered, while those originating higher in the vertebral column produce a syndrome of spinal cord compression. Some chordomas simulate a destructive lesion of the vertebral body. If the vertebral body is involved, the roentgenograms may show a rounded cavity (Fig. 304), mottled appearance or collapse of the vertebral body (Fig. 306). Richards and King (1940) reported a 52-year-old male with a chordoma arising in the third lumbar vertebra. Serial studies showed progressive destruction over a 5-year period, starting with a decalcified vertebral body and discoid intervertebral discs above and beneath the lesion. The tumor advanced until there was complete collapse of the vertebral body,

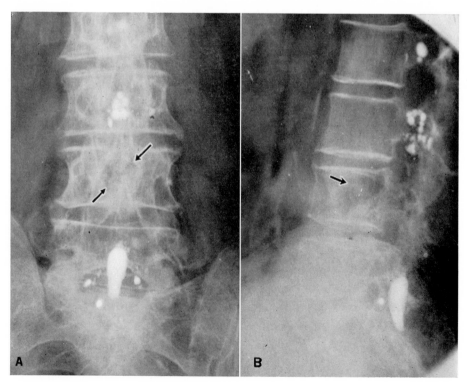

Fig. 304. *A*, Chordoma originating in the fourth lumbar vertebra. A central area of rarefaction is seen (arrows). *B*. The rarefaction within the vertebral body is better visualized on this projection (arrow).

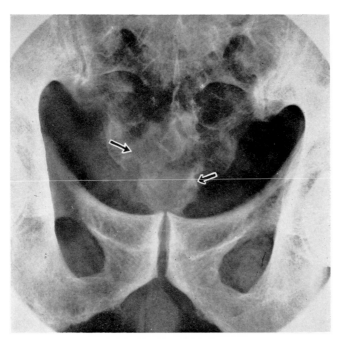

Fig. 305. Sacrococcygeal chordoma, with mottled bands and islands of bone within the area of the tumor in the lower sacrum (arrows).

marked decalcification of the adjacent vertebrae and distortion of the interposed discs. Nerve involvement was minimal for the size and location of the tumor. In the case reported by Robbins (1945), a 41-year-old man with a vertebral chordoma who died 9 days after laparotomy had a large mass adherent to many abdominal organs. Morris and Rabinovitch (1947) reported a chordoma in a 27-year-old woman with initial signs and symptoms of a herniated lower lumbar disc. Myelography disclosed a block and at operation an extradural mass was observed opposite the lumbosacral disc which could be followed into the body of the fifth lumbar vertebra.

Wood and Himadi (1950) described 5 cases of vertebral chordoma. Two or more adjacent vertebrae were involved, the tumor extending from the segment of origin to an adjoining vertebra by growth through the intervening intervertebral disc. Bone destruction was a prominent feature, the final stages being compression fractures. In 2 osteoblastic reactions were observed, and expansion of a vertebral body extending into its transverse processes was seen in 1. In 2 myelographic examination showed complete obstruction. The Pantopaque column tapered gradually to the point of obstruction seen with an epidural mass compressing the dural sac. Poppen and King (1952) in a report on 6 cases of spinal chordoma, observed 3 in the lumbar or sacral regions. In all the tumors were extensive, and the spinal cord, the cauda equina and the nerve roots were compressed by extradural masses. At times the dura was penetrated, with marked intradural extension. In these the tumors displayed an embryonal facility for easy penetration of bone, dura and nervous tissue. In 3 which occurred in the cervical region, the diagnosis was not made preoperatively. All were thought to have metastatic malignancy. Gentil and Coley (1948) mentioned that an analysis revealed that a correct x-ray diagnosis had been made in but 10 per cent.

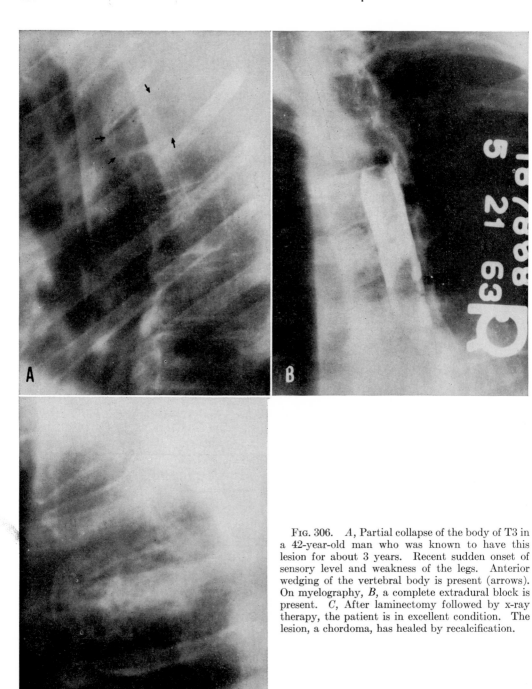

FIG. 306. *A,* Partial collapse of the body of T3 in a 42-year-old man who was known to have this lesion for about 3 years. Recent sudden onset of sensory level and weakness of the legs. Anterior wedging of the vertebral body is present (arrows). On myelography, *B,* a complete extradural block is present. *C,* After laminectomy followed by x-ray therapy, the patient is in excellent condition. The lesion, a chordoma, has healed by recalcification.

Chordomas in the thoracic region are rare. A case was described by Hansson (1941) in a 45-year-old man with a level of hyperaesthesia at the sixth and seventh thoracic segments. X-ray examination showed destruction of the neural arches, and operation revealed that the cartilage between the seventh and eighth thoracic vertebrae had been transformed into a bluish tumor mass which penetrated into the vertebral body. Bahlin and MacCarty (1952) mentioned that in their case of chordoma of the eleventh thoracic vertebra, decompression and subtotal removal were carried out. This resulted in a 6-year remission, and reoperation for recurrence was necessary $6\frac{1}{2}$ years after the original operation.

We observed two vertebral chordomas. One occurred in a 52-year-old woman with low back pain extending into the right lower leg. The clinical picture was compatible with a herniated disc. Myelographic examination, performed after plain roentgenograms showed no evidence of bony change, showed a defect at the fourth lumbar interspace. At operation tumor was noted epidurally. This was a soft, gelatinous, friable mass which involved the body of the third lumbar vertebra inferiorly and the fourth lumbar vertebra superiorly as well as the intervertebral disc. The tumor was removed as completely as possible. Histologic examination revealed changes characteristic of chordoma. X-ray therapy was given postoperatively, and the patient was relieved of symptoms. She returned about 1 year later complaining of pain in the back. Further radiographic examination then disclosed a circular rarefied area within the body of the fourth lumbar vertebra without any distortion of the contours of this segment (Fig. 304). X-ray therapy was again given and the patient improved again.

The second patient was a 46-year-old man who had been complaining of pain over the upper thoracic spine for about 18 months, at which time a destructive lesion of the fourth thoracic vertebra was found on x-ray examination. No neurologic symptoms were present. The pain varied in severity until about 3 weeks before admission, when it became intense. This was followed by severe paresis of the lower extremities and a sensory level at about T6. Plain film examination disclosed a grossly lytic lesion at T4, and myelography revealed an extradural block at this site. At operation a soft, pink extradural tumor was found within the canal extending from the body of the fourth thoracic vertebra. This proved to be a chordoma. The patient did very well after supervoltage x-ray therapy. Three years later he was in excellent condition and the fourth thoracic vertebra displayed a heavy, mottled calcification (Fig. 306).

Clivus chordomas occasionally are confused with nasopharyngeal tumors producing marked destruction of the sphenoid bone. This sometimes mimics pituitary adenoma (Epstein, 1966), or may present as a thickening of the dorsum sellae (Epstein and Davidoff, 1953).

While chordomas are known to be locally invasive, systemic metastases are relatively uncommon. In 1921 Lewis described 4 chordomas, in 3 of which there were extensive metastases. Stewart (1922) demonstrated invasion of the blood vessels. Willis (1930) reported a sacral chordoma with widespread metastases. Mabrey (1935) observed that metastases occurred only in sacrococcygeal chordomas. He reported 10 cases with metastases from a group of 16 sacrococcygeal chordomas with postportem examinations. The regional lymph nodes were involved most often and blood borne metastases to the liver, lungs, pleura, peritoneum and other organs were present.

The roentgenologic changes associated with chordomas are predominantly lytic. Those tumors originating in the upper cervical region may destroy the bodies and occasionally the neural arches, producing changes in alignment of the cervico-occipital area. A fairly common site of origin in this rare condition is the odontoid process. Soft tissue swelling anteriorly into the nasopharynx is an early manifestation, and ap-

30

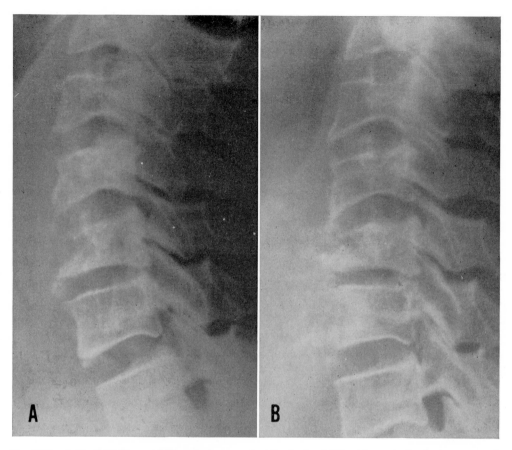

Fig. 307. *A*, Partial collapse of the anterior aspect of the body of C5, with marked soft tissue extension into the retropharyngeal and retrotracheal areas from a chordoma. *B*, About 8 months later extensive calcification is noted in the soft tissues. (Courtesy of M. Schechter, M.D., Albert Einstein College of Medicine.)

pears even when the destructive bone chagnes are minimal or even invisible. Calcification occasionally is present in the soft tissue extravertebral tumor (Fig. 307). In a case mentioned by Sennett (1953) the cervical esophagus was displaced anteriorly and to the right by a soft tissue mass emanating from a cervical chordoma. Myelographically, varying degrees of extradural block are noted when the spinal canal is compromised.

Chordomas in the thoracic or lumbar vertebrae usually produce bone destruction which cannot be differentiated accurately from other neoplasms. These growths are slowly progressive, and a tendency for dislocation or collapse of the vertebral body exists (Fig. 306). Osteoblastic reactions are infrequent. As noted in one of our cases, the plain films may be entirely normal, and vertebral and discal involvement be identified at operation for spinal cord compression.

Sacrococcygeal chordomas occur most frequently and present a varied roentgenographic appearance. Expansion of the sacrum as observed in the lateral view is a common feature in the early stages. The sacrum is slowly destroyed by the chordoma, and extension into the soft tissues as a relatively well-defined mass can be noted on appropriate roentgenograms. The destroyed edge of bone from which the tumor emerges leads to a correct interpretation in some cases. Remnants of calcification within the soft tissue mass may be present. Compression of the rectum and bladder by the soft tissue components of sacrococcygeal chordomas can produce symptoms, but as a rule the growths do not ulcerate through these structures.

Symptoms depend on the location and extent of the chordoma as well as its potential for entering the spinal canal. When considerable bone destruction is present the appearance often cannot be distinguished from that due to osteomyelitis or metastatic tumor. If paravertebral swelling is seen, it mimics that seen with osteomyelitis of infectious or granulomatous origin. Tumors low in the lumbar canal simulate herniated discs, and when little bone destruction exists, the diagnosis is made on histologic examination of tumor tissue removed from the epidural space. Similar tumors in the nasopharynx simulate primary tumors of this area such as lymphoepitheliomas or carcinomas, more so if there is destruction of the sphenoid. High cervical tumors, with or without intraspinal protrusion, likewise must be considered. Extension of chordoma into the pelvis and abdomen may simulate ovarian cysts or other tumors, and with spread a picture like that of peritoneal carcinosis of other origin appears. Tumors still confined within a capsule cannot be distinguished clinically from other presacral new growths. With destruction of the sacrum metastatic or primary tumors, presacral neurofibromas or meningoceles must be considered. The infrequent chordomas originating within the bodies of vertebrae may be confused with primary tumors, and diagnosis is established by biopsy.

References

Adson, A. W. Kernohan, J. W. and Woltman, H. W.: Cranial and Cervical Chordomas, Arch. Neurol. & Psychiat., *33*, 247, 1935.

Baker, H. W. and Coley, B. L.: Chordoma of Lumbar Vertebrae, J. Bone & Joint Surg., *35-A*, 403, 1953.

Dahlin, D. C. and MacCarty, C. S.: Chordoma, Cancer, *5*, 1170, 1952.

Epstein, B. S.: *Pneumoencephalography and Cerebral Angiography*, Chicago, The Year Book Medical Publishers, Inc., 1966.

Epstein, B. S. and Davidoff, L. M.: *An Atlas of Skull Roentgenograms*, Philadelphia, Lea & Febiger, 1953.

Faust, D. B., Gilmore, H. R., Jr. and Mudgett, C. S.: Chordomata, Ann. Int. Med., *21*, 678, 1944.

Gentil, F. and Coley, B. L.: Sacrococcygeal Chordoma, Ann. Surg., *127*, 432, 1948.

Greenwald, C. M., Meaney, T. F. and Hughes, C. R.: Chordoma—Uncommon Destructive Lesion of Cerebrospinal Axis, J.A.M.A., *163*, 1240, 1957.

Hansson, C. J.: Chordoma in a Thoracic Vertebra, Acta radiol., *22*, 598, 1941.

Horwitz, T.: Chordal Ectopia and its Possible Relation to Chordoma, Arch. Path., *31*, 354, 1941.

Hsieh, C. K. and Hsieh, H. H.: Sacrococcygeal Chordoma, Radiology, *27*, 101, 1936.

Husain, F.: Chordoma of the Thoracic Region, J. Bone & Joint Surg., *42-B*, 560, 1960.

Lewis, N. D. C.: Tumors from the Primitive Notochord, Arch. Int. Med., *28*, 434, 1921.

Littman, L.: Sacro-Coccygeal Chordoma, Ann. Surg., *137*, 80, 1953.

Mabrey, R. E.: Chordoma, Am. J. Cancer, *25*, 501, 1935.

McCormack, M. P.: Upper Lumbar Chordoma, J. Bone & Joint Surg., *42-B*, 565, 1960.

Mixter, C. G. and Mixter, W. J.: Surgical Management of Sacrococcygeal and Vertebral Chordoma, Arch. Surg., *41*, 408, 1940.

Morris, A. A. and Rabinovitch, R.: Malignant Chordoma of Lumbar Region, Arch. Neurol. & Psychiat., *57*, 547, 1947.

Poppen, J. L. and King, A. B.: Chordoma, J. Neurosurg., *9*, 139, 1952.

Reich, W. J. and Nechtwo, M. J.: Cystic Pelvic Chordoma Simulating an Ovarian Cyst, Am. J. Obst. & Gynec., *49*, 265, 1945.

Richards, V. and King, D.: Chordoma, Surgery, *8*, 409, 1040.

Robbins, S. L.: Lumbar Vertebra Chordoma, Arch. Path., *40*, 128, 1945.

Schmorl, G.: Über Chordareste in den Wirbelkörpern, Zentralbl. f. Chir., *55*, 2305, 1929.

Sennett, E. J.: Chordoma, Am. J. Roentgenol., *69*, 613, 1953.

Stewart, M. J.: Malignant Sacrococcygeal Chordoma, J. Path. & Bact., *25*, 40, 1922.

Utne, J. R. and Pugh, D. G.: The Roentgenologic Aspects of Chordoma, Am. J. Roentgenol., *74*, 593, 1955.

Willis, R. A.: Sacral Chordoma with Widespread Metastases, J. Path. & Bact., *33*, 1035, 1930.

Windeyer, B. W.: Chordoma, Proc. Royal Soc. Med., *52*, 1088, 1959.

Wood, E. H., Jr. and Himadi, G. M.: Chordomas, Radiology, *54*, 706, 1950.

Sacrococcygeal Teratomas

Sacrococcygeal teratomas arise from vestigial embryonic remnants of the primitive node, and have potentiality for development of a wide variety of tumors. They appear at birth as congenital malformations, some being large enough to interfere with delivery. Other teratomas do not become manifest until later in life. These are benign tumors which may become malignant. Early operation in infancy has been recommended to avoid this possibility.

As a rule sacrococcygeal teratomas arise from the dorsal aspect of the sacrum. Concomitant congenital malformations of the vertebrae occasionally are present, as are lipomatous tumors involving the spinal canal and the cauda equina. Displacement of the bladder and rectum occurs when the tumors are large and enter the pelvis. Characteristically the tumor is situated between the rectum and the sacrum, sharply displacing the rectum and bladder so that evacuation becomes impeded. Retroperitoneal teratomas without sacral involvement also occur, but the distinction is one mainly of site of origin. The presence of calcification within the tumor favors the possibility of teratoma. Outwards extension of teratomas varies considerably, so that in some only a swelling of the buttocks is evident, while in others a large ulcerating tumor mass is visible.

Other tumors originating within the sacral canal or the sacrum itself have to be distinguished from teratomas. Those tumors of ependymal origin within the canal cause smooth loculated erosion of bone. Chordomas destroy bone, and are not as a rule manifest early in life. Bone tumors such as the various sarcomas and metastatic tumors likewise are not seen in infancy. Tumors of adjacent soft tissues such as fibromas and neurofibromas have to be considered in differential diagnosis. Congenital malformations including partial sacral agenesis and sacrococcygeal meningoceles as a rule do not present intratumoral calcification, nor do they reach the size and outward extent often present with sacrococcygeal teratomas. Eklöf (1965) regards destruction of the sacrum and coccyx or aplasia of more than two distal sacral segments as against the diagnosis of teratoma.

References

Brindley, G. V.: Sacral and Presacral Tumors, Ann. Surg., *121*, 741, 1945.

Camp, J. D. and Good, C. A.: Roentgenologic Diagnosis of Tumors Involving the Sacrum, Radiology, *31*, 398, 1938.

Eklöf, O.: Roentgenologic Findings in Sacrococcygeal Teratoma, Acta radiol., *3*, 41, 1965.

Hatteland, K. and Knutrud, O.: Sacrococcygeal Teratoma in Children, Acta chir. scandinav., *119*, 444, 1960.

Hudson, C. C. and Ross, S. T.: Presacral Neurofibroma, Am. J. Surg., *90*, 1005, 1955.

Mayo, C. W., Baker, G. S. and Smith, R. L.: Presacral Tumors, Proc. Staff Meet., Mayo Clin., *28*, 616, 1953.

McCune, W. S.: Management of Sacrococcygeal Tumors, Ann. Surg., *159*, 911, 1964.

Schiffer, M. A. and Greenberg, E.: Sacrococcygeal Teratoma in Labor and the Newborn, Am. J. Obst. & Gynec., *72*, 1054, 1958.

Willox, G. L. and MacKenzie, W. C.: Sacrococcygeal Teratomas, Arch. Surg., *83*, 11, 1961.

GIANT CELL TUMOR (Osteoclastoma)

The term giant cell tumor has been used rather loosely, and there is still uncertainty as to what should be regarded as a giant cell tumor of bone. In Lichtenstein's (1965) opinion the growth is a distinctive neoplasm which apparently arises from non-bone-forming supporting connective tissue of the marrow and can be identified readily on the basis of cytologic details. The pattern consists of a vascularized network of ovoid or spindle-shaped cells interspersed with multinuclear giant cells. He separated these tumors from others which have been confused with them. Chief among these are the xanthic, spindle cell, or healing variety of giant cell tumors which are now designated as non-osteogenic fibromas of bone. The calcifying or chondromatous giant cell tumor is now designated as benign chondroblastoma of bone, probably representing an independent benign tumor of cartilage forming connective tissue, unrelated histogenetically to giant cell tumor. Another entity termed atypical subperiosteal giant cell tumor has been clearly identified as aneurysmal bone cyst. Giant cell tumors of the spine are rare. Some lesions so designated in the past probably represent aneurysmal bone cysts. In a group of 76 giant cell tumors of bone Hutter and his co-workers (1962) found none in the vertebrae and 5 in the sacrum. Of these 3 were benign and 2 malignant. Histologically benign giant cell tumor caused death in 2 because of uncontrollable local growth. The possibility of recurrence if the tumor is not removed completely is always present, and recurrent growths are likely to be malignant.

The usual locations of giant cell tumors are the distal end of the femur, the proximal end of the tibia and the distal end of the radius, but occasionally they have been observed in the upper humerus, the upper femur and fibula, and the patella. These tumors appear in individuals between 15 and 40 years of age, and are characterized by a lytic process with little or no bone production. The cortex of the bone on the side of the tumor may practically disappear. At one time it was believed that giant cell tumor characteristically presented a latticework of bony traversing strands across the lytic area, but this view has been abandoned. The difficulty of making a diagnosis of the histologic type of a tumor on the basis of the radiographic changes alone is apparent.

The question as to biopsy verification has largely been resolved in favor of such examination of any accessible lesion (Buschke and Cantril, 1949). However they do not consider the vertebrae in this group. There are others, notably Brailsford (1944), who believe that the characteristic picture of giant cell tumor may be recognized on the roentgenogram. In his opinion excellent results can be obtained by x-ray therapy alone, and biopsy may be hazardous because stability may be weakened, and there may be dissemination of tumor cells. He suggested that surgical trauma may incite malignant metastases in some cases. Others (Murphy, 1935; Gershon-Cohen, 1943; Cade, 1949;

Prossor, 1949) hold that x-ray therapy alone may be effective, but Lichtenstein pointed out that he knew of several cases of sarcoma which developed in an irradiated and ostensibly cured giant cell tumor after a long latent interval. Cahan, Woodward, Higgenbotham, Stewart and Coley (1948) have reported several cases of sarcomatous degeneration in irradiated bone as well.

While most giant cell tumors are benign, some are malignant even at their onset or eventually become malignant, particularly following some form of inadequate therapy. It is not possible to distinguish radiologically the so-called malignant giant cell tumor from one which might be benign. This constitutes another factor favoring the trend towards biopsy investigation before instituting therapy.

Coley (1935) reported cases diagnosed as benign giant cell tumor on biopsy and x-ray films which later underwent malignant change. He estimated that this might be expected in as high as 15 per cent of cases, a figure which is somewhat higher than reported by other observers.

It is possible that a pathologic fracture alone may result in healing of this lesion. A giant cell tumor of the lumbar vertebra was reported by Murphy (1935) in which operation was deemed inadvisable and x-ray therapy was refused by the patient. Healing followed a pathologic fracture.

Giant cell tumors of the spine affect the vertebral bodies or the neural arches, alone or in combination. As a rule there is decalcification of the involved area, the lesion being demarcated by smooth edges which merge with the adjacent normal bone. The lesion may produce expansion of the involved vertebra with thinning of the cortex, and linear traversing bands may be present. The paravertebral soft tissues may be invaded. These, however, cannot be considered as of definite diagnostic importance. If the giant cell tumor expands towards the spinal canal, it can cause spinal cord or cauda equina compression.

In view of the changing concepts of the pathology of bone tumors, it becomes difficult to accept without reservation reports of vertebral giant cell tumors in the literature. Mention may be made of several should the reader wish to investigate further (Murphy, 1935; Jenkinson, Hunter and Roberts, 1938; Gershon-Cohen, 1933; Brock and Bogart, 1945; Prossor, 1949; Hamsa and Campbell, 1953; Keplinger and Bucy, 1961 and Pan and MacKinnon, 1962).

The sharply outlined area of bone destruction, absence of adjacent bone reaction and the intact adjacent discs help distinguish giant cell tumors of the spine. However, this appearance is not unique, and collapse of the involved body and paravertebral swelling adds to the difficulty in distinguishing giant cell tumors from those with a similar picture such as aneurysmal bone cysts, myelomas, lymphomas and metastatic tumors.

References

Brock, E. H. and Bogart, F. B.: Benign Giant Cell Tumor of Spine, Am. J. Roentgenol., 54, 512, 1945.

Brailsford, J. F.: Diagnosis and Treatment of Osteoclastoma, Radiology, 43, 35, 1944.

Buschke, F. and Cantril, S. T.: Roentgenotherapy of Benign Giant-Cell Tumor of Bone, Cancer, 2, 293, 1949.

Cade, S.: Osteoclastoma or Giant Cell Tumor of Bone, J. Bone & Joint Surg., 31-B, 157, 1949.

Cahan, W. G., Woodward, H. Q., Higinbotham, N. L., Stewart, F. W. and Coley, B. L.: Sarcoma Arising in Irradiated Bone, Cancer, 1, 3, 1948.

Coley, W. B.: Malignant Changes in So-Called Giant Cell Tumor, Am. J. Surg., 28, 768, 1935.

Gee, V. R. and Pugh, D. G.: Giant-Cell Tumor of Bone, Radiology, 70, 33, 1958.

Gershon-Cohen, J.: Giant-Cell Tumors, Radiology, 41, 261, 1943.

Hamsa, W. R. and Campbell, L. S.: Giant-Cell Tumor of Spine, J. Bone & Joint Surg., 35-A, 476, 1953.

Hutter, V. P., Worcester, J. N., Jr., Francis, K. C., Foote, F. W., Jr. and Stewart, F. W.: Benign and Malignant Giant Cell Tumors of Bone, Cancer, 15, 653, 1962.

Jaffe, H. L., Lichtenstein, L. and Portis, R. B.: Giant Cell Tumor of Bone, Arch. Path., 30, 993, 1940.

Jenkinson, E. L., Hunter, A. F. and Roberts, E. W.: Giant Cell Tumor of the Vertebrae, Am. J. Roentgenol., 40, 344, 1938.

Johnson, E. W., Jr. and Dahlin, D. C.: Treatment of Giant-Cell Tumor of Bone, J. Bone & Joint Surg., 41-A, 895, 1959.

Keplinger, J. E. and Bucy, P. C.: Giant-Cell Tumors of the Spine, Ann. Surg., 154, 648, 1961.

Lichtenstein, L.: Bone Tumors, 3rd Ed., St. Louis, The C. V. Mosby Co., 1965.

Meyerding, H. W.: Treatment of Benign Giant-Cell Tumors by Resection or Excision and Bone Grafting, J. Bone & Joint Surg., 27, 196, 1945.

Murphy, W. G.: Giant Cell Tumor of Spine, Am. J. Roentgenol., 34, 386, 1935.

Pan, P. and MacKinnon, W. B.: "Benign" Giant Cell Tumour of Thoracic Vertebra with Pulmonary Metastasis, Canadian M. A. J., 87, 1026, 1962.

Prossor, T. M.: Treatment of Giant-Cell Tumors of Bone, J. Bone & Joint Surg., 31-B, 261, 1949.

Whally, N.: Vertebral Osteoclastoma with Spinal Cord Compression, Brit. J. Surg., 45, 364, 1958.

Windeyer, B. W. and Woodyatt, P. B.: Osteoclastoma, J. Bone & Joint Surg., 31-B, 252, 1949.

BENIGN CHONDROBLASTOMAS. (Epiphyseal chondromatous giant cell tumor of Codman)

While sometimes confused with osteoclastomas, these tumors are not related to them histogenetically. Benign chondroblastomas are classified with benign tumors of cartilage or cartilage forming connective tissue, occur mainly in young males under 20 years of age, and tend to involve the articular ends of long bones, especially the humerus, femur and tibia, and crosses the epiphyses. The tumor is lytic, has poorly demarcated margins and may bulge beyond the cortex without actually destroying it. Stippled calcific densities may be present within the tumor. It should not be confused with chondrosarcoma or osteogenic sarcoma. Chondroblastomas are curable, and do not undergo malignant degeneration. Its occurrence in the spine is rare, one such case being reported by Buraczewski, Lysakowska and Rudowski (1957).

References

Buraczewski, J., Lysakowska, J. and Rudowski, W.: Chondroblastoma (Codman's Tumor) of the Thoracic Spine, J. Bone & Joint Surg., 39-B, 705, 1957.

Lichtenstein, L. and Bernstein, D.: Unusual Benign and Malignant Chondroid Tumors of Bone, Cancer, 12, 1142, 1959.

Treasure, E. R.: Benign Chondroblastoma of Bone, J. Bone & Joint Surg., 37-B, 462, 1955.

ANEURYSMAL BONE CYSTS

As mentioned above, many bony lesions of the spine have been reported in the literature as primary giant cell tumors, giant cell variants, subperiosteal giant cell tumor, giant cell variants of bone cysts, osteitis fibrosa cystica, pulsating benign giant cell tumor, angioma, ossifying hematoma and even osteogenic sarcoma. Among these undoubtedly are many aneurysmal bone cysts (Besse, Dahlin, Bruwer, Svien and Ghormley, 1953), a condition first brought into prominence by Jaffe and Lichtenstein (1942).

Aneurysmal bone cysts occur in children and young adults as solitary, localized expanded fibrous tissue lesions honeycombed with an enormously dilated vascular bed. These appear in the long bones, in the short bones of the feet, the flat bones, the sacroiliac area, the calvarium and the spine (Jaffe, 1950; Lichtenstein, 1950). Of 17 mentioned by Lichtenstein (1953), 4 were encountered in the spine. The neural arches (Fig. 308) of one or perhaps two adjacent vertebrae may be involved, although occasionally the body may be cystically transformed with a thin cortex (Fig. 309). Trabeculae may be visible across the thinned bone. These probably represent endosteal ridges and spurs rather than true septae. The normal cancellous bone is replaced by fibrovascular tissue with numerous large dilated vascular pools and channels. Encroachment on the spinal canal may result in extradural spinal cord compression.

The radiographic appearance of vertebral aneurysmal bone cysts is one characterized by localized rarefaction and bulging of the involved bone, with thinned cortex and sometimes small focal deposits of new bone and calcifying osteoid tissue.

Aneurysmal bone cysts are amenable to surgical treatment or x-ray therapy. In 2 cases seen by us, and at first believed to be giant cell tumors, healing occurred after deep x-ray therapy. These patients were followed from 5 to 12 years. In 1 case, in which the spinous process and neural arch of the fourth cervical vertebra was involved, and which was not confirmed by biopsy, healing occurred within 3 months after the course of x-ray treatment had been concluded. At first a web-like stroma outlined the restored contours, and ultimately dense

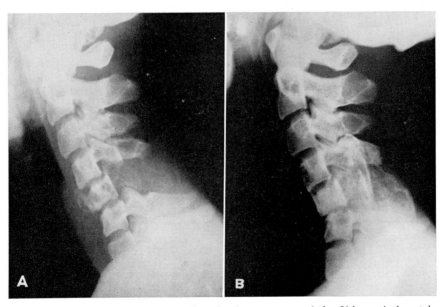

FIG. 308. *A*, Destruction of the neural arch and spinous process of the fifth cervical vertebra. The vertebral body is also affected. This was believed to be a giant-cell tumor or aneurysmal bone cyst. *B*, Same case, 4 months after x-ray therapy. Extensive recalcification of the fifth cervical vertebra has taken place, with complete relief of symptoms. The patient was a 19-year-old man.

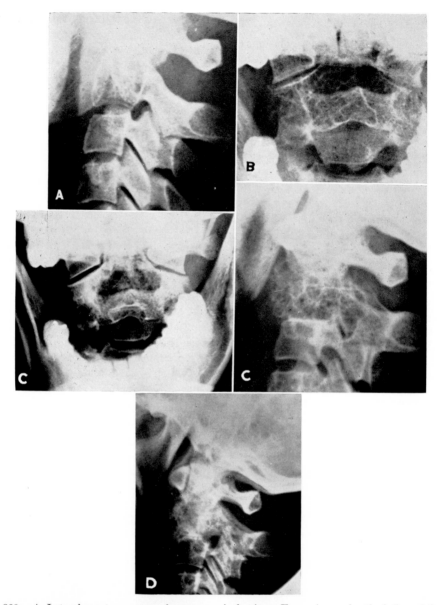

Fɪɢ. 309. *A*, Lateral roentgenogram of upper cervical spine. Expansion and reticulation of the second cervical vertebra. *B*, Same case, anteroposterior view. *C*, Same case. Progression of the lesion. Probable aneurysmal bone cyst. *D*, Same case, following x-ray therapy. The bone has recalcified. The patient was a 14-year-old girl.

calcification occurred in this 19-year-old male patient. The second patient was a 14-year-old girl in which the second cervical vertebra was markedly decalcified, bulging, and traversed by thin septa. X-ray therapy was followed by restoration of the bone, which remained relatively ballooned but re-assumed a good osseous density.

References

Beeler, J. W., Helman, C. H. and Campbell, J. A.: Aneurysmal Bone Cysts of Spine, J.A.M.A., *163*, 914, 1957.

Besse, B. E., Jr., Dahlin, D. C , Bruwer, A , Svien, H. J. and Ghormley, R. K.: Aneurysmal Bone Cyst, Proc. Staff Meet., Mayo Clin., *28*, 249, 1953.

Cruz, M. and Coley, B. L.: Aneurysmal Bone Cyst, Surg., Gynec. & Obst., *103*, 67, 1956.

Dahlin, D. C., Besse, B. E., Jr., Pugh, D. G. and Ghormley, R. K.: Aneurysmal Bone Cysts, Radiology *64*, 56, 1955.

Jaffe, H. L.: Aneurysmal Bone Cyst, Bull. Hosp. Joint Diseases, *11*, 3, 1950.

Jaffe, H. L. and Lichtenstein, L.: Solitary Unicameral Bone Cyst, Arch. Surg., *44*, 1004, 1942.

Lichtenstein, L.: Aneurysmal Bone Cyst, Cancer, *3*, 279, 1950.

————: Aneurysmal Bone Cyst, Cancer, *6*, 1228, 1953.

MacCarty, C. S., Dahlin, D. C., Doyle, J. B., Jr., Lipscomb, P. R. and Pugh, D. G.: Aneurysmal Bone Cysts of the Neural Axis, J. Neurosurg., *18*, 671, 1961.

Mayer, L. and Kestler, O. C.: Aneurysmal Bone Cyst of Spine, Bull. Hospital Joint Dis., *5*, 16, 1944.

Parrish, F. F. and Pevey, J. K.: Surgical Management of Aneurysmal Bone Cyst of the Vertebral Column, J. Bone & Joint Surg., *49-A*, 1597, 1967.

Sherman, R. S. and Soong, K. Y.: Aneurysmal Bone Cyst: Its Roentgen Diagnosis, Radiology, *68*, 54, 1957.

Taylor, F. W.: Aneurysmal Bone Cyst, J. Bone & Joint Surg., *38-B*, 293, 1956.

Verbiest, H.: Giant-Cell Tumours and Aneurysmal Bone Cysts of the Spine, J. Bone & Joint Surg., *47-B*, 699, 1965.

Winter, A. and Firtel, S.: Aneurysmal Bone Cyst of Vertebra with Compression Symptoms, J.A.M.A., *177*, 870, 1961.

Hemangiomas

Vertebral hemangiomas are among the more frequent tumors affecting the spine. Schmorl (1951) reported that of 3829 spinal columns examined, an incidence of 10.7 per cent of angiomas was noted. This series consisted of 1948 males and 1881 females, and the angiomas were more frequent in females. In 66.5 per cent of cases, only 1 angioma was demonstrated. In the remaining 32.8 per cent, 2 to 5 angiomas were seen, and in 3 cases even more were observed. In all, 579 different angiomas were encountered. Of these 32 occurred in the cervical region, 350 in the thoracic region, 170 in the lumbar region and 27 in the sacrum. The most frequent sites were the twelfth thoracic vertebra (47 cases), the fourth lumbar vertebra (38 cases), the first lumbar vertebra (37 cases), the second lumber vertebra (36 cases), and the third lumbar vertebra (36 cases). Most were incidental findings in routine necropsy examinations, and were without clinical symptoms. They varied in size from a pinhead to lesions involving almost the entire vertebra including the neural arches.

Töpfer (1928) reported that hemangiomas of the vertebral bodies were encountered in approximately 12 per cent of 200 patients examined at necropsy. However, Lichtenstein (1952) made the point that occasionally an incidental finding at autopsy was a circumscribed, roundish, bright red hemangioma-like focus within the spongiosa of a vertebral body. It was more likely that these represented venous localized spaces rather than true tumors. He indicated that lesions considered angiomatous may be aneurysmal bone cysts. If extensive enough, they cause expansion of the vertebra, with bulging into the epidural space. Angiomatous tissue destroys the horizontal trabeculae of the vertebra, so that the remaining trabecular structures become thickened, producing the vertically parallel appearance of the remaining cancellous strands noted radiologically (Figs. 310, 311).

Ghormley and Adson (1941) divided angiomas into four groups including those which were asymptomatic, those with local signs and symptoms without spinal cord compression, those with symptoms of spinal cord compression without paraplegia, and those with paraplegia. Compression myelopathy with vertebral hemangioma has been known for a long time. Soon after the original description of the radiologic appearance of hemangiomas by Perman (1927), Bailey and Bucy (1929) described a case of cavernous hemangioma of a vertebra with compression myelopathy. By 1942 Ferber and Lampe were able to collect 52 cases of vertebral hemangioma with spinal cord compression. In a discussion of the possible causes of compression of the spinal cord, Schlezinger and Ungar (1939) pointed out that this condition could be brought about by a ballooning of the vertebra caused by thrombosis and edema associated with osteoporosis and subsequent formation of bone, or by extension of angiomatous tissue to the epidural space.

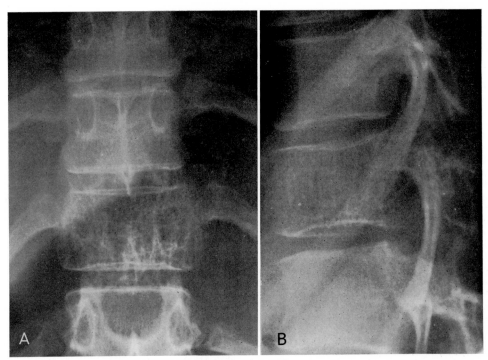

Fig. 310. *A*, Hemangioma of the body of T10 in a 19-year-old pregnant woman with back pain who became paraplegic about at term. *B*, Lateral view discloses involvement of the pedicles and the neural arch. Laminectomy was required for relief, followed by x-ray therapy after delivery.

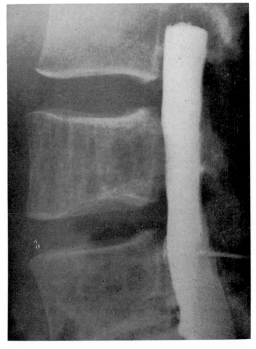

Fig. 311. A vertebral hemangioma with mild epidural compression incident to dorsal bulging of the vertebral body.

This occurred in 8 of the 40 cases reviewed by them. Fracture of the involved vertebra causing spinal cord compression was encountered in only 4 cases in the literature, indicating the rarity of this complication. Extradural hemorrhage from hemangiomas of the spine and cord also occur. Of about 100 such reported cases Nelson (1964) stated that 11 occurred during pregnancy, usually in the last trimester. However, epidural bleeding from vertebral hemangiomas alone is infrequent.

An interesting point was made by Karshner, Rand and Reeves (1939) who described an epidural hemangioma associated with a hemangioma of a dorsal vertebra giving rise to compression myelitis. In this patient there were hemangiomatous nevi in the same dorsal segment as the epidural hemangiomas. Brøbeck (1950) reported a 16-year-old male patient with a spastic paraparesis of the lower limbs due to a hemangioma of the seventh dorsal vertebra. Operation disclosed extradural vascular tumor which involved the neural arch, and compressed the spinal cord from its dorsal aspect. This patient had complained of prolonged insidious development of disturbance in gait, increasing disturbances in sensibility and severe pain. Brøbeck mentioned that pain was a rare and often a late symptom and may sometimes occur in periodic attacks, presumably brought about by congestion in the cavernous blood spaces of the tumor. Michon, Gergoire and Lafont (1935) stated that symptoms had been intensified during menstrual periods and pregnancy.

The incidence of fractures with vertebral hemangiomas is infrequent. Holta (1942) described such a case in the fourth cervical vertebra of a 66-year-old man with compression myelomalacia. On the other hand, Griep (1942) described a case of fracture of the eighth and twelfth dorsal vertebra and the second lumbar vertebra which were otherwise healthy, while the third lumbar vertebra was undamaged even though it showed characteristics of hemangioma.

Asymptomatic vertebral hemangiomas, which are most frequent, require no treatment. However, in the event of pain without central nervous symptoms, x-ray therapy alone may relieve distress. When symptoms of cord or cauda equina compression are minimal, x-ray therapy may be cautiously attempted. However, in the event of rapidly progressive symptoms, decompressive laminectomy followed by x-ray therapy is the method of choice. There are numerous reports of the efficiency of x-ray therapy in relieving the distress incident to hemangiomas of the vertebra, including those of Bucy and Capp (1930), Ferber and Lampe (1942), Kaplan (1946), Foster and Heublein (1947), Schlezinger and Ungar (1939), Brobeck (1950), Manning (1951) and Lindqvist (1951).

The plain film roentgen change seen most often with hemangiomas of the vertebra is a vertical, slightly wavy, parallel striated cancellous marking, most often seen in the vertebral body. The horizontal trabeculae also may be thickened, although diminished in number. This produces a web-like configuration of the trabecular pattern.

We have observed cases in which the vertical striations extended into the neural arches, and in 3 the changes were also present in the transverse and spinous processes. In 1 unusual case of a hemangioma of the second and third thoracic vertebrae (Fig. 312) the patient was paraplegic. The vertical striations in this case were more or less obliterated by a peculiar overlying increased density. Lateral to the vertebral body was a smoothly lobulated tumor mass made up of fairly dense tissue. At first it was believed that we were dealing with an osteochondromatous sarcoma with spinal cord compression. Myelography disclosed a complete block, and at laminectomy the tumor tissue removed was characteristic of vertebral hemangioma. The patient did well following decompression and x-ray therapy. This points out that hemangiomas may perforate the cortex of the vertebral body and extend into the adjacent soft tissues. By far the more common method of progression of the tumor, however, is extension into the spinal canal.

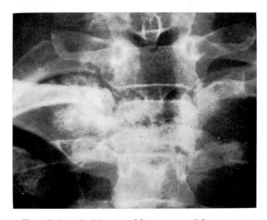

Fig. 312. A 56-year-old woman with a sensory level at T2 and 3, weakness of both legs and urinary and rectal incontinence. She had been under treatment for pernicious anemia. A hemangioma is present in the 2nd thoracic vertebra which has burst from the body into the adjacent soft tissues on the right side. At operation the tumor thickened the laminae and spinous process, and compressed the cord by thickened bone as if by a cuff.

Myelographic examination is indicated whenever there is a question of compression myelopathy. In 3 cases observed by us a complete block was encountered, an observation reported before by several of the observers mentioned previously in this section. Lindqvist (1951) mentioned that in his case a relative block was noted in the anterior aspect of the spinal canal at the level of the ninth dorsal vertebra, but contrast fluid was able to pass the obstacle in a thin band 3 mm in breadth.

One case observed by us appears to be worthy of record inasmuch as it confirms the observation of Michon, Gregoire and Lafont (1935). This patient was a 19-year-old girl, who, during the third trimester of pregnancy, suddenly began to complain of pain in the back followed by progressive weakness of the lower extremities which soon progressed to a paraplegia. In view of the urgent situation, laminectomy was done the day after demonstration of a hemangioma involving the neural arch as well as the body of the twelfth thoracic vertebra (Fig. 310). This was followed by slow improvement, and 1 month later, when the obstetrician judged the time propitious, a cesarean section was done and a normal infant delivered. X-ray therapy was instituted immediately after delivery of the infant. Slow, progressive improvement followed, and the patient was symptom free 6 months later.

References

Bailey, P. and Bucy, P. C.: Cavernous Hemangioma of the Vertebrae, J.A.M.A., *92*, 1748, 1929.
Bell, R. L.: Hemangioma of a Dorsal Vertebra with Collapse and Compression Myelopathy, J. Neurosurg., *12*, 570, 1955.
Brøbeck, O.: Haemangioma of Vertebra Associated with Compression of the Spinal Cord, Acta radiol., *34*, 235, 1950.
Czerniak, P. and Schorr, S.: Hereditary Hemorrhagic Telangiectasis with Involvement of Bone, Am. J. Roentgenol., *74*, 299, 1955.
Ferber, L. and Lampe, I.: Hemangioma of Vertebra Associated with Compression of the Cord, Arch. Neurol. & Psychiat., *47*, 19, 1942.
Ghormley, R. K. and Adson, A. W.: Hemangioma of Vertebrae, J. Bone & Joint Surg., *23*, 887, 1941.
Hoefnagel, D. and Wegner, W.: Vertebral Hemangioma with Spinal Cord Compression, Am. J. Dis. Child., *102*, 126, 1961.
Holta, O.: Hemangioma of the Cervical Vertebra with Fracture and Myelomalacia, Acta radiol., *23*, 423, 1942.
Kaplan, I. I.: Vertebral Hemangioma in Children, J. Pediat., *28*, 498, 1946.
Karschner, R. G., Rand, C. W. and Reeves, D. L.: Epidural Hemangioma Associated with Hemangioma of the Vertebrae, Arch. Surg., *39*, 942, 1939.
Lichtenstein, L.: *Bone Tumors*, 3rd ed., St. Louis, C. V. Mosby Co., 1965.
Manning, H. J.: Symptomatic Hemangioma of the Spine, Radiology, *56*, 58, 1951.
Michon, P., Gregoire and Lafont, J.: A Propos du Diagnostic de Compression Medullaire par Hâmangiome Vertêbral, Rev. Neurol., *53*, 565, 1935.
Nelson, D. A.: Spinal Cord Compression Due to Vertebral Angiomas During Pregnancy, Arch. Neural., *11*, 408, 1964.
Perman, E.: Hemangiomata in Spinal Column. Acta chir. scandinav., *61*, 91, 1926–1927.
Reeves, D. L.: Vertebral Hemangioma with Compression of the Spinal Cord. J. Neurosurg., *21*, 710, 1964.
Robbins, L. R. and Fountain, E. M.: Hemangioma of Cervical Vertebrae with Spinal-Cord Compression, New England J. Med., *258*, 685, 1958.
Schlezinger, N. S. and Ungar, H.: Hemangioma of Vertebra with Compression Myelopathy, Am. J. Roentgenol., *42*, 192, 1939.
Schmorl, G. and Junghanns, H.: *Die Gesunde und Kranke Wirbelsäule in Röntgenbild und Klinik*, 2nd ed., Stuttgart, Georg Thieme, 1951.
Sherman, R. S. and Wilner, D.: The Roentgen Diagnosis of Hemangioma of Bone, Am. J. Roentgenol., *86*, 1146, 1961.
Töpfer, D.: Über ein infiltrierend wachsene Hämangiom der Haut und multiple Kapillarektasien der Haut und inneren Organe; zur Kenntnis der Wirbelangiom, Frankf. Ztschr. f. Path., *36*, 337, 1928.

CYSTIC ANGIOMATOSIS OF BONE

The appearance of multiple skeletal cystic lesions together with scattered hemangiohamartomata is part of a picture of hamartomatous cystic vascular malformations. In most cases similar lesions appear in various viscera, including the spleen, lungs and pleura, kidneys, pericardium, thymus, liver, and retroperitoneal tissues. Nine cases have been reported in the English literature (Moseley and Starobin, 1964). The basic lesion is a cystic malformation lined with a single layer of endothelium. In bone the marrow is replaced by dilated thin-walled cysts which may be solitary or multiple and communicating. Some contain blood, others are filled with clear fluid and are designated as multiple lymphangiectasis of bone. In the long bones the epiphyses, metaphyses and diaphyses may be involved, and cystic areas expanding bone appear in the ribs. In the vertebrae and the skull the lesions tend to be round and cystic, without the striations or honeycomb appearance seen in hemangiomas of these bones.

References

Gramiak, R., Ruiz, G. and Campeti, F. L.: Cystic Angiomatosis of Bone, Radiology, *69*, 347, 1957.
Moseley, J. E. and Starobin, S. G.: Cystic Angiomatosis of Bone, Am. J. Roentgenol., *91*, 1114, 1964.
Nehrkorn, O. and Wolfert, E.: Generalisierte Knochenhämangiomatose mit Lungenbeteiligung, Fortschr. Röntgenstr., *104*, 107, 1966.

Massive Osteolysis

Decalcification of bone is a nonspecific phenomenon related to diverse causes such as infection, trauma, central nervous system disorders, metastatic tumors, metabolic conditions, the various reticuloses, and other processes. A remarkable, infrequent form of extensive osteoclasis is that associated with vascular changes of a benign nature with markedly prominent venous channels and without bone reaction. It has been attributed to a variant form of hemangioma in which the bone becomes weakened, soft and spongy, and filled with a benign proliferation of endothelial-lined channels which can be outlined radiologically after the injection of water soluble contrast material. The bone practically disappears progressively, giving rise to various appellations including phantom bone, vanishing bone, disappearing bone, cryptogenic osteolysis and essential osteolysis. The condition appears in patients from childhood to middle age, most often in children and young adults. There are no endocrine or chemical disturbances which might point to a causative mechanism.

Complaints are referable to pathologic fractures with pain, swelling and deformities predominating. The lesion can originate in almost any bone except the skull and phalanges, mostly in the pelvis, sacrum and shoulder girdles. The osteolytic process sometimes ceases spontaneously, but reossification does not take place. Absorption is first localized to one bone, and then extends to those adjacent to a degree which clinically is malignant even though the associated angiomas histologically are benign. Some of the tissue in this disease is lymphangioma rather than hemangioma, and clear fluid exudes from the involved tissue. Although the spine is involved infrequently, instances have been reported with extensive vertebral changes (Halliday, Dahlin, Pugh and Young, 1964; Lagier and Rutishauser, 1965).

References

Bickel, W. H. and Broders, A. C.: Primary Lymphangioma of the Ilium, J. Bone & Joint Surg., *29*, 517, 1947.
Gorham, L. W. and Stout, A. P.: Massive Osteolysis (Acute Spontaneous Absorption of Bone, Phantom Bone, Disappearing Bone): Its Relation to Hemangiomatosis, J. Bone & Joint Surg., *37-A*, 985, 1955.
Gorham, L. W., Wright, A. W. Schultz, H. and Maxon, F. C., Jr.: Disappearing Bones; A Rare Form of Massive Osteolysis, Am. J. Med., *17*, 674, 1954.
Halliday, D. R., Dahlin, D. C., Pugh, D. G. and Young, H. H.: Massive Osteolysis and Angiomatosis, Radiology, *82*, 637, 1964.
Hambach, R., Pujman, J. and Maly, V.: Massive Osteolysis Due to Hemangiomatosis, Radiology, *71*, 43, 1958.
Johnson, P. M. and McClure, J. G.: Observations on Massive Osteolysis, Radiology, *71*, 28, 1958.
Lagier, R. and Rutishauser, E.: Osteoarticular Changes in a Case of Essential Osteolysis, J. Bone & Joint Surg., *47-B*, 339, 1965.
Milner, S. M. and Baker, S. L.: Disappearing Bones, J. Bone & Joint Surg., *40-B*, 502, 1958.

Osteoid Osteoma

This lesion was designated by Jaffe (1935) as a benign osteoblastic tumor composed of osteoid tissue and atypical bone. As first reported, the tumor involved spongy bone.

In 1940 Jaffe and Lichtenstein observed the same lesion in the cortex of the shafts of long bones accompanied by a considerable degree of periosteal reaction. Pathologically the lesion is characterized by the presence of a nidus, which on cut sections stands out from the surrounding bony tissue as a slightly bulging, rather rubbery, circumscribed red nodule surrounded by thickened and sclerotic bone. This nidus is the osteoid osteoma itself. An osteoid osteoma within spongy bone provokes a thin rim of sclerotic reaction, quite different from the rather pronounced periosteal proliferation of bone observed with the same lesion developing in the cortex.

The lesion is one which affects relatively young people, from childhood to early adult life. It is accompanied by pain which often is more severe at night. The pain seems to respond quite readily to aspirin. Sharp tenderness over the involved area may be elicited on physical examination. Scoliosis and a radicular syndrome often are present. With cervical lesions torticollis may be the presenting symptom.

The usual sites of origin of these benign tumors are the shafts of the long bones, particularly the femurs and tibias. Lesions have also been identified in other long bones and in the feet. Occasional instances of involvement of the humeri have been reported. Osteoid osteomas appear in the vertebral column, and usually involve the neural arches or the articular facets. In a review of 62 cases the vertebrae were involved in 4 (Jaffe, 1945). In this paper Jaffe presented a roentgenogram showing an osteoid osteoma on the right side of the isthmus between the ascending and descending articular facets of the second lumbar vertebra. In a photomicrograph from another case of osteoid osteoma also in an articular facet of the second lumbar vertebra, Jaffe showed how the osteoid osteoma was sharply demarcated from the unaffected bone area.

Kleinberg (1944) reported a 10-year-old girl who had been treated for about a year for backache attributed to strain, scoliosis and osteochondritis. Lateral roentgenograms showed a slight kyphosis at the level of the first and second lumbar vertebra, with diminution in the size of the intervertebral disc. A diagnosis of possible Pott's disease was made. Later films showed an excavation and absorption of part of the right lamina of the second lumbar vertebra, which had been previously overlooked. At operation a red granular mass the size of a cherry was found between the laminae of the first and second lumbar vertebrae on the right side, with erosion of part of the lamina of the second lumbar vertebra. Complete recovery followed excision of this lesion, which proved to be an osteoid osteoma.

Lewis (1944) included a case in which a nidus with surrounding sclerotic reactive bone tissue was encountered in a small articulation between the tenth and eleventh thoracic vertebra in a 15-year-old male. Sherman (1947) mentioned that 128 reported cases of osteoid osteoma were available in the literature, 11 of which were in the vertebrae. In his series 7 additional cases were presented, making a total of 18 cases. An additional case of involvement of the right lamina of the third lumbar vertebra with clinical manifestations suggesting protrusion of an intervertebral disc was described by Jackson, Dockerty and Ghormley (1949). Two years later Dockerty, Ghormley and Jackson reported a clinical pathologic study of 20 cases in which the vertebrae were involved in 5. In 1 case the transverse process of a vertebra was destroyed with no surrounding sclerosis of bone. These authors mentioned a case with typical clinical and x-ray findings, in which successive roentgenograms demonstrated disappearance of the lesion without surgical intervention. Sabanas, Bickel and Moe (1956) also observed spontaneous disappearance in 3 cases observed from 4 to 8 years.

Osteoid osteoma affect chiefly the neural arches, particularly the isthmus and the articular facets, and the transverse proc-

esses. Walker (1952) in a description of
3 cases of osteoid osteoma in children from
9 to 14 years of age, mentioned that the
spinous process, pedicle and body were involved in 2. One was of interest in that the
spinous process of the fifth cervical vertebra
involved with relatively little was surrounding sclerosis of bone. In the second case
pedicle and the body of the fifth cervical
vertebra were affected. Maclellan and
Wilson (1967) found 36 documented cases in
the literature and added 6 more. Two additional cases are illustrated here (Figs. 313
and 314). In most the posterior elements
and the transverse processes were affected,
only 3 occurring in vertebral bodies. Of the
36 mentioned by Maclellan and Wilson 20
were in the lumbar vertebrae, 10 in the
cervical vertebrae, 5 in the thoracic vertebrae and one was located in the sacrum.

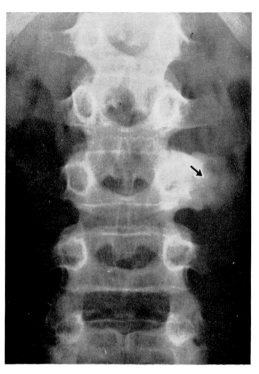

FIG. 314. Osteoid osteoma of the left transverse
process of the third lumbar vertebra. Note the
heavy bony reaction, and the small calcified central
core within a radiolucent circle (arrow).

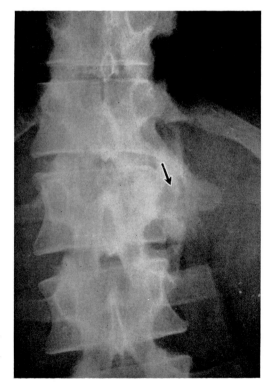

FIG. 313. Osteoid osteoma of the left transverse
process of the first lumbar vertebra. Considerable
bony reaction is present. A small central densely
calcified core is seen within a radiolucent focus
(arrow).

Radiologic changes indicative of osteoid
osteoma usually can be made out on conventional films, especially if the transverse
processes are affected. Lesions in the
neural arches or the vertebral bodies are
better observed on oblique stereoroentgenograms, and body section roentgenograms are
also helpful. Osteoid osteomas usually are
rather small, but at times the extent of the
adjacent sclerotic reaction is prominent.
The nidus is oval or circular in configuration,
and rarely exceeds 1 cm in diameter. The
radiolucent focus of osteoid becomes opaque
when calcification appears within it. The
lesion then appears as a central circular area
of increased density surrounded by a comparatively radiolucent halo. This in turn
may be enveloped in sclerosing reactive bone.

Usually the combination of symptoms and
the sclerotic reaction about a nidus permits

accurate diagnosis. However, in some instances a predominantly sclerotic process cannot be distinguished from a sclerosing bone tumor. Other diagnoses which have been made in some instances include herniated disc, tuberculosis, osteomyelitis, eosinophilic granuloma and osteochondritis. Not infrequently failure to identify the lesion has resulted in considering the patient to be hysterical. Giant osteoid osteoma presents a larger nidus and less apparent sclerotic change.

References

Dockerty, M. B., Ghormley, R. K. and Jackson, A. E.: Osteoid Osteoma, Ann. Surg., *133*, 77, 1951.

Fett, H. C., Sr. and Russo, V. P.: Osteoid Osteoma of a Cervical Vertebra, J. Bone & Joint Surg., *41-A*, 948, 1959.

Jackson, A. E., Dockerty, M. B. and Ghormley, R. K.: Osteoid Osteoma, Proc. Staff Meet., Mayo Clin., *24*, 380, 1949.

Jaffe, H. L.: Osteoid-Osteoma; Benign Osteoblastic Tumor Composed of Osteoid and Atypical Bone, Arch. Surg., *31*, 709, 1935.

————: Osteoid-Osteoma of Bone, Radiology, *45*, 319, 1965.

Jaffe, H. L. and Lichtenstein, L.: Osteoid-Osteoma, J. Bone & Joint Surg., *22*, 645, 1940.

Kleinberg, S.: Osteoid Osteoma, Am. J. Surg., *66*, 396, 1944.

Maclellan, D. I. and Wilson, F. C.: Osteoid Osteoma of the Spine, J. Bone & Joint Surg., *49-A*, 111, 1967.

Mustard, W. T. and DuVal, F. W.: Osteoid Osteoma of Vertebrae, J. Bone & Joint Surg., *41-B*, 132, 1959.

Sankaran, B.: Osteoid Osteoma, Surg., Gynec. & Obst., *99*, 193, 1954.

Sabanas, A. O., Bickel, W. H. and Moe, J. H.: Natural History of Osteoid Osteoma of the Spine, Am. J. Surg., *91*, 880, 1956.

Walker, J. W.: Benign Bone Tumors in Pediatric Practice, Radiology, 58, 662, 1952.

Benign Osteoblastoma (giant osteoid osteoma)

This benign bone tumor resembles osteoid osteoma in that it is an infrequent benign lesion which presents a nidus with surrounding sclerosed bone. However, the nidus usually is large, reaching from 1 to 2 cm in diameter, and the extent of the associated sclerotic change is less marked. The nidus tends to be softer and more hemorrhagic than that seen with osteoid osteoma. Vascularity of the tumor is more pronounced with benign osteoblastomas. The lesion is formed by osteoblasts which form osteoid tissue, with varying degrees of calcification, surrounded by a vascularized connective tissue stroma. Resorptive changes also may be present, and osteoclasts producing this change should not be confused with cells of a giant cell tumor (Otis and Scoville, 1961).

Benign osteoblastomas have a predilection for the neural arches and pedicles of the vertebrae, and may cause extradural compression (Fig. 315) or impinge on and widen the intervertebral foramina. This tumor also occurs in the tubular bones, including those of the hands and feet, where they often are eccentric in position. Occasionally benign osteoblastomas appear in the ribs and skull.

The radiologic picture is not entirely characteristic. The nidus is ill-defined and larger than that present with osteoid osteoma. There is expansion of the involved bone, and in the main the lesion is lytic (Fig. 316). The cortex is thinned and eroded, leaving an expanded, well circumscribed shell. In some a sclerosing, stippled deposition of bone is present. The lesion is amenable to surgery.

Fig. 315. *A*, An 8-year-old boy with neck pain radiating down both arms and weakness of the lower extremities. A diagnosis of dislocation of the second or the third cervical vertebra was made. The spinous process of C3 is bulbous and presents an area of radiolucency surrounded by a rim of condensed bone. The spinous process of C2 is tilted upwards so that its body is shifted downwards and anteriorly. *B* and *C*, On myelographic examination a diffuse widening of the cord is present, with a holdup in the cephalad and caudad flow of Pantopaque. *D*, On cross-table studies the cord is flattened markedly at C5. At operation a benign osteoblastoma originating from the spinous process of C2 was found extending into the canal, producing marked cord compression from C2 to 5.

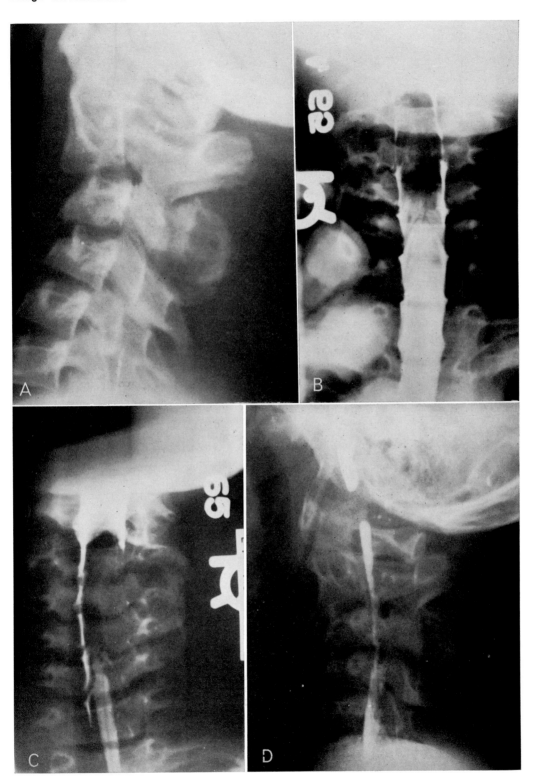

Fig. 315. (*Legend on opposite page.*)

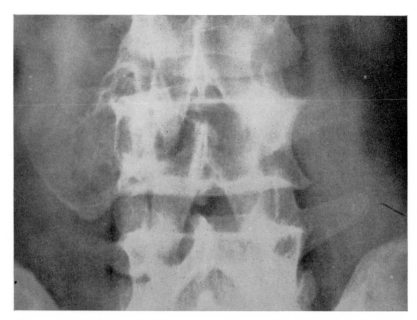

Fig. 316.   Benign osteoblastoma involving the right pedicle and transverse process of the fourth lumbar
vertebra, eroding the right lateral border of the body.

References

Crabbe, W. A. and Wardill, J. C.: Benign Osteo-
    blastoma of the Spine, Brit. J. Surg., *50*, 571, 1963.
Karlsberg, R. C. and Kittleson, A. C.: Osteoid
    Osteoma, Radiol. Clin. North America, *2*, 337,
    1964.
Lichtenstein, L.: Benign Osteoblastoma, Cancer, *9*,
    1044, 1956.
Otis, R. D. and Scoville, W. M.: Benign Osteo-
    blastoma of the Vertebra, J. Neurosurg., *18*, 700,
    1961.
Pochaczevsky, R., Yen, Y. M. and Sherman, R. S.:
    The Roentgen Appearance of Benign Osteoblas-
    toma, Radiology, *75*, 429, 1960.

NASOPHARYNGEAL NEOPLASMS

It is generally agreed that most nasopharyngeal tumors exclusive of chordomas
or those arising as primary or metastatic
growths in the subjacent bone originate in
the soft tissues. Among these tumors are
lympho-epitheliomas, transitional and squa-
mous cell carcinomas, lymphoblastomas and
sarcomas. As a rule these tumors manifest
themselves first by proliferation in the soft
tissue of the nasopharynx and then by invasion of the base of the skull, usually by way
of the basilar foramina. Involvement of the
cervical spine by these tumors is rare. Such
a case was reported by Geist and Portmann
(1952) who described destruction of the
first and second vertebral bodies by a nasopharyngeal malignancy. Occasionally a
nasopharyngeal tumor may be identified on
x-ray examination of the cervical spine because of soft tissue swelling in the upper prevertebral area, best seen on lateral projections.

Reference

Geist, R. M. and Portmann, U. V.: Primary Malig-
    nant Tumors of the Nasopharynx, Am. J. Roent-
    genol., *68*, 262, 1952.

6

Spinal Traumatic Changes

Industrial, automobile and sports accidents are the most frequent causes of injury
to the cervical spine. The vertebral bodies,
the neural arches, the intervertebral discs
and the contents of the spinal canal are
affected, depending on the direction, force,
duration of the blow and the posture and
muscular tone of the patient at the time of
injury. Often, the muscular and ligamentous structures are injured, but these are
difficult to evaluate in the absence of skeletal
changes. With displacement of affected
components of the vertebra and intervertebral disc, acute or chronic spinal cord or
nerve root compression supervenes, followed
by a clinical picture in accord with the compressive phenomena. These vary widely,
from immediate transection to the results of
more or less gradual compression of the cord.
Epidural, subarachnoid and intramedullary
hemorrhages may also occur. Damage to the
vertebral artery is another consequence of
injury of the neck (Carpenter, 1961).

In a review of 59 cases of cervical spine
trauma, Crooks and Birkett (1944) found
6 fractures of the sixth or seventh cervical
spinous processes or both. One fracture of
the transverse process of the seventh cervical
vertebra was seen. Fracture or fracture dislocation of the atlantoaxial region occurred
in 3, and there were 2 with displacement of
the atlas on the axis. Four fractures of the
dens were seen, with forward displacement
in 3 and backwards displacement in 1. The

second cervical vertebra was fractured or
displaced on the third in 6 cases. There
were 7 compression fractures, and 10 fracture
dislocations and subluxations. In 8 casee
there were dislocations with locking of the
articular facets, and in 5 of these complets
paraplegia appeared immediately after the
injury. In a review of 87 lesions in 77 patients Rogers (1957) found anterior dislocation and bursting fractures of the vertebral
body in 29 and 10 instances respectively.
Anterior fracture dislocation was present in
8 cases, fracture of the dens in 9 and 6 had
wedge-compression fractures.

Injuries of the cervical spine are classified
according to the forces of flexion, extension
and rotation involved, the resultant displacements, and compressive or disruptive changes.
Anterior dislocation, with and without fracture, occurs when a shearing force from
behind produces anterior displacement of the
affected vertebrae. The posterior segments
of the displaced vertebrae are tipped anteriorly and cephalad by the altered inclination
of the articular facets. Dislocation is complete when the inferior articular process of
the displaced vertebra becomes anterior to
the superior articular process of the subjacent vertebra. If the displacement is such
that the inferior articular process of the involved vertebra remains posterior, but is
displaced partly anteriorly and upwards,
partial dislocation is present. Fractures
occur when longitudinal compression is
added to this type of force. Compression of
the vertebral body or disruption of the

469

pedicles or laminae add considerably to the possibility of concomitant cord injuries. Careful neurologic examination should precede radiographic examination of the cervical spine to avoid endangering the patient. It is advisable to review the preliminary films before proceeding with more complete examinations. Our first films are made in the anteroposterior, lateral and open-mouth projections. If indicated, flexion and extension lateral studies, stereo oblique views and body sections examinations are made.

Posterior dislocation of a vertebra results when the shearing force is applied anteriorly, as in a fall on the face. The anterior spinal ligaments are torn and the intervertebral disc is disrupted. The ligamenta flava and interspinal ligaments partake in the injury, and the spinal cord and nerve roots may be injured severely. With this type of injury the elements involved can reassume a normal relationship, leaving a lacerated spinal cord.

The most frequent cause of injury of the first and second cervical vertebrae is a blow on the vertex of the head or a fall from a height, striking head first. The fracture results from pressure on the vertex and counterpressure from the spine squeezing the lateral masses of the atlas between the occipital condyles and the axis. The posterior and anterior arches are the weakest points of the atlas, and fractures through these result in lateral displacements of the lateral masses. Fractures also occur through the grooves for the vertebral arteries. Unilateral rotary dislocations follow forced lateral flexion and rotation away from the dislocated fragment.

The weakest point of the dens is its base. A force exerted from behind will result in a forward dislocation, while if force is applied to the forehead with the head in hyperextension a posterior dislocation follows. The forward dislocation is more frequent (Fig. 317), but paralysis is observed more often with backward displacement of the dens.

Other mechanisms for fracture of the atlas include extreme extension, causing a fracture at the weakest point of the posterior arch close to the lateral masses on one or both sides. Pressure of the odontoid against the anterior arch may result in a fracture of this area. There may be dislocation of the lateral masses towards the head in bilateral fractures of the posterior arch because of upward pulling of the rectus capitis posterior minor muscle. Plaut (1930), reporting 93 fractures of the atlas gathered from the literature, mentioned that an overwhelming majority recovered to full occupational activity (Fig. 318).

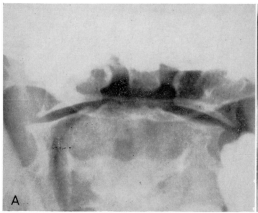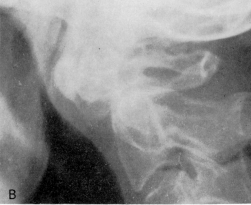

FIG. 317. *A*, Fracture dislocation involving the base of the dens, with a shift of the articular structures of C1 and 2 from right to left. *B*, The dens and the anterior arch of the atlas is displaced sharply anteriorly, causing a bulge in the soft tissues of the nasopharynx. The tip of the spinous process of C1 is also displaced anteriorly.

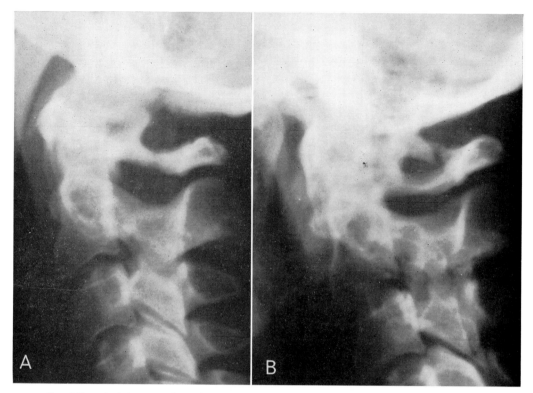

Fig. 318. *A*, A fracture through the neural arch of C1 is faintly seen on a true lateral film, but shows up better, *B*, on a tilted film.

Fractures and fracture dislocations of the second cervical vertebra occur quite frequently with accidents such as diving injuries which produce direct trauma on the occiput with a torsional force as the body swings over to the side when the head strikes the bottom. In these cases a lateral displacement of the atlas on the axis is seen, together with a fracture through the base of the odontoid process (Fig. 317). Davies (1945) reported a 38-year-old man who had fractured his first and second cervical vertebrae after diving into a swimming pool 23 years before admission to the hospital. An ununited fracture at the base of the odontoid with a false articulation was present. Movement occurred at this false joint which subjected the patient to attacks of unconsciousness, attributed to compression of the vertebral arteries.

The dens may be displaced dorsad with no gross displacement from its root if its posterior restraining ligament is torn. Observation of the distance between the dens and the anterior arch of the atlas is essential in identifying this dislocation. As a consequence of fracture of the dens it may subsequently disappear, leading to the question as to a possible congenital absence of this structure (Fielding, 1965; Freiberger, Wilson and Nichols, 1965). Associated with this, as well as with true congenital absence of the dens, is abnormal movement of the atlas on the axis. Backward displacement of the atlas also is present with congenital malformations, such as absence of its anterior arch.

A rare, but distinctive, fracture is bilateral fracture of the neural arch of the second cervical vertebra, with or without dislocation of the body of the axis on the third cervical vertebra. The fracture may involve the first intervertebral disc or the third cervical vertebra. The dens is unbroken, and the

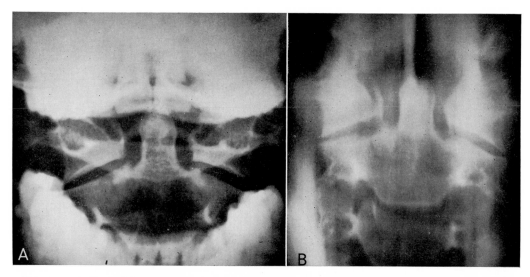

FIG. 319. *A*, Vertical fracture of the lateral aspect of the body of C2. The fracture line enters the joint space, but no displacement is present. *B*, Laminagram shows the fracture line passing medially under the dens. There were no symptoms attributable to this fracture, which was found during a neck examination for "a whiplash injury" after an automobile accident.

transverse atlantal ligament is intact. This type of fracture is observed in traffic accidents, and occurs in judicial hangings (Schneider and co-workers, 1965).

Occasionally a vertical fracture is noted in the body of the second cervical vertebra, unassociated with injury to the dens and without evidence of atlantoaxial joint derangement. This may follow a blow on the vertex of the skull, and is not accompanied by anything more than some pain which subsides fairly quickly (Fig. 319).

Malformations of the occipitocervical junction, when present, influence the type of fracture. With occipitalization of the atlas or basilar invagination the dens is high in the spinal canal in relation to the malformed foramen magnum. Therefore the dens is more likely to cause injury to the cord and the medulla oblongata. In children the dens may separate at its basilar epiphyseal line. One should not interpret a normal persistent epiphyseal line as a fracture.

Neurologic sequelae following fracture of the dens occur immediately or later. Hemorrhage into the spinal canal or outside the canal with disruption of adjacent nerves,

contusions of the greater occipital, glossopharyngeal, palatal or chorda tympani nerves may occur. Immediate paralysis below the lesion, hypalgesia and hypesthesia together with preserved position, touch, motion and vibratory sense after injury indicates the necessity for surgical relief. Myelography is contraindicated under these circumstances.

Delayed consequences of high cervical trauma include failure of healing of the fracture, with persistent abnormal mobility, excessive callus formation at the fracture site or necrosis of the dens. Compressive changes involving the anterior aspect of the spinal cord are important, and simulate various degenerative diseases with progressive weakness, spasticity, hyperreflexia and absence of sensory disturbances. Pain and numbness of the lower extremities can be produced by myelopathy incident to lower cervical spinal injuries, and in the absence of lumbar discal changes. The situation becomes confused when minor or no changes are found on lumbar myelography, and the cervical canal should always be studied carefully in such cases.

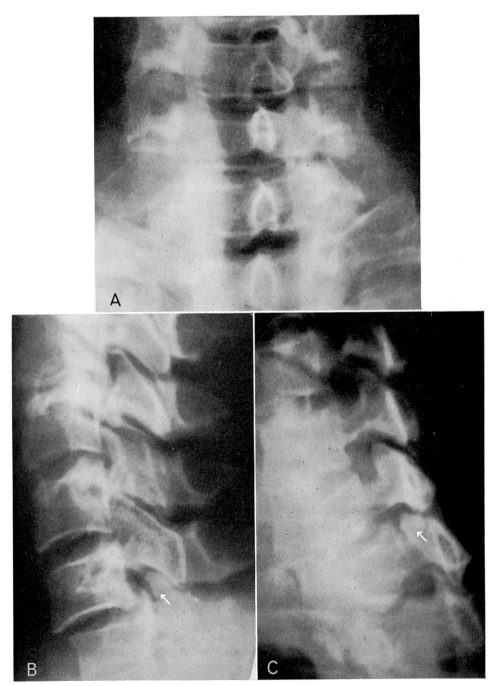

Fig. 320. *A*, AP study of the lower cervical spine in a 43-year-old man who had been in a diving accident. He complained of dizziness and neck pain. An irregularity and overlapping of the left transverse processes of C6 and 7 is present. *B*, On a lateral view a slight forward shift of C6 on C7 is present. A fracture is present in the superior articular facet of C7 (arrow). *C*, This fracture is better seen on an oblique view (arrow).

Injuries to the lower cervical spine frequently involve the bodies of the fourth, fifth, sixth and seventh cervical vertebrae. Many of these follow an injury which causes hyperflexion followed by a spontaneous extensor recoil. Head-on automobile collisions, or sudden stops, are common causes. This may result in partial compression of the anterior aspects of the lower cervical vertebral bodies. Injuries to the transverse and spinous processes, the laminae and pedicles also occur as a result of these injuries, together with subluxations of the articular facets. The clinical picture varies greatly, depending on the location and extent of the injury. These may be difficult to identify, considerable disparity may exist between so-called negative roentgenograms of the neck and a patient who appears to be painfully injured. In these cases the usual lordotic curve of the cervical spine is straightened, an observation which should induce detailed examinations. A so-called "sprain" may well be a subluxation, a fracture or both of an articular facet (Fig. 320) almost indistinguishable even on complete roentgenographic examination. In such cases stereoscopic lateral studies in flexion and extension, as well as oblique stereoroentgenograms are essential. Slight changes in the alignment of the articular facets, increased spacing between the spinous processes and minor alterations in the configurations of the apophyseal joints point towards minor dislocations which may be asymptomatic or productive of considerable discomfort. These are difficult to evaluate and often give rise to much discussion, particularly in medicolegal situations. The presence of bleeding into the adjacent soft tissues produces visible swelling at times. This may be present in the absence of a visible fracture. If so, further search for a bone injury is required.

Hyperflexion injuries to the cervical spine result in injury to the vertebral bodies and the intervertebral disc. In some a "teardrop" fracture appears at the anterosuperior aspect of one of the middle cervical vertebrae, associated at times with considerable

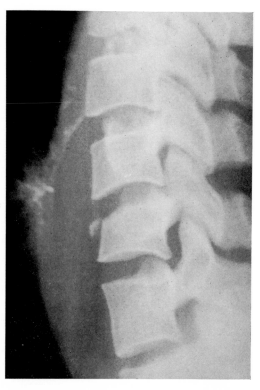

FIG. 321. A tear-drop fracture of the anterosuperior aspect of the body of C6 in a 21-year-old man who had been in a diving accident. The cervical curve is straightened. Considerable soft tissue swelling incident to a prevertebral hematoma is present.

swelling of the adjacent soft tissues (Fig. 321). More extensive damage occurs when the injury is severe, leading to gross dislocation of one vertebra on another because of disruption of the intervertebral disc usually associated with injury to the articular facets of the displaced vertebrae (Fig. 322). This also occurs when there is destruction of a vertebra and its neural arch by metastatic tumor. Epidural compression of the cord follows hemorrhage, intraspinal extension of tumor or alteration in the configuration of the canal caused by the dislocation.

In injuries of the cervical spine in which the intervertebral foramina are affected, one may encounter a syndrome simulating that of a herniated disc. Two such cases were reported by Kristoff and Dratz (1948) who observed that fracture of the margins of an

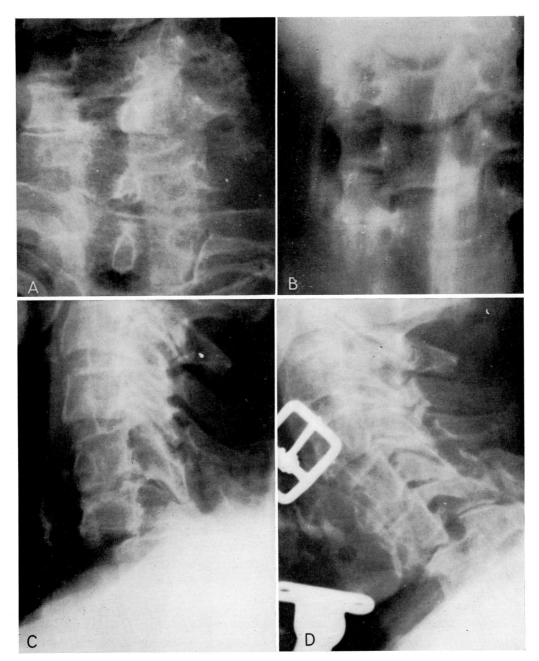

Fig. 322. *A*, A 76-year-old woman who was struck by an automobile. The alignment of C6 on C7 as seen on the AP view is abnormal. *B*, Laminagram shows a shift of the sixth on the seventh cervical vertebrae from left to right. There is a fracture through the right pedicle of C6. *C*, The lateral view shows a sharp anterior shift of C6 on C7. A fracture through the neural arch of C6 is visible. *D*, After traction and maintenance in a collar the dislocation is still evident, but the patient is ambulatory and relatively free from symptoms.

intervertebral foramen resulted in compression of the corresponding nerve root. The pain may be radicular and aggravated by motion of the head. Myelograms may or may not show a filling defect with such injuries.

The dramatic effect of hyperflexion injury on the intervertebral discs of the lower cervical spine has been the subject of several reports. Brooke (1944) reported quadriplegia with complete transverse cervical myelitis produced by traumatic herniation of an ossified nucleus pulposus. At necropsy 15 days after admission, a defective and frayed posterior longitudinal ligament was found, with posterior protrusion of a calcified nucleus pulposus between the fourth and fifth cervical vertebrae. The cord at this level was softened. In this patient, a 56-year-old male, the plain films revealed narrow interspaces between the fourth, fifth and sixth cervical vertebrae. The vertebrae were normally aligned. A soft defect was palpated in the spinal cord opposite the interspace between the fourth and fifth cervical vertebrae, and directly anterior to this was a hard, irregular calcified intervertebral disc which measured $1 \times 1.5 \times 0.5$ cm. On slight flexion of the head this bulged about 1 cm into the spinal canal. It appeared obvious that the herniated disc was responsible for the area of cord softening. The disc itself was readily lifted from its bed, and could be completely removed after cutting a few fibers of the posterior longitudinal ligament.

Cramer and McGowan (1944) pointed out that recoil injuries with extreme retroflexion may cause similar damage to the spinal cord by posterior discal displacement in the lower cervical spine. They described a case in which the cervical cord of a patient who died after a diving injury was almost completely severed anteriorly, without vertebral dislocation. Necropsy revealed that the intervertebral disc had protruded directly opposite the lesion in the spinal cord, and they postulated that violent protrusion of the nucleus pulposus due to compression of the

intervertebral disc was the mechanism for the spinal cord injury. These authors did not believe that the explanation could be extreme vertebral dislocation with immediate spontaneous reduction. This possibility was excluded because dislocation occurring under great stress must be associated with tearing of the ligaments, fractures, or both.

Another case of paraplegia following a hyperextension cervical spine injury was reported by Taylor and Blackwood (1948) who indicated that myelography may be required to demonstrate prolapse of the disc, particularly if the plain film roentgenograms were normal. In their opinion, spinal canal block may develop because of edema of the cord due to contusion, discal herniation, or dislocation with immediate spontaneous reduction. Rogers (1945) reported 4 patients who became paraplegic a few minutes to 48 hours after injury. All were able to walk during this interval.

An unusual case of fatal nucleus pulposus embolism involving a large segment of the spinal cord and medulla was reported by Naiman, Donohue and Prichard (1961) in a 15-year-old boy who died shortly after a minor injury with progressive quadriplegia, respiratory paralysis and sensory loss. Multiple microemboli of nucleus pulposus material were found in arteries of the spinal cord and medulla. Liss (1965) reported a 16-year-old boy who suffered fatal cervical cord injury while making a rapid underwater turn in a swimming race. As a result of hyperflexion, torsion and hyperextension a thin segment of his cord was injured at the C2-3 level in the form of acute petechial hemorrhages. There was no evidence of other injury.

The effect of injuries to the cervical spines of elderly individuals with arthritis was discussed by Barnes (1948). These patients have a tendency towards kyphosis of the thoracic spine, usually compensated for by a cervical lordosis. This results in a relatively fixed position of the cervical spine, and an injury may cause hyperextension because of the inability of the patient to flex his neck. Under such circumstances strain develops on the anterior spinal ligament, which may rupture and be accompanied by a chip fracture of the vertebral body. The intervertebral disc may be torn, but there is little chance for a posterior discal displacement. Kaplan (1953) postulated that hyperextension injuries might cause thrombosis of the spinal arteries with consequent cord damage, and reported a verified case in a 54-year-old male who had been overthrown by a wave while sea-bathing.

Patients with ankylosing spondylitis and rheumatoid arthritis with involvement of the cervical vertebrae suffer from rigidity of the neck, and the consequence of injury is complicated by this stiffness. Inasmuch as the neck cannot bend, a break may occur much in the same way as in a long bone. The weakest point usually will be at one of the intervertebral discs. The fracture line passes through the affected disc, and forward displacement of one vertebra occurs. For this to happen there must also be a break through the neural arch to permit forward movement of the body. This is an infrequent occurrence. Grisolia, Bell and Peltier (1967) reported 6 cases of fractures and dislocations of the spine complicating ankylosing spondylitis. They mentioned that in a review of 1646 patients an additional 6 were found who had old unrecognized fractures of the vertebral column. Injury to the cord is frequent. Varying degrees of neural involvement ranging from mild sensory loss to quadriplegia may be encountered.

Hyperextension injuries may produce serious damage in newborn infants, especially during breech deliveries. Leventhal (1960) reported these at the cervicothoracic junction, with injury to the brachial plexus. The spine itself is not damaged, but injury to the head and first cervical vertebra may occur. The development of meningeal adhesions might cause block, as in 2 cases reported by him.

In evaluating hyperextension injuries of the cervical spine, the ligamenta flava, the presence of spondylotic ridges and the sagittal diameter of the spinal canal all are important factors. During the moment of extreme hyperextension the combination of wrinkling of the ligamenta flava anteriorly and the increased dorsad bulging of spondylotic ridges combine to cause compression of the cord. This is enhanced when the diameter of the spinal canal is reduced either as a developmental change, consequent to increased thickness of the neural arches, because of associated hypertrophic spondylosis or a combination of these factors.

Some hyperextension injuries damage the central area of the cord, but more often the anterior aspect is affected. The dentate ligaments in checking dorsal protrusion of the cord against the neural arches enhances the probability for injury to its anterior aspect. Considerable time may elapse before these injuries manifest themselves clinically, and their association with previous trauma sometimes is overlooked. Schneider and Knighton (1959) pointed out that the syndrome of chronic injury to the central zone is characterized by weakness of the fingers, hands and arms to a greater extent than seen in the lower extremities. The sensory pattern is erratic, and the picture can be confused with syringomyelia. Acute injury to the central zone also damages the vicinity of the central canal, with involvement of the nerve supply to the neck, shoulders and upper extremities and lesser damage to the nerves of the trunk and lower extremities. To the degree in which permanent damage exists, the chronic picture develops later. Considerable recovery occurs if the damage is reversible.

Injuries to the spinous processes of the lower cervical and upper thoracic spine have been referred to as "clay-shoveler's" fractures, and may occur in one or several vertebrae, upper from the sixth cervical to the thoracic segments. The fracture line appears mainly at the narrowest part of the spinous process about 2 cm from its end but also occurs at its base (Fig. 323). This type of injury is attributed to muscular pull caused by a sudden jerk. Undernutrition and fatigue are contributing factors. These

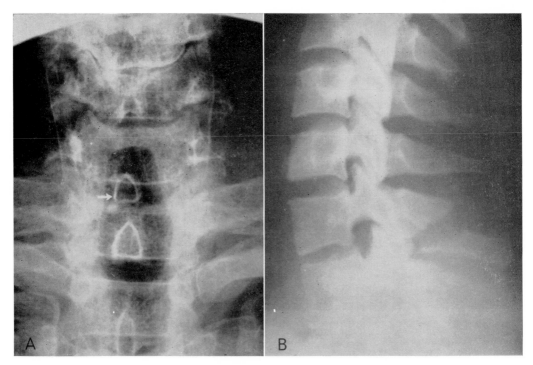

Fig. 323. *A*, Fracture through the base of the spinous process of C7. As seen on the AP view the involved tip is displaced downwards (arrow). *B*, Lateral view.

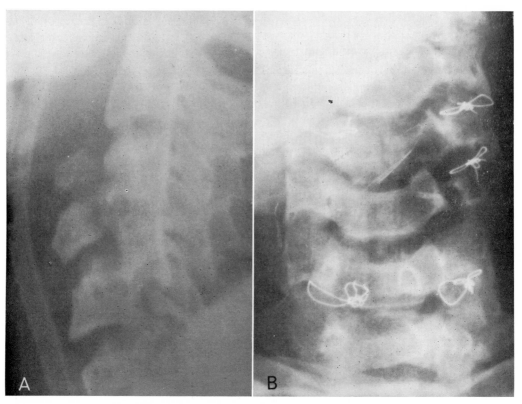

Fig. 324. *A*, Multiple shearing vertical fractures of C3, 4 and 5, lateral view. *B*, AP view after attempt at reduction. The fracture lines pass through the left pedicles of C4 and 5.

stress fractures are best seen on lateral roentgenograms. They may be identified in the anteroposterior view by a downward displacement of the tip of the spinous process as seen on an overexposed film. With some hyperflexion injuries fractures of the spinous processes of the lower cervical and uppermost thoracic vertebrae occur. These tend not to heal, and may be followed by calcifications in the adjacent soft tissues due to the laying down of calcium in an accompanying hematoma (Gershon-Cohen, Budin and Glauser, 1954).

Vertical fractures of the cervical vertebrae are infrequent. Fissure fractures of this variety are difficult to identify. Body section roentgenograms are useful for this purpose (Fig. 319). When there is no neural involvement, vertical fractures are not threatening. However, severe trauma can produce a shearing force producing multiple oblique and vertical fractures associated with severe damage to the soft tissues, the cord and the meninges (Fig. 324).

Fractures of the cervical transverse processes likewise are infrequent. Occasionally the seventh cervical transverse process is broken and is accompanied by pain aggravated by motion or pressure which radiates down the arm. These patients may be referred for radiographic examination of the shoulder and the transverse process fracture is then discovered incidentally (Fig. 325). Probably the most important factor in the identification of this lesion is a high index of suspicion.

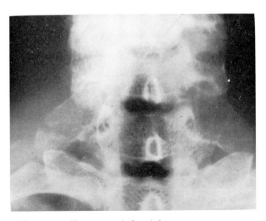

FIG. 325. Fracture of the right transverse process of C7 after an automobile accident. Exquisite tenderness on slight pressure elicited over the fracture.

References

Amyes, E. W. and Anderson, F. M.: Fracture of the Odontoid Process, Arch. Surg., *72*, 377, 1956.

Annan, J. H.: Shoveller's Fracture, Lancet, *1*, 174, 1945.

Barnes, R.: Paraplegia in Cervical Spine Injuries, J. Bone & Joint Surg., *30-B*, 234, 1948.

Blockley, N. J. and Purser, D. W.: Fractures of the Odontoid Process of the Axis, J. Bone & Joint Surg., *38-B*, 794, 1956.

Brooke, W. S.: Complete Transverse Cervical Myelitis Caused by Traumatic Herniation of an Ossified Nucleus Pulposus, J.A.M.A., *125*, 117, 1944.

Carpenter, S.: Injury of Neck as Cause of Vertebral Artery Thrombosis, J. Neurosurg., *18*, 849, 1961.

Cramer, F. and McGowan, F. J.: Nucleus Pulposus in Pathogenesis of So-Called "Recoil" Injuries of Spinal Cord, Surg., Gynec. & Obst., *79*, 516, 1944.

Crooks, F. and Birkett, A. N.: Fractures and Dislocations of the Cervical Spine, Brit. J. Surg., *31*, 252, 1944.

Davies, H.: Unusual Sequel to Fracture of the Odontoid Process, Brit. J. Radiol., *18*, 132, 1945.

Davis, A. G.: Injuries of Cervical Spine, J.A.M.A., *127*, 149, 1945.

Durbin, F. C.: Fracture-Dislocations of the Cervical Spine, J. Bone & Joint Surg., *39-B*, 23, 1957.

Fielding, J. W.: Disappearance of the Central Portion of the Odontoid Process, J. Bone & Joint Surg., *47-A*, 1228, 1965.

Freiberger, R. H., Wilson, P. D., Jr. and Nicholas, J. A.: Acquired Absence of the Odontoid Process, J. Bone & Joint Surg., *47-A*, 1231, 1965.

Gershon-Cohen, J., Budin, E. and Glauser, F.: Whiplash Fractures of Cervico-Dorsal Spinous Processes; Resemblance to Shoveller's Fracture, J.A.M.A., *155*, 560, 1954.

Grisolia, A., Bell, R. L. and Peltier, L. F.: Fractures and Dislocations of the Spine Complicating Ankylosing Spondylitis, J. Bone & Joint Surg., *49-A*, 339, 1967.

Hall, R. D. McKellar: Clay-Shoveller's Fracture, J. Bone & Joint Surg., *22*, 63, 1940.

Helfer, L. M.: Prolonged Spinal Cord Compression of Traumatic Origin, Southern M. J., *43*, 1027, 1950.

Hinchley, K. J. and Bickel, W. H.: Fracture of Atlas, Ann. Surg., *121*, 826, 1945.

Jefferson, G.: Fracture of the Atlas Vertebra, Brit. J. Surg., *7*, 407, 1920.

Kaplan, C. J.: Cervical Hyperextension Injuries with Paraplegia, J. Bone & Joint Surg., *35-B*, 97, 1953.

Kristoff, F. V. and Dratz, M.: Minor Fractures of Cervical Laminae Simulating Ruptured Cervical Disk, J. Neurosurg., *5*, 95, 1948.

Leventhal, H. R.: Birth Injuries of the Spinal Cord, J. Pediat., *56*, 447, 1960.

Liss, L.: Fatal Cervical Cord Injury in a Swimmer, Neurology, *15*, 675, 1965.

Mansfield, C. M.: A Vertical Fracture of the Fifth Cervical Vertebra Without Neurologic Symptoms, Am. J. Roentgenol., *86*, 277, 1961.

Morrison, A.: Hyperextension Injury of the Cervical Spine with Rupture of the Esophagus, J. Bone & Joint Surg., *42-B*, 356, 1960.

Naiman, J. L., Donohue, W. L. and Prichard, J. .S: Fatal Nucleus Pulposus Embolism of Spinal Cord After Trauma, Neurology, *11*, 83, 1961.

Plaut, H. F.: Fractures of Atlas Resulting from Automobile Accidents, Am. J. Roentgenol., *40*, 867, 1938.

Richman, S. and Friedman, R. L.: Vertical Fracture of Cervical Bodies, Radiology, *62*, 536, 1954.

Roaf, R.: A Study of the Mechanics of Spinal Injury, J. Bone & Joint Surg., *42-B*, 810, 1960.

Rodgers, W. A.: Fractures and Dislocations of the Cervical Spine, J. Bone & Joint Surg., *39-A*, 341, 1957.

Rogers, L.: Delayed Paraplegia Following Fractures of Vertebrae, Brit. J. Surg., *32*, 514, 1945.

Taylor, A. R.: The Mechanism of Injury to the Spinal Cord in the Neck Without Damage to the Vertebral Column, J. Bone & Joint Surg., *33-B*, 543, 1951.

————: Mechanism and Treatment of Spinal Cord Disorders Associated with Cervical Spondylosis, Lancet, *1*, 717, 1953.

Taylor, A. R. and Blackwood, W.: Paraplegia in Hyperextension Cervical Injuries with Normal Radiographic Appearances, J. Bone & Joint Surg., *30-B*, 245, 1948.

Schneider, R. C.: The Syndrome of Acute Anterior Spinal Cord Injury, J. Neurosurg., *12*, 95, 1955.

————: Chronic Neurologic Sequelae of Acute Trauma to the Spine and Spine Cord. Part II. The Syndrome of Chronic Anterior Spinal Cord Injury or Compression. Herniated Intervertebral Discs, J. Bone & Joint Surg., *41-A*, 449, 1959.

————: Chronic Neurological Sequelae of Acute Trauma to the Spine and Spinal Cord. Part V. The Syndrome of Acute Central Cervical Spinal-Cord Injury Followed by Chronic Anterior Cervical-Cord Injury (or Compression) Syndrome, J. Bone & Joint Surg., *42-A*, 253, 1960.

Schneider, R. C. and Crosby, E. C.: Vascular Insufficiency of Brain Stem and Spinal Cord in Spinal Trauma, Neurology, *9*, 643, 1959.

Schneider, R. C. and Kahn, E. A.: Chronic Neurological Sequelae of Acute Trauma to the Spine and Spinal Cord. Part I. The Significance of the Acute-Flexion or Tear-Drop Fracture-Dislocation of the Cervical Spine, J. Bone & Joint Surg., *38-A*, 985, 1956.

Schneider, R. C. and Knighton, R.: Chronic Neurological Sequelae of Acute Trauma to the Spine and Spinal Cord. Part III. The Syndrome of Chronic Injury to the Cervical Spinal Cord in the Region of the Central Canal. J. Bone & Joint Surg., *41-A*, 905, 1959.

Schneider, R. C., Livingston, K. E., Cave, A. J. E. and Hamilton, G.: "Hangman's Fracture" of the Cervical Spine, J. Neurosurg., *22*, 141, 1965.

Venable, J. R., Flake, R. E. and Kilian, D. J.: Stress Fracture of the Spinous Process, J.A.M.A., *190*, 881, 1964.

Whiteley, J. E. and Forsyth, H. F.: The Classification of Cervical Spine Injuries, Am. J. Roentgenol., *83*, 633, 1960.

Zanca, P. and Lodmell, E. A.: Fracture of Spinous Process, Radiology, *56*, 427, 1951.

ATLANTOAXIAL DISLOCATIONS

The normal atlantoaxial articulation consists of four joints, two pivotal and two arthrodial, or gliding joints. One pivot joint is between the posterior surface of the anterior arch of the atlas and the front of the odontoid process, and the second is between the anterior surface of the transverse ligament of the atlas and the posterior aspect of the odontoid process. The two gliding joints are those on either side of the articular processes between the atlas and the axis. On either side of the odontoid process is a bursa which separates it anteriorly from the transverse ligament of the atlas. All four joints are lined with synovial membrane.

The structures connecting the atlas and axis consist of the articular capsules, which unite the margins of the lateral masses of the atlas with those of the posterior articular surface of the axis. In front is the anterior atlantoaxial ligament, which extends from the inferior margin of the anterior arch of the atlas to the anterior aspect of the body of the axis. The posterior atlantoaxial ligament is attached from the lower border of the posterior arch of the atlas to the upper edge of the laminae of the axis. The transverse ligament of the axis extends across the ring, keeping the odontoid process in contact with the anterior arch. Arising from either side of the upper portion of the odontoid process are the alar ligaments, two strong rounded ligaments, which insert into the occipital condyles on their medial aspects. These limit the motion of the head, and are referred to as check ligaments. Between the two alar ligaments lies the apical odontoid ligament, which extends from the tip of the odontoid process to the anterior margin of the foramen magnum, and unites with the deep portion of the anterior atlanto-occipital membrane and the superior crus of the transverse ligament of the atlas. This is regarded as a rudimentary intervertebral fibrocartilage, and traces of notochord may persist within it.

Radiologic investigations of the atlanto-occipital articulations include lateral and anteroposterior views projecting the atlas and axis through the open mouth. In addition submento-vertical or vertical-submental views aid in visualizing the atlanto-occipital articulations. The latter are sometimes difficult to obtain, particularly in patients with symptoms of atlantoaxial dislocation. Body section radiography brings out the articular surfaces between the occipital condyles and the first and second cervical vertebrae better than routine methods. This is particularly important in individuals who are unable to move their necks or open their mouths widely.

In patients who can cooperate observation of the movement of the atlas and axis by means of image intensification fluoroscopy is rewarding. Spot film roentgenograms and cineradiographic studies at that time are important in evaluating the possibility of dislocation (Fig. 326). The cineradiographic records are particularly helpful in that they permit detailed study of movement, and sometimes are almost essential in the identification of subluxations which appear only during movement. The displacement of the first on the second cervical vertebrae occurring with rheumatoid arthritis or ankylosing spondylitis is mainly a separation of the dens and the anterior arch of the atlas (Sharp and Purser, 1961). Cineradiographic examination is particularly useful for bringing this out.

There is a wide range in the normal configuration of the atlanto-occipital joints, with considerable asymmetry in the lateral aspects of the articulations between the first and second cervical vertebrae. A distinct lateral motion of the atlas on the axis can be demonstrated on lateral flexion of the head, or by forceful pressure by the examiner against muscular resistance on the part of the patient. Such lateral mobility of the atlas in relationship to the axis should not be mistaken for subluxation.

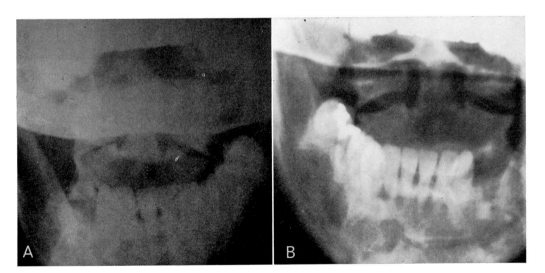

FIG. 326. *A*, AP study of the atlas and axis through the open mouth with the patient recumbent. An asymmetry in the articulations on the right and left is noted, and the possibility of subluxation was considered. *B*, Spot film made under image intensification control shows no dislocation.

Alterations in the normal cervical curve are likely to appear when there is muscle spasm. This can occur with atlantoaxial displacements, with a reversal of the usual lordotic curve and limitation of movement in flexion and extension. The possibility that such alteration in alignment of the cervical vertebrae is produced by spasm incident to other injuries involving the articular facets or the laminae must be investigated. In patients with torticollis incident to trauma the alignment of the atlas on the axis as seen on anteroposterior roentgenograms may reveal some lateral displacement on the superior or the inferior articular surfaces of these vertebrae, and the dens may be slightly to one side. However, the distance between the dens and the anterior arch of the atlas is not grossly altered. There may be some forward displacement of the second on the third vertebra, and distinct limitation of motion be seen on flexion and extension films. However, this malalignment usually clears with a few days of conservative treatment. During the acute phase of torticollis the angle of the jaw deviates to the side opposite the lateral curve of the spastic cervical spine. This, too, returns to normal.

The usefulness of cineradiographic studies of the neck lies in the fact that a permanent record of movement is made. Another factor is that the radiologist himself makes the cineradiographic run, and personally evaluates the range of movement which the patient can perform. This is not always accurate when a technician routinely positions the patient for filming. It is unfortunate, but nevertheless true, that some peculiar alignments of the cervical vertebrae can be obtained when the patient does not cooperate fully in the procurement of movement studies.

Not infrequently straightening of the usual cervical curve is observed in patients who have had recent trauma. In some of these patients pain of a temporary nature will restrict movement. However, demonstration of such a change should not be regarded as indicative of bony injury with the assumption that small fractures cannot be demonstrated. A recheck examination a few days later under the personal observation of the radiologist often is helpful. If prevertebral or supraclavicular hematoma also is present, careful and detailed search for a small fracture can be rewarding.

Rotary movement of the atlas and axis is best recorded on spot films made in the course of image intensification fluoroscopy and cineradiographic examination. At this time one can also obtain oblique views of the atlas and axis, particularly useful for demonstrating fractures of the posterior arches (Fig. 318).

The width of the atlantoaxial joint in the lateral position is an important index to its condition. The normal width is between 1 to 2 mm, and the normal upper range of the inclination of the atlas against the axis is about 10 degrees. This angle is determined by a line joining the inferior borders of the anterior and posterior atlantic arches, and a second line joining the inferior border of the articular processes of the axis with the inferior border of its spinous process. The distance between the anterior aspect of the dens and the posterior articular surface of the atlas, in flexion and extension, in children varies from 2 to 3 mm, but can reach 4.5 mm. In flexion or extension in adults the space does not exceed 2.5 mm, the measurement being greatest in flexion.

In normal individuals the tip of the spinous process of the first cervical vertebra is short, and is in a direct line with that of the second cervical vertebra. With subluxation the tip of the first cervical spinous process moves forward. The jaw is displaced forward as well, and deviates to the opposite side. The arch of the atlas is moved anterior in relationship to the arches below (Fig. 327).

Dislocations of the atlantoaxial joints may occur unilateraly or bilaterally. Anterior or posterior displacement of one of the lateral masses of the first cervical vertebra in relation to the subjacent articular surface of the second cervical vertebra is the most frequent subluxation noted. This may or may not be

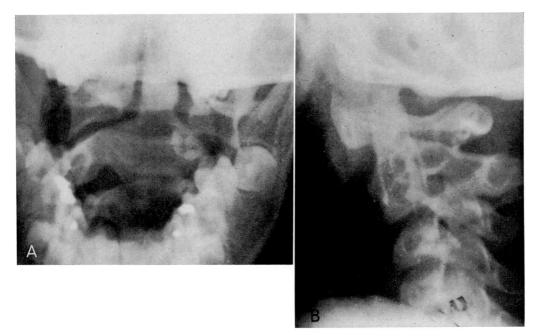

Fig. 327. *A,* Atlantoaxial dislocation in a 12-year-old boy who had a wry neck for 10 days after a sore throat and cervical adenitis. The left articulation is displaced sideways. *B,* The anterior arch of the atlas is shifted anteriorly. The tip of the dens is elevated. Note the change in the alignment of C2 and 3.

accompanied by displacement of the anterior arch of the atlas in relation to the dens. Such a change is best identified cineradiographically and on flexion and extension roentgenograms (Fig. 327). Both articular surfaces of the atlas may rotate in relationship to those of the axis, one directed anteriorly and the other posteriorly. Such a rotary displacement may be quite extensive, so much so that one lateral mass disappears and can be seen only on body section examinations. The tip of the dens projects upwards, but may retain its usual relationship to the anterior arch of the atlas (Fig. 328).

There may be right or left lateral dislocation of the atlas on the axis. In this circumstance a fracture of the odontoid process usually accompanies the lesion, and a history of trauma is generally obtained (Fig. 329).

The etiologic factors associated with atlanto-occipital dislocations include trauma, congenital defects of the cervico-occipital junction, absence or incomplete fusion of the odontoid process with the body of the second cervical vertebra (Clark, 1941; Weiler, 1942;

Nievergelt, 1948), inflammatory diseases such as acute tonsillitis, cervical adenitis or the various exanthematous diseases (Sullivan, 1949). Cases have also been reported following mastoid infections (Frank, 1936), rheumatic fever (Evans, 1941), and after tonsillectomy (Swanberg, 1919). Tuberculosis, syphilis, or more often metastases, of the cervical spine, by destroying structures comprising the atlanto-occipital articulations, may be followed by dislocations following an unguarded sudden movement of the head or other trauma (Willard and Nicholson, 1941). Kyphoscoliosis in children might be a causative factor (Hess, Abelson and Bronstein, 1942). Poliomyelitis, ankylosing spondylitis and rheumatoid arthritis and steroid therapy are additional factors.

Excluding cases of obviously traumatic origin, those due to tuberculosis, syphilis, or other bone-destroying lesions such as osseous metastases, or to congenital anomalies of the atlas and axis, the etiology of spontaneous atlantoaxial subluxation has been ascribed (Wittek, 1908) to effusion into the joint

32

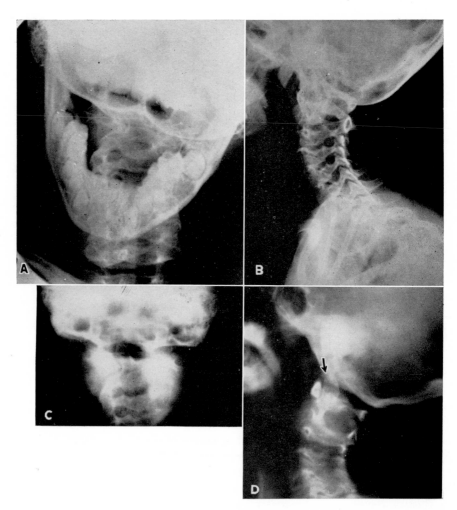

Fig. 328. *A,* Atlantoaxial dislocation incident to a mild attack of measles. The head is tilted to the left. Note the tilting of the dens to the right. The left cervical mass of the first cervical vertebra is rotated out of view. *B,* Lateral view. Because of the tilt of the head true laterals could not be obtained. *C,* Antero-posterior body section roentgenogram. Note the tilt of the dens and the absence of the left lateral mass of the first cervical vertebra. *D,* Same case, lateral body section roentgenogram. The tip of the dens is well above the anterior arch of the atlas (arrow).

capsule, with overdistention of the liga-ments. A diffuse tissue hyperemia results, which produces decalcification of the adja-cent bone and loosening of the intervertebral ligaments, particularly those between the atlas and axis. This permits the skull and first cervical vertebra to dislocate anteriorly, or there may be a backward slipping of one articular facet of the atlas on the axis. This hyperemia is not accompanied by destruc-tion of bone, and is difficult to identify roentgenologically. An inflammatory proc-

ess anywhere in the upper cervical region may cause this condition, particularly in children (Greig, 1931) (Watson-Jones, 1932).

Frank (1936) compared dislocation of the atlas to subluxation of the hips, which some-times complicates various exanthematous diseases, typhoid and mastoiditis. A case of an associated spontaneous dislocation of the hip with a spontaneous dislocation of the atlas was described by Steele (1937). Stein, Bloch and Kenin (1953) in a report of a non-traumatic subluxation of the atlanto-

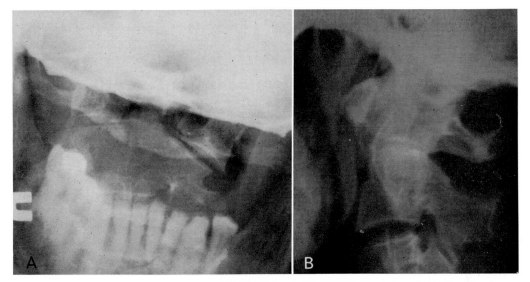

FIG. 329. *A*, Dislocation of the atlas and axis. A sharp lateral shift of the atlas is present towards the left. The base of the dens is fractured. *B*, The atlas is shifted anteriorly and the dens is inclined dorsally.

axial articulation suggested that joint effusion as a result of hypersensitivity might be a causative factor, comparing the change to that described by Edwards (1952) in transient synovitis of the hip joint in children.

Most atlantoaxial dislocations occur in children. The disease usually appears about 2 weeks after the onset of an inflammatory lesion involving the nose and throat. The patient holds his head in a torticollis position, with the chin pressed closely against the neck and pointed to the side opposite the dislocation if a unilateral dislocation exists. The patient may find it difficult to open his mouth and complains of pain in the occipital and mastoid areas. Some degree of flexion may be obtained, but extension of the head usually produces pain. Rotation of the head from side to side is impaired, and the chin cannot be rotated beyond the midline. Considerable spasm of the posterior spinal muscles of the neck is present.

Central nervous system symptoms referable to atlanto-occipital dislocations are infrequent in cases of the spontaneous variety. Wilson, Michele and Jacobson (1940) reported an elderly patient who had pneu-

monia followed by atlanto-occipital dislocation resulting in quadriplegia. This patient recovered following treatment by head traction. Another case with nontraumatic atlanto-occipital dislocation accompanied by quadriplegia was reported by Titrud, McKinlay, Camp and Hewitt (1949) in a 40-year-old woman who recovered after surgical decompression followed by spinal fusion. Alexander, Masland and Harris (1953) reported an infant with anterior dislocation of the first cervical vertebra simulating cerebral birth injury. Myelography in this case revealed obstruction at the level of the first cervical interspace. Myelopathy following atlantoaxial dislocation is uncommon. However, such instances have been reported not only immediately after the onset of the displacement, but long thereafter (Dunbar and Ray, 1961; Stratford, 1957; Dzenitis, 1966).

A review of our cases of atlanto-occipital dislocation indicates findings much the same as reported by others. In 7 of our cases, however, we noted no gross forward displacement of the body of the atlas anteriorly, while the odontoid process was tilted dorsally and laterally, opposite to the dislocated lateral mass. The space between the dens and the undisplaced lateral mass was narrowed. The space between the anterior aspect of the odontoid and the arch of the first cervical vertebra was within normal limits in 7 of the 12 cases observed, and appreciably widened in 3.

Atlantoaxial dislocations were observed in 7 patients with metastases to the upper cervical vertebrae from carcinoma of the breast and 4 from bronchogenic carcinomas. In each a forward displacement of the head was observed, with loss of rotary motion and extension. Roentgenologic investigations disclosed destruction of the atlas or the axis or both, with disruption of the joints at the atlanto-occipital and atlantoaxial junctions. Forward displacement of the first or second cervical vertebral bodies was present in 7.

References

Alexander, E., Masland, R. and Harris, C.: Anterior Dislocation of First Cervical Vertebra Simulating Cerebral Birth Injury in Infancy, Am. J. Dis. Child., 85, 173, 1953.

Askenasy, H. M., Braham, J. and Kosary, I. Z.: Delayed Spinal Myelopathy Following Atlanto-Axial Fracture Dislocation, J. Neurosurg., 17, 1100, 1960.

Cattell, H. S. and Filtzer, D.: Pseudosubluxation and Other Normal Variations in the Cervical Spine in Children, J. Bone & Joint Surg., 47-A, 1295, 1965.

Clark, W. A.: Fractures and Dislocations of Cervical Portion of Spine, A.M.A. Arch. Surg., 42, 537, 1941.

Colsen, K.: Atlanto-Axial Fracture Dislocation, J. Bone & Joint Surg., 31-B, 395, 1949.

Coutts, M. B.: Atlanto-Epistropheal Subluxations, Arch. Surg., 29, 297, 1934.

Dankmeijer, J. and Rothmeier, B. J.: Lateral Movement of Atlantoaxial Joints, Acta radiol., 24, 55, 1943.

Dunbar, H. S. and Ray, B. S.: Chronic Atlanto-Axial Dislocations with Late Neurologic Manifestations, Surg., Gynec. & Obst., 113, 757, 1961.

Dzenitis, A. J.: Spontaneous Atlanto-Axial Dislocation in a Mongoloid Child with Spinal Cord Compression, J. Neurosurg., 25, 458, 1966.

Edwards, E.: Transient Synovitis of Hip Joint in Children, J.A.M.A., 148, 30, 1952.

Englander, O.: Non-Traumatic Occipito-Atlanto-Axial Dislocations, Brit. J. Radiol., 15, 341, 1942.

Epstein, B. S.: Skull Laminagraphy, Radiology, 38, 22, 1942.

Epstein, B. S. and Kulick, M.: Body Section Radiography in Some Orthopedic Problems, Radiography & Clin. Photog., No. 2, 1945.

Evans, W. A., Jr.: Pathologic Dislocation of Atlanto-Axial Joint, Radiology, 37, 347, 1941.

Frank, I.: Spontaneous (Non-Traumatic) Atlanto-Axial Subluxation, Ann. Otol., Rhinol., and Layrngol., 45, 405, 1936.

Gabrielsen, T. O. and Maxwell, J. A.: Traumatic Atlanto-Occipital Dislocation, Am. J. Roentgenol., 97, 624, 1966.

Gelehrter, G.: Differentialdiagnose der Halswirbelverletzungen im Kindesalter, Fortschr. Röntgenstrah., 99, 506, 1963.

Greig, D. M.: Clinical Observations on the Surgical Pathology of Bone, Edinburgh, Oliver & Boyd, 1931.

Hadley, L. A.: Cervical Spine, Am. J. Roentgenol., 52, 173, 1944.

Hess, J. H., Abelson, S. M. and Bronstein, I. P.: Spontaneous Atlanto-Axial Dislocations; Possible Relationship to Deformity of Spine, Am. J. Dis. Child., 64, 51, 1942.

Hess, J. H., Bronstein, I. P. and Abelson, S. M.: Atlanto-Axial Dislocations Unassociated with Trauma and Secondary to Inflammatory Foci in the Neck, Am. J. Dis. Child., 49, 1137, 1935.

Jackson, H.: Minimal Atlanto-Axial Subluxation, Brit. J. Radiol., 23, 672, 1950.

Jones, M. D.: Cervical Spine Cineradiography after Traffic Accidents, Arch. Surg., 85, 974, 1962.

Makon, R. F. and Lovell, W. W.: Spontaneous Atlantoaxial Subluxation Accompanied by Severe Neurologic Deficits, Surgery, 40, 770, 1956.

Martin, R. C.: Atlas-Axis Dislocation Following Cervical Infection, J.A.M.A., 118, 874, 1942.

Nievergelt, K.: Luxatio Atlanto-Epistrophica bei Aplasie des Dens epistrophei, Schweiz. med. Wchnschr., 78, 653, 1948.

Paul, L. W. and Moir, W. W.: Non-Pathologic Variations in Relationship of the Upper Cervical Vertebrae, Am. J. Roentgenol., 62, 519, 1949.

Sharp, J. and Purser, D. W.: Spontaneous Atlanto-Axial Dislocation in Ankylosing Spondylitis and Rheumatoid Arthritis, Ann. Rheum. Dis., 20, 47, 1961.

Stratford, J.: Myelopathy Caused by Atlanto-Axial Dislocation, J.. Neurosurg., 14, 97, 1957.

Sullivan, A. W.: Subluxation of Atlanto-Axial Joint; Sequel to Inflammatory Processes of the Neck, J. Pediat., 35, 451, 1949.

Swanberg, H.: Anterior Dislocation of Atlas Following Tonsillectomy, J.A.M.A., 72, 107, 1919.

Titrud, L. A., McKinlay, C. A., Camp, W. E. and Hewitt, H. B.: Non-Traumatic Atlanto-Axial Dislocation, J. Neurosurg., 6, 174, 1949.

Washington, E. R.: Non-Traumatic Atlanto-Occipital and Atlanto-Axial Dislocation, J. Bone & Joint Surg., 41-A, 341, 1959.

Weiler, H. G.: Congenital Absence of Odontoid Process of Axis with Atlanto-Axial Dislocation, J. Bone & Joint Surg., 24, 161, 1942.

Willard, D. P. and Nicholson, J. T.: Dislocation of First Cervical Vertebra, Ann. Surg., 113, 464, 1941.

Wilson, M. J., Michele, A. A. and Jacobson, E. W.: Spontaneous Dislocation of Atlanto-Axial Articulation, J. Bone & Joint Surg., *22*, 698, 1940.

Wittek, A.: Ein Fall von Distentionluxation im Atlanto-epistropheal Gelenke, München. med. Wchnschr., *55*, 1837, 1908.

Wollin, D. G. and Botterell, E. H.: Symmetrical Forward Luxation of the Atlas, Am. J. Roentgenol., *79*, 575, 1958.

FRACTURES OF THE THORACIC SPINE

Fractures of the thoracic vertebrae follow injuries causing sudden severe hyperflexion, as may occur during an automobile accident, a fall or in games. Infrequently, fractures of the upper thoracic spine occurs if an individual is struck with a heavy object in a stooped position while his head is bent forward. Thoracic vertebral fractures usually are of the compression variety, with narrowing of the anterior aspect of the involved bodies. The posterior aspect tends to retain its normal height in the event of mild compression fractures. Pathologic fractures are quite frequent, and collapse of vertebrae incident to eosinophilic granulomas in children similarly require consideration in differential diagnosis. Osteoporosis and osteomalacia, hyperparathyroidism and Paget's disease have been mentioned before.

The most frequent site is the lower thoracic spine. Upper and middle thoracic vertebral fractures occur less commonly. Fractures of the neural arches and of the transverse and spinous processes are infrequent. Usually the superior aspect of the vertebrae are affected, and multiple fractures are likely to occur. Compaction of cancellous bone results in increased density of the injured vertebrae. This may increase in the course of healing (Fig. 330). If multiple segments are affected, the middle body may present compaction of bone both in the upper and lower surfaces (Fig. 330). When the trauma includes a lateral and rotary force as well as hyperflexion, the resultant fracture presents lateral wedging together with injury to the pedicles, laminae and adjacent rib heads. This occurs more often in the lower thoracic region, and is associated with severe injury. The soft tissues are affected, with paravertebral hemorrhage and laceration of the adjacent ligamentous structures. The intervertebral disc may be torn, so that a lateral and anterior shift of the upper vertebra is produced. Together with this may be intraspinal hemorrhage, displacement of bony and discal fragments into the spinal canal and edema all contributing to spinal cord compression (Fig. 331). Occasionally vertical fractures through the long axis of a vertebral body are seen, usually with severe trauma and compression fractures of several segments (Fig. 332).

Simple minor fractures of a vertebral body usually are of little concern. When comminution of fracture fragments occurs, particularly with injuries of the neural arches and pedicles, or when dislocations are superimposed, serious difficulty may arise because of intrusion into the spinal canal. Myelography may be required.

Dislocations of the thoracic vertebrae are relatively uncommon and are usually seen with fractures. Stanger (1947) in a review of 43 patients, noted a relatively high incidence of paraplegia with such injuries to the thoraco-lumbar junction. His patients were coal miners who worked in a crouched position. In 30, the eleventh and twelfth dorsal and first lumbar vertebrae were involved. In our experience there were 4 patients with a foward displacement of the body of the tenth thoracic on the eleventh thoracic vertebra, together with fractures of the eleventh ribs and of the laminae of the tenth dorsal vertebra. In addition to the forward displacement of the tenth on the eleventh dorsal vertebrae there was lateral displacement of approximately 0.5 cm. The intervertebral discs were torn, permitting the sliding displacement of the involved vertebrae while the height of the discs were somewhat diminished. These patients all had severe pain, but no central nervous system complications. Three had been in head-on automobile collisions, and one had fallen from a scaffold.

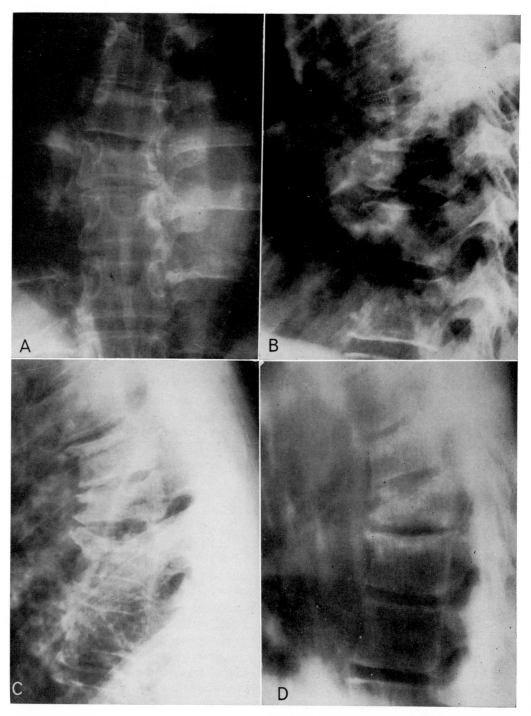

Fig. 330. A, Fracture of the thoracic spine following a convulsion. The left side of T7 is compressed. On the lateral view, B, the body is flattened. C, Five weeks later sclerotic changes are visible in the superior aspect of C7. A fracture of the superior aspect of C8 is now visible. D, Laminagram shows the sclerotic changes and deformities of C7 and 8.

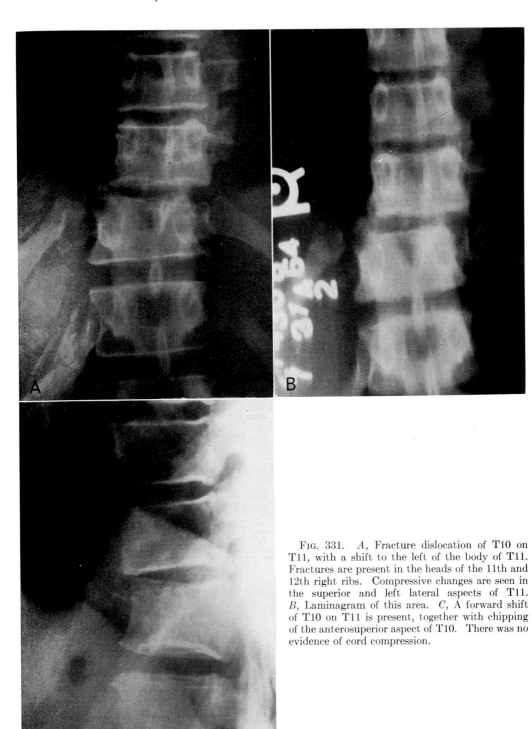

Fig. 331. *A*, Fracture dislocation of T10 on T11, with a shift to the left of the body of T11. Fractures are present in the heads of the 11th and 12th right ribs. Compressive changes are seen in the superior and left lateral aspects of T11. *B*, Laminagram of this area. *C*, A forward shift of T10 on T11 is present, together with chipping of the anterosuperior aspect of T10. There was no evidence of cord compression.

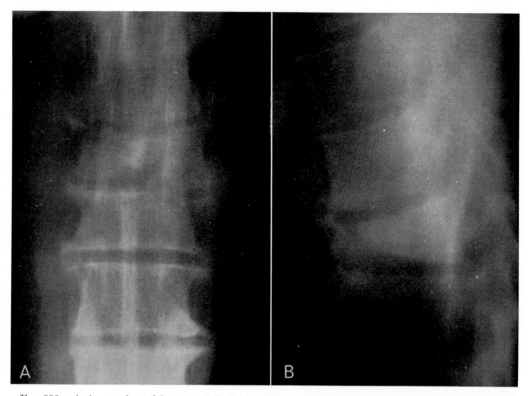

FIG. 332. *A*, A comminuted fracture of the body of T7, including a vertical fracture through the middle of the body. There is also a fracture of the left lateral aspect of the superior portion of T9. *B*, Laminagram shows compression of T8, together with a fracture of the anterosuperior portion of the underlying ninth thoracic vertebra.

A more frequent group of fractures of the thoracic vertebrae occurs in patients undergoing shock treatment. Forceful anterior flexion during the convulsive episode may produce compression fractures of the anterior aspects of one or several upper thoracic vertebrae, usually the fourth, fifth or sixth. No changes of the intervertebral discs are associated with these compressions. Alterations in vertebral contour usually are more readily identified on the lateral than the frontal views. However, lateral compression can be seen only on frontal roentgenograms. Such fractures were reported by Vogl and Osborn (1940) during convulsions following metrazol therapy. Similar changes were reported by Krause and Langsam (1941), both indicating that the fractures were more common in the upper dorsal spine. The latter authors reported an incidence of 42.6 per

cent out of 75 consecutive cases. Fractures following electric shock therapy were reported by Lingley and Robbins (1947) in 23 per cent of 230 cases. Meschan, Scruggs and Calhoun (1950) reported an incidence of vertebral injury of the thoracic spine in 35.4 per cent of their cases, with an average of 2.6 vertebrae involved per patient. Funkhouser and Davis (1952), in a review of 50 spinal fractures due to electric shock treatments, noted an incidence of approximately 20 per cent, and that men were affected more frequently. Pain with these fractures is absent or mild. Similarly, stress fractures associated with fatigue may occur (Hartley, 1943).

It has long been known that major epileptic convulsions can cause fractures of the dorsal spine by acute hyperflexion. In 1938 Rand reported on post-tetanic gibbus in 3 children with varying degrees of collapse of the bodies of the midthoracic vertebrae. Radiographic examination 6 months later showed kyphosis with marked narrowing of the fifth, sixth and seventh thoracic vertebrae in a 12-old-year-old girl who recovered after anti-tetanus serum convulsions, and similar observations were made in 2 other children.

Dietrich, Karshner and Stewart (1940) reported on 28 cases of tetanus with characteristic compression fractures of the midthoracic vertebrae, with wedge-shaped appearance of the involved vertebrae, and intact intervertebral discs. Zurcher (1948) also noted that the intervertebral discs remained unaltered following postconvulsive fractures. In marked cases the vertebrae may be divided into fragments (Sujoy, 1962).

References

Baab, O. D. and Howorth, M. B.: Fractures of Dorsal and Lumbar Vertebrae, J.A.M.A., *146*, 97, 1951.

Bohrer, S. P.: Spinal Fractures in Tetanus, Radiology, *85*, 1111, 1965.

Davis, P. R. and Rowland, H. A. K.: Vertebral Fractures in West Africans Suffering from Tetanus. J. Bone & Joint Surg., *47-B*, 61, 1965.

DeWald, P. A., Margolis, N. M. and Weiner, H.: Vertebral Fractures as a Complication of Electroconvulsive Therapy, J.A.M.A., *154*, 981, 1954.

Dietrich, H. F., Karshner, R. G. and Stewart, S. F.: Tetanus and Lesions of Spine in Childhood, J. Bone & Joint Surg., *22*, 43, 1940.

Ellis, J. D.: Compression Fractures of the Vertebral Bodies and Other Changes Mistaken for Them, J. Bone & Joint Surg., *26*, 139, 1944.

Funkhouser, J. B. and Davis, H. W.: Spinal Fractures Due to Electric Shock Treatments, J. Nerv. & Ment. Dis., *116*, 131, 1952.

Griffith, H. B., Gleave, J. R. W. and Taylor, R. G.: Changing Patterns in Fracture in the Dorsal and Lumbar Spine, Brit. Med. J., *1*, 891, 1966.

Hartley, J. B.: "Stress" or "Fatigue" Fractures of Bone, Brit. J. Radiol., *16*, 255, 1943.

Howorth, M. B.: Fracture of the Spine, Am. J. Surg., *92*, 573, 1956.

Isard, H. J.: A Roentgen Evaluation of Vertebral Fractures Resulting from Convulsive Shock Therapy, Am. J. Roentgenol., *68*, 247, 1952.

Krause, G. R. and Langsam, C. L.: Fractures of Vertebrae Following Metrazol Therapy, Radiology, *36*, 725, 1941.

Lingley, J. R. and Robbins, L. L.: Fractures Following Electroshock Therapy, Radiology, *48*, 124, 1947.

Meschan, I., Scruggs, J. B., Jr. and Calhoun, J. D.: Convulsive Fractures of Dorsal Spine Following Electro-Shock Therapy, Radiology, *43*, 180, 1950.

Newbury, C. L. and Etter, L. E.: Clarification of the Problem of Vertebral Fractures from Convulsive Therapy. II. Roentgenologcial Considerations, Arch. Neurol. & Psychiat., *74*, 479, 1955.

Nicholas, J. A., Wilson, P. D. and Freiberger, R.: Pathological Fractures of the Spine, J. Bone & Joint Surg., *42-A*, 127, 1960.

Norcross, J. R.: Compression Fractures of the Spine Complicated by Injury to the Spinal Cord, Surg. Clin. North America, *29*, 189, 1949.

Quinlan, A. G.: Post-Tetanic Kyphosis, J. Bone & Joint Surg., *36-B*, 80, 1954.

Rand, C. W.: Post-Tetanic Gibbus, Bull. Los Angeles Neurol. Soc., *3*, 141, 1938.

Stanger, J. K.: Fracture-Dislocation of Thoracolumbar Spine, J. Bone & Joint Surg., *29*, 107, 1947.

Sujoy, E.: Spinal Lesions in Tetanus in Children, Pediatrics, *29*, 629, 1962.

Vogl, A. and Osborne, R. L.: Fracture of the Column after Treatment of Psychoses with Cardiazol Shock, Acta radiol., *21*, 538, 1940.

Watson-Jones, R.: *Fractures and Joint Injuries*, 6th ed., Edinburgh, E. & S. Livingstone, Ltd., 1955.

Zürcher, P.: Die Posttetaniche Kyphose, Ann. Paediat., *170*, 42, 1948.

FRACTURES OF THE LUMBAR SPINE

Fractures of the upper lumbar spine are frequently accompanied by fractures of the eleventh and twelfth thoracic vertebrae. The mechanism for such injuries most often is hyperflexion incurred during various accidents. While only a single vertebra may be involved, it is more common to observe compressions of two or sometimes three segments, particularly if the thoracolumbar junction is involved. Compaction of cancellous bone often is present (Fig. 335). Concomitant injury to the ligaments, capsular structure, soft tissues and intervertebral discs are frequent. Symptoms depend on the effects of local hemorrhage, laceration and cauda equina and nerve root distortions. There is a higher incidence of paraplegia associated with injuries to the thoracolumbar junction than observed in the lower lumbar region, ascribed to the difference in the configuration of the spinal cord at the thoracolumbar level. The extent of skeletal damage is not indicative of the degree of cord trauma.

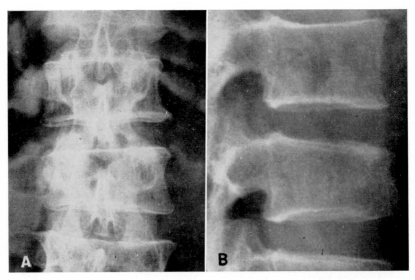

Fig. 333. Compression fracture involving the right lateral and anterior aspects of the body of the third lumbar vertebra. The vertebral body is wedged anteriorly, with no change in the height of its posterior aspect as seen on the lateral projection.

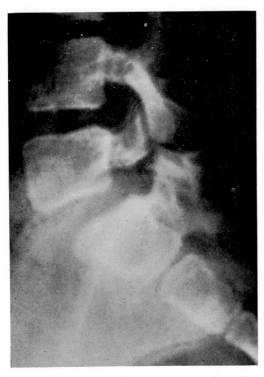

Fig. 334. Fracture of the pars interarticularis of a 12-year-old girl who fell from a swing.

Lumbar fractures usually are of the compression variety, with narrowing of the anterior aspect of the affected vertebral bodies. Depending on the torsional force, fractures of the lateral aspects of the bodies also occur (Fig. 333). When pronounced rotational injury is encountered, fractures also involve the neural arches. Anomalous fissures at the distal tips of the inferior articular processes may simulate such fractures. However, fractures of the articular processes without associated injuries of the vertebral bodies are rare. Nevertheless, in a patient who has suffered a recent injury followed immediately by disabling pain, small fractures of the neural arches may be identified. Body section and oblique stereo-roentgenographic study of the lumbar spine is almost essential in identifying these injuries. Fractures through the pars interarticularis are infrequent. They may follow torsional trauma (Fig. 334), and often are associated with stress or fatigue. Multiple such fractures are observed, for example, in ballet dancers or athletes. These may heal with union of bone or the visible break may persist.

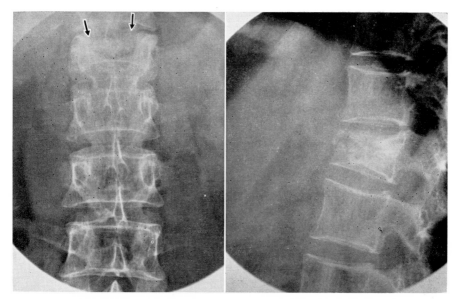

FIG. 335.   Impacted fracture through the superior surface of the body of the first lumbar
vertebra (arrows), with condensation of bone of the superior surface.

Occasionally one encounters what appears like small avulsion fractures of the anterior aspect of a vertebral body. These are usually accompanied by narrowing of the anterior or anterolateral aspect of that vertebra. In such instances, even though there is a history of recent trauma, the change is one associated with anterior discal herniation rather than a fracture, and is of no clinical importance most of the time.

Baab and Howorth (1951) mentioned that a majority of patients with mild compression fractures in the thoracolumbar region, and all with severe fractures eventually had spontaneous anterior bony ankylosis. They also noted posttraumatic thinning of the intervertebral discs. Osteophyte formation at the fracture sites could not be correlated with symptoms. Patients with spur formations prior to fracture had their symptoms somewhat longer, but the end-results were the same as with other patients.

Fractures of the transverse processes of the lumbar spine are readily identified when there is displacement of fracture fragments. However, in many the fracture line is difficult to identify because of overlying soft tissue and gas shadows. In such instances

the study should be repeated, preferably with a compression band to help eliminate confusing gas shadows. Spinous process fractures of the lumbar spine are infrequent, but should be considered whenever a point of tenderness is found over one of these structures. It is helpful to view all lateral lumbar spine films through a bright light to check on the spinous processes, inasmuch as these are usually obscured because of relative overpenetration. Special cone-down views with a lighter technic may be of assistance.

A case in which pseudarthrosis followed fractures of the transverse processes of the second to fifth lumbar vertebrae was reported by Hyman (1945). This patient had pain 3 months after having been immobilized for this injury. Re-examination showed joint formations at the fracture sites. At operation these joints were enclosed in a capsule, and section through the pseudarthrosis showed a fibrous band between the bony masses which prevented union. A comparatively well-organized hyalin cartilage covered the joint surfaces.

Subluxations of the apophyseal articulations of the lumbar spine are considered a cause of pain because of the production of

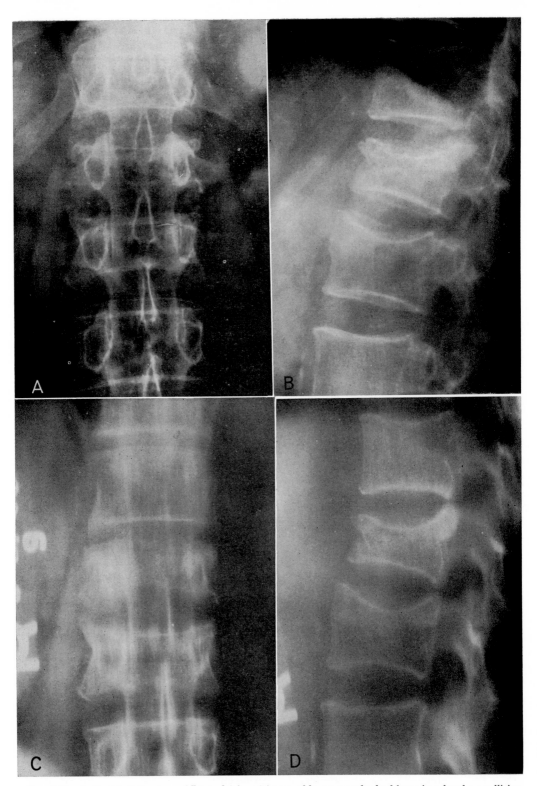

Fig. 336. *A*, Seat-belt fracture of L1 and 2 in a 54-year-old woman who had been in a head-on collision. The superior aspect of L1 is depressed, and the L1 disc is driven downwards into the body of L2, *B*. AP and lateral laminagrams *C* and *D*, reveal condensation of bone in the fracture area, and bulging of the anterior aspect of the body of L2.

494

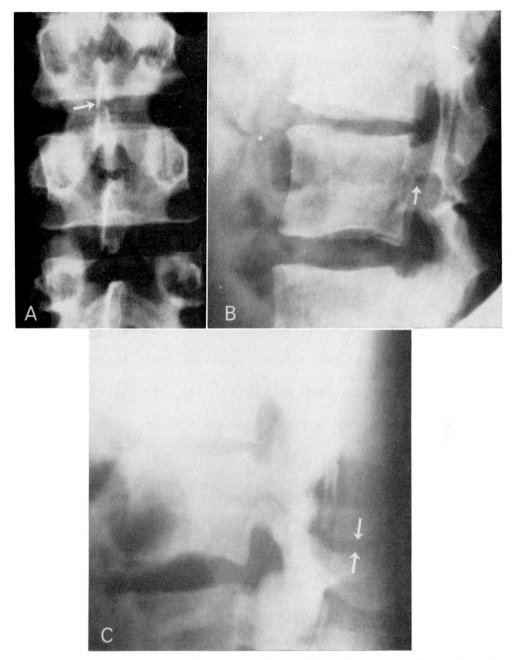

Fig. 337. *A*, Seat-belt fracture of L2 in a 23-year-old man. The AP view reveals a discontinuity of bone through the spinous process overlying the 2nd lumbar interspace (arrow). *B*, On the lateral view the fracture passes through the pedicles (arrow). A lighter film, *C*, discloses the fracture passing horizontally through the spinous process (arrows).

tension on the capsular ligaments, encroachment of the articular facets on the lumen of the intervertebral foramina, and because of erosion and sclerosis of the apposing joint surfaces (Hadley, 1935).

The advantages of myelography in investigating penetrating wounds of the spinal canal were discussed by Hinkel and Nichols (1946). They advocated this procedure because of information made available concerning the location and nature of an injury. Only a small number of patients suffering from penetrating wounds have actual perforation of the dura and extensive cord damage. More often the injury is in the nature of a hemorrhage, dislodged bone chips and infection. All of these may be remedied and present a better prognosis than does destruction of the cord or cauda equina. Included among myelographic defects observed after spinal trauma are sharply localized, clearly marginated indentations, angulations of the dural sac with displacement, and feathery irregular filling defects which may be part of the picture of an arachnoiditis. Complete spinal canal block may be observed. Passage of Pantopaque outside of the spinal canal which might be interpreted as due to faulty technic can be due to a tear in the arachnoid. In their cases the escaping contrast medium never flowed freely into any other space, but outlined a blind pocket. This extra-arachnoid puddle is located with its long axis parallel to that of the neural canal. When myelography disclosed a diverticulum-like contour, the possibility of a local collection of fluid causing compression of the spinal canal or the nerve roots had to be considered. Avulsion of nerve roots produces a similar change, and is discussed later (Fig. 341).

Unusual fractures of the lumbar vertebrae occur after a variety of relatively new traumas. The use of seat belts in automobiles, for instance, may cause a markedly localized hyperflexion injury, with compression of an upper lumbar segment and biconvex deformity of the intervertebral discs above and below (Fig. 336). Another patient involved in a head-on collision suffered a transverse fracture through the spinous process and the neural arch of the second lumbar vertebra with no gross change in the height of that vertebra (Fig. 337). In another patient recently seen there was a fracture dislocation of the second on the third lumbar vertebra, together with a forward flexion type of fracture of the anterosuperior aspect of the third lumbar vertebra. The involved discal interspaces were actually widened. This patient had rapidly become paraplegic, and was operated upon within an hour after the accident. Surgery disclosed a considerable epidural hemorrhage, a tear in the dura and a few nerve roots were severed. The cauda equina was intact. Following closure of the dura and reduction of the fracture there was no perceptible improvement during the first few days after the injury, at the time when this paragraph was written. Concomitant soft tissue injuries, such as rupture of the duodenum or jejunum or other abdominal injuries may take place (Campbell, 1964).

References

Bailey, W.: Anomalies and Fractures of the Vertebral Articular Processes, J.A.M.A., *108*, 266, 1937.

Campbell, H. E.: The Automobile Seat Belt and Abdominal Injury, Surg. Gynec. & Obst., *119*, 591, 1964.

Ellis, J. D.: Compression Fractures of the Vertebral Bodies and Other Changes Mistaken for Them, J. Bone & Joint Surg., *26*, 139, 1944.

Hadley, L.: Subluxation of Apophyseal Articulations with Bony Impingement as a Cause of Back Pain, Am. J. Roentgenol., *33*, 209, 1935.

Hinkel, C. L. and Nichols, R. L.: Opaque Myelography in Penetrating Wounds of Spinal Canal, Am. J. Roentgenol., *55*, 689, 1946.

Howland, W. I., Curry, J. L. and Buffington, C. B.: Fulcrum Fractures of the Lumbar Spine. Transverse Fracture Induced by an Improperly Placed Seat Belt, J.A.M.A., *193*, 240, 1965.

Hyman, G.: Pseudarthrosis Following Fractures of Lumbar Transverse Processes, Brit. J. Surg., *32*, 503, 1945.

Melamed, A.: Fracture of Pars Interarticularis of Lumbar Vertebra, Am. J. Roentgenol., *94*, 584, 1965.

Roche, M. B.: Bilateral Fracture of Pars Interarticularis of a Lumbar Neural Arch, J. Bone & Joint Surg., *30-A*, 1005, 1948.

Stanger, J. K.: Fracture-Dislocation of Thoracolumbar Spine, J. Bone & Joint Surg., *29*, 107, 1946.

FRACTURES OF THE SACRUM AND COCCYX

These usually follow direct trauma, most often secondary to a fall or a direct blow. Characteristically, these patients complain of pain which is exaggerated by attempting to walk or stand, and becomes acute when the patient places weight on the injured area. It is advantageous to make antero-posterior studies in several angles of projection in order to bring out the sacral and coccygeal segments. The fracture lines may be difficult to identify because of overlying gas and fecal shadows, even after adequate preparation of the patient. The lateral views have proved to be of more help in diagnosing such fractures. Tears of the sacrospinous and sacrotuberous ligaments may be diagnosed when there is avulsion of their insertions into the lower sacrum (Burman, 1952).

In addition to the bony injuries incurred in fractures of the sacrum there may be neurologic complications because of trauma to the sacral nerves. Bonnin (1945) in a review of 44 pelvic fractures, noted that the sacrum was involved in 45 per cent. He mentioned that the weakest portion of the sacrum was at the first and second foramina,

where the fracture lines usually were found (Fig. 338). He also observed that the fractures sometimes were not visible until several weeks after injury. The neurologic manifestations included evidence of damage to the first and second sacral nerves, with weakness of plantar flexion of the ankle, loss of ankle jerk reflexes and loss of the power of the hamstrings and glutei muscles. Marked paralysis of the biceps femori is frequent, and the calf and hamstring muscles may be tender. Altered sensations and referred pain to the outer side of the calf and foot may be present.

Vertical fractures of the sacrum are rare (Fig. 339), and usually are associated with ischiopubic fractures. Traumatic separation of the sacro-iliac joints occur with severe torsion, and also are related to ischiopubic fractures.

An unusual complication of a sacral fracture was described by Dobrzaniecki and Haak (1942) in a 26-year-old man who fell from a tree, striking the ground in a sitting posture. A fracture of the right side of the sacrum was found. Intrathecal injection of lipiodol showed globules along the line of fracture, gathering within a protuberance

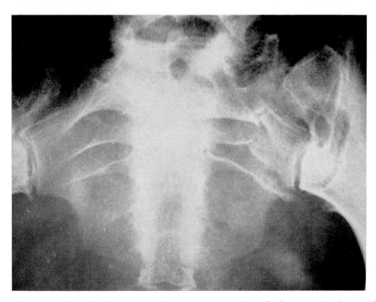

FIG. 338. Fracture through the left sacral wing passing through the superior first and second foraminal margins and the left side of the sacrum just beneath the sacro-iliac joint.

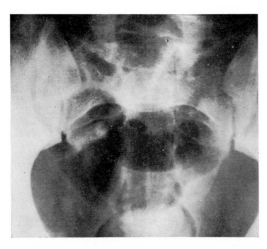

FIG. 339. A vertical fracture through the left side of the sacrum just lateral to the midline in a 19-year-old man who was struck by an automobile. There was also a fracture through the ischiopubic bones.

descending into the intragluteal furrow. Rectal examination revealed an elastic projection of the posterior wall, and the finger could palpate the fracture line. This was considered to be a spurious meningocele following trauma. The mass-like lesion disappeared under conservative treatment, and no operation was necessary.

A fracture dislocation of the sacro-iliac joint associated with rupture of the symphysis pubis, presumably produced by the force of uterine contraction during labor was reported by Urist (1953). In this patient an associated injury to the first sacral nerve root was produced. The plain roentgenograms showed the fracture line in the superior aspect of the left side of the sacrum adjacent to the sacro-iliac joint. Myelography showed a displacement of the caudal sac contralaterally.

Fractures and fracture dislocations of the sacro-coccygeal area are frequent. They usually follow trauma, and are painful out of proportion to the degree of osseous injury. The fracture lines sometimes are difficult to identify, and may become more apparent on roentgenograms made some time after the accident. Pain can be persistent and require surgical relief.

References

Bonnin, J. G.: Sacral Fractures and Injuries to the Cauda Equina, J. Bone & Joint Surg., 27, 113, 1945.
Burman, M.: Tear of Sacrospinous and Sacrotuberous Ligaments, J. Bone & Joint Surg., 34-A, 441, 1952.
Dobrzaniecki, W. and Haak, E.: Meniningocele Traumatica Spuria, Ann. Surg., 116, 150, 1942.
Urist, M. R.: Obstetric Fracture-Dislocation of Pelvis, J.A.M.A., 152, 126, 1953.

TRAUMATIC AVULSION OF NERVE ROOTS

Murphy, Hartung and Kirklin (1947) reported 3 cases in which cervical myelography revealed lateral collections of Pantopaque which were not extensions of the nerve sheaths, but rather Pantopaque extending into an area created by rupture of the meninges which permitted escape of the opaque medium into the adjacent tissues. The term "traumatic meningocele" was suggested even though they had no way of stating that the outpouchings were lined by meninges. No operative confirmation was available. In 1950, Whiteleather and Clayton reported 3 additional cases, 1 of which was confirmed at operation. This patient, a 14-year-old boy, had been struck on the left shoulder and upper arm in a downward direction by a whirling airplane propeller, resulting in considerable injury to the soft tissues, fracture of the left clavicle and humerus, and loss of motor and sensory functions in the area innervated by the left brachial plexus. Myelography revealed an oval collection of Pantopaque lateral to the interspace between the fifth and sixth cervical vertebrae, the collection being separated from the main column by a hiatus of about 1 cm. A preoperative diagnosis of traumatic avulsion of the left seventh and eighth cervical and first thoracic nerve roots was made, with formation of a traumatic meningocele at the sixth interspace. Exploration of the left brachial plexus revealed that the sixth and seventh cervical nerve roots were surrounded by a hard, dense scar. The eighth root had been pulled through the seventh intervertebral foramen and the torn end was found

1 cm lateral to the foramen. In the other 2 cases, lateral collections of Pantopaque were seen outside of the spinal canal, extending into the intervertebral foramen. It was deemed inadvisable to operate on the other 2 patients.

The subarachnoid space in the cervical region does not extend beyond the axillary pouch. If there is a tear of the pouch, the Pantopaque passes through the intervertebral foramen into a diverticulum-like cavity (Fig. 340). With avulsion of a nerve root, that structure or its rootlets are torn from the spinal cord. Separation of a nerve root implies rupture of its continuity. Inasmuch as the nerve roots are more fragile than their investing membranes, situations can occur in which the roots are torn but the investing membrane remains intact. In such cases myelographic examinations are likely to be normal (Jaeger and Whitley, 1953).

Donald McRae has pointed out that myelographic evidence of a recent disruption of continuity of the dura and arachnoid incident to cervical trauma is an irregular extravasation of Pantopaque parallel to the long axis of the cord, with small collections of the contrast material in pool-like accumu-

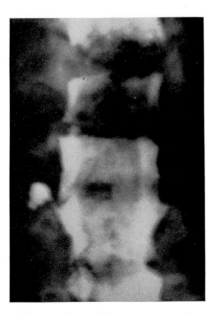

FIG. 340. Avulsion of the nerve root of the right sixth cervical nerve. Note the pooling of Pantopaque lateral to the column.

33

lations. This pattern is quite different from the normal smooth lateral rivulets interrupted by the axillary pouches at regular intervals. It is only later that the better known pattern of accumulations of Pantopaque lateral to the main column becomes evident. Identification of a nerve trunk in a laterally placed pouch is evidence against the possibility of traumatic extravasation.

Brachial plexus injuries are associated with traction traumas in older children and adults. In newborn infants brachial plexus injuries follow difficult deliveries, and obstetrical paralysis is attributed to tearing or stretching of the brachial plexus or avulsion of nerve roots from the cord. Injury to the cord itself is not rare, the principal damage found at necropsy being subdural or extradural hemorrhage, laceration or rupture of the cord, or hematomyelia (Adams and Cameron, 1965).

The usual cause of brachial plexus injury is a motor or industrial accident or a fall. The upper nerve roots are torn if the arm is adducted at the time of impact. If the arm is abducted, the main injury is to the lower roots. Most of the time the upper roots are affected more often than the lower ones. If the lower roots are torn, the upper ones also are involved. The fifth and sixth roots are most affected. The root fibers usually tear before either the nerve trunk or perineurium give way. Partial or complete tear occurs in either the dorsal or ventral nerve root or both. After a tear the dura over the root pouch may remain intact, or be torn so that cerebrospinal fluid leaks into the soft tissues and spreads beyond the intervertebral foramen. When cerebrospinal fluid escapes, it produces a reaction so that it becomes confined by a dense, impervious membrane with a smooth glistening inner surface. Proliferation of meninges may seal the dural sac altogether or obliterate the root pouches.

The usual picture of a laterally situated, irregular pool of Pantopaque is seen when there is continuity with the subarachnoid space. If, however, this is sealed off the lateral margin of the column may remain smooth or become convex medially. Rarely

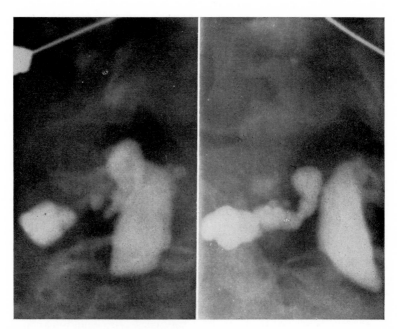

Fig. 341.   Traumatic avulsion of fourth lumbar nerve root.   The Pantopaque collects in an irregular cavity on the lateral aspect of the column, and can flow freely back into the subarachnoid space.   (From Finney, L. A. and Wulfman, W. A., Am. J. Roentgenol., *84*, 952, 1960.)

a cystic collection of cerebrospinal fluid remains in the canal and extends axially. This may or may not fill with Pantopaque (Davies, Sutton and Bligh, 1966).

In differential diagnosis the presence of an abnormally long axillary sleeve may cause some difficulty. These occasionally terminate in a sac-like structure, adding to the difficulty in diagnosis, especially if Pantopaque remains entrapped. Lateral intrathoracic or cervical meningoceles must be considered. The dilated sleeves associated with neurofibromatosis offer another possibility. Subdural or extradural extension of Pantopaque are recognized without difficulty in most instances.

Traumatic avulsions of the lumbar nerve roots are rare. Finney and Wulfman (1960) reported such a case secondary to a flexion-abduction injury to the hip with concomitant traction damage to the common peroneal nerve and the intradural fourth lumbar nerve roots. The myelographic picture was comparable to that seen with brachial plexus avulsions (Fig. 341).

References

Adams, J. H. and Cameron, H. M.:   Obstetrical Paralysis Due to Ischaemia of the Spinal Cord, Arch. Dis. Childhood, *40*, 93, 1965.

Davies, E. R., Sutton, D. and Bligh, A. S.:   Myelography in Brachial Plexus Injury, Brit. J. Radiol., *39*, 362, 1966.

Finney, L. A. and Wulfman, W. A.:   Traumatic Intradural Lumbar Nerve Root Avulsion with with Associated Traction Injury to the Common Perneal Nerve, Am. J. Roentgenol., *84*, 952, 1960.

Jaeger, R. and Whiteley, W. H.:   Avulsion of the Brachial Plexus, J.A.M.A., *153*, 644, 1953.

Lester, J.:   Pantopaque Myelography in Avulsion of the Brachial Plexus, Acta radiol., *55*, 186, 1961.

McRae, D.:   Personal communication.

Mendelsohn, R. A., Weiner, I. H. and Keegan, J. M.:   Myelographic Demonstration of Brachial Plexus Avulsion, Arch. Surg., *75*, 102, 1957.

Murphy, F., Hartung, W. and Kirklin, J. W.:   Myelographic Demonstration of Avulsing Injury of the Brachial Plexus, Am. J. Roentgenol., *58*, 102, 1947.

Rayle, A. A., Gay, B. B., Jr. and Meadors, J. L.:   The Myelogram in Avulsion of the Brachial Plexus, Radiology, *65*, 65, 1955.

Whiteleather, J. E.:   Roentgen Demonstration of Cervical Nerve Root Avulsion, Am. J. Roentgenol., *72*, 1017, 1954.

Whiteleather, J. E. and Clayton, R. S.:   Traumatic Avulsion of Nerve Roots, Med. Radiography & Photography, *26*, 27, 1950.

POSTLAMINECTOMY DEFORMITIES

Following multiple laminectomies changes may appear in the intervertebral discs and the margins of the involved vertebral bodies. Horowitz (1941) reported obvious deformities following laminectomy of from 2 to 5 vertebrae in which the spinous processes and both laminae had been removed, but in which the articular facets had been preserved. Over a period of from 8 months to 15 years narrowing of the discs, kyphosis and bony proliferations of the margins of the vertebrae were found.

Multiple laminectomies of the cervical vertebrae are done for relief of cord and nerve root compression produced by spondylotic ridging. Sometimes the operation is extensive, four or five neural arches being removed together with foraminotomies for freeing the nerve trunks. In our experience during the past 5 years we have not encountered any serious difficulty after this procedure in over 35 patients. Postoperative examinations of the cervical spine in flexion and extension and cineradiographic studies revealed a surprisingly normal range of motion (Fig. 342A and B). In 3 instances we have had the opportunity of performing myelographic examinations after multiple laminectomies had been done before. These patients had developed symptoms or continued to have symptoms referable to the lower spine, so that lumbar myelography was indicated. On filling the cervical canal bulging of the dura towards the defect occurred with the neck held in mild flexion. In extension indentations of the yellow ligaments into the dorsal aspect of the Pantopaque column appear in the upper cervical region where the neural arches were still present. No gross change appeared at the operative site.

In 1 patient who had a wide cervical laminectomy for removal of a giant osteoid osteoma with severe cord compression a reversal of the usual cervical curve appeared. This patient had weakness of his shoulders and arms prior to operation. This persisted

after operation as followed for 2 years (Fig. 342C and D). It is of interest that 3 months prior to the identification of the tumor of the spinous process of the third cervical vertebra an x-ray examination failed to reveal this lesion. At the time the tumor was discovered the cervical curve had already altered perceptibly, and the study 2 years later revealed that the change in this malalignment was at most only moderate. Flexion and extension examinations, including cineradiography, revealed an excellent range of motion without pain. During this interval the third and fourth cervical bodies had become flattened, with a wedge-shaped configuration prominent anteriorly. On the conventional as well as on the cineradiographic examinations no specific slipping of these vertebrae was seen. The laminae were well preserved and the apophyseal joints permit an adequate range of movement.

Multiple lumbar laminectomies also are done for patients who have symptoms produced by multiple lumbar ridges and spondylo-arthritis with marked thickening of the laminae. These patients have had no untoward reactions after operation. Postoperative myelograms were obtained in a few of these individuals. These disclosed bulging of the dura towards the operative defect. In an occasional instance this posterior bulging assumes almost a cyst-like proportion.

The absence of postoperative complications in our patients is attributed to the fact that the operation is performed so that the laminae are removed for adequate decompression, but the articular facets are spared.

Following bilateral laminectomies changes appear in the intervertebral discs and the cervical vertebrae associated with weakness and pain (Taylor, 1927). Horowitz (1941) reported obvious deformities following laminectomy of from 2 to 5 vertebrae in which the spinous processes and laminae on both sides had been removed, but in which the articular facets had been preserved. Over a period of from 8 months to 15 years, changes

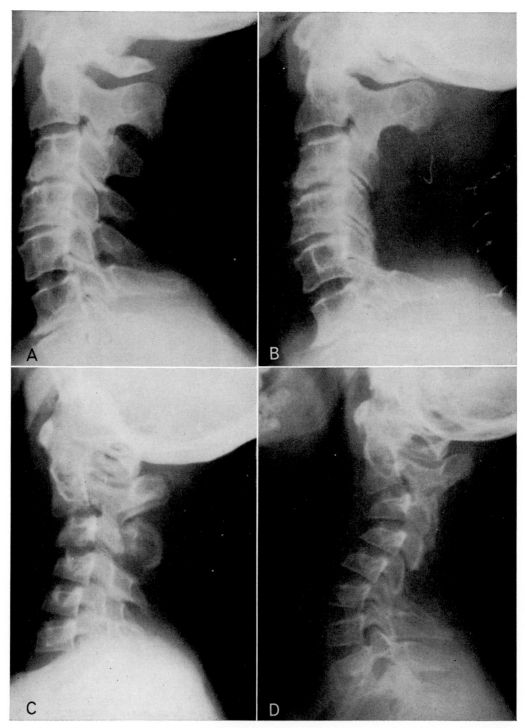

Fig. 342. *A,* Lateral roentgenogram of the cervical spine of a 62-year-old man with multiple ridges producing myelopathic changes. There is narrowing of the canal at the third, fourth and fifth levels. *B,* Three years after laminectomies of these vertebrae the alignment of the cervical spine is well maintained. Cineradiographic examination and clinical inspection showed normal movement. *C,* Lateral cervical spine of the patient with a giant osteoid osteoma of the spinous process of C2. Note the altered curve. Following operation the altered curve persists, but there is a good range of motion clinically and on cineradiographic examination. Same patient as Figure 315.

appeared in the intervertebral discs and vertebral bodies in the region of lumbar laminectomies, including narrowing of the discs, kyphosis and bony proliferations at the margins of the vertebral bodies.

In 1 of our patients cervical laminectomy was done for relief of an Arnold-Chiari malformation, and the patient developed severe pain after operation. Radiographic examinations over a period of 1 year showed progressive decalcification and irregularity of the bodies of the second to fifth cervical vertebrae. The usual lordotic curve vanished, the intervertebral spaces became irregularly narrowed, and the margins of the involved vertebrae became irregular. However, with conservative orthopedic treatment the cervical curve straightened and the vertebral bodies regained their osseous densities. Spur formation between the bodies resulted in a stable cervical spine after about 3 years.

References

Horwitz, T.: Structural Deformities of the Spine Following Bilateral Laminectomy, Am. J. Roentgenol., 46, 836, 1941.

Taylor, A. S.: Hemilaminectomy, Tr. Am. Neurol. Assn., 53, 524, 1927.

KÜMMEL'S DISEASE

This condition refers to posttraumatic compression of a vertebral body either in the thoracic or lumbar region, which usually is unidentifiable immediately after the injury. The degree of collapse is usually mild, and becomes apparent only several months after the injury (Kümmel, 1895, 1928). The process is believed to be secondary to decalcification of bone because of interference with its blood supply. According to Schinz and his co-workers (1952) this lesion is of practical importance. They mentioned that histologic examination of the affected vertebrae may reveal infractions of the cartilaginous laminae, hemorrhages into the medullary tissues and microfractures and necrosis of the trabeculae. The intervertebral discs may also be fragmented, with protrusions of cartilaginous material into the cancellous tissue. They also mentioned that the intervertebral disc eventually may undergo calcification, simulating synostosis of the adjacent vertebral bodies.

There is difference of opinion as to whether Kümmel's disease actually represents a true clinical entity. Morton (1943) stated that there was doubt as to its existence, and cautioned against the diagnosis unless one were sure of the facts involved in the history. He stressed the sequence of injury, normal roentgenographic examination of the spine followed by slow, progressive wedging of an involved vertebra associated with pain.

Fletcher (1947) pointed out that wedging of vertebral bodies occurs as a normal variation, and regarded epiphysitis as a more common cause of wedging than compression fractures. While he made no direct reference to Kümmel's disease, his statistical study of uncomplicated wedging in a group of 550 adult male veterans under 50 years of age is of interest when a diagnosis of Kümmel's disease is considered.

In our experience we frequently encounter wedging of the thoracic or upper lumbar vertebrae in individuals referred for examination of the spine for reasons other than trauma. In such cases we mention that the wedging is present, and further state that the process is most probably the result of a discal disturbance or incident to osteoporosis if this is evident.

References

Fletcher, G. H.: Anterior Vertebral Wedging, Am. J. Roentgenol., 57, 232, 1947.

Kümmel, H.: Über die Traumatischen Erkrankungen der Wirbelsaule, Deutsch. med. Wchnschr., 21, 180, 1895.

————: Der heutige Standpunkt der posttraumatischen Wirbelkrankung (Kümmelsche Krankheit), Arch. orthop. u. Unfall.-Chir., 26, 491, 1928.

Morton, S. A.: Differential Diagnosis of Traumatic Lesions of Spine, Radiology, 41, 560, 1943.

Schinz, H. R., Baensch, W. E., Friedl, L. and Uehlinger, E.: Roentgen Diagnostics, New York, Grune & Stratton, 1952, Vol. 2, p. 1556.

PARAPLEGIC NEUROARTHROPATHY

Following injuries to the spine with consequent paraplegia, neuropathic articular and periarticular changes occur in the lower extremities. Solovay and Solovay (1949) included intraarticular destructive and productive changes, and extra-articular soft tissue ossification. They described changes in the lower extremities like those of Charcot's neuroarthropathy. The mechanism postulated was a long continued pressure over an anesthetic bony prominence and lack of warning sensations.

Abramson and Kamberg (1949) noted similar changes in the soft tissues, chiefly about the hips, and erosive bone changes around the trochanters. They pointed out an additional change, a spondylitis which in many ways was like rheumatoid arthritis, with frequent involvement of the diarthrodial joints. Lesions below the first lumbar vertebra were not associated with such changes. With lesions above the first lumbar level the apophyseal joints showed varying degrees of fusion, some with osteoporosis and some with osteosclerosis of the vertebral bodies, others with a combination of both. They believed that the cause of this was hyperemia of bone followed by decalcification, diminished circulation, and that the osteosclerosis followed loss of blood supply due to necrosis of bone.

Subjective complaints in these patients were not striking because of the cord lesions. Heilbrun and Kuhn (1947) pointed out that erosive lesions developed where the soft tissues over bony prominences such as the trochanters became devitalized. Pathologically, subacute and chronic infection of the tissues appeared overlying the bone, with extension to the superficial layers of bone. This leads to resorption of the cortex and the underlying trabeculae, and the bone marrow becomes replaced by fibrovascular tissue which accompanies a low grade inflammatory process. They recognized that the neurogenic influences were probably of major importance, even though soft tissue trauma has an important role in the appearance of these changes.

References

Abramson, D. J. and Kamberg, S.: Spondylitis, J. Bone & Joint Surg., *31-A*, 275, 1949.

Heilbrun, N. and Kuhn, W. G., Jr.: Erosive Bone Lesions and Soft-Tissue Ossifications Associated with Spinal Cord Injuries (Paraplegia), Radiology, *48*, 579, 1947.

Solovay, J. and Solovay, H. U.: Paraplegia Neuroarthropathy, Am. J. Roentgenol., *61*, 473, 1949.

LUMBAR SPONDYLOLISTHESIS

Spondylolisthesis indicates displacement of one vertebral body on another, usually with disruption of the neural arch of the involved vertebra at the pars interarticularis. This occurs most often at the fourth and fifth lumbar articulations. Meyerding (1938) noted displacement at the lumbosacral interspace in 82.1 per cent of 583 cases. In 11.3 per cent the fourth lumbar vertebra was displaced. Spondylolisthesis of the third lumbar vertebra occurred in 0.5 per cent, and displacement of the second lumbar vertebra in 0.3 per cent. He observed two with the fifth lumbar vertebra displaced on a sixth lumbar vertebra (0.3 per cent) and another with a sixth lumbar segment displaced anteriorly on the first sacral vertebra. In 5 cases (0.9 per cent) there was a double spondylolisthesis with displacement of both the fourth and fifth lumbar vertebrae. Reverse spondylolisthesis, with posterior displacement of the involved vertebra, was observed in 26 cases (4.4 per cent), usually at the lumbosacral interspace. Spondylolisthesis occurring in the cervical spine will be considered later. Thoracic spondylolisthesis is of traumatic origin, or is part of a widespread congenital malformation once in a while.

In a limited number of cases spondylolisthesis occurs without a defect in the neural arch. This appears in patients with exaggerated lumbar lordotic curves together with malacic diseases, osteoporosis and spondy-

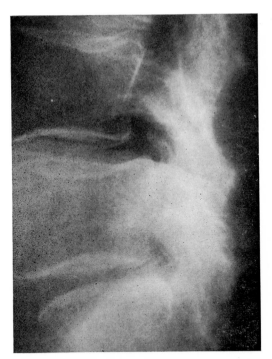

FIG. 343. There is a forward slip of L4 on L5 due to an anterior inclination of the superior lamina of L5. The patient is a 56-year-old woman with no symptoms referable to this change (Jünghanns spondylolisthesis).

losis. Changes in the inclination of the articular facets permits a forward displacement of one vertebra on another (Fig. 343).

The origin of the defect in the pars interarticularis with spondylolisthesis still causes speculation. Present evidence favors traumatic origin rather than a failure of fusion of two centers of ossification. Bowman and Goin (1926) believed that infantile or birth trauma with actual fractures or local osteochondrovascular disturbances of the neural arch were the initiating factors. Chandler (1931) mentioned that ossification of the pars interarticularis progressed by the formation of cyst-like spaces within a thin shell of bone. The pars interarticularis, consisting mainly of cartilage and a large lake of blood vessels during the period of early ossification, was considered particularly susceptible to fracture. In an investigation of two hundred fetal spines Batts (1939) found none with

separated neural arches, and postulated that if the lesions were congenital such defects might be anticipated in about the same number of fetal spines as seen later in life, approximately 5 per cent. Rowe and Roche (1953) did not find a single example of a defective neural arch in over 500 stillborn and neonatal cadavers. Lerner and Gazine (1946) favored the idea that isthmic defects from trauma in early life, and commented that fracture through cartilage heals by pseudoarthrosis rather than by callus formation. Hadley (1945) mentioned that bony callus was frequently seen as a mass projecting into the spinal canal from the lamina, and believed this to be derived from a break in the lamina. Mutch (1956) described the pattern of ossification in the vertebral arches, noting that the fifth ossifies later than the first. He, too, favored the traumatic etiology of defects in the pars interarticularis.

Clefts in the pars interarticularis, while often associated with spondylolisthesis, occur without displacement of the involved vertebral body (Fig. 344). This condition is referred to as spondylolysis or spondyloschysis (Rhodes and Colangelo, 1946). The term prespondylolisthesis has sometimes been applied to this situation. An interesting mechanism for the production of spondylolysis was postulated by Nathan (1959). He found 19 cases in a series of 450 skeletons. In typical instances the lower lumbar vertebrae were involved. The clefts in the isthmus were located between the downward projecting inferior articular processes of the vertebra above and the upward projecting superior articular processes of the vertebra below. Such clefts appeared to be produced by compression of the isthmuses between these articular processes by a sort of pincers mechanism. Preceding bony abnormalities or congenital lesions were not found. He observed skeletons in which the development of the spondylolysis stopped before total separation of the vertebral arch occurred, with marked depression on the

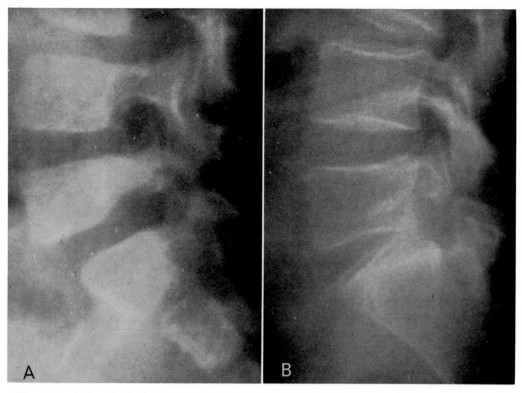

FIG. 344. *A*, Spondylolysis in a 2-year-old girl with a dermal sinus. There is a slight forward slip of L5 on S1. At operation the sinus tract traversed the rudimentary spinous process of S1 (film magnified 1.5 ×). *B*, Asymptomatic spondylolysis of L5 in a 58-year-old woman. Note the smooth edges of the defect of the pars interarticularis.

upper and lower surfaces of isthmuses precisely at the site of contact with the articular processes of the adjacent vertebrae. We have observed 6 instances in which lumbar spine roentgenograms in children from 3 months to 3 years of age disclosed similar waist-like narrowing in the pars interarticularis of the fifth lumbar vertebra (Fig. 344).

Wiltse (1962) suggested that a defect in the pars interarticularis was a hereditary dysplasia characterized by a lack of normal ability of the bone to repair itself. The dysplasia probably exists in the cartilaginous model of the affected vertebral arch, and usually is present in several other vertebrae. With strain on the pars interarticularis in the lower lumbar spine incident to the erect posture and the lordotic curve characteristic in man, stress results in the bony defect. However, stress or strain alone on the pars

interarticularis will not of itself produce this lesion unless the dysplasia is present. Occasionally the dysplasia is such that resorption of bone occurs without strain or trauma. If the degree of dysplasia is unequal, one side may undergo resorption while the other remains intact. Bailey (1947) believed that heredity played a definite part, and added 3 cases of hereditary transmission to the case reported by George (1939). The combination of hereditary spondylolisthesis and spina bifida in a family in which the lesion was transmitted as an autosomal dominant through three generations was reported by Amuso and Mankin (1967). They noted that it is generally conceded that if a genetic lesion is present it is transmitted as an autosomal recessive with incomplete penetrance, and that their example was unique.

According to Brailsford (1933) the term "prespondylolisthesis," as described by Armitage Whitman, also may be applied when the lumbosacral angle approaches 90 degrees. It was considered that such an exaggerated lordotic curve may precede dislocation. Brailsford felt that this term was unfortunately chosen because exaggerated lumbosacral angles occur in a wide variety of conditions unassociated with spondylolisthesis, such as neglected rickets, osteomalacia and osteogenesis imperfecta. The use of the term "prespondylolisthesis" to refer either to a cleft neural arch or to an exaggerated lumbar lordotic curve is unsuitable, inasmuch as in neither is spondylolisthesis a necessary concomitant. An anatomic reference is a better way of describing such changes, and avoids the unfounded supposition that another pathologic entity may in time be superimposed.

Spondylolysis can be regarded as an acquired defect in the nature of a stress fracture (Fig. 334) which may affect a single or several pars interarticularis. It may appear after multiple small traumas of a recurrent nature, as for example in ballet dancers or athletes. Moreton (1966), in a review of 32,600 examinations, noted that instances of such defects varied from 7 to 7.6 per cent, were bilateral in from 72 to 88 per cent, and involved the fifth lumbar vertebra in 91.2 per cent. In most patients such stress fractures remain ununited insofar as radiologic examination shows no bony union or callus formation. However, instances of visible healing are observed occasionally. Calabrese and Freiberger (1963) reported acquired spondylolysis in a child treated by spinal fusion for tuberculous spondylitis. Films taken over a 9-year period thereafter revealed a defect in the pars interarticularis of the fifth lumbar vertebra which progressively increased in size.

The anatomic changes present with spondylolisthesis include looseness of the lamina, permitting it to be rocked back and forth to a variable degree. Some, with lesser or no mobility, are bound down by fibrous ankyloses, with ill-defined masses of fibrous tissue merging with the adjacent ligaments. Mucoid degeneration occurs at these sites, and bulging of soft tissue towards the intervertebral foramina and spinal canal may be considerable. The foramina become distorted, and the nerve roots in proximity to the displaced inferomedial wall of the superior pedicle may be bound down by adhesions. A step formation results as the vertebra is displaced. The disc often is considerably narrowed. The dura makes a double bend as it follows the angulated spinal canal, and becomes adherent to the lamina and ligamenta flava (Fig. 345). The cauda equina may be stretched quite tautly across the step. When this is accompanied by a narrow lumbar canal and distorted lateral recesses of the spinal foramen, small discal herniations or spondylotic spurs may produce disproportionate symptoms (Fig. 346).

The incidence of spondylolisthesis has been reported as between 3.5 per cent (George, 1939) and 5 per cent (Bailey, 1947). Bailey mentioned that among 2080 lateral lumbosacral roentgenograms in unselected cases, 4.4 per cent showed isthmic defects. Only 0.5 per cent complained of low back pain. He concluded that spondylolisthesis or its presumed precursors were not connected with recent trauma. Garland and Thomas (1946) mentioned that in army and navy personnel spondylolisthesis occurred in as many as 10 per cent of cases of low back pain referred for roentgen examination.

Spondylolisthesis also has been reported with infrequent congenital defects of the neural arches, including congenital lengthening and shortening of the pars interarticularis and defects involving only one side of a neural arch (Roche and Bryan, 1946) and anomalies of the articular facets (Brocher, 1950).

Kleinberg (1934) reported spondylolisthesis in a 17-month-old infant. No symptoms were present, and it was presumed that the defect was congenital. This patient also had bilateral dislocated hips. Kierulf (1951)

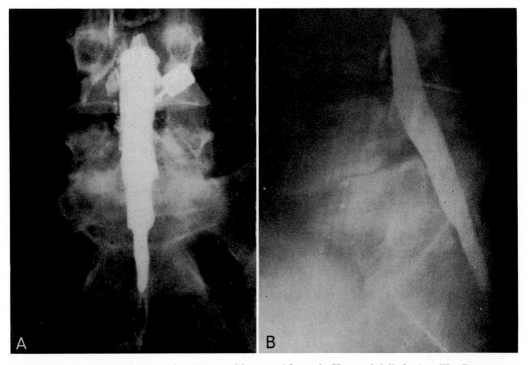

FIG. 345. *A*, AP myelogram of a 46-year-old man with grade II spondylolisthesis. The Pantopaque column is narrow, but otherwise not remarkable. *B*, On lateral examination the spondylolisthesis is apparent, with narrowing of the L5 interspace. A slight step formation is present in the Pantopaque column as it crosses the spondylolisthetic segment.

quoted Hammerbeck as mentioning a case of spondylolisthesis in a 40-cm long fetus described by Blum. Hitchcock (1940) reported a case of a 4-year-old child. Most patients are seen from adolescence to adult life, the greatest incidence being between 20 and 50 years of age. In Meyerding's series of 876 cases (1943), the average age was 34.7 years. The youngest was 14 years and the oldest 59 years. I have seen spondylolisthesis in a child 2 years old, and in patients over 65 years of age.

The relationship of spondylolisthesis to congenital malformations of the neural arches has not been clearly defined. In several reports it has been noted that a developmental defect involving the spinous processes was seen 5 to 10 times more often than in normal adults (Meyerding, 1931), (Rowe and Roche, 1953) (Wiltse, 1962). The 2-year-old child mentioned here had a dermal sinus. When excised, the tract was followed down to

and through the dura. Attachments to the filum terminale had to be severed. The spinous process of S1 was unfused (Fig. 344).

The clinical picture of symptomatic spondylolisthesis is one of low back pain, with or without sciatica often associated with trauma. However, it occurs even in advanced form without clinical manifestations. When the condition is mild, physical examination discloses nothing characteristic. With advanced spondylolisthesis a characteristic dimple often is present in the lower lumbar region, due to depression of the spinous process of the fourth or fifth lumbar vertebra. In Meyerding's (1938) cases, 63.1 per cent of the 583 patients complained of backache, 17 per cent had backache and pains in the legs, 7.7 per cent had hip pain also. Paralysis was observed in 1.9 per cent.

Meyerding divided spondylolisthesis into four groups. Stage 1 indicates only spondylolysis, with no displacement of the vertebral

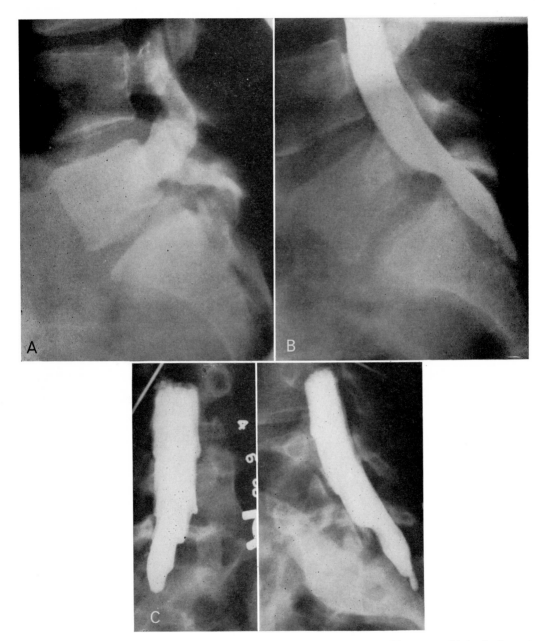

FIG. 346. *A*, Lateral examination of the lumbosacral spine of a 32-year-old woman with backache and left sciatic pain intermittent for about 7 years. A grade I spondylolisthesis is present. *B*, Lateral myelogram reveals an indentation into the column at the lumbosacral interspace. *C*, The oblique views show the right side to be normal, but a discal intrusion is visible on the left. At operation a spur was present. This projected upwards from the superior surface of S1 and extended to compromise the left intervertebral foramen. A small discal herniation also was present, intruding into the left foramen. Relief followed decompression.

body. Stages 2, 3 and 4 respectively refer to the degree to which the body of the sliding vertebra has been displaced forward. The underlying surface is divided into three parts, and forward slip of up to one third is considered stage 2, slip between one and two thirds is considered stage 3 and from two thirds forward to a complete displacement is regarded as stage 4. Others regard spondylolysis as a separate entity, and

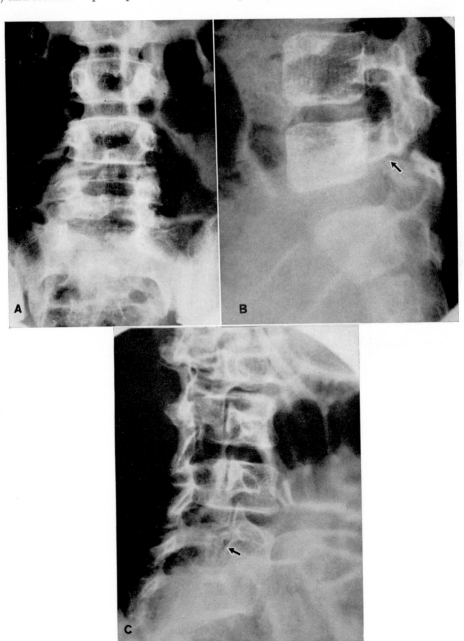

Fig. 347. *A*, Grade I spondylolisthesis in a 12-year-old girl. The anteroposterior view is not diagnostic. *B*, Lateral view. A defect is present in the pars interarticularis (arrows). *C*, Oblique view. The articular facets at the lumbosacral joint are inclined forward (arrows). The defect in the pars interarticularis is not as well seen as in *B*.

divided the degree of forward displacement into four grades, each representing one quarter of the surface of the underlying vertebra, a system which I prefer.

The question whether spondylolisthesis is progressive often arises. Hitchcock (1940) presented 3 patients, 4, 13 and 45 years of age, in whom progressive slipping occurred. In the first the initial films showed an isthmic defect without displacement. Over 8 years this progressed to frank spondylolisthesis. In the 13-year-old patient a grade 3 spondylolisthesis progressed to grade 4 in 2 years. In the 45-year-old woman a grade 1 became a grade 2 spondylolisthesis in 3 years. In none was trauma involved. Kierulf (1951) reported a 30-year-old man who in 1939 had spondylolysis. In 1950

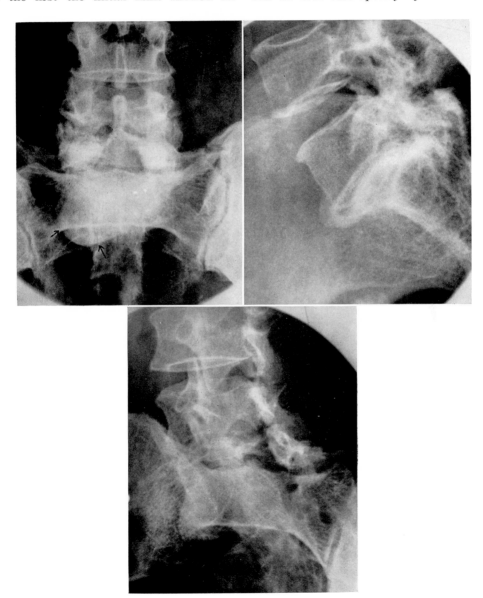

Fig. 348. Grade II lumbosacral spondylolisthesis with heavy bone bridging on anterolateral aspect of the joint. This produces a bow-like density in the anteroposterior view (arrows). The interspace is markedly narrowed, with sclerotic changes. The bony defect in the pars interarticularis is overshadowed by the bony proliferation. Arthritic changes are present in the lower apophyseal joints.

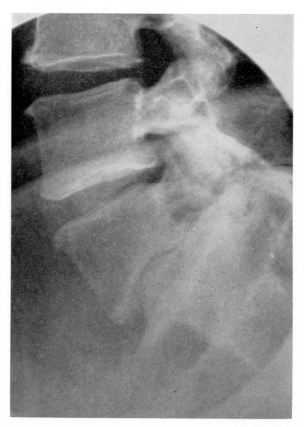

Fig. 349.   Grade III spondylolisthesis with ball and socket arrangement of the articulation.
Note arthritic changes in the lowermost two apophyseal joints.

a definite spondylolisthesis was present, with decrease in the intervertebral space, narrowing of the intervertebral foramina and forward slipping of the fifth lumbar vertebra.

The radiologic investigation of spondylolisthesis should include, in addition to the usual anteroposterior and lateral fims, cone-down views of the lumbar segments in oblique and lateral positions. The oblique views are desirable for portrayal of the articular facets and the pars interarticularis. Lateral roentgenograms often disclose defects in the pars interarticularis, and a review of our material showed that these defects are seen as often on the lateral as on the oblique films, and sometimes to better advantage (Fig. 347). Laminagrams occasionally are helpful, particularly in elderly patients who have pronounced spondylotic overgrowth.

Spondylolisthesis is frequently associated with a varying degree of narrowing of the intervertebral disc and sclerotic changes of the apposing vertebral surfaces. In about a third of our cases, particularly in patients over 30, such hypertrophic changes are seen (Fig. 348). In an equal number of cases sclerotic changes were observed along the articular facets of the lower lumbosacral spine. In some, bony bridging between the anterior aspects of the fifth lumbar and first sacral segments was extensive, and served as a supporting buttress. Such spur formation usually was encountered with grade 3 or 4 spondylolisthesis (Fig. 349). In 11 cases with pronounced narrowing of the involved interspace, a concavity developed in the inferior aspect of the fourth or fifth lumbar vertebra into which projected a semicircular prominence from the upper aspect of the

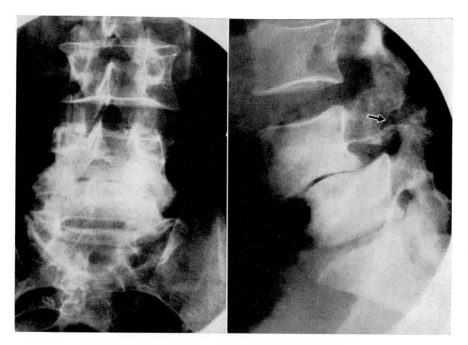

FIG. 350.   Grade III lumbosacral spondylolisthesis with heavy bony bridging on the
left anterolateral aspect of the joint (arrows).

subjacent segment, forming a ball and socket joint which blocked further displacement of the vertebra. This corresponds to the term "Torus Promontoralis Sustentaculum" mentioned by Turner and Tchirkin (quoted by Hitchcock, 1940) (Figs. 349 and 352).

In advanced spondylolisthesis, the body of the fifth lumbar vertebra projects below the level of the anterosuperior aspect of the first sacral segment. An anteroposterior roentgenogram will reveal a "bow-line" (Brailsford, 1929). This line is simulated when the fifth lumbar segment is not displaced far anteriorly, but has a large bony excrescence between the anterior aspect of the fifth lumbar and the first sacral vertebrae. In several of our cases this line involved only half of the anterior aspect of the upper sacrum as studied in the anteroposterior view, an observation which led to the identification of the large calcific spur as differentiated from the true bow-line of Brailsford (Fig. 350).

Displacement of the fourth on the fifth lumbar vertebra rarely is as extensive as occurs at the lumbosacral articulation. I have not observed any in which the spondylolisthesis was more than grade 2, and most corresponded to grade 1 (Fig. 351). A ball-and-socket deformity is occasionally seen (Fig. 352).

Practically all those with grade 2 spondylolisthesis had localized spondylosis and thinning of the intervertebral disc. In grades 3 and 4 spondylolistheses, subdivided into two groups according to whether or not new bone formation was present, a buttress at the anterior aspect of the sacrum was present in most cases. In some the sacrum and the body of the fifth lumbar vertebra were fused. When new bone formation did not take place, rounding off of the anterior border of the sacrum and occasionally arching of the inferior surface of the fifth lumbar vertebra occurred, forming a joint-like structure between the fifth lumbar vertebra and the sacrum (Fig. 349).

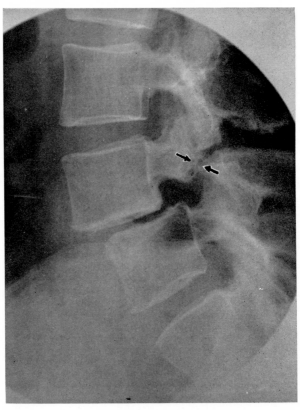

FIG. 351. Spondylolisthesis of the fourth on the fifth lumbar vertebrae, with marked narrowing of the intervertebral space. The defect in the pars interarticularis is prominent (arrows).

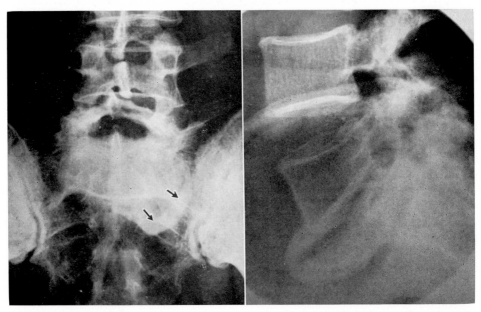

FIG. 352. Grade II spondylolisthesis of the fourth on the fifth lumbar vertebrae, with ball and socket arrangement of the articular surfaces. The laminar defect is seen in the lateral view (arrows). Note the deformity of the intervertebral foramen. A mild reverse spondylolisthesis is present at the lumbosacral interspace.

514

Spondylolisthesis of the fourth on the fifth lumbar vertebra usually was associated with less localized bony overgrowth than lumbosacral spondylolisthesis. Thinning of the intervertebral disc was commonly present (Figs. 351 and 352).

Arthritic changes of the articular facets of the lumbosacral articulation, and less frequently, of those between the fourth and fifth lumbar vertebrae are frequently present in adult patients. On oblique roentgenograms increased bony densities at the margins of the defect in the pars interarticularis and occasionally small spur-like formations appear at these margins. It is possible that arthritis of the apophyseal joints of the fourth and fifth lumbar vertebrae causes low back pain in a fairly large number of patients (Figs. 348 and 349).

The appearance of the intervertebral disc with spondylolisthesis is of interest. In grade 1 spondylolisthesis, the disc frequently is normal. However, with wear and tear, progressive degeneration of the annulus fibrosus and disruption of the fibrocartilage is followed by narrowing, first manifest in the posterior aspect of the disc. Later, the disc becomes reduced in height. Discal degeneration is one of the factors in progressive slipping of an involved vertebra.

In cases of spondylolisthesis which have come to surgery, there is variability in the degree of fixation of the supposedly separated neural arch. In some my orthopedic colleagues have found that the neural arch was readily moved about after the spinous process has been exposed, and this was believed to indicate instability. In other instances

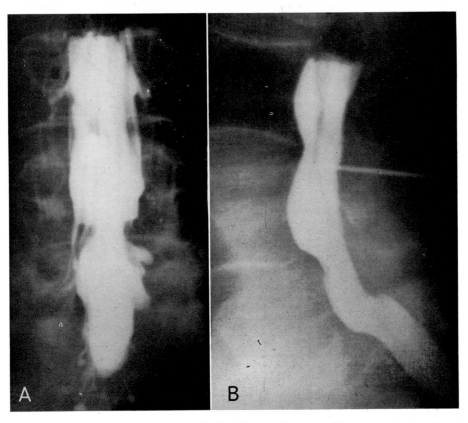

Fig. 353. *A*, AP and lateral myelograms, *B*, of a 67-year-old woman diagnosed as having disseminated spinal cord disease. An S-shaped configuration of the caudal sac is noted at the fourth and fifth lumbar interspaces. These changes were not considered as significant because they did not fit the clinical picture.

little, if any, instability existed because traction and pulling on the exposed spinous process barely moved the neural arch. Woolsey (1954) reported relief of pain in 7 cases of spondylolisthesis after surgical excision of the movable neural arch. Todd and Gardner (1958) favor simple excision of the unattached lamina as the operation of choice, and regard fusion as unnecessary. Lance (1966) advocated reduction and maintenance of reduction in selected cases of severe spondylolisthesis.

It is well known that many with a first degree spondylolisthesis have no pain, and that following trauma or prolonged strain symptoms become apparent. A radiologic picture of spondylolysis and spondylolis-thesis occurs with fractures of the pedicles and laminae. One of our patients fell off a scaffold and suffered fractures of the laminae of the fourth lumbar vertebra. Soon there-after he developed a grade 2 spondylolisthe-sis. This patient probably had a weak inter-vertebral disc which facilitated the gliding of the fourth over the fifth lumbar vertebra. The fifth lumbar interspace was narrowed, and there was posterior displacement of the fifth on the first sacral vertebra measuring 0.5 cm. The latter probably predated the injury (Fig. 352). Another 7-year-old boy who fell under a roller coaster suffered a fracture of the pars interarticularis of the fourth lumbar vertebra, and had a grade 2 spondylolisthesis.

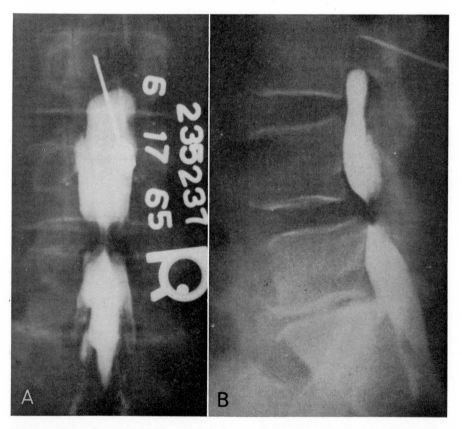

FIG. 354. *A,* AP myelogram in a 65-year-old woman with severe pain referable to the back and both legs. There is a marked pinch defect at L4. On the lateral myelogram, *B,* a tapered defect is present. There is a grade I spondylolisthesis of L4 on L5. The neural arch and apophyseal joints of L4 and L5 are heavy. At operation marked hypertrophy of the neural arch and of the ligamentum flavum together with an extruded L4 disc practically closed the canal at that level.

Spondylolisthesis is accompanied by deformity of the spinal canal varying with the sagittal diameter as well as with the extent of slippage. With grade 1 spondylolisthesis in normal canals there is only a slight angulation of the anterior aspect of the dural sac as it passes over the lip of the subjacent vertebra. The axillary pouches are indented slightly or not at all. With further forward displacement a more pronounced step deformity appears in the anterior aspect of the Pantopaque column, and its dorsal aspect becomes deformed in an opposite direction because of pressure from the neural arches. This results in a waist-like deformity, with a relatively narrow channel at the level of the involved intervertebral disc. In the frontal projection bilateral indentation into the Pantopaque column sometimes is apparent (Fig. 353), or the axillary pouches may be undisturbed. It is important to realize that spondylolisthesis producing such a deformity may exist without symptoms in normal or wide canals. On the other hand, even small intrusions into a narrow canal at the level of spondylolisthesis can cause marked compressive changes on the cauda equina and nerve roots, with consequent clinical manifestations. The association of herniations of the intervertebral disc with spondylolisthesis requires careful investigation (Fig. 354), especially in patients with narrow canals. Spurs projecting into the canal can compromise the adjacent nerve roots severely (Fig. 355). Compression of the cauda equina and nerve roots at the level of the spondylolisthesis is due mainly to pinching of the dural envelope by the displaced vertebra. Flexion and extension can influence the extent of compression, being less apparent when the trunk is flexed. This is heightened by the presence of a narrow spinal canal, spondylotic ridges, thickening of the ligamentum flavum and any hyper-

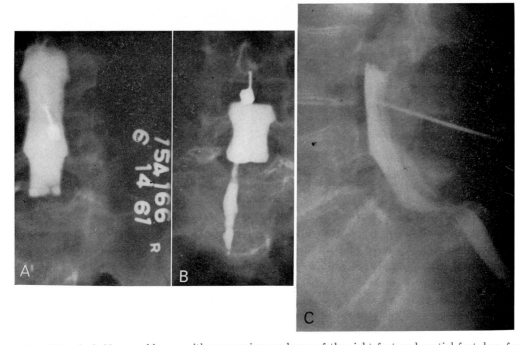

Fig. 355. *A*, A 29-year-old man with progressive weakness of the right foot and partial foot-drop for a month, together with tingling of both legs. A holdup in the descent of Pantopaque is noted at L5. Within a few moments, *B*, a thin trickle into the caudal sac occurs. *C*, A grade II spondylolisthesis is present. There is a sharp angulation of the column with indentations dorsally and ventrally.

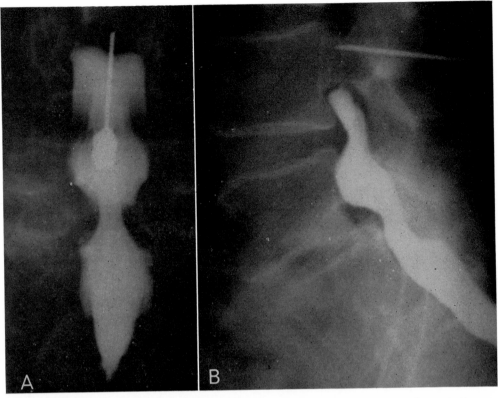

FIG. 356. *A*, A 68-year-old man with back pain, weakness and ataxia for 4 years, increasingly severe. Neck pain down both arms for 2 years. Large lumbar ridges causing bilateral defects at L4 and 5. Spondylolisthesis grade I, *B*, with intrusions into canal anteriorly. Cervical myelogram revealed advanced ridging at C4, 5 and 6. Question as to which should be attacked first was considered, but the patient refused surgery.

trophic change present at the region of the cleft in the pars interarticularis or thickening of the neural arch (Figs. 356 and 357). At times a pronounced block can be found in grades 1 or 2 spondylolisthesis in a patient with a narrow canal, a thickened neural arch and minimal or no discal herniation (Fig. 355). Preoperative myelography is advisable if there is question as to caudal sac compression, and should be done before operation if fusion is contemplated.

References

Adkins, E. W. O.: Spondylolisthesis, J. Bone & Joint Surg., *37-B*, 48, 1955.

Amuso, S. J. and Mankin, H. J.: Hereditary Spondylolisthesis and Spina Bifida, J. Bone & Joint Surg., *49-A*, 507, 1967.

Bailey, W.: Etiology and Frequency of Spondylolisthesis and its Precursors, Radiology, *48*, 107, 1947.

Batts, M., Jr.: Etiology of Spondylolisthesis, J. Bone & Joint Surg., *21*, 879, 1939.

Bowman, W. B. and Goin, L. S.: Traumatic Lesions of the Spine, Am. J. Roentgenol., *16*, 111, 1926.

Brailsford, J. F.: Deformities of Lumbosacral Region of Spine, Brit. J. Surg., *16*, 562, 1929.

————: Spondylolisthesis, Brit. J. Radiol., *6*, 666, 1933.

Brocher, J. E. W.: Die Dysplasie des Wirbelbogens, Fortschr. Röntgenstr., *73*, 719, 1950.

Chandler, F. A.: Lesions of the "Isthmus" (Pars Interarticularis) of Laminae of Lower Lumbar Vertebrae and their Relation to Spondylolisthesis, Surg., Gynec. & Obst., *53*, 273, 1931.

Galluccio, A. C.: Spondylolisthesis, Radiology, *42*, 143, 1944.

————: Spondylolisthesis, Radiology, *46*, 356, 1946.

Garland, L. H. and Thomas, S. F.: Spondylolisthesis, Am. J. Roentgenol., *55*, 275, 1946.

George, E. M.: Spondylolisthesis, Surg., Gynec. & Obst., *68*, 774, 1939.

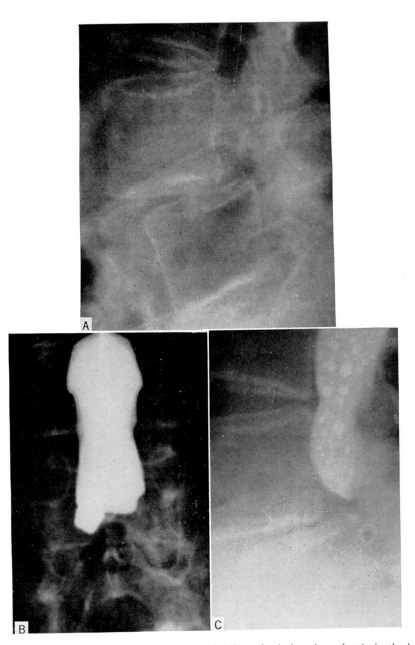

Fig. 357.   Grade II spondylolisthesis in patient with bilateral sciatic pain and pain in the lower back. The fourth intervertebral disc is reduced in height and the intervertebral foramina are encroached upon. A complete myelographic block was found (B and C). In addition to the spondylolisthesis a definite ridge was encountered together with only a modest discal herniation. The combination of spondylolisthesis, ridge and disc deformities caused the block.

Gill, G. G., Manning, J. G. and White, H. L.: Surgical Treatment of Spondylolisthesis Without Spine Fusion. Excision of the Loose Lamina with Decompression of the Nerve Roots, J. Bone & Joint Surg., *37-A*, 493, 1955.

Guri, J. P.: Treatment of Painful Spondylolisthesis, Surg., Gynec. & Obst., *83*, 797, 1946.

Hitchcock, H. H.: Spondylolisthesis: Observations on its Development, Progression and Genesis, J. Bone & Joint Surg., *22*, 1, 1940.

Kierulf, E.: Spondylolysis-Spondylolisthesis, Acta radiol., *36*, 253, 1951.

Kleinberg, S.: Spondylolisthesis in an Infant, J. Bone & Joint Surg., *16*, 441, 1934.

Kleinberg, S. and Burman, M. S.: Spondylolisthesis, J. Bone & Joint Surg., *24*, 899, 1942.

Lance, E. M.: Treatment of Severe Spondylolisthesis with Neural Involvement, J. Bone & Joint Surg., *48-A*, 883, 1966.

Lerner, H. H. and Gazin, A. I.: Interarticular Isthmus Hiatus, Radiology, *46*, 573, 1946.

Meschan, I.: Spondylolisthesis, Am. J. Roentgenol., *53*, 230, 1945.

Meyerding, H. W.: Spondylolisthesis as Etiologic Factor in Backache, J.A.M.A., *111*, 1971, 1938.

————: Low Backache and Sciatic Pain Associated with Spondylolisthesis and Protruded Intervertebral Disk, J. Bone & Joint Surg., *23*, 461, 1941.

————: Spondylolisthesis, J. Bone & Joint Surg., *25*, 65, 1943.

Meyerding, H. W. and Flashman, F. L.: Backache, J.A.M.A., *130*, 75, 1946.

Moreton, R. D.: Spondylolysis, J.A.M.A., *195*, 671, 1966.

Nathan, H.: Spondylolysis, Its Anatomy and Mechanism of Development, J. Bone & Joint Surg., *41-A*, 303, 1959.

Newman, P. H.: With a Special Investigation by K. H. Stone. The Etiology of Spondylolisthesis, J. Bone & Joint Surg., *45-B*, 39, 1963.

Niemeyer, Th. and Penning, L.: Functional Roentgenographic Examination in a Case of Cervical Spondylolisthesis, J. Bone & Joint Surg., *45-A*, 1671, 1963.

Rhodes, M. P. and Colangelo, C.: Spondylolysis and its Relation to Spondylolisthesis, Am. J. Surg., *72*, 20, 1946.

Roche, M. B. and Bryan, C. S.: Spondylolisthesis, Additional Variations in Anomalies of the Pars Interarticularis, Arch. Surg., *53*, 675, 1946.

Rowe, G. G. and Roche, M. B.: The Etiology of Separate Neural Arch, J. Bone & Joint Surg., *35-A*, 102, 1953.

Sullivan, C. R. and Bickel, W. H.: The Problem of Traumatic Spondylolysis, Am. J. Surg., *100*, 698, 1960.

Todd, E. M., Jr. and Gardner, W. J.: Simple Excision of the Unattached Lamina for Spondylolisthesis, Surg., Gynec. & Obst., *106*, 724, 1958.

Wigby, P. E. and Thomas, J. R.: Spondylolisthesis: An Autopsy Study, Radiology, *68*, 94, 1957.

Willis, T. A.: Separate Neural Arch, J. Bone & Joint Surg., *13*, 709, 1931.

————: Backward Displacement of 5th Lumbar Vertebra, J. Bone & Joint Surg., *17*, 347, 1935.

Wiltse, L. L.: Spondylolisthesis in Children, Clinical Orthopedics, *21*, 156, 1961.

————: The Etiology of Spondylolisthesis, J. Bone & Joint Surg., *44-A*, 539, 1962.

Woolsey, R. D.: Neurological Symptoms and Signs in Spondylolisthesis at the Fifth Lumbar, First Sacral Level, J. Neurosurg., *11*, 67, 1954.

REVERSE SPONDYLOLISTHESIS

In this condition a posterior displacement of the body of a lumbar vertebra on the vertebra beneath results from an anatomic variation in their articular facets. As a rule, the displacement occurs at the fourth or fifth lumbar interspaces, and is only moderate. It is associated with downward and posterior alteration in the alignment of the lumbosacral articular facets. Johnson (1934) reported 12 such cases out of 126 with spondylolisthesis and estimated the incidence as about 10 per cent. Seven of his 12 cases had narrowed intervertebral discs. Smith (1934) also believed that the displacement was the consequence of anatomic variations in the lumbosacral articular facets. Both agreed that if displacement was sufficient, sciatica might result from nerve root pressure. Smith, who reported 56 cases, mentioned that trauma played a secondary role. Degeneration of the intervertebral disc as well as loosening of the associated ligaments and frequent small traumas were considered by De Veer (1935) as important in the development of reverse spondylolisthesis. Fletcher (1947) noted a high incidence of degenerative changes in the posterior fibers of the annulus fibrosus as well as advanced degenerative disc disease with this condition. He observed no exaggeration of the lumbosacral angle, and that the apophyseal joints were principally of a frontal type directed downwards and backwards.

A group of 77 cases of vertebral retroposition was reported by Gillespie (1951). These were encountered in a series of 493 cases of lumbosacral disc protrusions confirmed at operation. All involved the lumbosacral articulation. Thirty-five had detailed examinations, and it was found that the average backwards displacement ranged from 0.3 to 0.9 cm. The majority of his cases showed an anteroposterior type of articular facet. Gillespie noted that retroposition occurs at any level, most often the lumbosacral and the cervical regions, and appears with arthritis, herniated discs, degeneration of the intervertebral cartilages, infection and trauma. He did not consider it a cause of backache.

Willis (1935) reported on the examination of 50 consecutive museum skeletons. From analysis of the apposing lumbar and sacral surfaces he noted that a frequent difference existed in the anteroposterior depth of the fifth lumbar vertebra and the first sacral vertebra. The anteroposterior diameters were equal in 34 per cent of his cases, while the remaining 66 per cent showed that the sacral diameter was from $\frac{1}{16}$ to $\frac{1}{4}$ inch shorter than the lumbar diameter. Posterior displacement of the lumbar segment could therefore be attributed to the relative shortening of the sacral diameter. Melamed and Ansfield (1947) found that technical errors might simulate this condition. Nevertheless, they considered it a true pathologic entity, the origin of which may lie in degenerative processes, trauma, various inflammatory diseases or congenital anomalies. Roche and Bryan (1946) commented that a reverse spondylolisthesis in the presence of an intact neural arch and posterior articulation may be the result of congenital shortening of the pars interarticularis.

Posterior displacement of a vertebra was mentioned as an early sign of tuberculous spondylitis of the lumbar spine by Hagel-

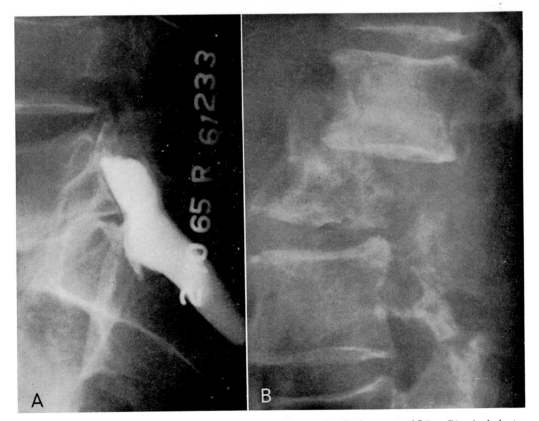

Fig. 358. *A*, Asymptomatic retrospondylolisthesis with posterior displacement of L5 on S1. An indentation into the anterior aspect of the Pantopaque column is present. *B*, Retrospondylolisthesis in a patient with myeloma and gross destruction of the body of L3. A sharp posterior displacement of L2 is present.

stam (1947). He observed that laxity of vertebral fixation which results from destruction of a disc permits slight displacement of the vertebra in the horizontal plane. A retroposition of less than 1 cm of one or more vertebrae appeared in 5 out of 45 patients with lumbar spine tuberculosis. In all cases except 1 narrowing of the intervertebral disc also was present. In 1 case of tuberculosis in an osteoporotic spine the vertebral retroposition was the only diagnostic radiographic sign. Hagelstam also reported a case in which the causative disc lesion was due to staphylococcic infection.

Retrospondylolisthesis is not uncommon, and usually is unassociated with symptoms.

However, when present in a patient who has a narrow spinal canal, the possibility of small discal herniations causing nerve root damage is increased. This also is true if spondylotic ridges or spurs are present. With gross vertebral destruction such as occurs with metastases, myeloma or granulomas a pronounced displacement sometimes is noted (Fig. 358). Rather marked lateral as well as as forward displacement sometimes is observed (Fig. 359), usually associated with marked discal degeneration. Congenital malformations of the neural arch sometimes permit posterior displacement of a vertebral body (Fig. 360).

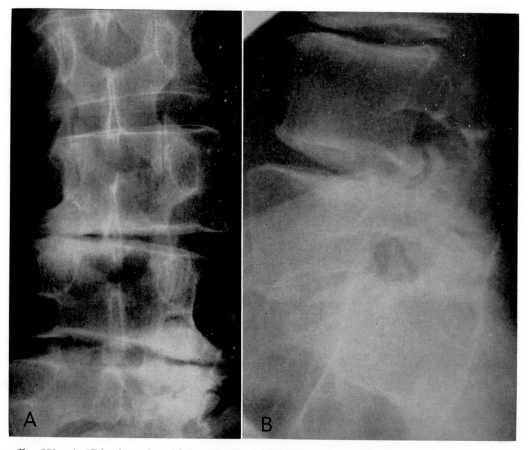

Fig. 359. A, AP lumbar spine with lateral shift of the third on the fourth lumbar vertebra and narrowing of the right lateral side of the third and fourth discs. Spurring and osteosclerotic reactions are present at the articular margins. B, Retrospondylolisthesis of L4 on L5. Note the curved configuration of the superior articular facet of L5.

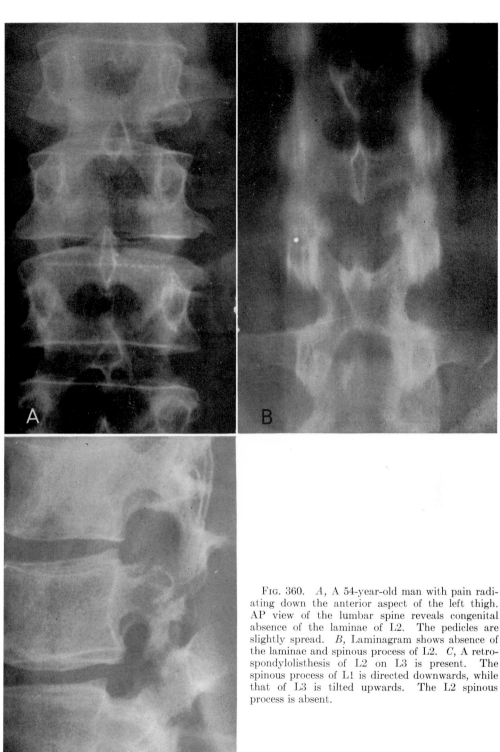

FIG. 360. *A*, A 54-year-old man with pain radiating down the anterior aspect of the left thigh. AP view of the lumbar spine reveals congenital absence of the laminae of L2. The pedicles are slightly spread. *B*, Laminagram shows absence of the laminae and spinous process of L2. *C*, A retro-spondylolisthesis of L2 on L3 is present. The spinous process of L1 is directed downwards, while that of L3 is tilted upwards. The L2 spinous process is absent.

References

DeVeer, A.: Wirbelverschiebung nach hinten unter dem Bilde schwerer Ischias, Röntgenpraxis, *7*, 27, 1935.

Fletcher, G. H.: Backward Displacement of Fifth Lumbar Vertebra in Degenerative Disc Disease, J. Bone & Joint Surg., *29*, 1019, 1947.

Gillespie, H. W.: Vertebral Retroposition, Brit. J. Radiol., *24*, 193, 1951.

Hagelstam, L.: Retroposition of Vertebrae as an Early Sign of Tuberculous Spondylitis of the Lumbar Spine, Acta orth. scandinav., *17*, 31, 1947.

Johnson, R. W.: Posterior Luxations of Lumbosacral Joint, J. Bone & Joint Surg., *16*, 867, 1934.

Melamed, A. and Ansfield, D. J.: Posterior Displacement of Lumbar Vertebrae, Am. J. Roentgenol., *58*, 307, 1947.

Roche, M. B. and Bryan, C. S.: Spondylolisthesis. Additional Variations in Anomalies of the Pars Interarticularis, Arch. Surg., *53*, 675, 1946.

Smith, A. D.: Posterior Displacement of the Fifth Lumbar Vertebra, J. Bone & Joint Surg., *16*, 877, 1934.

Willis, T. A.: Backward Displacement of 5th Lumber Vertebra, J. Bone & Joint Surg., *17*, 347, 1935.

PSEUDOSPONDYLOLISTHESIS OF JUNGHANNS

Pseudospondylolisthesis of Junghanns is predicated on displacement of a vertebral body anteriorly because of weakening of the apophyseal joints and a forward inclination of the inferior articular facets, with consequent forward displacement of the suprajacent vertebra. The neural arch remains intact, and no isthmic defect is present. The condition is usually accompanied by spondylosis and weakening of the intervertebral disc. Occasionally a definite anterior shift takes place when there is no visible spondylosis. However, the articular facets are inclined anteriorly and narrowing of the apophyseal joints together with elongation of the pars interarticularis of the displaced vertebra is present (Fig. 361). Paget's disease also produces changes which permit a forward slip (Fig. 362). It occurs more often in females, and the usual site is at the

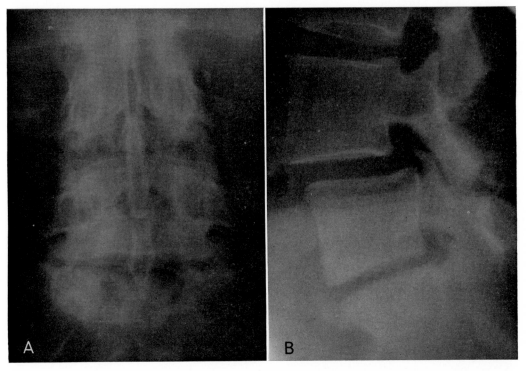

Fig. 361. *A*, AP view of the lower lumbar spine reveals a mild spondylotic reaction. *B*, The forward slip of L4 on L5 is incident to anterior inclination of the superior articular facet of L5. This was asymptomatic in a 60-year-old woman.

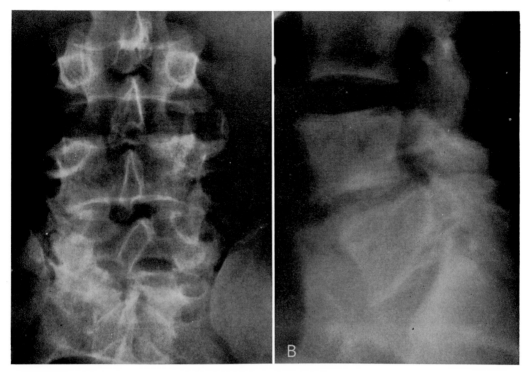

Fig. 362. *A*, Junghanns spondylolisthesis of L4 on L5 in a 58-year-old man with Paget's disease. An extensive involvement of the neural arches of L3, 4 and 5 is seen on the lateral projection, *B*.

fourth on the fifth lumbar vertebra. Although brought into prominence by Junghanns (1931), its existence had been known for a long time (Friberg, 1939). Guri (1946) mentioned that according to Sisefski the term "pseudospondylolisthesis" was first used by Neugebauer for cases of violent vertebral dislocations secondary to fracture.

In a collection of Eskimo and Indian skeletons (Stewart, 1935) found 3 specimens with first or second degree spondylolisthesis without separated neural arches. This was shown to be due to arthritic erosion of the articular facets. McNab (1950) reported 22 such cases in a series of 142 patients with spondylolisthesis. The roentgenograms in this series revealed an increase in the angle between the articular facets and the pedicles which permitted subluxations at the inferior joints. The anterior displacement averaged less than 1 cm. McNab observed an increased range of motion of the vertebral bodies with flexion and extension. Degenerative discal changes, spondylosis, osteoporosis and arthritic changes in the apophyseal joints were described.

References

Friberg, S.: Spondylolisthesis, Acta chir. scandinav., *82*, 1, 1939. (suppl. 55).

Guri, J. P.: Treatment of Painful Spondylolisthesis, Surg., Gynec. & Obst., *83*, 797, 1946.

Junghanns, H.: Spondylolisthesis, pseudo-spondylolisthesis und Wirbelverschiebung nach hinten, Beitr. path. Anat., *151*, 376, 1931.

McNab, I.: Spondylolisthesis with Intact Neural Arch, J. Bone & Joint Surg., *32-B*, 325, 1950.

CERVICAL SPONDYLOLISTHESIS

Spondylolisthesis of the sixth on the seventh cervical vertebra was reported by Perlman and Hawes (1951) in an adult patient with bilateral pedicle defects. Kornblum, Clayton and Nash (1952) observed that the acute stage of rheumatoid arthritis might be accompanied by hyperemia and capsular distention of the cervical joints, together with deforming muscle spasm. This may produce dislocations of the various cervical segments. They reported 4 cases to stress that lower cervical as well as atlantoaxial dislocations occur with this condition (Fig. 363). In 1 case (case 3) they described a slight anterior dislocation of the fifth on the sixth cervical segment. The initial displacement was only 2 or 3 mm, but 6 months later it was a full 2 cm forward, with about a 30-degree kyphotic and right lateral angulation and marked encroachment on the neural canal. Wide separation of the apposing articular surfaces of the posterior articulations at this level were noted, with marked erosion of the superior articular

facets of the sixth vertebra. This was reduced by skull traction, and repeat roentgenograms 1 year later showed only minimal posterior displacement of the fifth cervical vertebra, with narrowing of the fifth cervical interspace. The articular facets were recalcified, with partial fusion of their surfaces.

Advanced cervical spondylosis, with increased cervical lordosis and prominent dorsum rotundum not infrequently is accompanied by a slight but fairly definite forward slip of the fifth or sixth cervical vertebra. This represents the cervical equivalent of the pseudospondylolisthesis seen in the lower lumbar spine. Another

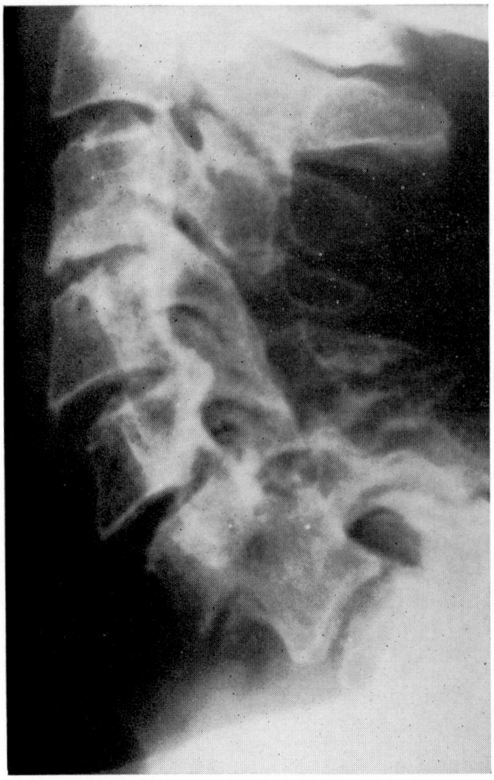

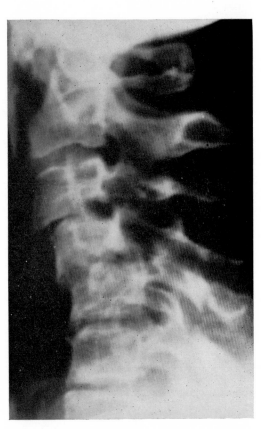

FIG. 363. Spondylolisthesis of C6 on C7 in a 48-year-old woman with rheumatoid arthritis. Narrowing of the intervertebral disc and erosive changes along the apposing bony margins are evident.

FIG. 364. Cervical spondylolisthesis in a 51-year-old woman with rheumatoid arthritis and progressive weakness of the hands and legs which advanced to tetraplegia. A forward slip of the third, fourth and fifth cervical vertebrae is present, with erosive changes at the intervertebral discs. This was considered to be due to granulomatous changes. A decompressive laminectomy was required for relief.

cause of cervical spondylolisthesis is fracture of the pars interarticularis or malignant disease with destruction of the pedicles or neural arches.

While this condition is usually asymptomatic, instances of cord compression are occasionally encountered. In 1 of our patients with rheumatoid arthritis, a 51-year-old woman who had the disease for more than 15 years, progressive weakness of the hands and legs was followed by tetraplegia. Roentgenograms of her cervical spine revealed forward displacement of the third, fourth and fifth vertebrae with considerable erosion of the intervertebral discs. She improved considerably after multiple laminectomies were performed as an urgent procedure (Fig. 364).

In patients with spurring along the dorsal aspect of the discs such a slip is important when symptoms of cord pressure appear. The so-called ridge syndrome of spondylosis may be heightened if a forward displacement of one of the lower cervical segments appears.

References

Kornblum, D., Clayton, M. L. and Nash, H. W.: Nontraumatic Cervical Dislocations in Rheumatoid Spondylitis, J.A.M.A., *149*, 431, 1952.

Perlman, R. and Hawes, L. E.: Cervical Spondylolisthesis, J. Bone & Joint Surg., *33-A*, 1012, 1951.

PSEUDOARTHROSIS

When spinal fusion is done for relief of spondylolisthesis, a method for checking the effect of the operation is useful. Cleveland, Bosworth and Thompson (1948) found that pseudarthrosis could best be demonstrated on films made in flexion and extension, and with bending to the right and left. Superimposition of identical films was the best way of evaluating untoward movement. Thompson and Ralston (1949) used flexion and extension films, but mentioned that at times the condition could be diagnosed only at operation. In the present author's experience body section roentgenograms through the fused areas have sometimes been helpful. At best, however, these methods are of doubtful reliability. Cineradiographic examinations have given rise to as many arguments as agreement in several cases.

References

Adkins, E. W. O.: Lumbo-sacral Arthrodesis after Laminectomy, J. Bone & Joint Surg., *37-B*, 208, 1955.

Cleveland, M., Bosworth, D. M. and Thompson, F. R.: Pseudarthrosis in Lumbosacral Spine, J. Bone & Joint Surg., *30-A*, 302, 1948.

Thompson, W. A. L. and Ralston, E. L.: Pseudarthrosis Following Spine Fusion, J. Bone & Joint Surg., *31-A*, 400, 1949.

7

Diseases of the Intervertebral Discs

JUVENILE KYPHOSIS DORSALIS (Scheuermann's disease) (Vertebral epiphysitis)

This condition was first described by Scheuermann (1921) as an osteochondrosis, predominantly of the middle, lower thoracic, and upper lumbar vertebrae. He ascribed this to deficient epiphyseal growth of the vertebrae, occurring more often in females between the ages of 10 and 14 years. Schmorl objected to the term "vertebral epiphysitis" as designating the apophyseal line as an epiphyseal line, inasmuch as it is not a true growth epiphysis. Schmorl pointed out that vertebral growth occurred on the spongiosa side of the cartilage end plates, which are the true growth zones. He held that weakening and thinning of this growth zone together with herniations of the intervertebral disc, with resultant decrease in the anterior height of the vertebral body, was the primary cause of this disease. It has been held that the ring apophyses play no part in the growth of the vertebral body, and that disturbances in this structure visualized roentgenologically are the result rather than the cause of juvenile kyphosis.

Beadle (1931) attributed vertebral epiphysitis to an inborn weakness of developmental error which produces minute fissures in the cartilaginous plates. These serve as passageways for prolapse of nuclear material into the spongiosa following strain or small traumas. With continued intrusion of nuclear substance into the end plates, defective growth follows. Diminution of the efficiency of the intervertebral disc as an equalizing mechanism results in undue strain on the anterior aspect of the involved vertebrae, with consequent wedging and appearance of the characteristic curve.

MacGowan (1944) pointed out that with adolescent kyphosis the nucleus pulposus is disrupted before ossification of the vertebral body is complete. This may be caused by failure of the cartilaginous disc to retain the nucleus, or by softening of the vertebral body. The weight-bearing function is then transferred to the vertebral bodies anteriorly and the axis of motion to the posterior vertebral elements. Increased pressure results at the anterior borders when the spine is in flexion. If the patient is adolescent, the epiphyses will be subjected to trauma and abnormal ossification follows. Premature closure of the epiphyses, failure of anterior vertebral ossification and wedging of the bodies constitute the end results. MacGowan's experience differed from others in that his patients were predominantly male. Knuttson (1948) studied juvenile kyphosis by means of serial films in growing children. He concluded that there was retarded vertical growth of the vertebral bodies involved. This resulted in an intact rectangular shape with diminished height in some, while in others narrowing anteriorly produced wedge-shaped deformities. He considered Scheuermann's disease as an obscure disturbance of growth involving either the entire surface or only a portion of the vertebral body.

The association of spinal extradural cysts and kyphosis dorsalis juvenalis was described by Cloward and Bucy (1937). These authors believed that the changes in the vertebrae were not inflammatory, and did not predominantly or selectively involve the vertebral epiphyses. They stated that the many vascular channels in the epidural space comprising the vertebral circulation may become occluded by the pressure of a cyst wedged between the bony walls of the spinal canal and the dura mater. The changes in the vertebral bodies could then be explained on the basis of venous congestion. The partial collapse of the contiguous vertebral bodies resulted in the rounded and fixed deformity. While this may occur with spinal extradural cysts, which are not common, the frequency of juvenile kyphosis suggests that this mechanism is not a major factor.

The clinical picture of juvenile kyphosis varies considerably. In the early stages the diagnosis may be made accidentally by discovery of characteristic changes of the articular surfaces of the vertebral bodies. Symptoms are mild or even absent during the acute stage of the disease in some patients. In others persistent mild pain between the shoulder blades is associated with a stooping posture. There may be tenderness on pressure over the involved area and pain may be aggravated after exercise. Symptoms referable to compression of the spinal cord are infrequent. However, Wretblad (1939) reported 6 patients, all young

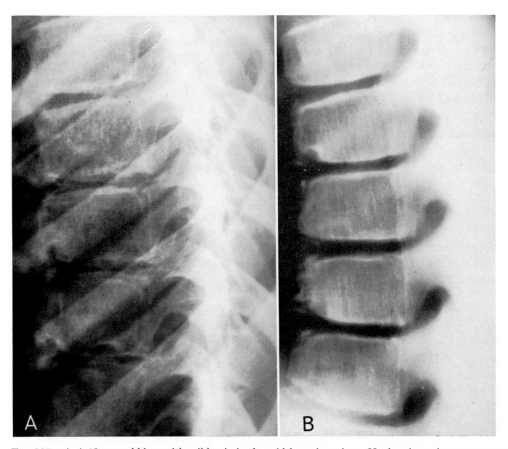

Fig. 365. A, A 12-year-old boy with mild pain in the midthoracic region. Nuclear intrusions are present in the midthoracic vertebrae, particularly along the inferior and anterior aspects of the vertebral bodies. B, Laminagrams reveal the changes more clearly. The apophyseal rings are forming normally, but their positions are altered by the nuclear prolapses.

men engaged in hard physical labor, who had numbness, weakness, and unsteadiness in the legs. Spastic paralysis of the legs appeared in several cases. Myelograms showed a block at the apex of the curve and improvement followed laminectomy. In 1 patient in whom symptoms had been present for several years and who died after laminectomy, autopsy showed irreparable damage in the spinal cord. Van Landingham (1954) reported a 17-year-old male in whom herniated discs in the mid-dorsal spine was associated with Scheuermann's disease. These were demonstrated myelographically, and the spinal cord compression had to be relieved surgically. More often myelography discloses only a gradual narrowing of the subarachnoid space at the apex of the curve (Lindgren, 1941).

The radiologic appearance of juvenile kyphosis is variable, depending on the stage and extent of the disease. In the early stages the roentgenograms show only a slight irregularity of the vertebral end plates associated with slight decalcification of the peripheries of the vertebral bodies immediately adjacent to the apophyseal rings. At this stage there may be no alteration in the usual alignment of the thoracolumbar spine (Fig. 365). As the disease progresses the marginal irregularities become more marked and decalcification of the vertebral body appears.

The intervertebral discs between the involved vertebrae become narrowed and irregular, with nuclear extrusions projecting through the end plates into the vertebral bodies. There may be decalcification of the

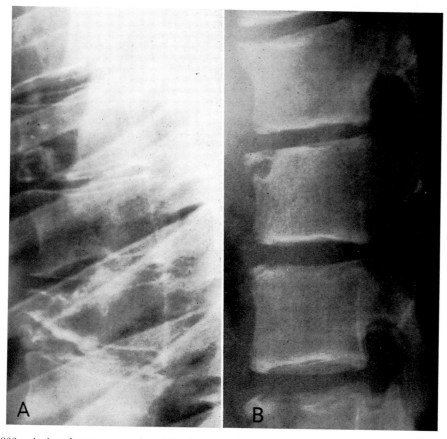

Fig. 366. *A,* A rather pronounced wedging is present in the anterior aspect of T-9 in this asymptomatic 30-year-old man. *B,* Localized epiphyseal discal herniations in the anterior aspects of L3, 4 and 5 in an asymptomatic 14-year-old boy.

anterior aspects of the vertebral bodies. In more advanced cases deficiency of bone appears, with resultant irregular tongue-like projections into the anterior aspect of the involved vertebral body.

The apophyseal rings in early Scheuermann's disease may be small, fragmented and irregular. Later they become thickened and appear in grooves along the vertebral margins in a discontinuous pattern. Fusion of the apophyseal rings may be delayed. The nuclear intrusions are most prominent in the anterior and middle thirds of the involved vertebrae. The posterior height of the vertebral bodies is maintained. The intervertebral discs are uniformly narrowed. The extent of reactive calcification around the nuclear intrusions varies from slight to considerable, and is best seen on laminagrams (Fig. 366). Associated with advanced

changes are progressive wedging and notching of the anterior aspects of the vertebrae, producing a kyphotic deformity. Scoliosis may be observed if the vertebral wedging is irregular, leading to a diminished height on one side. As the disease passes into a healing stage, and eventual cure, the fragmented appearance of the end plates and the associated irregular decalcifications in the vertebral bodies disappear. By the age of 18 to 20 years union of these elements occurs, resulting in a well-calcified vertebral body with an anterior wedge-like deformity. Persistent bits of calcification remaining at the anterior aspects of the vertebral bodies have been referred to as Scheuermann's nodes, and sometimes are mistaken for fractures. Occasionally similar bony changes occur in the lumbar and the cervical spine. Ununited fragments of bone may be residual from the

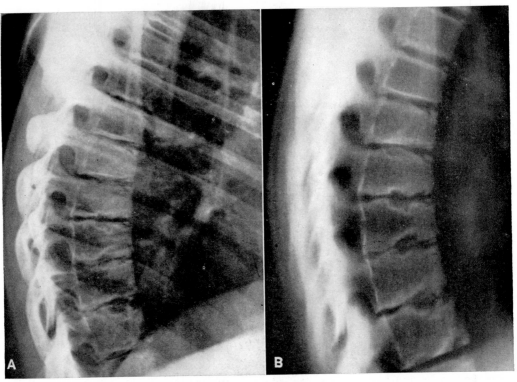

Fig. 367. *A*, Moderately advanced case of kyphosis dorsalis juvenalis. Note the nuclear protrusions into the superior and inferior surfaces of the vertebrae. *B*, Same case, lateral body section roentgenogram. The nuclear protrusions with some bony reaction around them are well demonstrated. The ring apophyses in the midthoracic vertebrae are rather large but intact. In the lower thoracic vertebrae the ring apophyses are widened, irregular and have bony rarefaction immediately beneath them.

pathologic process associated with juvenile kyphosis. It has been established by discography that these bony changes are due to anterior discal herniations and represent bits of bone separated from the main body of the vertebra by intervening islands of cartilage. They are sometimes referred to as "limbus bones" (Fig. 378).

Scheuermann's disease usually can be distinguished from tuberculous spondylitis without difficulty because of the nuclear intrusions, the reactive changes about these lesions and the intact narrowed intervertebral discs (Fig. 368). Other infections affecting the discal surfaces, such as acute infectious discitis or osteomyelitis usually present evidence of bone destruction adjacent to the narrowed involved interspace.

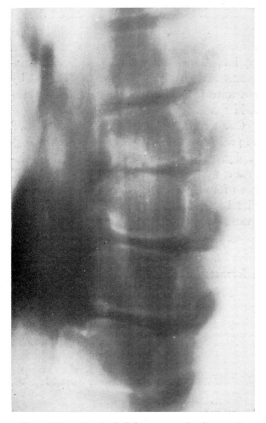

FIG. 368. Atypical Scheuermann's disease in a 14-year-old boy with midthoracic pain. There are step-like deformities in the anterior aspect of several of the vertebral bodies. The patient had been referred with a diagnosis of tuberculous spondylitis.

References

Bauer, W.: Zur Ätiologie der juvenilen Kyphose (M. Scheuermann), Fortschr. Röntgenstr., *83*, 839, 1955.

Beadle, O. A.: The Intervertebral Discs: Observations on Their Normal and Morbid Anatomy in Relation to Certain Spinal Deformities, M. Res. Council, *161*, 1, 1931.

Cloward, R. B. and Bucy, P. C.: Spinal Extradural Cysts and Kyphosis Dorsalis Juvenalis, Am. J. Roentgenol, *38*, 681, 1937.

Cole, W. H.: Epiphyseal Disturbances in Childhood, J.A.M.A., *127*, 318, 1945.

Knuttson, F.: Growth of Vertebral Body in Scheuermann's Disease, Acta radiol., *30*, 97, 1948.

Lindblom, K.: Discography of Dissecting Transosseous Ruptures of Intervertebral Discs in Lumbar Region, Acta radiol., *36*, 12, 1951.

Lindgren, E.: Myelographic Changes in Kyphosis Dorsalis Juvenalis, Acta radiol., *22*, 461, 1941.

MacGowan, T. J. B. A.: Adolescent Kyphosis, Lancet, *1*, 211, 1944.

Scheuermann, H.: Kyphosis Dorsalis Juvenalis, Ztschr. f. orthop. Chir., *41*, 305, 1921.

————: Kyphosis Dorsalis Juvenalis, Fortschr. Röntgenstr., *53*, 1, 1936.

Schmorl, G.: Die Pathogeneses der juvenilen Kyphose, Fortschr. Röntgenstr., *41*, 359, 1930.

Schmorl, G. and Junghanns, H.: *The Human Spine in Health and Disease*, New York, Grune & Stratton, 1959.

Stammel, C. A.: Juvenile Osteochondrosis, Radiology, *35*, 413, 1940.

Van Landinghan, J. H.: Herniation of Thoracic Intervertebral Discs with Spinal Cord Compression in Kyphosis Dorsalis Juvenalis (Scheuermann's Disease), J. Neurosurg., *11*, 327, 1954.

Williams H. J. and Pugh, D. G.: Vertebral Epiphysitis, Am. J. Roentgenol., *90*, 1236, 1963.

Wretblad, G.: Spatschadilungen des Ruckenmarks bei Wirbelsaulanverk Rummungen besonders Solchen zum Typus des Juvenile Kyphose Scheuermann, Acta psychiat. et neurol., *14*, 617, 1939.

INTERVERTEBRAL DISC INJURIES

Disc Puncture. In view of the frequency with which lumbar puncture is performed for myelography and discography, it is worth reviewing the possible hazards of this procedure. It has been reported that perforation of the posterior spinal ligament may be followed by changes in the intervertebral disc (Pease, 1935). Progressive narrowing of a lower lumbar intervertebral space and Schmorl's nodes were noted by Gellman (1940) on successive roentgenograms of a 14-year-old girl who had had a spinal tap. Epps (1942) described degeneration and collapse of an intervertebral disc following lumbar puncture, which he attributed to aseptic degeneration. Three similar cases were described by Everett (1942). Downing (1944) reported 2 cases in which the intervertebral disc collapsed following operation under spinal anesthesia. He mentioned that if the needle were inserted so that it did not enter the subarachnoid space, and was further advanced so that it penetrated the annulus fibrosus and entered the disc in its lateral aspect, escape of nuclear material sometimes was followed by discal degeneration and collapse. Baker (1947) observed narrowing of an intervertebral disc in a 4-year-old boy after a spinal tap. Severe backache and rigidity of the spine appeared within a few days after lumbar puncture. Serial roentgenograms showed relatively rapid narrowing of the intervertebral disc. In some opinions these changes represent the effect of infection rather than simple trauma.

In an experimental investigation of intervertebral disc lesions in dogs, Key and Ford (1948) found that after the discs had been punctured once by a 20-gauge needle, an atypical protrusion of the nucleus pulposus occurred in one instance. Congdon (1952) punctured the intervertebral discs in 13 rabbits, and observed that this was followed by regeneration of nucleus pulposus cells which presented some resemblance to neoplasm. In rabbits which survived from 6 to over 10 months after such puncture, gelatinous nodules of nucleus pulposus cells were found in the adjacent soft tissues. Dripps and Vandam (1952) concurred that trauma to the annulus fibrosus may be followed by herniation of the nucleus pulposus. They stated that they had seen gelatinous material drop from the needle which had entered the nucleus pulposus of a 14-year-old girl who moved inadvertently as the needle was being advanced during a spinal tap.

On the other hand, Gardner, Weiss, Hughes, O'Connell and Weiford (1952) asserted that the small bore of the needle used to perforate the posterior spinal ligament for discography was not likely to damage either the ligament, the annulus fibrosus or the nucleus pulposus. Erlacher (1952), who suggested a lateral approach to the nucleus pulposus, bypassing the neural sac, also was of the opinion that the small gauge of the needle used did not increase the danger of nuclear protrusion. Cloward (1959) reported that no case of rupture of a normal intact disc followed discography in his series of over 450 lumbar discograms over an 8-year period, and he regarded the fear of injury to a normal disc by needle puncture as unfounded. De Seze and Levernieux (1952) reported that a review of 59 patients who had had discography showed that 13 had collapsed discs attributed to necrosis due to puncture and instillation of contrast material.

Among other hazards encountered during lumbar puncture, but which are quite uncommon, are hemorrhage into the cauda equina, the formation of epidural hematomas and meningeal irritations caused by entrance of blood into the spinal subarachnoid space.

Our experience in this respect is limited to patients who had spinal taps for myelography. Included in the over 3000 myelograms were several in which the needle had been forcibly pushed into the intervertebral disc because of sudden uncontrolled movements by the patient. None developed untoward reactions to this trauma.

References

Baker, A. H.: Lesion of the Intervertebral Disk Caused by Lumbar Puncture, Brit. J. Surg., *34*, 385, 1947.
Cloward, R. B.: Cervical Diskography, Ann. Surg., *150*, 1052, 1959.
Congdon, C. C.: Proliferative Lesions Resembling Chordoma Following Puncute of Nucleus Pulposus in Rabbits, J. National Cancer Inst., *12*, 893, 1952.
De Seze, S. and Levernieux, J.: Les Accidentes de la Discographie, Rev. Rheum., *19*, 1027, 1952.
Downing, F. H.: Collapse of Intervertebral Disc Following Spinal Puncture, U. S. Naval Bull., *43*, 666, 1944.
Dripps, R. D. and Vandam, L. D.: Hazards of Lumbar Puncture, J.A.M.A., *147*, 1118, 1952.

Erlacher, P. R.: Nucleography, J. Bone & Joint
  Surg., *34-B*, 204, 1952.
Everett, A. D.: Lumbar Puncture Injuries, Proc.
  Royal Soc. Med., *35*, 208, 1942.
Gardner, W. J., Wise, R. E., Hughes, C. R., O'Connell,
  F. B., Jr. and Weiford, E. C.: X-Ray Visualiza-
  tion of the Intervertebral Disk, Arch. Surg., *64*,
  355, 1952.
Gellman, M.: Injury to Intervertebral Discs
  During Spinal Puncture, J. Bone & Joint Surg.,
  22, 980, 1940.
Key, J. A. and Ford, L. T.: Experimental Interver-
  tebral Disc Lesions, J. Bone & Joint Surg., *30-A*,
  621, 1948.
Pease, C. N.: Injuries to Vertebrae and Interverte-
  bral Disks Following Lumbar Puncture, Am. J.
  Dis. Child., *49*, 849, 1935.

Disc Infections

Inasmuch as the normal intervertebral disc is avascular, hematogenous infections are rare. However, extension of an inflammatory process from adjacent bone through a crevice in the cartilaginous plate may occur, and probably explains the rapid degeneration of disc tissue seen with extensive osteomyelitis. When some vascularization of the disc is present because of a degenerative process, it is conceivable that a hematogenous infection may occur. However, no such cases have been clearly identified. It is generally agreed that discal infection is incident to infection in the adjacent bone. From the radiologic point of view, it may be difficult, if not impossible, to detect minimal osteomyelitis, so that the initial change may be a progressively decreasing discal height.

In tuberculosis of the spine the intervertebral discs are resistant, put eventually succumb to the destructive process. The progress of such destruction is variable, and may be accompanied by a wide variety of change in which bone destruction is first seen. Then, as the lesion progresses, various discal deformities appear. Finally the disc practically disappears. At the end stages, when bony fusion occurs, the intervertebral disc may no longer be identified. When a tuberculous focus is initially implanted adjacent to the anterior spinal ligament, the intervertebral disc may become involved relatively early by spread of the infection behind these ligaments.

Brucellosis may cause relatively rapid destruction of an intervertebral disc which may proceed to total disappearance (Di Rienzo, 1944).

Direct infection can be introduced into the intervertebral disc during lumbar puncture for diagnostic purposes or discography. Another more frequent association of intervertebral disc infection is that with surgery for herniated discs. The rate of progression of the infection varies considerably, and is preceded by severe lumbar pain for a few days to several weeks after operation. At first no specific changes can be identified radiologically. As the infection progresses the involved intervertebral disc becomes narrowed, and the bone on either side loses its trabeculation, assuming a washed-out appearance. It is presumed that the original infection in postoperative discal herniation patients is in the bone. Healing is slow and is accompanied by later development of peripheral osteophytes, mainly on the anterolateral aspect of the involved vertebrae.

A benign form of osteitis of the vertebrae in children was reported by Bremner and Neligan (1953). They described 7 patients, all under 3 years of age, with fever, limp, stiff back with painful spasm and limited hip motion. Symptoms increased in severity for about 5 to 6 weeks, then became stationary or improved. Radiographic examination of the spine disclosed narrowing of the disc space, with erosion of the adjacent margins of one or both vertebrae. Recalcification was observed on serial study. Ghormley, Bickel and Dickson (1940) described a presumable acute infectious lesion of the intervertebral discs, characterized by clinical signs of infection of a mild nature, with backache, spasm and tenderness over the affected areas. These authors stated that the intervertebral disc at first remained unaltered, but later diminished in height. The narrowing persisted for several months, and then bony proliferation appeared at the margins of the involved vertebrae. In some of their cases bony fusion occurred. In others paravertebral soft sissue thickening appeared. They believed that if osseous involvement became evident, osteomyelitis probably was the diagnosis. The infectious nature of discitis in children has been established by positive cultures of Staphylococcus aureus in biopsy material (Milone, Bianco and Ivins, 1962; Möes, 1964; Menelaus, 1964).

References

Bremner, A. E. and Neligan, G. A.: Benign Form of Acute Osteitis of the Spine in Young Children, Brit. Med. J., *1*, 856, 1953.

Bromley, L. L., Craig, J. D. and Kessel, A. W. L.: Infected Intervertebral Disk after Lumbar Puncture, Brit. Med. J., *1*, 132, 1949.

DiRienzo, S.: Die brucellose Spondylitis, Fortschr. Röntgenstr., *73*, 333, 1950.

Doyle, J. R.: Narrowing of the Intervertebral-Disc Space in Children, J. Bone & Joint Surg., *42-A*, 1191, 1960.

Ghormley, R. K., Bickel, W. H. and Dickson, D. D.: Acute Infectious Lesions of Intervertebral Disks, Southern M. J., *33*, 347, 1940.

Key, J. A.: Intervertebral-Disc Lesions in Children and Adolescents, J. Bone & Joint Surg., *32-A*, 97, 1950.

Lowman, R. M. and Robinson, F.: Progressive Vertebral Interspace Changes Following Lumbar Disk Surgery, Am. J. Roentgenol., *97*, 664, 1966.

Milone, F. P., Bianco, A. J., Jr. and Ivins, J. C.: Infections of the Intervertebral Disk in Children, J.A.M.A., *181*, 1029, 1962.

Menelaus, M. B.: Discitis. An Inflammation Affecting the Intervertebral Discs in Children, J. Bone & Joint Surg., *46-B*, 16, 1964.

Möes, C. A. F.: Spondylarthritis in Childhood, Am. J. Roentgenol., *91*, 578, 1964.

Scherbel, A. L. and Gardner, W. J.: Infections Involving the Intervertebral Discs, J.A.M.A., *174*, 370, 1960.

Sullivan, C. R., Bickel, W. H. and Svien, H. J.: Infections of Vertebral Interspace after Operations on Intervertebral Disks, J.A.M.A., *166*, 1973, 1958.

Sullivan, C. R. and Symmonds, R. E.: Disk Infections and Abdominal Pain, J.A.M.A., *188*, 655, 1964.

Turnbull, F.: Postoperative Inflammatory Disease of Lumbar Discs, J. Neurosurg., *10*, 469, 1953.

THE EFFECTS OF TRAUMA ON THE INTERVERTEBRAL DISC

Because of the elasticity of the intervertebral fibrocartilage and the cushioning action of the intact nucleus pulposus, the intervertebral disc usually is not affected by mild trauma. However, repeated or violent injury may produce rupture and fissure of the cartilaginous plates and consequent extrusion of nuclear material through such rents. Rotary or compressive trauma may injure the lateral aspects of the annulus fibrosus and be accompanied by fracture of the adjacent bone. Injuries to the posterior spinal ligament as a cause of posterior protrusion of the nucleus pulposus and discal material is well recognized.

Progressive degeneration and narrowing of the intervertebral disc may follow extrusion of nuclear material. Part of the picture of healing is the development of osteophytes along the lateral and anterior margins of the involved vertebrae. Sclerosis of the apposing bony surfaces of a narrowed disc, particularly in the lower lumbar area, is frequent. Such changes were produced experimentally by Compere and Keyes (1933). They reported that in dog operations in which the intervertebral disc was opened and nuclear material curetted, the discs completely disappeared. The adjacent bony surfaces became markedly sclerosed, with spur formation and lipping of the anterior edges. These dogs were sacrificed 3 months after operation, and histologic study revealed that the discs at the site of injury had vanished. The bone had become dense, with marked hyperostosis and new bone formation similar to that seen clinically in cases of marked hypertrophic spondylitis.

With severe trauma to the spine, there may be a complete break through the fibrocartilage with shifting of the vertebral bodies for an appreciable distance, as with fracture dislocations of the vertebrae. Wright and Gardner (1952) reported a case of traumatic chylothorax incident to dislocation of the sixth on the seventh thoracic vertebra. A complete transection of the spinal cord caused the death of this patient.

It is known that in hyperflexion injuries of the neck retropulsion of the nucleus pulposus through the posterior spinal ligament into the spinal canal occurs, with damage to the cervical cord (Gay and Abbot, 1953). The displaced nucleus pulposus may return to its normal position. Such cases have been reported by Taylor and Blackwood (1948), Schneider (1951), and Cramer and McGowan (1944). It is worth recounting the case reported by Brooke (1944), in which a patient was admitted with a complete flaccid paralysis below the fifth cervical segment, with loss of sensation of all modalities below the sixth cervical segment. Necropsy 15 days after admission showed defective and frayed posterior spinal ligaments, with posterior protrusion of a calcified nucleus pulposus which had impinged against the spinal cord, producing a soft defect in the lower cervical region. These authors noted that when the head was flexed slightly, this irregularly calcified intervertebral disc bulged about 1 cm into the spinal canal.

References

Brooke, W. S.: Complete Transverse Cervical Myelitis Caused by Traumatic Herniation of an Ossified Nucleus Pulposus, J.A.M.A., *125*, 117, 1944.

Cramer, F. and McGowan, F. J.: Nucleus Pulposus in Pathogenesis of So-called "Recoil" Injuries of Spinal Cord, Surg., Gynec. & Obst., *79*, 516, 1944.

Gay, J. R. and Abbott, K. H.: Common Whiplash Injuries of the Neck, J.A.M.A., *152*, 1698, 1953.

Key, J. A.: Intervertebral-disc Lesions in Children and Adolescents, J. Bone & Joint Surg., *32-A*, 97, 1950.

Keyes, D. C. and Compere, E. L.: Normal and Pathological Physiology of Nucleus Pulposus of Intervertebral Disc. J. Bone & Joint Surg., *14*, 897, 1932.

Schneider, R. C.: A Syndrome in Acute Cervical Spine Injuries for Which Early Operation is Indicated, J. Neurosurg., *8*, 360, 1951.

Taylor, A. R. and Blackwood, W.: Paraplegia in Hyperextension Cervical Injuries with Normal Radiographic Appearances, J. Bone & Joint Surg., *30-B*, 245, 1948.

Degenerative Changes in Intervertebral Discs

Although degeneration of intervertebral discs has been considered in the chapter on spondylosis, the importance of these changes makes it advisable to review briefly their anatomic and radiologic characteristics. The intervertebral discs are enveloped by the annulus fibrosus, which is thickest in its anterior portion where it blends with the anterior spinal ligament. The annulus is formed by fibrous and elastic lamellae, with irregularly scattered cartilaginous cells attached to the adjacent bone by Sharpey's fibers. These are arranged in an oblique and spiral fashion, extending from one vertebral body to another, with considerable variation in the anatomic placement of their lateral aspects. The posterior portion of the annulus fibrosus is its weakest, and in some is so poorly defined as to present breaks in continuity. Encased within the annulus fibrosus is the nucleus pulposus, an elastic, gelatinous, almost lozenge-shaped structure which merges imperceptibly with the annulus fibrosus. In childhood and early adult life this structure is relatively smooth and homogeneous. Its turgor and elasticity are greatest during the early life. The cellular components of the nucleus pulposus are mostly fibroblasts, cartilage cells and notochordal remnants. Above and beneath the nucleus pulposus, forming respectively the superior and inferior surfaces of the vertebrae, are the cartilage plates. These are thickest centrally, and merge with the annulus fibrosus peripherally. Usually the plates are complete, but small crack-like defects are quite frequent. Through these perforating fissures may project bits of cancellous bone, or fragments of the nucleus pulposus may enter the vertebral bodies. Normally the disc is avascular, receiving its nutrition by means of perfusion, a process aided by the presence of lymphatics at the junction of bone and cartilage. With advancing age and in the presence of degeneration, vascular intrusion appears.

Although degenerative changes of the intervertebral disc have long been known, today's knowledge stems mainly from the work of Schmorl and his co-workers. This was recounted in detail in the classical monograph by Schmorl and Junghanns (1957). An excellent brief review of the normal and pathologic intervertebral disc was published by Coventry, Ghormley and Kernohan (1945).

Progressive degenerative discal changes are closely related to fluid loss, with consequent alterations of turgor and elasticity. The hydration of intervertebral discs is greatest in the neonatal period, and diminishes slowly thereafter. A relatively more rapid loss of fluid content is noted for a short time during infancy. Thereafter the rate of dehydration is relatively slow until about the third decade, when the process becomes accelerated. The borderline between the normal and abnormal at this stage is incident to the wear and tear of living. With advancing degeneration of the intervertebral disc there is gradual dissolution and atrophy of the annulus fibrosus with progressive softening and weakening of its structure. Necrotic changes appear in the anterior portion of the annulus fibrosus weakening the ring and permitting prolapse of nuclear material. The nucleus pulposus likewise loses its gelatinous turgor because of loss of fluid. In association with weaken-

ing of the annulus fibrosus and changes in the cartilaginous plates, the lozenge shape of the nucleus pulposus alters. Erlacher (1952) correlated the anatomic and radiologic appearance of the nucleus pulposus by means of a staining technic combined with radiography. He identified five principal forms, including a normal globular nucleus, a lobed nucleus with a few large lobulations considered normal in adults, a simple branched nucleus with long narrow limbs, which appeared to be predisposed towards herniation. He also mentioned a multiple branched nucleus with a small central shadow and several extensions considered a transitory form of degeneration in which prolapse was likely to occur. The fifth form was the spread nucleus with many branches in all directions instead of a single central shadow. This last type represented a typical degenerated disc, and was most often associated with a narrow intervertebral disc space.

The association of changes in the intervertebral discs with alterations in spina

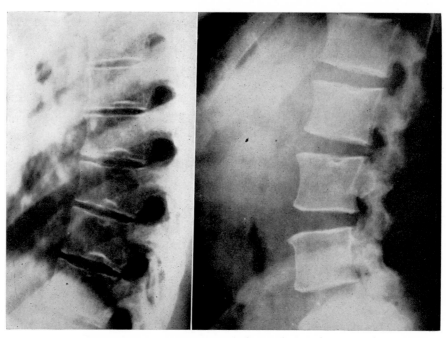

Fig. 369. Throacolumbar spine with multiple Schmorl's nodes in an athletic, 19-year-old girl who was symptom free.

curvature is exemplified by adolescent kyphosis.

Senile kyphosis occurs as a curvature of the upper and middle portions of the dorsal spine late in life. This condition is attributed to degenerative changes in the anterior aspects of the involved intervertebral discs, which assume a tapered appearance with the narrow end directed anteriorly. With progressive narrowing, the edges of the vertebrae eventually touch, and actual bony fusion occurs. The posterior aspects of the discs may be narrowed, but usually remain identifiable even with advanced senile kyphosis. The vertebral bodies become cuneiform in shape, with some osteophyte production at the lateral aspects. It is not uncommon to observe a considerable degree of osteoporosis with senile kyphosis. The wide biconvex appearance of the discs associated with the swelling of the nucleus pulposus usually seen with osteoporosis does not occur when senile kyphosis is present.

References

Beadle, O. A.: The Intervertebral Discs, His Majesty's Stationery Office, London, 1931.

Compere, E. L. and Keyes, D. C.: Roentgenological Studies of Intervertebral Disc, Am. J. Roentgenol., *29*, 774, 1933.

Coventry, M. B., Ghormley, R. K. and Kernohan. J. W.: The Intervertebral Disc., J. Bone & Joint Surg., *27*, 105, 223, 460, 1945.

Erlacher, P. R.: Nucleography, J. Bone & Joint Surg., *34-B*, 204, 1952.

Mooney, A. C.: Disc Lesions in Relation to Pain, Brit. J. Radiol., *18*, 153, 1945.

Oppenheimer, A.: Lesions of Intervertebral Disks, New England J. Med., *230*, 95, 1944.

Saunders, J. B. de C. and Inman, V. T.: Intervertebral Disc., Surg., Gynec. & Obst., *69*, 14, 1939.

Schmorl, G.: Die gesunde und kranke Wirbelsäule im Röntgenbild, Fortschr. Röntgenstr., Erganzungsband XLIII, Leipzig, Georg Thieme Verlag, 1932.

Schmorl, G. and Junghanns, H.: Die Gesunde und die Kranke Wirbelsäule in Röntgenbild und Klinik, Stuttgart, Georg Thieme Verlag, 1957. (First American edition, 1959, Grune & Stratton, New York, Translated and edited by Wilk, S. P. and Goin, L. S.)

Scheuermann, H.: Kyphosis dorsalis juvenalis, Ztschr. f. orthop. Chir., *41*, 305, 1921.

————: Kyphosis dorsalis juvenalis, Fortschr. Röntgenstr., *53*, 1, 1936.

Calcification of the Intervertebral Discs

According to Sandström (1951) calcification of the intervertebral discs was mentioned by Luschka (1858), and was first demonstrated roentgenologically in cadavers by Beneke (1897). In 1930 Calvé and Galland described them during life. The pathologic aspects of the condition were investigated by Schmorl (1929), who believed that calcification followed small discal ruptures followed by necrosis. Other etiologies proposed include persistent overloading of the spine beyond its work capacity, degenerative changes, inflammations, senile alterations and disturbances in calcium metabolism.

Intervertebral disc calcifications occur in the nucleus pulposus, the annulus fibrosus or both. Calcifications also appear in the cartilaginous end plates of the vertebral bodies, sometimes by extension from the annulus fibrosus. The most common location is the annulus fibrosus. The radiologic differentiation of these sites can be made with some degree of accuracy. Calcifications of uniform density in the middle of the intervertebral disc are more likely to be nuclear calcifications (Fig. 370). These may be ovoid in configuration, and sometimes extend to the posterior third of the intervertebral space. Calcifications in the annulus fibrosus are more frequent in its anterior, superior and inferior portions. Occasionally calcium deposits occur in both areas, and cannot be differentiated one from the other (Fig. 371). Calcifications in the cartilaginous end plates alone are infrequent.

Intervertebral discal calcifications in adults as a rule are symptomless, while those in children may be associated with painful syndromes. Adult intervertebral discal calcifications do not as a rule disappear, while those in children may or may not vanish. The reason for the occurrence of calcifications of the intervertebral discs in children, as well as for their disappearance and association with symptoms, is not known.

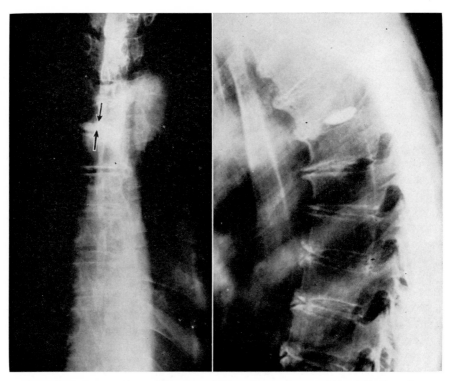

Fig. 370. Symptomless calcification of the nucleus pulposus of the sixth thoracic
intervertebral disc (arrows).

Calcification of the intervertebral discs in children is infrequent. In a report on discal calcifications in childhood, Weens (1945) described a 5-year-old girl with pain in the lower cervical spine radiating to the back of her head. Roentgenograms revealed dense calcification in the sixth cervical interspace extending from the anterior to the midportion of the disc. Apparently these had been present for some time, inasmuch as a review of films made prior to hospitalization showed the lesion present then. Disappearance of the calcification was noted over a period of about 4 months. There is a predilection for this condition to involve the lower cervical or upper thoracic spine at multiple levels. Of particular interest is the fact that the calcifications have been known to disappear over a period of from several weeks to a few months, or may persist for a period of years. Melnick and Silverman (1963) collected 48 cases from the available literature, and added 5 of their own. The youngest was 7 days

old, and the size and density of the lesion suggested that it may have been present at or before birth. The oldest patient was 16 years old. The incidence varied from the newborn period to adolescence, with decreasing frequency as adulthood was approached. In the 53 cases reviewed there were 90 discal calcifications. In 31 only a single disc was calcified, and in 18 multiple lesions were present. The largest number of calcified discs in a single patient was 8. The cervical region was most frequently affected, most often at the second to sixth interspaces. In the thoracic region the sixth interspace was involved most often. The lumbar region was least involved, four being observed at the first lumbar interspace and one at the fifth interspace. In 3 patients seen by us persistence of the calcifications in the cervical spine was observed over an 18-month period, during which time neck pain disappeared and recurred several times (Fig. 372). The second patient (Fig. 373) was

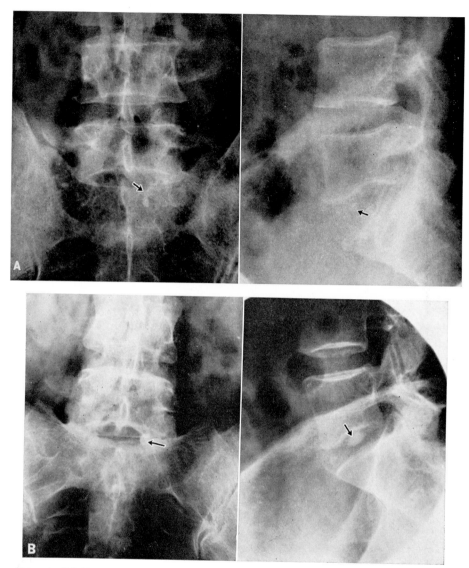

Fig. 371. *A*, Calcification in the lateral aspect of the nucleus pulposus and adjoining annulus fibrosus at the lumbosacral interspace (arrows). *B*, Another case of local calcification of the annulus fibrosus (arrows). The calcification is excentric, and is smooth.

seen because of neck pain and torticollis which disappeared spontaneously in about a month. The third patient was asymptomatic, the discal calcifications being observed on a chest film.

Sandström (1951) reported a 59-year-old woman in whom calcifications in the first lumbar interspace disappeared, and another 59-year-old male in whom calcifications were present in several of the lower thoracic intervertebral discs. Both had pain which was acute at the onset, with sensitivity to pressure and limitation of motion. A rapid sedimentation rate was present during the acute phase. Both patients benefited from x-ray therapy. Calcifications in the annulus fibrosus are usually permanent. Calcifications of the nucleus pulposus and the adjoining annulus fibrosus, which may be transitory, probably are caused by an inflammatory

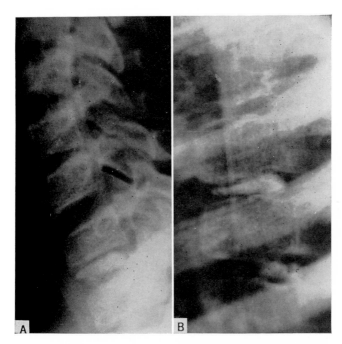

Fig. 372. Calcification of nucleus pulposus between the sixth and seventh cervical vertebrae, *A*, and the fourth and fifth thoracic vertebrae and the fifth and sixth thoracic vertebrae, *B*. Severe pain was present in the lower neck and between the shoulder blades at the time these films were made. Subsequent examinations over a period of 18 months showed no change in the discal calcifications even though pain disappeared completely.

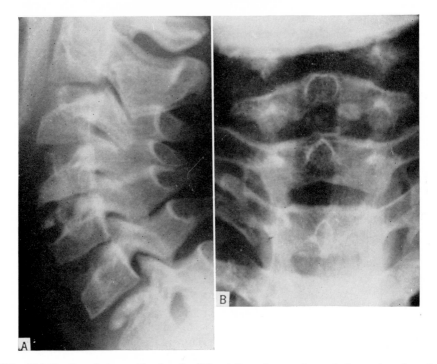

Fig. 373. Calcifications between the fourth, fifth, sixth and seventh cervical vertebrae in a 4-year-old child with severe neck pain. There is an atypical wedging of the anterior aspect of the fourth cervical vertebra. (Courtesy of Dr. M. Boorstein, The Long Island Jewish Hospital.)

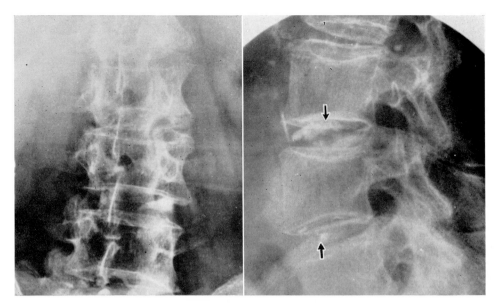

Fig. 374. Multiple intervertebral discal calcifications (arrows), mainly of the annulus fibrosus.

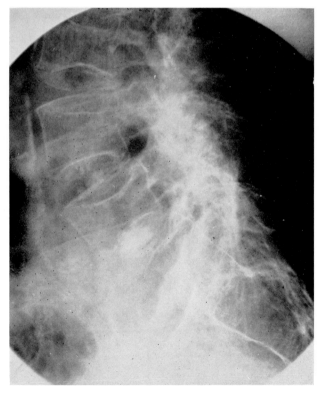

Fig. 375. Multiple intervertebral discal calcifications in patient with
myeloma and extensive osteoporosis.

process which Sandström termed myo-tendonitis calcarea, occurring in areas where tendons are attached to bone. The adjoining muscular tissue may also show such changes. When the disease is localized exclusively to tendinous tissues, such as the intervertebral disc, the name "tendonitis calcarea" is suggested by him. Sandström also mentioned that calcification induced by overdosage with vitamin D may be associated with transitory intervertebral disc calcification.

Calcification of the annulus fibrosus (Fig. 374), or less commonly, of the nucleus pulposus in adults is of no clinical significance. It occurs most frequently in the middorsal (Fig. 375) and lower lumbar regions, less often in the other parts of the spine. Calvé and Galland (1930) described a case of calcified intervertebral disc in which the entire nucleus pulposus was converted into a mass of lime salt. Microscopically the calcium could not be seen, having been dissolved out during the preparation of the slide. In its place only strands of an amorphous residue could be observed. We have examined several cases of nucleus pulposus calcification at necropsy. In these, all resiliency was lost, and the usual glistening appearance was replaced by a dull, grey discoloration. The nucleus pulposus was converted into a gritty, inelastic fissured rubbery substance which merged imperceptibly with the surrounding tissue. The calcification was more readily identified on roentgenograms. With weakening of the posterior spinal ligament protrusion of a calcified nucleus pulposus may occur and severely damage the spinal cord. This is of special importance in the cervical and thoracic spine.

Calcifications in the intervertebral discs of osteoporotic spines is not uncommon. It occurs not only in the benign forms of osteoporosis, but also in multiple myeloma.

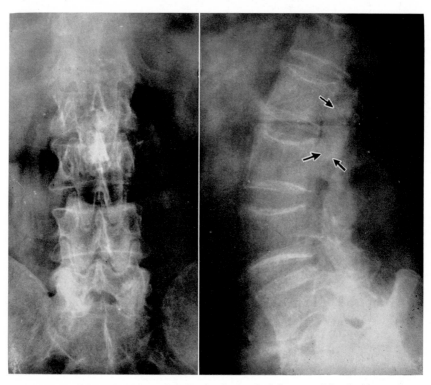

Fig. 376. Calcified old extruded disc at the level of the second lumbar interspace (arrows) producing paraplegia.

Rarely an intervertebral disc which has herniated into the spinal canal will further calcify. We saw one such patient (Fig. 376), a 65-year-old woman who had a slowly progressing paraplegia attributed to a spinal cord tumor. Because the calcification within the spinal canal was quite apparent on plain films, it was assumed that she had a large spinal cord tumor, probably a meningioma. At operation a large, irregularly calcified mass identified as an old prolapsed disc was encountered. This was fixed firmly in position, and could not be dislodged. Only a decompressive laminectomy was done.

References

Asadi, A.: Calcification of Intervertebral Discs in Children, J. Dis. Childhood, 97, 282, 1959.

Bjelkhagen, I. and Gladnikoff, H.: Calcified Disc Protrusion in Children, Acta radiol, 48, 151, 1957.

Calvé, J. and Galland, M.: Intervertebral Nucleus Pulposus, J. Bone & Joint Surg., 12, 555, 1930.

Melnick, J. C. and Silverman, F. N.: Intervertebral Disk Calcification in Childhood, Radiology, 80, 399, 1963.

Newton, T. H.: Cervical Intervertebral-Disc Calcification in Children, J. Bone & Joint Surg., 40-A, 107, 1958.

Peacher, W. G. and Storrs, R. P.: Cervical Disc Calcification in Childhood, Radiology, 67, 396, 1956.

Sandström, C.: Calcifications of the Intervertebral Discs and the Relationship Between Various Types of Calcifications in the Soft Tissues of the Body, Acta radiol., 36, 217, 1951.

Silverman, F. N.: Calcification of Intervertebral Disks in Childhood, Radiology, 62, 801, 1954.

Walker, C. S.: Calcification of Intervertebral Discs in Children, J. Bone & Joint Surg., 36-B, 601, 1954.

Weens, H. S.: Calcification of Intervertebral Discs in Childhood, J. Pediat., 26, 178, 1945.

"VACUUM PHENOMENON" IN INTERVERTEBRAL DISCS

Knuttson (1942) first called attention to the presence of a radiolucent streak at the lumbosacral intervertebral space, usually associated with a marked narrowing of the disc. He attributed this to desiccation of the disc in cases of spondylitis deformans. Inasmuch as the annulus fibrosus remains intact,

irregular gas streaks corresponding to cracks in the dried portion of the disc appear. This was more apparent on roentgenograms made with the spine in extension, because widening of the intervertebral space increases the radiolucent area. The accentuation of the vacuum phenomenon in the hyperextended position also was described by Gershon-Cohen (1946). He too attributed this change to degeneration in the nucleus pulposus, and observed that no herniation of nuclear material into the vertebral bodies occurred when the vacuum phenomenon existed. Samuel (1948) attributed the presence of gas in the disc "vacuum" to diffusion from the blood.

In a survey of 2419 lumbosacral roentgenograms Marr (1953) found gas in the intervertebral discs in 2.026 per cent of cases, mostly in the lumbosacral interspace. This was associated with discal narrowing, marginal spurring and eburnation of the bony surfaces. He attributed the presence of gas to vaporization from surrounding fluids as a result of a partial vacuum presumed present in the intervertebral disc. These radiolucent streaks were found mostly in the central portion of the disc. If the narrowing of the interspace was asymmetric, the gas seemed to collect in the narrowest portion. Raines (1953) attributed no clinical significance to this change. Gershon-Cohen, Schraer, Sklaroff and Blumberg (1954) observed that the vacuum phenomenon also occurred in multiple discs.

The largest number of discs with the vacuum phenomenon in our series was three, at the three lowermost lumbar interspaces (Fig. 377). A similar phenomenon is seen in the lower cervical spine occasionally, and somewhat more often in the small anterior spur formations present in the cervical (Fig. 378A, B) and lumbar spine. Since the latter are due to intervertebral discal intrusions, a similar mechanism probably exists. The same change also has been observed in the symphysis pubis during and immediately after pregnancy.

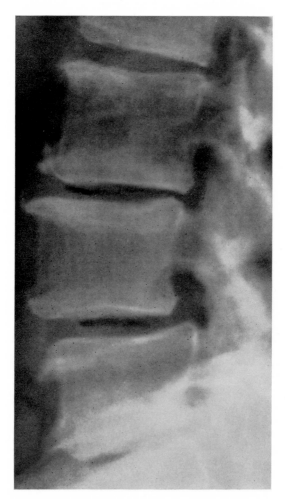

Fig. 377. "Vacuum phenomenon" in the intervertebral discs between the third, fourth and fifth lumbar vertebrae and the first sacral vertebra. Incidental finding in a 59-year-old woman. Note slight anterior displacement of the fourth lumbar vertebra.

Fig. 378, opposite page. *A,* Flexion film of the cervical spine with anterior discal herniation of the antero-superior aspect of C6 (limbic bone). *B,* With the neck in extension a vacuum phenomenon appears at the small bony chip, which moves slightly upwards and posteriorly. *C,* An asymptomatic limbic bone of the anterosuperior aspect of T12. *D,* A larger limbic bone with a surrounding sclerotic reaction is present in the anterosuperior aspect of the body of L3.

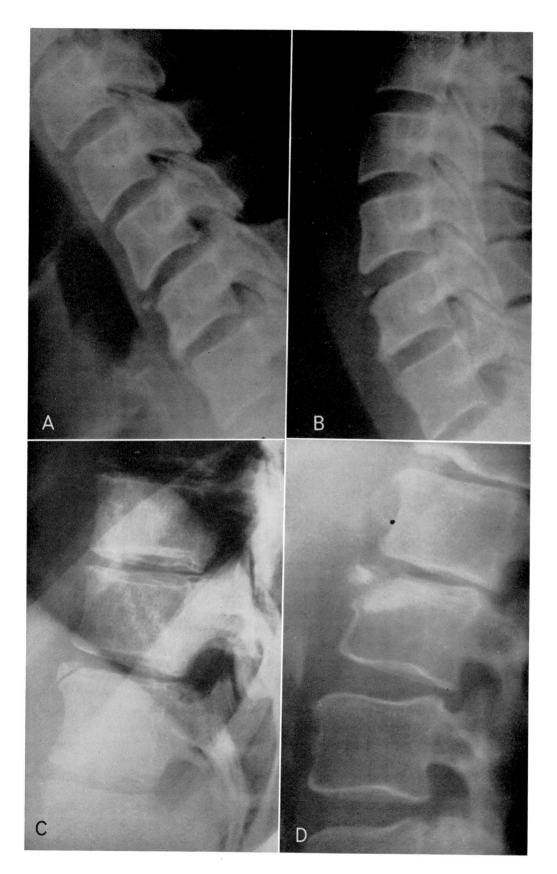

References

Camiel, M. R. and Aaron, J. B.: The Gas or Vacuum Phenomenon in the Pubic Symphysis during Pregnancy, Radiology, *66*, 548, 1956.

Fiebelkorn, H.-J.: Über Aufhellungssteifen (sog. Vakuum-Phänomen) in lumbalen Zwischenwirbelscheiben, Fortschr. Röntgenstr., *81*, 601, 1954.

Gershon-Cohen, J.: Phantom Nucleus Pulposus, Am. J. Roentgenol., *56*, 43, 1946.

Gershon-Cohen, J., Schraer, H., Sklaroff, D. M. and Blumberg, N.: Dissolution of the Intervertebral Disk in the Aged Normal. The Phantom Nucleus Pulposus, Radiology, *62*, 383, 1954.

Knuttson, F.: Vaccum Phenomenon in Intervertebral Discs, Acta radiol., *23*, 173, 1942.

Marr, J. T.: Gas in the Intervertebral Discs, Am. J. Roentgenol., *70*, 804, 1953.

Raines, J. R.: Intervertebral Disc Fissures (Vacuum Intervertebral Disc). Am. J. Roentgenol., *70*, 964, 1953.

Samuel, E.: Vacuum Intervertebral Discs, Brit. J. Radiol, *21*, 337, 1948.

Vollmar, K.: Über das Vakuumphänomen an der Randleisten der Lendenwirbel, Radiol. clin., *26*, 75, 1957.

HERNIATED DISCS

According to Mixter (1949) one of the earliest illustrations of a ruptured disc was that published by Charles Bell in 1824. This was described as a fracture, which undoubtedly was present. The illustration, reproduced in Mixter's paper, shows a fragment apparently partly disc and partly bone impinging against the spinal cord. Lindblom (1951) mentioned drawings of ruptured intervertebral discs in two earlier texts, one by Weitbrecht in 1742, and the other by Henle in 1856. These had been made to illustrate the normal anatomy of the disc, and the pathologic nature of the lesion had not been recognized. Disc protrusion was described in 1857 by Virchow, who mentioned a cervical "ecchondrosis" with lethal compression of the spinal cord. In 1896, Kocher reported the case of a man who fell 100 feet, landing on his lower limbs. Death occurred because of rupture of the jejunum. Necropsy revealed intraspinal protrusion of the first lumbar intervertebral disc, with no evidence of fracture. In 1911, Middleton and Teacher reported a case of spinal cord injury due to rupture of an intervertebral disc in a man who felt a sudden sharp pain while lifting a metal plate. Paralysis soon developed and the patient died a few hours thereafter. Necropsy revealed softening and hemorrhage about the lumbar enlargement in addition to a mass of cartilage lying in the spinal canal.

During the following years there were isolated reports of injuries to the spinal cord attributed to "enchondroma." now known to be herniated discs, such as those published by Frazier, Elsberg, Stookey, Ott and Adson, and Mixter (Mixter, 1949). Of particular interest is Dandy's report (1929) of 2 cases of transverse lesions of the cauda equina caused by free fragments of the intervertebral disc in the spinal canal. This report apparently was the first in which surgical treatment for ruptured discs was described, and the first to postulate that such fragments could cause sciatica. In 1930 Bucy collected 15 similar cases from the literature, and included 1 of his own. He regarded the lesions as chondromas of the intervertebral disc.

Recognition for attributing the syndrome of sciatica and low back pain to discal herniations belongs to Mixter and Barr (1934). Mixter's account of the events leading to recognition of this syndrome should be read in the original (1949). In this communication he mentioned that Barr had read a paper on the same subject in 1933, but this had received such an indifferent reception that it was not published. Mixter mentioned the work of Mauric, published in 1933, which came to the same conclusions.

Lumbar Intervertebral Disc Herniations. Herniation of lumbar discs occurs most often in males in the third and fourth decades. The youngest patient was reported by Fernström (1956) in an 11-year-old girl. Love (1947) mentioned that of 1217 patients with herniated discs, 25 were between the ages of 10 and 19 years. Webb, Svien and Kennedy (1954) reported 5 patients 15 years old or less at the time of operation. Herniated discs in patients beyond the fifth decade is by no means uncommon. The oldest patient in our series was

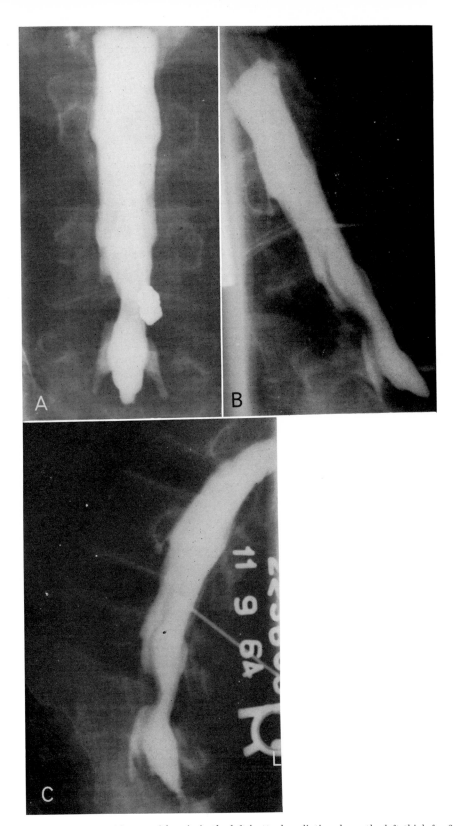

FIG. 379. *A*, A 52-year-old man with pain in the left buttock radiating down the left thigh for 6 months which became intense and did not respond to conservative treatment. A large herniated disc is present on the left side of the fourth lumbar interspace. With the patient in flexion, *B*, the defect diminishes somewhat in size, but in extension, *C*, it is more prominent. At operation a large extruded fragment of disc lay in the lateral recess humping the remnant of the posterior longitudinal ligament over it.

well over 70 and the youngest was a 15-year-old boy (Epstein and Levine, 1964).

The history of the patient is helpful. Not infrequently, particularly in a young active person, a history of trauma will be elicited. However, many patients, particularly females, have no history of obvious trauma. The type of pain varies with the extent and situation of the herniation as well as the patient's sensitivity to pain. Lateral and anterolateral displacements may compress the ipsilateral nerve roots, producing unilateral sciatica (Fig. 379). This is the most frequent complaint, occurring in about two-thirds to three-quarters of patients. Bilateral sciatica occurs in approximately 15 per cent, and may indicate a bilateral or a central protrusion with impingement against both sides (Fig. 380). In the remaining individuals the distribution of pain may be

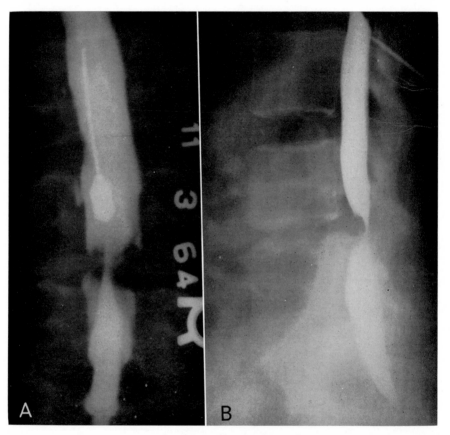

Fig. 380. *A*, An hour-glass defect is present at the 4th lumbar interspace in this 40-year-old woman with a history of bilateral sciatica for 6 months. *B*, A sharp indentation is present in the anterior aspect of the Pantopaque column, leaving a dorsally placed midline channel for the passage of fluid. At operation an extruded disc together with osteophytic spurs were present bilaterally, more marked on the right side.

Fig. 381. *A*, A 48-year-old woman with rheumatic heart disease and low back pain radiating down the right leg, thought to be embolic in origin. Pantopaque introduced at L3 dripped slowly into the caudal sac, filling it from below upwards, *B*. The canal filled to the L3 level with 9 ml of Pantopaque. When filled, a bilateral defect was seen at the L4 interspace, with a deep indentation into the anterior aspect of the column, *C* and *D*. At operation a huge extruded disc was removed.

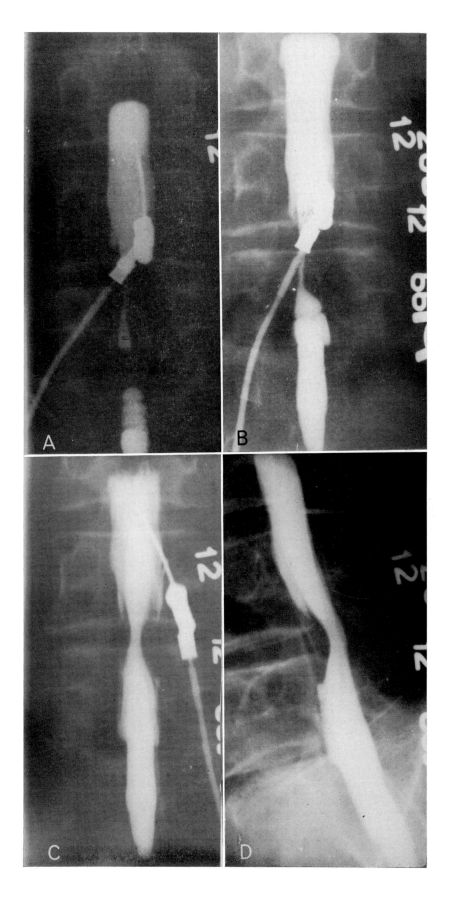

atypical, shifting from side to side or involving only the low back. Pain may be exaggerated by straining, coughing or sneezing. Low back pain without sciatic radiation appears with small midline discal protrusions. The onset of pain may be almost instantaneous, or gradual and progressive. In some the protrusion develops so rapidly that the acute compression of the cauda equina requires emergency care (Fig. 381).

Physical examination may disclose loss of the usual lumbar lordotic curve, tilting of the spine away from the side of the lesion, tenderness over the spinous processes of the lower lumbar vertebrae, painful straight leg raising with the patient in the dorsal recumbent position, and tenderness on pressure over the sciatic nerve. Diminished or absent ankle jerk or knee jerk reflexes, muscular weakness and atrophy of the affected limb may be present. Evaluation of the neurologic changes depends on understanding the peripheral nerve distribution. Thus, with discal protrusions involving the third lumbar interspace alteration in knee jerk reflexes may be encountered. Knee jerk reflex changes are uncommon in lesions involving the fourth or fifth lumbar interspaces. Diminution or absence of the ankle jerk reflex are common with herniated discs of the lumbosacral interspace, and are relatively infrequent at other levels. Areas of hypesthesia may be demonstrated depending on the level involved. Keegan (1943, 1944, 1947) presented dermatome charts for the trunk and extremities based on a study of the hypalgesic areas accompanying damage to a single nerve root. He pointed out that the neurologic deficits associated with lumbosacral disc herniations are easier to identify than those at the fourth lumbar interspace with compression of the fifth lumbar root. In the latter he found no reflex loss and the sensory changes were not easily found. McKenzie and Botterell (1942) concluded that 95 per cent of sciatica is associated with pressure on the roots of the first sacral or the fifth lumbar nerve. They were unable to distinguish between lesions of the fourth or

fifth lumbar discs in 15 per cent of their cases.

Young (1947) considered neurologic signs of little help in the localization of herniated discs, and regarded such changes as only confirmatory in importance. Parrella and Zovickian (1950) pointed out that the neurologic changes seen with herniated discs were not constant. For example, 8 of their cases had hypesthesia of the fifth lumbar dermatome according to Keegan's chart. Of these, 3 had herniation of the fourth lumbar disc, 1 had a large disc protruding at the third lumbar interspace and the remaining 4 had fifth lumbar discal herniations. Absence or diminution of ankle jerk reflexes were encountered in 43 per cent of their cases. Sixteen had a lumbosacral protruded disc, and 4 had herniated discs at the fourth lumbar interspace. Davis, Martin and Goldstein (1952) reviewed the sensory pattern in 500 cases, and found no correlation between this and the level of the lesion.

Our experience corresponds with the inconstancy of clinical localization observed by others. A review of 50 verified herniated discs at the fourth lumbar interspace revealed diminished ankle jerks on the side of the lesion in 17 cases. In 4 others, bilateral diminished ankle jerks were present, and this occurred when the lesion did not approach the opposite nerve root. Diminution of the knee jerk reflexes on the ipsilateral side was observed in 5 cases. No changes in the ankle or knee jerk reflexes were present in 24 instances. In 50 other herniations at the lumbosacral interspace, knee jerk reflex changes were observed in 6 cases. Ankle jerk reflexes occurred in 35 others, and the remainder had no such changes. It becomes evident that while reflex alterations, when present, are of considerable diagnostic significance, they are neither constant nor entirely reliable.

Patients with massive extrusions of the nucleus pulposus may present a syndrome of cauda equina compression indistinguishable from that caused by tumors. Symptoms of cord compression are accompanied by sciatic pain if the disc protrudes laterally as well as centrally. Ver Brugghen (1945) reported that out of 300 consecutive cases of herniated discs there were 9 with acute compression of the cauda equina by massive lumbar disc protrusions. These patients had saddle anesthesia, weakness of the legs below the knees, sphincter disturbances, and changes in the ankle reflexes in all and knee jerk reflex changes in some. Eight were operated upon. In 3 the lesion occurred at the lumbosacral interspace, in 3 at the fourth lumbar interspace, and in 2 at the third lumbar interspace. French and Payne (1944) reported that cauda equina compression due to herniation of the nucleus pulposus was accompanied by bilateral sensory disturbances and reflex changes in 8 of their cases. The fact that massive extrusions of the disc may occur without the usual picture of cauda equina compression was brought out by Epstein (1949), who reported that of 150 lumbar myelograms there were 5 with complete spinal canal block. Only 1 of these patients had a syndrome suggestive of cauda equina compression. Robinson (1965) also observed large discal extrusions with minimal symptoms.

Fernström reported on the association of herniated lumbar discs with abdominal or anogenital pain, noting that pain may arise in the disc itself. This type of discogenic pain is conveyed by way of the sinuvertebral nerve, and is interpreted as deep somatic pain, spreading to the sclerotome and myotome of the afferent nerve fibers affected. He differentiates this type of pain from that which arises in a nerve root, which he terms neurogenic pain. Both discogenic and neurogenic pain from all lumbar disc levels can be appreciated in the abdominal and anogenital regions. Fernström noted that pain may be entirely discogenic, and in that case the signs and symptoms characteristic of root compression are absent, so that the condition can be mistaken for visceral disease.

Bladder paralysis caused by cauda equina lesions incident to discal prolapse occasionally occur in the absence of more familiar symptoms (Love and Emmett, 1967). More often bladder paralysis is associated with other symptoms of cauda equina compression, particularly pain. However, occasionally severe bladder and limb paralysis are present with minimal pain (Robinson, 1965).

Another manifestation of cauda equina compression is intermittent claudication which simulates peripheral vascular disease. This may be produced either by discal herniations or stenosis of the lumbar spinal canal with or without concomitant discal protrusions. The syndrome is attributed to a temporary but recurring disturbance to the blood supply of the cauda equina. Usually this can be distinguished from peripheral vascular disease by noting adequate pulsations in the femoral arteries and normal oscillometric measurements. Some patients have associated sciatic pain as well as low back pain. The discal herniations appear centrally (Joffe, Appleby and Arjona, 1966) or laterally (Spanos and Andrew, 1966).

The possibility that a herniated disc is associated with another intraspinal lesion at another level must be kept in mind. For this reason it is advisable to investigate the entire spinal canal even though an obviously herniated disk is seen. Love and Rivers (1962) commented that patients with intractable root pain after operation for a herniated disc require careful re-evaluation to rule out a coexisting intraspinal tumor. If this is done prior to surgery, a recurrent disc at the same or another level still has to be ruled out by means of myelography. Another possibility which must be kept in mind is concerned with the presence of a myelographic defect which does not fit in with the clinical picture. Such defects may be of no clinical importance, and serve to mask the possibility of another lesion elsewhere in the spinal canal. This is particularly true in elderly patients with prominent defects incident to spondylotic changes (Fig. 382).

Back pain, sometimes with a radicular distribution, also occurs with porphyruria. These patients present themselves with con-

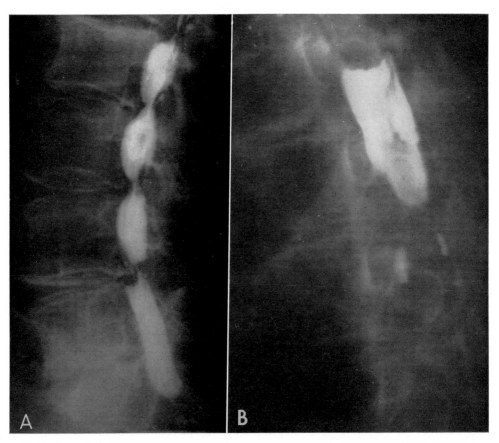

FIG. 382. *A*, A 69-year-old woman with 18 months' progressive weakness and numbness of both lower extremities and a sensory level at T3. She had been falling repeatedly. On lumber myelography numerous deeply indented ridges were seen at L2, 3 and 4 interspaces. When the column was brought up to the thoracic canal, a cup-like defect appeared at T3. This proved to be caused by a meningioma.

fusing clinical pictures, and at times a diagnosis of discal herniation appears reasonable. Myelographic examination is normal. It is surprising how long some of these patients are treated before someone comes up with the suggestion that porphyruria might be present. In one such patient seen recently the patient had undergone a wide variety of diagnostic tests and was currently under psychiatric treatment.

The reasons for the wide variation of symptoms in patients with herniated discs are not entirely understood. Deucher and Love (1939) described edematous changes in protruded portions of intervertebral discs, and proposed that this may in part be responsible for the clinical recession of symp-

toms. Lindblom and Hultqvist (1950) suggested that protruded disc tissue might be absorbed. This was based on 160 necropsies, in which they observed all stages of change in the intervertebral disc from radial rupture with beginning loss of tissue to almost complete disappearance of the nucleus pulposus and the annulus fibrosus. Absorption of prolapsed portions of an intervertebral disc might, in their opinion, result in the disappearance of symptoms.

Lateral, cephalad, caudad, intradural or subligamentous migrations of fragments of protruded disc material may occur and give rise to perplexing clinical pictures (Fig. 383). Tucker (1956) mentioned 2 cases in which disc herniations at the first lumbar interspace

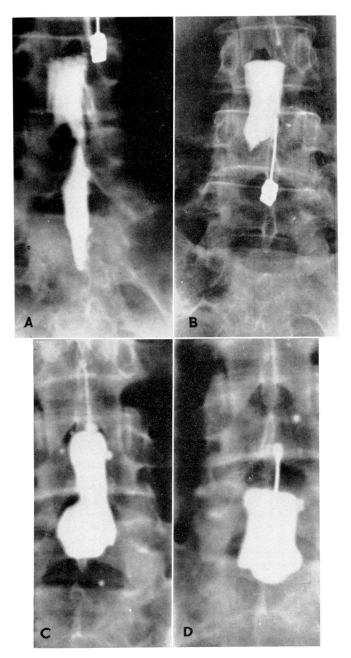

Fig. 383. Three cases of massive discal herniation with intraspinal migration. *A*, Large extruded disc from the fifth lumbar interspace rotated in the spinal canal, producing an elongated defect extending well above the level of that interspace. No defect is seen at the lumbosacral interspace. *B*, Extruded disc from the fourth lumbar interspace migrating cephalad, producing obstruction well above the involved interspace. *C* and *D*, Extruded disc from the third lumbar interspace migrating caudad, producing defect at the level of the fourth lumbar interspace.

entered the dural sac, causing a complete block. Kessler and Stein (1961) reported complete spinal canal block by posterior migration of a herniated lumbar disc. Greenwood, McGuire and Kimbell (1952) made special mention of a case in which herniated discal material from the third lumbar interspace had migrated downward to compress the fifth lumbar nerve root. Paterson and Gray (1952) reported that of 91 cases, 11 had fragments of disc tissue between the annulus fibrosus and the posterior spinal ligaments. In 8 others pieces of fibrocartilage passed through the posterior spinal ligament and lay free in the spinal canal. In 2 still further displacements had occurred, the ventral dura being torn and the fragment entering the thecal sac. Paterson and Gray mentioned that the clinical pictures in these

cases were atypical, and were suggestive of a cauda equina tumor. Involvement of several nerve roots and of bladder function was common. If a hole is found in the annulus fibrosus at operation, and discal tissue is not readily observed, further search may be required until the prolapsed material is discovered and removed. Even after removal, discal herniations can recur at the same interspace (Fig. 384), or additional lesions may appear at other interspaces. (Epstein and co-workers, 1967).

Intradural herniations of lumbar intervertebral discs can follow a long-standing protrusion. Wilson (1962) noted that dense arachnoidal adhesions may appear, complicating the presence of an extrathecal disc protrusion and causing intractable compression of the cauda equina. In a 56-year-old

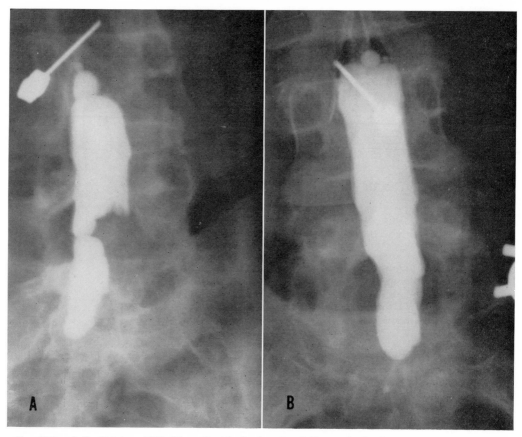

FIG. 384. *A*, In October, 1961 this patient had a herniated disc at the lumbosacral interspace situated anterolaterally on the left side. *B*, Eight years later symptoms recurred on the opposite side, and myelography disclosed a recurrent discal herniation at the lumbosacral interspace.

patient he found a complete block with a tapered distal end on myelographic examination. At operation no discal extrusion was found outside the dural sac. When the dura was incised from L4 to S1, a ragged and tangled mass of whitish degenerated disc material was found among the roots of the cauda equina. This mass measured $3 \times 1 \times 1$ cm, and had mushroomed into the subarachnoid space through a gap in the dura anteriorly, which was adherent to the fourth lumbar disc. Slater, Pineda and Porter (1965) reported 2 similar cases, and observed that intradural exploration is required when the extradural findings do not account for the clinical and radiologic changes.

Transvertebral rupture of an intervertebral disc was reported by Smith (1962). Cartilage prolapses into a vertebral body, and then breaks through the posterior wall of the involved body producing an intraspinal neurologic problem. This was associated with defective osseous structure, which was osteoporosis in his 3 cases. It may occur with other bony deficiencies, even conceivably with tumors.

It is possible for discal herniations to exist without causing symptoms, provided they do not intrude into the spinal canal or intervertebral foramina sufficiently to compromise the nerve roots or cauda equina. Not infrequently relatively large discal protrusions or spondylotic ridges produce myelographic defects unassociated with clinical manifestations. On the other hand, strategically situated spurs or small herniated discs can produce intense symptoms even though the myelographic defect is slight. One must keep in mind the concept of available space in the intervertebral foramina and the spinal canal, and realize that not only herniated discs but spondylotic spurs, bulging, softened but intact discs, thickening of the ligamenta flava, hypertrophy of the neural arches and variations in the sagittal diameter of spinal canals greatly influence pressure effects (Fig. 385). Of great importance is the configuration of the lateral recesses of the spinal foramina,

especially in the lowermost three lumbar vertebrae. The nerve trunk passing through the intervertebral foramen is in close proximity to the superior lip of the vertebral body and the inner aspect of the base of the pedicle. When this groove is constricted by thickening of the adjacent bone, the available space for the nerve root is diminished and the effect of small protrusions is enhanced (Fig. 227). Unfortunately, the configuration of these lateral recesses cannot be directly estimated radiologically. It appears that narrowing of the sagittal diameter of the lumbar spinal canal to less than 1.5 cm is associated with the possibility of constriction of the lateral recesses (Epstein, Epstein and Lavine, 1964).

The great sensitivity of the sciatic nerve to touch or pressure was verified by Smyth and Wright (1958). These workers experimentally pulled on the sciatic nerve after passing a suture around it at operation, controlling their observations by doing the same to the ligamentum flavum, the interspinous ligaments and the annulus fibrosus. They found that a simple pull on the thread sufficient to bring it in contact with the nerve root closely simulated the irritation and pressure of a herniated disc. The nerve need only be touched to cause sciatica, and if touched repeatedly or continuously the nerve root becomes hypersensitive. Dr. Joseph A. Epstein has repeatedly demonstrated at operation edematous, flattened and hemorrhagic nerve roots caught in constricted canals when discal herniation or osteophytic spur formation was disproportionately small in relation to the severity of the clinical syndrome. These patients were relieved only after decompression of the intervertebral foramen and the narrowed lateral aspects of the canal was obtained surgically.

An investigation into the changes associated with degeneration of the intervertebral disc in a group of 100 spines of humans between 40 and 80 years of age was reported by Horwitz (1943). Posterior bulging of the entire intervertebral disc without localized

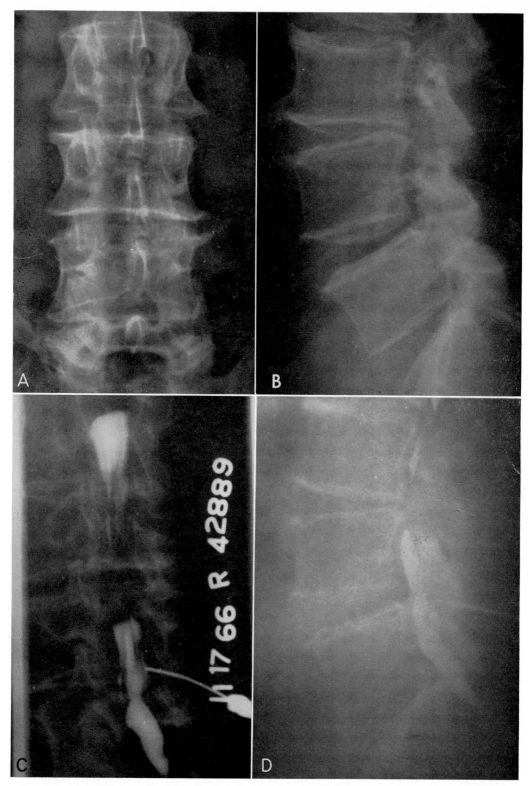

Fig. 385. *A*, A 62-year-old man with severe low back pain, weakness of both lower extremities and sphincteric disturbances. Plain film examination shows heavy spondylotic reaction and narrowed lumbar interspaces. *B*, The spinal canal is narrowed. *C*, Spinal tap accomplished with difficulty, and only 2 ml of Pantopaque were instilled. This revealed multiple spondylotic ridges, particularly at the L3 and 4 levels. The canal was practically obliterated by extrinsic compression, *D*. At operation the laminae were thickened and overgrown, and the ligamenta flava also were prominent. Large, dense spondylotic ridges intruded into the anterior aspect of the canal at L3 and 4. Exploration of the second lumbar interspace revealed a large discal herniation as well.

herniation was a common finding. The posterior protrusions were formed not only by the dorsal bulge of the degenerated disc, but also by the hypertrophied posterior margins of the adjacent vertebrae. Softening of the intervertebral disc may be associated with its narrowing, together with a downward and backward settling of the upper vertebral body, further exaggerated by bony overgrowth at the postero-inferior margin. Proliferation of bone on the inferior surfaces of the articular facets of the apophyseal joints also occurs. Such changes may be associated with myelographic defects indistinguishable from herniated discs. In the lumbar spinal canal these may be asymptomatic because of the width of the available space, but in the cervical and thoracic regions significant pressure on the cord and nerve roots may be produced.

The anatomic effects of compression of the spinal nerves and ganglia by herniated discs were described by Lindblom and Rexed (1948), who removed specimens from 160 cadavers from 14 to 87 years of age. Among these were 60 instances of nerve compression, mostly caused by dorsolateral protrusions. Evidence of serious damage to the nervous structures was found, consistent with the degree of compression. Forty-four of the damaged nerves and of the corresponding normal nerves were examined histologically by serial sectioning. The compression produced serious deformity and atrophy of the spinal ganglion cells, fibrosis, and gross alterations of internal structure. Osteophytic enlargement of the intervertebral joint was an accessory factor in causing nerve damage.

Protrusion of the Intervertebral Disc on the Side Opposite Clinical Symptoms. In 1949 Murphy reported 2 cases in which the clinical impression was that of a herniated disc on the left side, and myelograms disclosed right-sided protrusions. In both it was felt that if the exploration had been carried out on the affected side the offending lesion would have been missed. Wycis (1950) reported 4 cases in which contralateral sciatic pain appeared after removal of a ruptured disc, the contralateral recurrence being at the same interspace. Three were verified at operation, and relief followed exploration of the contralateral side. He also reported a case in which ipsilateral symptoms were relieved by contralateral removal of a partly herniated disc. Wycis believed that bilateral exploration might be required in view of the fact that a disc may herniate bilaterally, resulting in a dumb-bell deformity. Kaplan (1949) also reported 2 cases in which herniated discs were associated with signs and symptoms on the opposite side. We, too, have observed several cases in which exploration on the side of long-standing pain did not disclose the lesion, while myelography correctly indicated its location.

Atypical myelographic defects may be due to migration of herniated discal material (Fig. 383). In the presence of a midline herniation, symptoms may vary from side to side. Due precaution must be exercised in evaluating clinical as well as myelographic observations to make sure that the proper, or both sides, are explored when necessary. In this regard, it is well to recall that with midline large protrusions, the lesion may be missed if only the lateral aspects of the spinal canal are explored, and a transdural exploration may be required.

Lumbo-Sacral Herniated Discs. Plain film roentgenograms of the spine should routinely precede myelography. Their importance lies more in the elimination of other causes of back and radicular pain than as an indication of disc herniation.

In a review of 300 verified cases of lumbosacral herniated discs, the plain film roentgenograms were normal in 64 per cent. The lumbosacral interspace was markedly narrowed in 16 per cent, and in the remaining 20 per cent slight to moderate narrowing was seen. In 12 per cent of the cases narrowing of the fourth lumbar interspace was observed. Osteophytic reaction at the lumbosacral interspace was present in about one-third of our cases, and in most the extent of the change was considered within normal limits for the age groups. Lateral films revealed straightening of the lordotic curve in one-third of the patients. Tilting of the spine towards the side of the lesion was relatively infrequent, being seen in 10 per cent of cases. In occasional instances the lumbar spine was tilted away from the side of the lesion.

Data were available in 50 cases in which more elaborate plain film studies had been made. Films were taken in flexion and extension in the erect lateral posture and in the anteroposterior position with the patient bent sharply to the right and left. These examinations were not helpful in identifying either the presence or location of a herniated disc. In more than half the cases changes at the articular facets of the lumbosacral joint were seen. The facets were either asymmetric or coronally placed. It was not believed that this was of diagnostic help, inasmuch as similar changes were observed regularly in patients without any back complaint. This concept is at variance with that expressed by Gillespie (1949), who reviewed 500 normal patients and 500 others in whom laminectomy had been done for disc protrusions. He found that 34.2 per cent of the laminectomy series showed congenital spinal instability as compared with 8.8 per cent of the control series. On the other hand, Peyton and Simmons (1947) and Splitthoff (1953) noted no significant roentgenographic difference in the lumbosacral junction of patients with and without backache. Gage and Shafer (1953) also concluded that plain films were unsatisfactory in the diagnosis of herniation of the lumbar intervertebral discs. Armstrong and his co-workers (1950) asserted that abnormalities in the planes of the articular facets were not an important cause of low back pain.

Herniation of the Fourth Lumbar Intervertebral Disc. The plain film roentgenograms may be somewhat more helpful in the identification of discal protrusions at the fourth lumbar interspace. In a review of 125 consecutive cases in our series, the plain films were normal in 55 per cent. In 25 per cent there was a significant narrowing at the fourth lumbar interspace. In the others a slight narrowing was present, but this was not sufficient to warrant any definite conclusions. In 18 patients there was marked narrowing at the lumbosacral interspace, and in 10, all over 45 years of age, significant arthritic changes were present. Of this group, 3 also had a slight narrowing of the fourth lumbar interspace. In 4 others, narrowing of the third lumbar interspace was seen.

Straightening of the lumbar lordotic curve was observed in one-fourth of this series, and when present, was presumed to be of some diagnostic help. The absence of a straightened lumbar lordotic curve was not considered significant. In 4 cases the lumbar spine was tilted contralateral to the affected side, and in 2 the spine was inclined towards the affected side.

In 12 cases the narrowing of the fourth lumbar interspace as observed in anteroposterior views was irregular. In 7 of these patients the narrowing was more marked on the side towards which the nucleus pulposus was herniated. In 4 instances there was a shifting of the fourth on the fifth lumbar vertebra laterally. In all these the shift was towards the side of symptoms. On reviewing the operative findings no relationship could be established between the size of the herniated disc and the degree of change noted on the plain films. Subsequent observations presented similar data.

Roentgenography of the articular facets, the intervertebral foramina and films made in flexion, extension, and bending to the right and left were not helpful in the diagnosis of fourth lumbar herniated discs.

Herniated Discs in the Upper Lumbar Spine. There were 27 such cases in our series, 6 at the first lumbar interspace, 8 at the second and 13 at the third lumbar interspace. The plain films in most patients were normal. In 8 instances there was narrowing of the affected disc, but in others discal changes were observed at levels which at myelography were normal. In 7 instances discal herniations of the upper lumbar levels were associated with other discal and spondylotic deformities. They noted that of 90 patients examined, 16 had narrowing of the corresponding interspace. However, similar narrowing was seen at other levels as well. In a discussion of a paper by Graf and Hamby (1953) Beswick incidentally mentioned a case which had a striking narrowing of one interspace. He felt this to be a reasonable localization without myelographic confirmation. Myelography, however, showed the lesion to lie two interspaces higher, and this was confirmed at operation. We have had similar experiences.

Myelographic Diagnosis of Herniated Lumbar Discs. Although in the opinion of many, an accurate diagnosis of a herniated disc can be reasonably established on the clinical aspects alone, myelography should not be disregarded. In the same way and for the same reasons that colon roentgenograms, for instance, are made before operation for a bowel lesion, so should myelography be done when surgery of the spinal canal is contemplated. In my opinion exploration of the spinal canal without preliminary myelography even when the clinical picture is presumably complete, is comparable to laparotomy without previous adequate investigation. To carry this a bit further, there are instances when x-ray examinations fail to reveal an intra-abdominal lesion, and laparotomy is done nevertheless. Similarly, myelography may fail to disclose a definite lesion, and still surgical intervention is required because of the over-all picture. In either case operation is not contraindicated by a presumably negative x-ray study.

It should be routine to investigate the spinal canal well above the site of the suspected lesion. The upper level for lumbar myelography should be at the cervical region. I have in mind a number of instances in which symptoms referable to the lower extremities were caused by lesions in the thoracolumbar-cervical spinal canal, and which had been misdiagnosed because adequate myelography was not done.

Unless fluoroscopy is carefully performed,

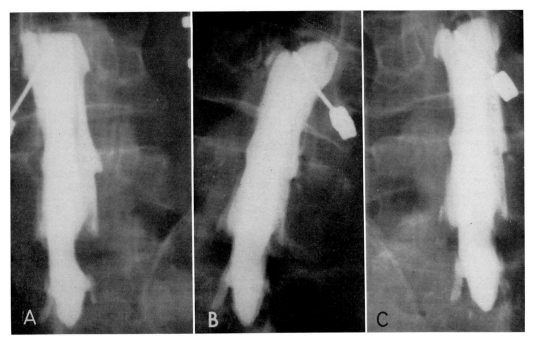

Fig. 386. *A,* A large discal herniation is present at the lumbosacral interspace on the right side. *B,* With the patient bent sharply to the right the defect is practically obliterated. With the patient erect and turned slightly towards the left, *C,* the defect is again seen, but has changed in configuration.

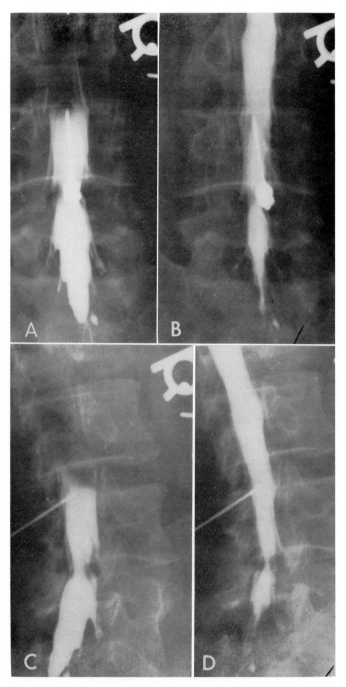

FIG. 387. *A,* A 64-year-old man with intermittent right lower extremity pain for a year. A defect is present at the fourth lumbar interspace on the right side. *B,* When the patient strains vigorously, the column rises for about two vertebral levels, and the caudal sac thins out. The discal deformity is diminished. *C* and *D,* Similar changes take place with the patient turned towards the left, bringing the right side into view. These studies were made with the patient erect.

there is a possibility of overlooking a small defect because of overdistention of the thecal sac or of missing a lateral or midline small defect. Cinemyelography is of the greatest help in recording fluoroscopic information, and I use this routinely. It has been seen repeatedly that small defects are detected most readily fluoroscopically and by cineradiographic and spot film roentgenograms made at the time when a lateral or veil defect appears in the Pantopaque column. Such lesions may be obliterated by distention of the thecal sac, and the need for watching the ends of the Pantopaque column in oblique and lateral as well as frontal positions during its flow is re-emphasized. Cross-table roentgenograms and lateral decubitus films are routine. The cineradiographic recording of the flow of Pantopaque in the oblique and lateral positions are essential in the investigation of the thoracic and cervical regions. In the lumbar region erect laterals

and lateral cineradiographic studies of the ascending and descending Pantopaque column has been found most helpful. The effect of bending and straining on the Pantopaque column are first recorded on cineradiographic examinations, and can be recorded on spot films as well. The dynamics of the fluid filled thecal sac are indeed interesting, and the effect on increasing or diminishing a defect can be important (Figs. 386, 387, 388).

The illustrations presented here depict some of the many filling defects seen with herniated lumbar discs. The absence of a defect does not in itself rule out a herniated disc, especially when the thecal sac is relatively narrow or high and the spinal canal is wide (Fig. 389). In such instances a herniated disc may not impinge against the dura and the myelogram appears normal. Careful review of the clinical aspects may lead to surgical intervention nevertheless.

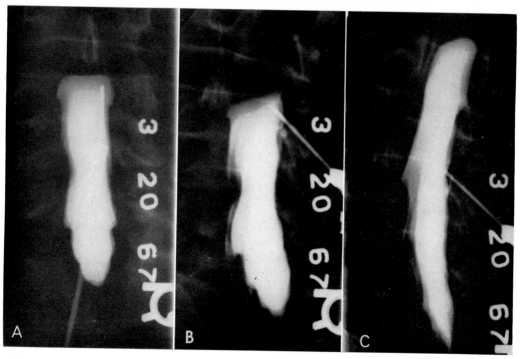

Fig. 388. *A,* A 57-year-old man with low back pain radiating down the left leg. In the AP position a shallow defect is present at the fourth lumbar interspace on the left side. With the patient turned into the right anterior oblique position, *B,* the defect is more prominent. *C,* Keeping this position, and having the patient strain, the defect is practically obliterated when the column rises about a vertebral segment. At operation a large laterally placed herniated disc was found.

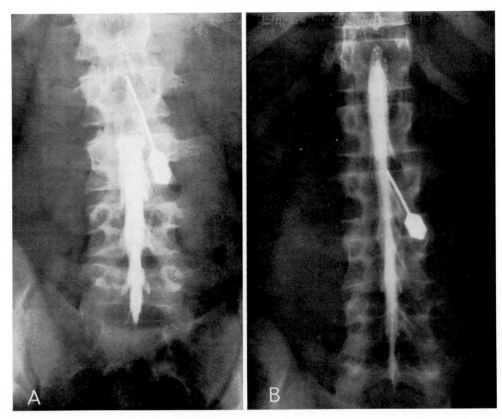

Fig. 389. *A*, A 17-year-old boy with right sciatic and low back pain. Four ml of Pantopaque fill the canal to the level of the upper margin of L3, indicating a narrow canal. The caudal sac is small, and terminates in a high position. When the patient strains, *B*, the height of the column reaches the body of T12. A shallow defect is present on the left side of the fourth interspace. At operation there was a fairly large herniated disc which extended into the intervertebral foramen and sharply compromised the nerve root.

Depending on the location and extent of a lesion, four major varieties of filling defects appear. When the protruded disc lies laterally, the defect is merely an obliteration of the corresponding axillary pouch. This may be so slight that the Pantopaque column remains unindented. In most instances, however, a slight convexity of the opaque column is co-existent with obliteration or elevation of the axillary pouch (Figs. 389 and 390). More obvious lesions are manifested by a greater indentation, varying from smooth shallow defects to elongated, oval or semicircular impressions which may be scalloped. In these the axillary pouch usually is obliterated, particularly with the larger lesions. The elongated defects are

observed when an extruded disc rotates upon itself within the spinal canal and comes to lie parallel to the thecal sac. In some the deformity extends across the midline and indents the contralateral side, particularly when nuclear extrusion is through multiple breaks in the posterior spinal ligament (Fig. 391).

Occasionally a horizontal, veil-like defect appears because of discal degeneration without rupture bulging against the posterior spinal ligament. Fluoroscopic study and spot roentgenograms in the lateral and various oblique positions are necessary to see whether a relatively deeper indentation is present on the anterior or the lateral margins of the column.

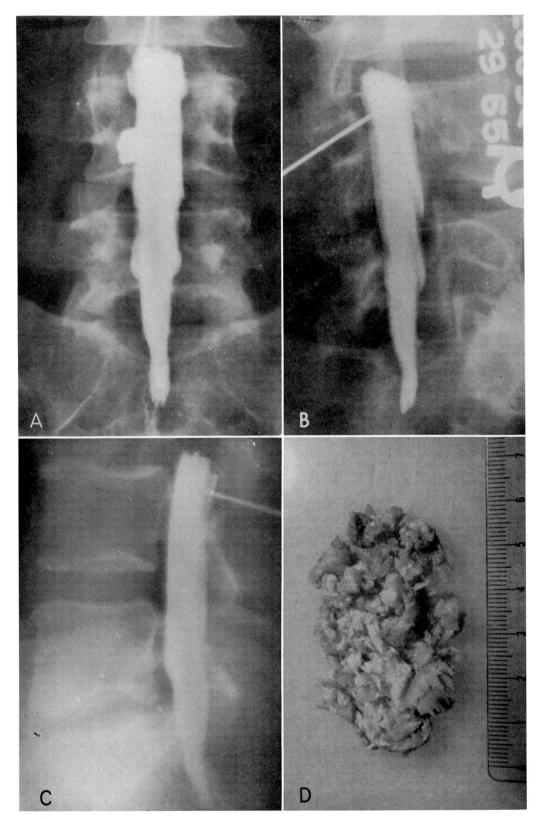

Fig. 390. *A*, A 45-year-old man with a right sciatic syndrome. On myelographic examination the caudal sac is narrowed and an elongated, flattened deformity is present on its right side. *B*, On oblique views the defect is more prominent. *C*, On lateral views the caudal sac is elevated from the floor of the canal. At operation a large herniated disc was found which extruded into the spinal canal under the thecal sac, elevating it from the floor, *D*.

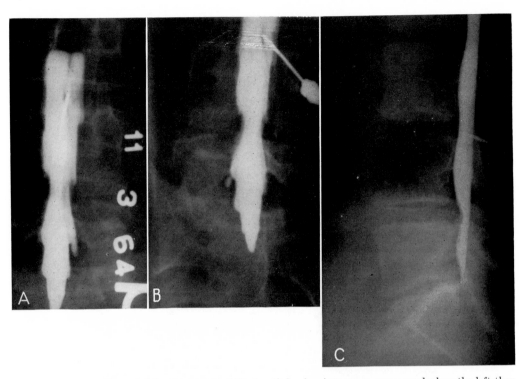

Fig. 391. *A*, A bilateral defect is present at the fourth lumbar interspace, more marked on the left than on the right side. The left fifth axillary pouch is blunted. *B*, On the oblique view the lumbosacral right sleeve is seen to be normal. *C*, On transabdominal views elevation of the thecal sac from the floor of the canal is seen at the fourth lumbar interspace. At operation a discal extrusion was present on the left side. On the right side a softened, bulging disc was found.

A fourth variety of defect, observed with massive herniation of the intervertebral disc is complete spinal canal obstruction. The entire degenerated disc with a rim of fibrocartilage may be extruded into the epidural space (Fig. 392). It is sometimes possible to predict this when xanthochromic fluid is obtained on lumbar tap. A protein content well above 100 mg per cent is not uncommon in this situation, particularly if the extruded disc is high in the lumbar canal. With high extruded discs multiple dry lumbar taps may be encountered even though the myelographer is quite positive that the needle is in the subarachnoid space. It may become advisable to make the puncture at the second lumbar interspace and introduce only a few drops of Pantopaque. Fluoroscopic examination in the erect posture will quickly disclose whether or not a block exists. Rarely it may become necessary to introduce the contrast medium through a cisternal tap.

A pronounced partial block to the flow of Pantopaque may occur even when manometric measurements are normal and the cerebrospinal fluid is crystal clear. The protein content may be moderately elevated, but normal values are not uncommon. Fluoroscopic study under these conditions often discloses a lateral or posterior channel through which the Pantopaque passes (Figs. 380 and 381).

In cases with partial or complete block, and sometimes when no block at all is present, linear vertical and somewhat oblique radiolucent streaks appear within the Pantopaque column above, and sometimes below the lesion. These have been noted at operation to be due to swelling of the roots of the cauda equina (Fig. 393). Medial displacement of nerve roots, either normal or edematous, by laterally placed herniated discs is seen relatively often. Upward displacement by midline herniated discs is best

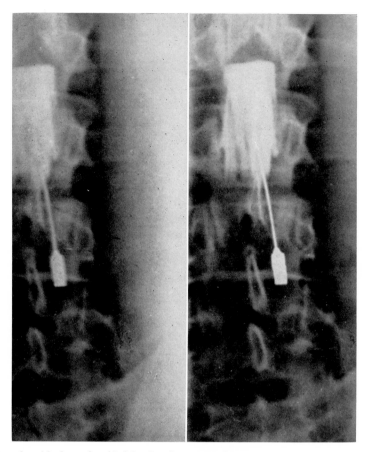

FIG. 392. Complete block at the third lumbar interspace due to extruded herniated disc. The lumbar punctures in the third and fourth interspaces were unsatisfactory, and a good flow was obtained at the second. The linear radiolucent streaks represent prominent nerve roots. (From Epstein, B. S., Am. J. Roentgenol., *61*, 778, 1949.)

demonstrated on transabdominal films, and constitutes an important observation. It may be present in the absence of any lateral deformity.

Redundant nerve roots have been reported as rarely producing serpentine shadows quite similar to those caused by vascular anomalies and tumors. Similar markings appear in individuals with spinal canal block incident to tumor or herniated discs, with venous engorgement above the level of the lesion (Fig. 226). It is difficult to distinguish these, particularly if sinuous shadows appear in immediate proximity to an obstructive lesion. Cressman and Pawl (1968) describe a 63-year-old man with a serpentine defect caused by a redundant nerve root at the L3-4 level who had an incomplete block at the L4-5 level due to an osteoarthritic bar. Schut and Groff (1968) reported a patient with a complete block at the L3 level caused by compression from three redundant nerve roots which had been considered on myelograms to be vascular channels.

The effects of postural variation and exertion on the available space in the spinal canal becomes more apparent on examinations made after filling the canal with sufficient Pantopaque to opacify it up to the level of the third lumbar vertebra with the patient erect. Studies in flexion and extension indicate the effect of wrinkling of the ligamentum flavum, and the indentations so produced on the dorsal aspect of the Pantopaque column occasionally are striking. However, the clinical implications of such changes must

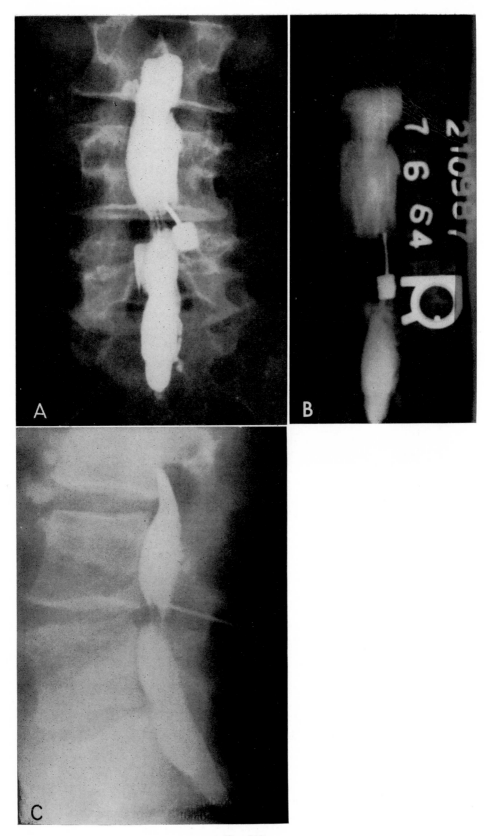

FIG. 393.

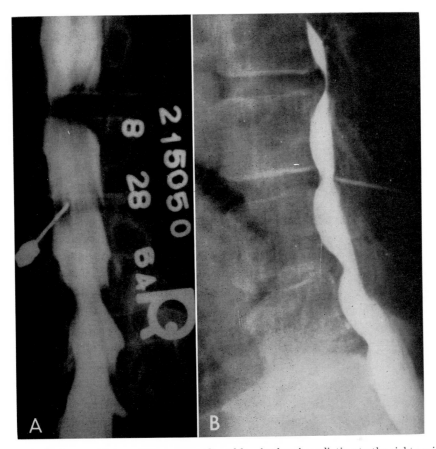

Fig. 394. *A*, A 63-year-old man with severe mid- and low-back pain radiating to the right groin. The tap was done with difficulty because of the narrow canal. After 15 ml of Pantopaque were instilled, multiple defects were found at the second, third, fourth and fifth lumbar levels. Pantopaque was removed after reinserting the needle at L5 interspace. At operation multiple ridges were found. An extruded disc was present at L3, which had rotated laterally and migrated downwards, impinging sharply on the left lateral aspect of the fourth interspace.

Fig. 393. *A*, A 53-year-old man with a 6-year history of low back pain with left sciatic radiation. The spinal tap is at the fourth interspace. A defect is present on the right side at the third lumbar interspace, and a transverse defect is seen at the fourth interspace. A third defect is present on the right side of the lumbosacral level. *B*, On overexposed films the fila of the cauda equina are seen. Delay in the caudal flow was present as the patient was placed erect. A serrated appearance of the column is observed at the fourth interspace. *C*, Indentations into the Pantopaque column are seen at the third and fourth interspaces, less marked at the fifth. At operation an almost complete block was found at L4, due to heavy ridge formation with overgrowth of the laminae and thickening of the yellow ligament. At the third interspace a lateral ridge was present, together with a bulging midline disc. At the fifth interspace a laterally situated herniated disc with a concomitant spur was found on the right side. At all three interspaces the canal was markedly narrowed.

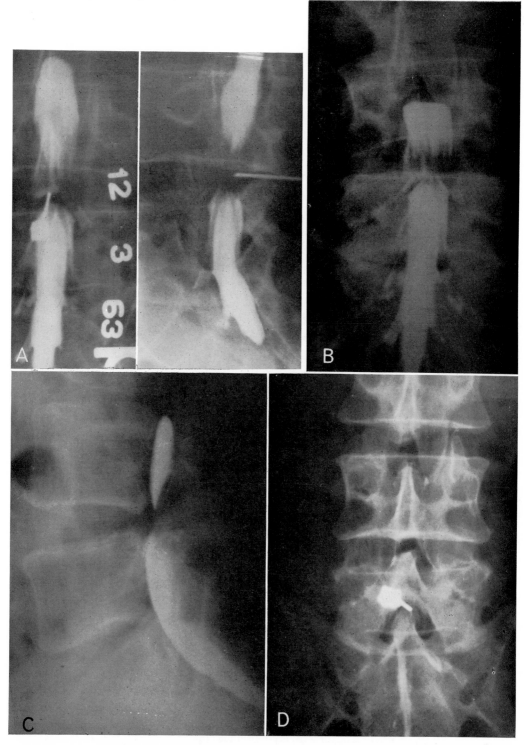

Fig. 395. *A*, Spinal puncture at the fourth interspace was accomplished with difficulty in this 46-year-old man with severe low back pain after an automobile accident. Pantopaque injected under image intensification control flowed smoothly cephalad and caudad. A total of 6 ml was injected. A large transverse defect is present at L4. *B*, After the needle was removed the defect was unchanged, and a "paint brush effect" of the column at the upper margin of the L4 disc is noted. *C*, A tapered defect is seen on the lateral view, the column being reduced to a thin thread-like configuration. In order to remove the Pantopaque an L5 tap was done, *D*. At operation a large L4 herniated disc was found. At the point of major compression there was absence of epidural fat. The canal was markedly compressed dorsally and ventrally.

be considered with regard to the available space in the canal. If the canal is deep, and if there is no osteophytic or spondylotic ridging or bulging of softened intervertebral discs, a moderate degree of dorsal indentation is not necessarily significant. However, when the canal is less than about 1.5 cm in its sagittal diameter, and when there is some ridging or discal bulging, such protrusions may assume clinical importance. Narrowing of the spinal canal is accompanied fairly often by thick laminae, short heavy pedicles and elongation and narrowing of the intervertebral foramina which can be seen on plain film examinations.

The concurrence of herniated discs with degenerative lesions is significantly frequent in older age groups. These bony spurs and cartilaginous ridges cannot be clearly distinguished in some cases from discal herniations. The presence of multiple ridges on lumbar myelograms is indicative of degenerative changes. The coexistence of discal herniation cannot be excluded. By the same token, a small bony protrusion may indent the Pantopaque column in exactly the same way as a herniated disc. The presence of multiple ridges in the lumbar canal, particularly together with sagittal narrowing, can be suspected when lumbar punctures are difficult, and often either blood-stained fluid or a poor flow of clear fluid is obtained (Fig. 394). It is advisable under these conditions to inject only about 1 ml of Pantopaque under image intensification fluoroscopic control. Removal of the Pantopaque may require reinsertion of the needle at another level (Fig. 395).

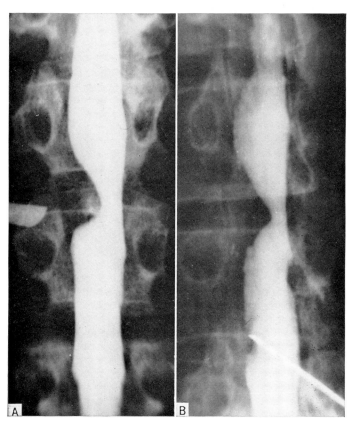

FIG. 396. Lateral defect at the second lumbar interspace on the right side due to a herniated disc, *A*. Four months later symptoms had recurred, and a repeat myelogram, *B*, showed an almost identical defect. Recurrent herniated disc found at operation.

Occasionally a patient who had been relieved of symptoms after removal of a herniated disc returns with complaints similar to those present before operation. This may occur without cause or after trauma, exertion or strain. The diagnosis of a new or recurrent herniated disc must be considered, and myelographic examination is again indicated if further surgery is planned. Recurrence of symptoms has been observed within a few days to many years after operation (Fig. 396) (Epstein, Levine and Epstein, 1967).

Plain film study is required to exclude some other cause for postoperative recurrent or persistent backache and radicular pain. Among these are arachnoiditis, dural scarring (Fig. 397), infection or an aseptic necrosis at the operative site. Progressive narrowing of the disc space and erosive bony changes followed by sclerosis and ultimate fusion of adjoining vertebral bodies are indications of the latter two possibilities.

If Pantopaque is still present in the spinal canal from a previous study, its flow should be checked fluoroscopically. Restriction of its passage and dispersal into fixed droplets may point to arachnoiditis. However, even when this is present the possibility of a recur-

rent or new discal herniation cannot be excluded. The addition of more Pantopaque into an already inflamed area should not be undertaken unless absolutely necessary. If it is decided to do this, it is advisable not to inject more than $\frac{1}{2}$ to 1 c.cm. If this does not flow freely the diagnosis of arachnoiditis may be made on the basis of the typical scattered droplets.

If the original myelographic study had been performed without leaving a useful residual, it is advisable to first inject about 1 c.cm and check its flow. Only after free movement has been ascertained should the remaining quantity be added, and the examination is then continued in the usual manner. The presence of lateral or anterior defects must be regarded as evidence of recurrent or further discal herniations if it occurs at the site of the first lesion. Additional herniated discs sometimes occur at other interspaces, presenting characteristic myelographic malformations. The possibility of scarring incident to previous surgery also must be recognized. This sometimes deforms the dorsal aspect of the dural sac, and can be checked only if adequate quantities of Pantopaque are used to permit visualization of the area immediately under

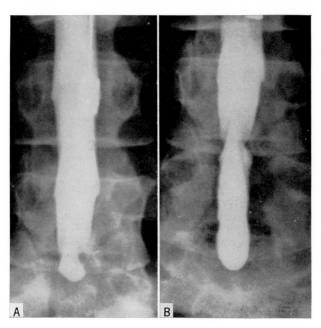

Fig. 397. Recurrent back pain with bilateral fluctuating sciatic radiation in a 52-year-old woman who had had a herniated disc at the fourth lumbar interspace operated on 4 years ago. The present myelogram revealed a hesitation at the fourth lumbar interspace in the passage of Pantopaque, A, and a waist-like defect when the patient was erect and the Pantopaque filled the lumbar canal, B. Re-operation revealed a markedly thickened ligamentum flavum and a thick ridge of inflammatory tissue encircling the dura. No recurrent discal herniation was found.

the ligamenta flava. Films in hyperextension should be obtained. Scarring of the ligamentum flavum at the operative site can result in thick bars of epidural and peridural tissue which project downwards towards the canal causing partial obstruction (Fig. 397). Postoperative bleeding or hematoma formation likewise may be associated with arachnoidal or epidural changes.

References

Armstrong, J. R., Golding, F. C., Gillespie, H. W. and Freeman, B.: Congenital Abnormalities of the Lumbosacral Region, Proc. Royal Soc. Med., 43, 635, 1950.

Begg, A. C.: Nuclear Herniations of the Intervertebral Disc, J. Bone & Joint Surg., 36-B, 180, 1954.

Begg, A. C. and Falconer, M. A.: Plain Radiography in Intraspinal Protrusion of Lumbar Intervertebral Discs, Brit. J. Surg., 36, 225, 1949.

Blau, J. N. and Logue, V.: Intermittent Claudication of the Cauda Equina. An Unusual Syndrome Resulting from Central Protrusion of a Lumbar Intervertebral Disc, Lancet, 1, 1081, 1961.

Breig, A. and Marions, O.: Biomechanics of the Lumbosacral Nerve Roots, Acta radiol., 1, 1141, 1963.

Brish, A., Lerner, M. A. and Graham, J.: Intermittent Claudication from Compression of Cauda Equina by a Narrowed Spinal Canal, J. Neurosurg., 21, 207, 1964.

Childe, A. E.: X-ray in Diagnosis of Posterior Herniation of Intervertebral Disc, Canad. M.A.J., 52, 458, 1945.

Cloward, R. B.: Multiple Ruptured Lumbar Discs, Ann. Surg., 142, 190, 1955.

Colonna, P. C. and Friedenberg, Z. B.: Disc Syndrome, J. Bone & Joint Surg., 31-A, 614, 1949.

Copleman, B.: Roentgenographic Diagnosis of Small Central Protruded Intervertebral Disc, Am. J. Roentgenol., 52, 245, 1944.

Cressman, M. R. and Pawl, R. P.: Serpentine Myelographic Defect Caused by a Redundant Nerve Root, J. Neurosurg., 28, 391, 1968.

Cronqvist, S.: The Postoperative Myelogram, Acta radiol., 52, 45, 1959.

Cronqvist, S. and Fuchs, W.: Lumbar Myelography in Complete Obstruction of the Spinal Canal, Acta radiol., 2, 145, 1964.

Davis, L., Martin, J. and Goldstein, S. L.: Sensory Changes with Herniated Nucleus Pulposus, J. Neurosurg., 9, 133, 1952.

Deucher, W. G. and Love, G. J.: Pathologic Aspect of Posterior Protrusions of the Intervertebral Disks, Arch. Path., 27, 201, 1939.

Echlin, F. A., Selverstone, B. and Scribner, W. E.: Bilateral and Multiple Ruptured Disks as One of Persistent Symptoms Following Operation for Herniated Disk, Surg., Gynec. & Obst., 83, 485, 1946.

Echolds, D. H. and Rehfeldt, F. C.: Failure to Disclose Ruptured Intervertebral Disks in 32 Operations for Sciatica, J. Neurosurg., 6, 376, 1949.

Eck, D. B.: Rupture of Intervertebral Disc, Am. J. Surg., 58, 3, 1942.

Epstein, B. S.: Complete Block of Lumbar Spinal Canal Due to Herniation of Nucleus Pulposus, Am. J. Roentgenol., 61, 775, 1949.

Epstein, B. S., Epstein, J. A. and Lavine, L.: The Effect of Anatomic Variations in the Lumbar Vertebrae and Spinal Canal on Cauda Equina and Nerve Root Syndrome, Am. J. Roentgenol., 91, 1055, 1964.

Epstein, J. A. and Lavine, L.: Herniated Lumbar Intervertebral Discs in Teen-age Children, J. Neurosurg., 21, 1070, 1964.

Epstein, J. A., Lavine, L. S. and Epstein, B. S.: Recurrent Herniation of the Lumbar Intervertebral Disk, Clin. Orthop., May-June, 1967, p. 169.

Fairburn, B. and Stewart, J. M.: Lumbar Disc Protrusion as a Surgical Emergency, Lancet, 2, 319, 1955.

Fernström, U.: Protruded Lumbar Intervertebral Disc in Children, Acta chirurg. scandinav., 111, 71, 1956.

————: Ruptured Lumbar Discs Causing Diagnostic Difficulties in Abdominal or Anogenital Pain, Acta Obst. et Gynecol. Scandinav., 41, 435, 1962.

French, J. D. and Payne, J. T.: Cauda Equina Compression Syndrome with Herniated Nucleus Pulposus, Ann. Surg., 120, 73, 1944.

Gage, E. L., Martin, J. and Goldstein, S. L.: Sensory Changes with Herniated Nucleus Pulposus, J. Neurosurg., 9, 133, 1952.

Gage, E. L. and Shafer, W. A.: Herniation of Lumbar Intervertebral Disks in Coal Miners, Am. J. Surg., 19, 577, 1953.

Gillespie, H. W.: Lumbar Intervertebral Disc Lesions, Brit. J. Radiol., 22, 270, 1949.

Graf, C. J. and Hamby, W. B.: Paraplegia in Lumbar Intervertebral Disk Protrusions, with Remarks on High Lumbar Disk Herniation, N. Y. State J. Med., 53, 2346, 1953.

Grant, F. C., Austin, G., Friedenberg, Z. and Hansen, A.: Neurologic, Orthopedic and Roentgenographic Findings in Displaced Intervertebral Discs, Surg., Gynec. & Obst., 87, 561, 1948.

Greenwood, J., Jr., McGuire, T. H. and Kimbell, F.: Causes of Failure in Herniated Intervertebral Disc Operation, J. Neurosurg., 8, 15, 1952.

Gurdjian, E. S., Ostrowski, A. Z., Hardy, W. G., Lindner, D. W. and Thomas, L. M.: Results of Operative Treatment of Protruded and Ruptured Lumbar Discs. Based on 1176 Operative Cases with 82 per cent Follow-up of 3 to 13 Years, J. Neurosurg., 18, 783, 1961.

Harris, R. I. and Macnab, I.: Structural Changes in the Lumbar Intervertebral Discs, J. Bone & Joint Surg., 36-B, 304, 1954.

Hirsch, C.: Studies on the Pathology of Low Back Pain, J. Bone & Joint Surg., 41-B, 237, 1959.

Horwitz, T.: The Diagnosis of Posterior Protrusion of the Intervertebral Disc, Am. J. Roentgenol., 49, 199, 1943.

Joffe, R., Appleby, A. and Arjona, V.: 'Intermittent Ischaemia' of the Cauda Equina Due to Stenosis of the Lumbar Canal, J. Neurol., Neurosurg & Psychiat., *29*, 315, 1966.

Jonck, L. M.: The Mechanical Disturbances Resulting from Lumbar Disc Space Narrowing, J. Bone & Joint Surg., *43-B*, 362, 1961.

Kaplan, A.: Herniated Intervertebral Discs Producing Contralateral Symptoms and Signs, Bull. Hosp. Joint Dis., *10*, 207, 1949.

Keegan, J. J.: Relations of Nerve Roots to Abnormalities of Lumbar and Cervical Portions of Spine, Arch. Surg., *55*, 246, 1947.

Kessler, L. A. and Stein, W. Z.: Posterior Migration of a Herniated Disk, Radiology, *76*, 104, 1961.

Lansche, W. E. and Ford, L. T.: Correlation of the Myelogram with Clinical and Operative Findings in Lumbar Disc Lesions, J. Bone & Joint Surg., *42-A*, 193, 1960.

Leader, S. A. and Rassell, M. J.: Pantopaque Myelography in Diagnosis of Herniation of Nucleus Pulposus in Lumbosacral Spine, Am. J. Roentgenol., *69*, 231, 1953.

Lindblom, K.: Technique and Results in Myelography and Disc Puncture, Acta radiol., *34*, 321, 1950.

————: Intervertebral-Disk Degeneration Considered as a Pressure Atrophy, J. Bone & Joint Surg., *39-A*, 933, 1957.

Lindblom, K. and Hultqvist, G.: Absorption of Protruded Disk Tissue, J. Bone & Joint Surg., *32-A*, 557, 1950.

Lindblom, K. and Rexed, B.: Spinal Nerve Injury in Dorso-Lateral Protrusions of Lumbar Disks, J. Neurosurg., *5*, 413, 1948.

Lindgren, S.: Herniated Intervertebral Disk, Acta chir. scandinav., *98*, 295, 1949.

Love, J. G.: Disc Factor in Low-Back Pain with or without Sciatica, J. Bone & Joint Surg., *29*, 438, 1947.

Love, J. G. and Emmett, J. L.: "Asymptomatic" Protruded Lumbar Disk as a Cause of Urinary Retention, Proceed. Staff Meet., Mayo Clinic, *42*, 249, 1967.

Love, J. G. and Rivers, M. H.: Intractable Pain Due to Associated Protruded Intervertebral Disk and Intraspinal Neoplasm, Neurology, *12*, 60, 1962.

Maltby, G. and Pendergrass, R. C.: Pantopaque Myelography, Radiology, *47*, 35, 1946.

Mandell, A. J.: Lumbosacral Intervertebral Disc Disease in Children, Calif. Med., *93*, 307, 1960.

McKenzie, K. G. and Botterell, E. H.: Common Neurological Syndromes Produced by Pressure from Extrusion of Intervertebral Disk, Canad. M.A.J., *46*, 424, 1942.

McRae, D. L.: Asymptomatic Intervertebral Disc Protrusions, Acta radiol., *46*, 9, 1956.

Munro, D.: Lumbar and Sacral Compression Radiculitis (Herniated Disk Syndrome), New England J. Med., *254*, 243, 1956.

Murphy, J. P.: Lumbar Intervertebral Disc Protrusion Contralateral to the Side of Symptoms and Signs, Am. J. Roentgenol., *61*, 77, 1949.

O'Connell, J. E. A.: Involvement of the Spinal Cord by Intervertebral Disk Protrusions, Brit. J. Surg., *43*, 16, 1955.

Odell, R. T. and Key, J. A.: Lumbar Disk Syndrome Caused by Malignant Tumors of Bone, J.A.M.A., *157*, 213, 1955.

Patterson, J. E. and Gray, W.: Herniated Nucleus Pulposus, Brit. J. Surg., *39*, 509, 1952.

Peyton, W. T. and Simmons, D. R.: Herniated Intervertebral Disk, Arch. Surg., *55*, 271, 1947.

Robinson, R. G.: Massive Protrusions of Lumbar Disks, Brit. J. Surg., *52*, 858, 1965.

Rubinstein, B. M., Stern, W. Z. and Jacobson, H. G.: Block of the Spinal Canal Caused by Herniated Disk, Am. J. Roentgenol., *81*, 1011, 1959.

Schultz, E. C.: Postoperative Bone Changes Following Lumbar Disc Removal, J. Neurosurg., *15*, 537, 1958.

Schut, L. and Groff, R. A.: Redundant Nerve Roots as a Cause of Complete Myelographic Block, J. Neurosurg., *28*, 394, 1968.

Scott, P. J.: Bladder Paralysis in Cauda Equina Lesions from Disc Prolapse, J. Bone & Joint Surg., *47-B*, 224, 1965.

Scoville, W. B., Moretz, W. H. and Hankins, W. D.: Discrepancies in Myelography, Surg., Gynec. & Obst., *86*, 559, 1948.

Silver, M. L., Field, E. A., Silver, C. M. and Simon, S. D.: The Postoperative Lumbar Myelogram, Radiology, *72*, 344, 1959.

Slater, R. A., Pineda, A. and Porter, R. W.: Intradural Herniation of Lumbar Intervertebral Discs, Arch. Surg., *90*, 266, 1965.

Smith, F. P.: Transvertebral Rupture of Intervertebral Disc, J. Neurosurg., *19*, 594, 1962.

Smyth, M. J. and Wright, V.: Sciatica and the Intervertebral Disc, J. Bone & Joint Surg., *40-A*, 1401, 1958.

Spanos, N. C. and Andrew, J.: Intermittent Claudication and Lateral Lumbar Disc Protrusions, J. Neurol., Neurosurg. & Psychiat., *29*, 273, 1966.

Splitthoff, C. A.: Lumbosacral Junction in Patients with and without Bachache, J.A.M.A., *152*, 610, 1953.

Svien, H. J., Dodge, H. W., Jr. and Camp, J. D.: Importance of Spinal Fluid Analysis and Contrast Myelography When Protruded Disc is Suspected, Surg., Gynec. & Obst., *93*, 623, 1951.

Tucker, A. S.: Myelography of Complete Spinal Obstruction, Am. J. Roentgenol., *76*, 248, 1956.

Ver Brugghen, A.: Massive Extrusions of Lumbar Intervertebral Discs, Surg., Gynec. & Obst., *81*, 269, 1945.

Wahren, H.: Herniated Nucleus Pulposus in Child of 12 Years, Acta orthop. scandinav., *16*, 40, 1945.

Walker, H. R.: Extradural Osseous Lesions Simulating Disk Syndrome, J.A.M.A., *172*, 691, 1960.

Webster, F. S. and Smiley, D. P.: End Result Study of Operations for Herniated Intervertebral Lumbar Discs, Am. J. Surg., *99*, 27, 1960.

Wilson, P. J. E.: Cauda Equina Compression Due to Intrathecal Herniation of an Intervertebral Disk: a Case Report, Brit. J. Surg., *49*, 423, 1962.

Wycis, H. T.: Contralateral Recurrent Herniated Disks, Arch. Surg., *60*, 274, 1950.

Young, H. H.: Non-Neurological Lesions Simulating Protruded Intervertebral Disk, J.A.M.A., *148*, 1101, 1952.

Herniated thoracic intervertebral discs are uncommon, occurring from 2 to 3 times per thousand cases, equally frequent in men and women. Apparently trauma plays no part in the occurrence of this lesion. Symptoms depend on the degree of compression of the cord and nerve roots, and whether the lesion lies laterally or centrally. These vary from a relatively acute onset with rapid progression requiring urgent attention to longstanding complaints which may have been present for as long as 20 years. In the upper dorsal area the clinical picture may simulate that seen with herniated low cervical discs. In the midthoracic spine radicular pains predominate, and in the lower thoracic area atypical symptoms referable to the abdominal viscera, the flanks and the inguinal regions appear. The usual course of spinal cord compressive symptoms including pain, tingling, burning, coldness or numbness, followed by symptoms referable to the motor tracts and sphincter control were observed in the 11 cases reported by Logue (1952). These were progressive and fairly rapid, so that the time between the appearance of symptoms and the indications for surgery was less than 7 months in 8 of his patients. In 3 paraplegia developed acutely. In 2 the protrusion had apparently existed for a long time because the prolapsed disc was bony hard. It was believed that the paraplegia was due to circulatory disturbances in the spinal cord. In the third case the prolapsed disc was soft, and believed to be of recent origin. Symptoms referable to the legs appeared first. Additional complaints referable to one side or the other, presenting a Brown-Séquard syndrome, may be caused by lateral compression of the cord.

The sensory manifestations follow the pattern caused by compression of the anterior tracts, with pain and temperature sense chiefly affected. Occasionally the dermatome distribution of sensory disturbance does not correspond with the level of the lesion. Logue mentioned 1 case in which the dermatome level was four segments higher than that of the compressed spinal segment. Sphincter disturbances occurred in 5 cases, and were mild. Three had slight urgency or dribbling, and in 2 others with paraplegia loss of sphincter control occurred. Love and Kiefer (1950) noted that in 5 of their 17 cases the neurologic examination was negative. They commented on the paucity of signs. In 8 of their cases the initial diagnosis was spinal cord tumor.

Investigation of the spinal fluid shows variable results, from completely normal observations both as to pressure and protein content to complete block with marked elevation of protein. Normal observations are by no means uncommon. Of the 8 cases seen by us manometric evidence of block or elevated protein content was absent in 4 instances.

By 1964 Arseni and Nash gathered a total of 94 previously reported cases of herniated thoracic intervertebral discs, and added 12 more out of a series of 2544 discs operated upon, an incidence of 4.72 per cent. Love and Schorn (1965) reported 61 cases, with an incidence of 0.5 per cent, and Baker, Love and Uhlein (1965) reported the radiologic changes associated with 43 cases. More than half failed to reveal any abnormality on plain film examination, and the majority of the remaining patients had nonspecific changes including calcification of the nucleus pulposus at one or more levels, narrowing of one or more interspaces, scoliosis and hypertrophic bony changes. Direct visualization of the calcified protruded disc fragment in the spinal canal was seen in 5 cases. These were the only ones in which plain films contributed to the diagnosis. The location of the protruded discal material into the spinal canal was either central or centrolateral in 77 per cent of the 61 cases presented by Love and Schorn.

Narrowing of an intervertebral disc is not necessarily indicative of discal herniation,

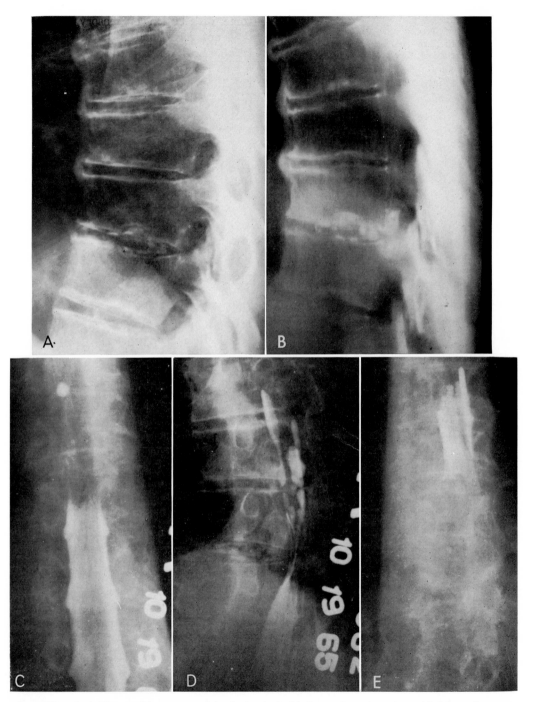

Fig. 398. *A*, A 58-year-old man complained of pain in his lower thoracic region with bilateral sensory disturbances and weakness of both legs. He was able to continue work even though his gait had become impaired. Lateral examination of the thoracic spine revealed narrow thoracic interspaces, and calcification of the ninth disc. *B*, Laminagram revealed a portion of the calcified disc to be within the spinal canal. *C, D* and *E*, Myelography revealed a hold up in cephalad flow, with a concave defect in the head of the column. On lateral examination the defect corresponds with the discal calcification. On caudad flow a cap-like defect is visible at the upper margin of the lesion. Diagnosis confirmed at operation.

but in the event of symptoms might be a helpful hint. Laminagraphic examination in the lateral position occasionally is useful in demonstrating calcified discal extrusion into the spinal canal (Fig. 398).

Transdural herniation of a thoracic intervertebral disc is a rare phenomenon. Fisher (1965) reported erosion of the dura mater in 2 cases, with serious circulatory damage in one. In one instance, there was dorsal erosion of the dura mater, apparently following an automobile accident in which a 35-year-old man was thrust forward vigorously. This was followed by vague complaints referred to the head, back, neck and abdomen lasting 6 months. Weakness of the legs was observed, with hypalgesia in the groin. Myelography revealed an hour-glass deformity at the eleventh interspace. At operation there was extensive dorsal erosion of the dura mater. The disc was removed by an intradural approach without complication. In the second case, a 47-year-old man, it was found that sequestrated hard disc was imbeded in the anterior substance of the cord. The cord was so discolored that a diagnosis of an angioma was made at first. The dura mater was left open, but because of persistence of symptoms he was reoperated 48 hours later. It was then that radical rotation of the cord disclosed a sequestered hard disc imbedded in the anterior substance of the cord. Tovi and Strang (1960) reported a 45-year-old woman who had had pain and weakness of the right leg for 2 years. At operation it was found that the disc penetrated the anterior aspect of the dura and was adherent to the cord, and both soft and bony hard material were removed from the intradural region.

We have encountered 1 patient who had transdural herniation of discal material. This 42-year-old woman had been in an automobile accident about 6 weeks before the onset of paresthesias in both legs. She had an unsteady gait, loss of heat and cold sensation on the right side and loss of proprioception in the right foot. For 10 days she had been dragging her left foot. A positive right Babinski reflex was present. Bilateral ankle clonus was also elicited. Myelographic examination revealed a cup-like defect at the interspace between the tenth and eleventh thoracic vertebrae. Preliminary plain film roentgenograms were normal. A diagnosis of a possible extradural tumor was offered, but in view of the history a thoracic herniated disc was considered more likely. At operation a rent in the dura was found, with extension of grumous and sandy material into the anterior aspect of the intradural space. The cord was flattened; and there was a cup-like depression in its anterior aspect. The dorsal aspect of the cord was discolored blue-black, and the cord was swollen. Engorged vessels were present in an abnormal pattern over the dorsal aspect of the cord. A wide laminectomy and facetectomy was performed. There was little improvement after operation (Fig. 399).

Peck (1957) reported a calcified thoracic intervertebral disc with spinal cord compression in a 12-year-old boy. Laminagrams revealed extension of the calcified sixth thoracic disc into the spinal canal after a fall. At operation the cord was humped over a soft bulging extradural mass which was situated outside the annulus and consisted of amorphous calcific material like that seen with peritendinitis calcarea. Exploration of the interspace yielded more of this toothpaste like material. Six months later only a residual trace of calcium was observed on re-examination.

The location of herniated thoracic discs are fairly evenly distributed from the fourth to the twelfth interspace. Young (1946) mentioned 1 of 4 cases at the third thoracic disc. Of a total of 43 cases, Logue found most to occur in the lower half of the thoracic spine. Kroll and Reiss (1951) also encountered a predominance of thoracic disc herniations in the lower thoracic spine, and observed that such lesions had a tendency to be multiple.

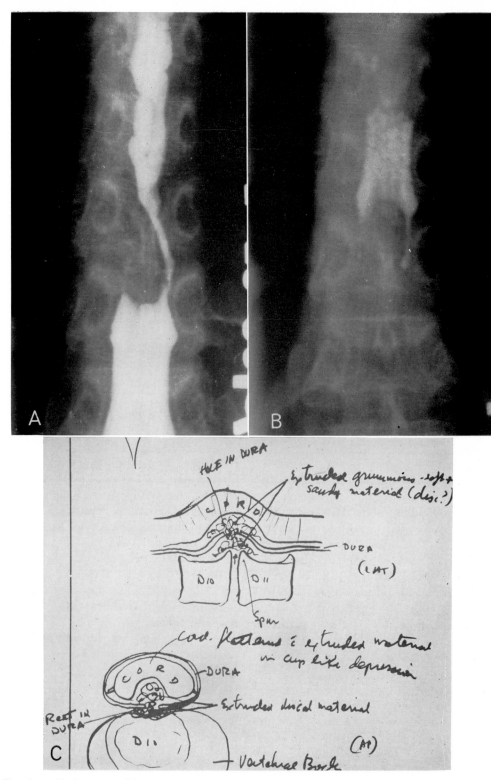

FIG. 399. *A,* A 42-year-old woman admitted with paresthesias in both legs for 5 weeks. Unsteady gait and loss of heat and cold sensation also noted. Plain film examination of the spine was normal. Myelography revealed a holdup at the T10 interspace, with the Pantopaque passing through a thin channel on the right side. *B,* On return flow a cap-like defect is observed at T10. *C,* At operation a herniated thoracic disc was found intruding into the spinal canal. The dura was penetrated and discal material projected against the cord.

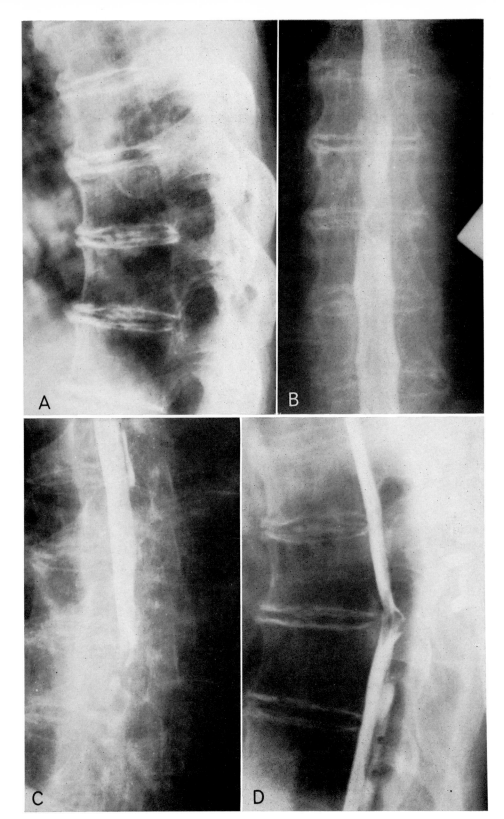

FIG. 400. *A*, A 60-year-old woman with weakness of both legs. Calcification is present in the ninth thoracic disc. *B*, Myelography reveals an oval midline defect at the tenth thoracic interspace. *C*, On caudad flow a definite delay in the descent of Pantopaque occurs. *D*, Transthoracic films reveal an indentation into the anterior aspect of the column. The myelographic defect is one interspace below the calcified disc.

Myelography is important in establishing the level and extent of the protrusion. The lumbar approach is advisable, and the most frequent change seen is a partial or complete block with a semicircular or oval defect in the Pantopaque column. Usually some of the Pantopaque passes to one side of the defect, permitting visualization of the canal above the level of the lesion. The uppermost aspect of the lesion can then be identified by returning the patient to a semi-erect position (Fig. 399). In the lateral view the Pantopaque is seen enveloping the lesion, resulting in a fork-like appearance of the column at the level of the prolapse (Fig. 400). While it is relatively easy to identify the lesion in the presence of a definite block, it is considerably more difficult to make the diagnosis when the Pantopaque flows freely through the thoracic spinal canal. This was well emphasized by 1 of our cases, a 43-year-old man with weakness of the lower limb together with neurologic deficits referable to the sixth thoracic interspace. Myelographic examination showed no obstruction. However, at the suspected interspace there was a momentary hesitation in the passage of the contrast medium, with a deviation of the column to the right side resulting in a small lateral hollow. When the entire column was over the lesion, it could not be identified. At operation the posterior spinal ligament was intact but bulging. When it was incised, degenerated material protruded. Cinemyelographic records of passage of Pantopaque through the thoracic canal in the frontal and oblique portions is especially useful. Good cross-table myelograms are also required, and at times convincing evidence of a herniated thoracic disc requires all these measures.

References

Arseni, C. and Nash, F.: Thoracic Intervertebral Disc Protrusions, J. Neurosurg., 17, 418, 1960.

Baker, H. L., Love, J. G. and Uhlein, A.: Roentgenologic Features of Protruded Thoracic Intervertebral Disks, Radiology, 84, 1059, 1965.

Epstein, J. A.: The Syndrome of Herniation of the Lower Thoracic Intervertebral Discs with Nerve Root and Spinal Cord Compression, J. Neurosurg., 11, 525, 1954.

Fisher, R. G.: Protrusions of Thoracic Disc. The Factor of Herniation through the Dura Mater, J. Neurosurg., 22, 591, 1965.

Hawk, W. A.: Spinal Compression Caused by Ecchondrosis of the Intervertebral Fibrocartilage, Brain, 59, 204, 1936.

Horwitz, N. H., Whitcomb, B. B. and Reilly, F. G.: Ruptured Thoracic Discs, Yale J. Biol. & Med., 28, 322, 1955–1956.

Kite, W. C., Jr., Whitfield, R. D. and Campbell, E.: The Thoracic Herniated Intervertebral Disc Syndrome, J. Neurosurg., 14, 61, 1957.

Kroll, F-W. and Reiss, E.: Der thorakale Bandscheibprolaps, Deutsch. med. Wchnschr., 76, 600, 1951.

LaSorte, A. F. and Brown, N.: Ruptured Anterior Nucleus Pulposus Between T 1 and T 2 Causing a Discrete Esophageal Defect and Minimal Dysphagia, Am. J. Surg., 98, 631, 1959.

Logue, V.: Thoracic Intervertebral Disc Prolapse with Spinal Cord Compression, J. Neurol., Neurosurg. & Psychiat., 15, 227, 1952.

Love, J. G. and Kiefer, E. J.: Root Pain and Paraplegia Due to Protrusion of Thoracic Intervertebral Disks, J. Neurosurg., 7, 62, 1950.

Love, J. G. and Schorn, V. G.: Thoracic-Disc Protrusions, J.A.M.A., 191, 627, 1965.

O'Connell, J. E. A.: Involvement of the Spinal Cord by Intervertebral Disk Protrusions, Brit. J. Surg., 43, 16, 1955.

Peck, F. C., Jr.: A Calcified Thoracic Intervertebral Disk with Herniation and Spinal Cord Compression in a Child, J. Neurosurg., 14, 105, 1957.

Tovi, D. and Strang, R. R.: Thoracic Intervertebral Disk Protrusions, Acta chir. scand., 1960, Supp. 267.

Williams, R.: Complete Protrusion of a Calcified Nucleus Pulposus in the Thoracic Spine, J. Bone & Joint Surg., 36-B, 597, 1954.

Young, J. H.: Cervical and Thoracic Intervertebral Disk Disease, Med. J. Australia, 2, 833, 1946.

Cervical Herniated Discs. Stookey (1928) first reported on compression of the spinal cord due to "ventral extradural cervical chondromas." Dandy (1929) included 1 case of cervical cord compression due to a protruded intervertebral disc. In 1940 Stookey recognized that these "chondromas" were herniated discs, and depending on size and location, compressed the spinal cord. Bilateral ventral pressure results in a clinical picture resembling a spinal cord tumor with pain, numbness, spasticity and weakness of the upper and lower extremities as well as atrophy, fibrillation and bilateral sensory disturbances. With more lateral lesions pressure is exerted against half of the cord. This produces focal atrophy of the lower motor neuron type at the level of the lesion, together with spasticity and ipsilateral pyramidal tract signs below the lesion and dissociated changes on the opposite side. Lateral pressure produces nerve root compression with radicular pain.

It was soon recognized that cervical disc herniations were less common than lumbar protrusions. However, from an anatomic viewpoint, Haley and Perry (1950) observed in 90 cadavers that cervical protrusions were twice as frequent as lumbar herniations. By 1936, Hawk collected 16 cases of cervical herniated discs and reported an additional case. Over the years larger series have been accumulated, such as the 22 cases reported by Browder and Watson (1945), 20 cases reported by Kristoff and Odom (1947), 26 cases reported by Poole (1953) and a series of 33 verified cases out of 110 patients with cervical foraminal root compression reported by Spurling and Segerberg (1953). Scoville (1966) reviewed 741 consecutive operable cervical disc lesions which he divided into five categories. These included (1) the lateral "soft" disc, (2) the lateral "hard" or osteophyte disc, (3) the central-bar or ridge-disc lesions, misnamed "spondylosis," (4) the rare central "soft" disc and (5) fracture-dislocations with disc protrusions. If this inclusive approach is taken, one would have to consider all ridge syndromes as part of that produced by herniated discs. Taking into consideration the fact that herniated discs and ridge syndromes both represent intervertebral disc disease, such an attitude is reasonable. However, we prefer to consider the ridge syndrome of spondylotic change (however misnamed) separately from that produced by herniations of the intervertebral disc into the spinal canal and intervertebral foramina. Due regard should be taken to remember that there are many examples of both ridge and disc lesions which affect either one or multiple cervical levels, and that these are difficult to catalogue. In reviewing our material there were less than 50 instances of pure discal herniations without concomitant ridge defects. The "hard disc" we considered part of the picture of spondylotic ridging. Nevertheless, it is fair to say that radiologically and clinically one cannot clearly recognize a discal lesion confined to a single level as being either a "hard" or a "soft" discal herniation or osteophyte, and that multiple lesions in which both herniated discs and spondylotic spurs coexist are by no means uncommon.

The most common site for cervical herniated discs is at the fifth and sixth interspaces. Of the 33 cases reported by Spurling and Segerberg, 30 per cent were at the fifth and 60 per cent at the sixth cervical level. Ten per cent occurred at both the fifth and sixth cervical interspaces. These authors mentioned a personal communication from Scoville, Whitcomb and McLaurin regarding 126 verified herniated cervical discs. Thirty per cent were at the fifth cervical level, 60 per cent at the sixth and 7 per cent at the seventh cervical levels. The remaining 3 per cent were found at the fourth cervical interspace.

Herniated cervical discs occur predominantly in males, with the highest incidence in the third and fourth decades. An appreciable number also are found in the decade between 50 to 60 years. While it is often possible to elicit a history of trauma, no specific correlation with a specific injury can be established. With lateral lesions pain in the shoulder and arm of the affected side is the presenting complaint. With central lesions and block of the spinal canal, the clinical picture is variable, including difficulty in moving the legs together with weakness, paresthesias and pain in the arms, symptoms referable to the dorsal funiculi, the pyramidal tracts and the lateral and ventral spinothalamic tracts. The clinical levels of neurologic disturbance may be different from those anticipated from the location of the herniated discs. Root pain is relatively inconspicuous, with the picture suggesting a spinal cord tumor in some and degenerative disease in others. The role of dentate ligaments in the production of compression effects against the anterior aspect of the spinal cord was discussed by Kahn

(1947). He presented stress analysis diagrams of mass lesions protruding into the spinal canal, demonstrating the role of the dentate ligaments in the distribution of pressure effects. He showed that the pressure of herniated discs on the anterior columns of the cord may produce relatively little in the way of symptoms. However, with pressure forcing the cord backwards, traction is produced against the dentate ligaments so that stress is exerted against the posterolateral columns, resulting in spasticity, weakness and disturbance of gait and balance. On the other hand, the posterior columns and the spinothalamic pathways are spared. There is considerable question as to whether the dentate ligaments really are that important, and today section of the dentate ligaments is not regarded as necessary in the operative management of this condition.

The wide variation in clinical pictures has been commented upon by many observers. Raney and Raney (1948) pointed out that headache may be a prominent symptom of cervical disc herniations. Semmes and Murphey (1943) and Josey (1949) reported cases in which pain in the chest and arm simulated angina pectoris. Pain along the course of the brachial plexus, especially in the shoulder and down the back of the arm, along the radial border of the forearm, and sometimes in the upper pectoral region was described by Elliott and Kramer (1945). They also observed paresthesias in the thumb, index and middle fingers. In some cases the patients complained of acute onset of a stiff neck. The pain was aggravated by movements of the neck and downward pressure of the head. Tenderness, weakness and wasting of the pectoralis major, triceps and extensor muscles of the wrist and fingers were also observed, together with hypalgesia over the thumb and index finger. Pain directly over the lower cervical spine is rather infrequent, although the spinous process of an involved segment sometimes is sensitive to pressure (Michelsen and Mixter, 1944). It has long

been recognized that herniated discs, particularly large ones in the midline, may produce syndromes indistinguishable from spinal cord tumors or obscure neurologic disturbances such as syringomyelia, multiple sclerosis, amyotrophic lateral sclerosis or combined system disease (Epstein and Davidoff, 1944; Bucy, Heimburger and Oberhill, 1948; Strully, Gross, Schwartzman and von Storch, 1951; Yuhl, Hanna, Rasmussen and Richter, 1955). Rarely involvement of the descending trigeminal tract may be seen with herniation of the fourth cervical disc (Elvidge and Li, 1950).

The cerebrospinal fluid changes associated with herniations of the cervical discs are variable. Manometric observations may be normal except when block exists. It is not uncommon to obtain normal manometric readings in the presence of a significant partial cervical spinal canal block as demonstrated on myelograms. The cerebrospinal fluid protein content varies from normal to considerably elevated figures when compression exists.

The cerebrospinal fluid circulation may be impaired by intrusions into the spinal canal from cervical ridges or herniated discs. Morton (1936) demonstrated 3 cases in which manometric measurements showed subarachnoid block when the patients' heads were extended to the point where they complained of numbness in the fingers. We have observed transitory Pantopaque block while the head was so maneuvered during myelography in patients with large herniated discs or prominent ridges. This phenomenon is well demonstrated on cervical cinemyelograms. Interruption of the Pantopaque column on hyperextension of the neck because of wrinkling of the ligamentum flavum also may be significant, especially if the sagittal diameter of the canal is narrow.

Because of anatomic conditions, symptoms of cervical discal herniations usually differ from those in the thoracic or lumbar regions. The cervical spinal cord almost fills the available space in the canal. The nerve roots emerge horizontally to enter the intervertebral foramina. The amount of epidural fat is scant. The cervical nerve roots are relatively large, and the intervertebral foramina are small, so that direct compression against the bony walls may result from relatively small protrusions. The posterior spinal longitudinal ligament expands opposite each intervertebral disc, but does not reach the lateral margins. The annulus fibrosus is weakest at the posterolateral margins, so that rupture at these points is facilitated. The intervertebral discs in the lower cervical spine are small. Bull (1948) observed that the volume of the cervical disc nucleus pulposus varied from 1.0 to 1.4 ml, as compared with lumbar discal contents up to 10 ml.

The mobility of the cervical spine is a significant factor in damage to the intervertebral discs. Herniations may occur acutely as a result of hyperflexion injuries, and be associated with compression fractures of the vertebrae or minor derangements of the small joints. Discal tissue can protrude through a weakening of the posterior spinal ligament, so that the nodule projects into the anterolateral aspects of the spinal canal, compressing the cord laterally, or impinging on the nerve roots. This change also takes place as part of a degenerative process with no gross change on plain film roentgenograms, but the appearance of narrowed intervertebral discs and spur formations at the uncovertebral joints directed anterolaterally and towards the intervertebral foramina is more frequent. It is often difficult to ascertain whether the primary condition is a degenerative spondylosis or a herniated disc.

The clinical and radiologic aspects of spondylosis with bulging and spurring of the cervical intervertebral discs were considered in Chapter 4. The compressive effects of these ridges are more prominent in the cervical than in the lumbar spine. Ridging of the thoracic intervertebral discs rarely is associated with intraspinal pressure effects. Narrowing of the cervical spinal canal reduces the available space, so that minor ridges or herniated discs produce disproportionate neurologic effects. Thickening of the neural arches, particularly of their posteroinferior margins, together with hypertrophy of the ligamenta flava, likewise produce abnormal pressures in narrow canals. Changes in the neural arches and ligamenta flava affect the dorsal aspect of the cervical cord, and pressures are augmented when the ligamenta flava are wrinkled inwards on extension of the neck. If spondylotic ridges also are present, they may act as anvils against which the anterior aspect of the cord is pressed. The movement of the spinal cord and nerve roots during activity enhances the pressure effects of these enveloping structures.

Differentiation between a herniated cervical disc or osteophytic changes affecting a single interspace is difficult even with myelographic evidence. The presence of multiple ridges points more towards spondylotic change. The importance of correlating clinical and radiographic changes is again emphasized because of the frequency with which apparently extensive bony changes are unaccompanied by symptoms, especially in the middle and later age groups. Herniated discs or single spurs occur at levels which apparently are normal on plain film investigations. In these individuals myelography is required for diagnosis, but should not be utilized unless surgery is considered.

The same objections raised in consideration of lumbar discography apply to the cervical adaptation, and we do not, except in unusual circumstances, perform this examination.

For reasons mentioned before, cinemyelographic examination of the cervical spinal canal provides information not available from conventional fluoroscopic and spot film observations. The pattern of flow of the opaque medium into the cervical canal, the deviation of the column by intraluminal lesions, the almost instantaneous changes in pattern as the canal fills can best be studied on cinemyelographic examination. Defects

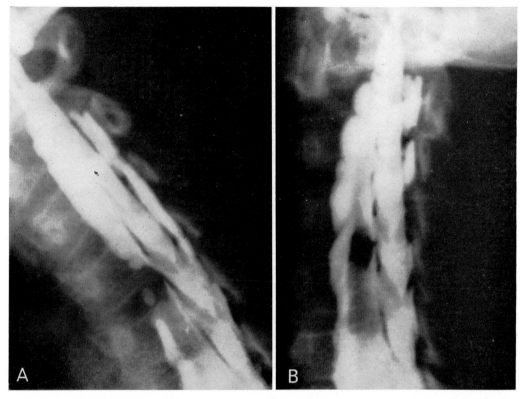

FIG. 401. *A*, A transitory defect is seen at the fifth cervical interspace when the neck is flexed. On elevating the head, *B*, the defect vanishes. This change is seen more graphically on the cinemyelographic study.

which on spot films appear almost diagnostic can be differentiated from momentary failure of filling (Fig. 401). The displacement of Pantopaque which may be questionable on conventional examinations can, on cinemyelograms in an adequately filled canal, be identified as produced by small but definite lateral protrusions. The effect of movement of the head, of flexion and extension of the neck, and of straining and coughing can all be recorded and studied. The caudad flow of Pantopaque can also be recorded, and the effect of ridges or discal herniations in holding the opaque medium above the lesion sometimes is helpful in diagnosis. Above all, one gets a record of the dynamic changes in the canal which cannot be obtained any other way.

Depending on the location and extent of the protrusion, myelographic examination may reveal only a small defect on the lateral aspect of the Pantopaque column. This sometimes is so small that difficulty is encountered in differentiating this indentation from an axillary pouch. The movement of the column in relation to the defect must then be investigated in frontal and oblique projections, and here cinemyelographic records are important. The variability of the fixed film examinations sometimes is quite striking (Fig. 402). With laterally placed lesions the transcervical roentgenograms are not necessarily helpful. However, if there is midline extension of the lesion indentation into the anterior aspect of the column is revealed (Fig. 403). This may be technically difficult in patients with discal herniations involving the sixth and seventh cervical and the first thoracic interspace. In these patients the oblique "swimmer's position" sometimes is useful (Fig. 404).

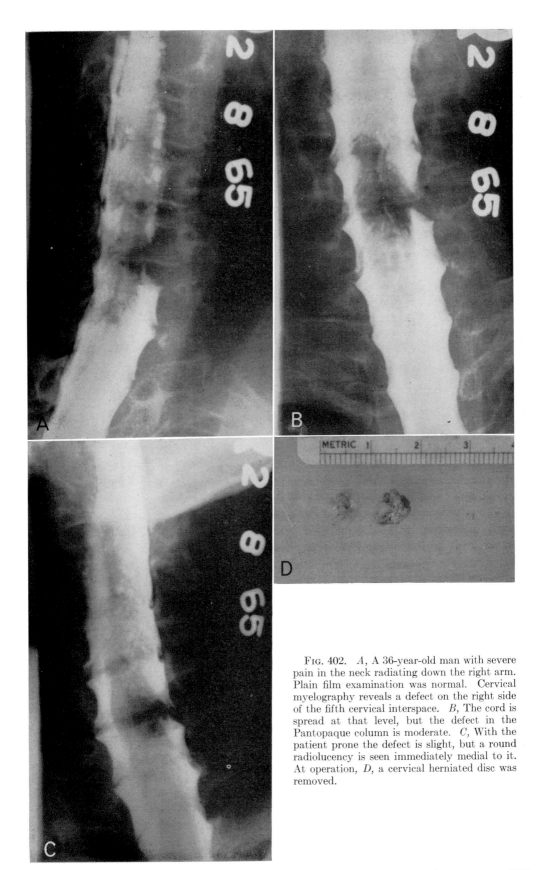

FIG. 402. *A*, A 36-year-old man with severe pain in the neck radiating down the right arm. Plain film examination was normal. Cervical myelography reveals a defect on the right side of the fifth cervical interspace. *B*, The cord is spread at that level, but the defect in the Pantopaque column is moderate. *C*, With the patient prone the defect is slight, but a round radiolucency is seen immediately medial to it. At operation, *D*, a cervical herniated disc was removed.

585

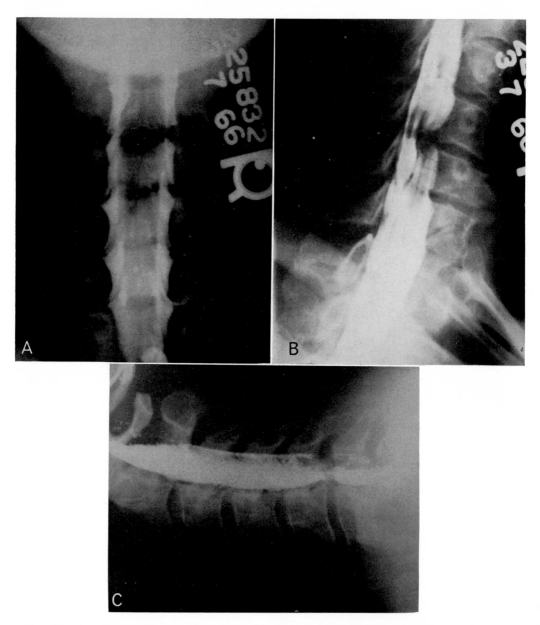

Fig. 403. *A*, A 35-year-old man with weakness of both arms and a right Horner's syndrome. Spondylosis at C5 and 6 present on plain film examination. Myelogram reveals a flattening of the axillary pouch of the right 5th nerve root. The defect is more prominent in the oblique view, *B*. A transcervical study, *C*, reveals pinching of the cord at C5. At operation a large midline ridge was present, together with a discal herniation on the right side of the C5 interspace.

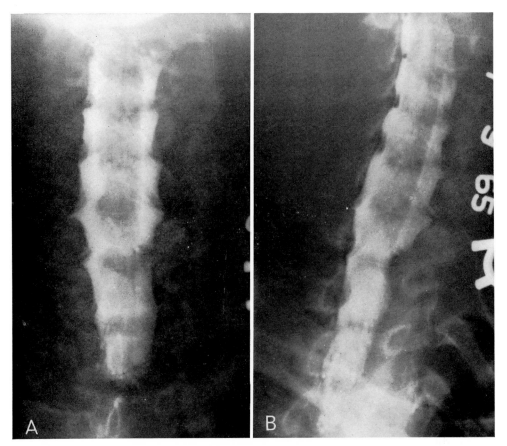

Fig. 404. *A*, A 64-year-old man with right shoulder and arm pain for 7 months. Plain cervical spine films showed multiple spondylotic changes. Myelography revealed a defect on the right side of the seventh cervical interspace, more marked with the patient in the oblique position, *B*. At operation a large herniated disc was found.

Midline lesions are difficult to identify, particularly when small. Nevertheless, they sometimes produce symptoms out of proportion to their size, particularly when the sagittal diameter of the cervical spinal canal is diminished. Observation of the advancing head of the Pantopaque column is important in identifying these lesions, the column being deviated laterally for a moment as it passes over the intrusion (Fig. 405). Oblique and transcervical views are best obtained under fluoroscopic control, and here again, cine-myelographic records prove their importance.

Large midline herniated discs produce a partial obstruction, with deviation of the Pantopaque column to one or both sides re-sulting in a "U" or "L" configuration. With marked obstruction this deformity is easily observed (Fig. 406), but with lesser obstruction it may be mistaken for the normal displacement of the opaque column as it passes the cervical bulge. Complete obstruction of the cervical spinal canal, of course, is readily recognized. As a rule, herniated discs at one interspace will not diffusely widen the cord, so that the elongated ovoid bulging negative shadow associated with intramedullary tumors is not observed as it sometimes is with multiple large spondylotic ridges. The caudad flow of Pantopaque usually is not retarded except with large obstructive lesions, and is more likely to occur with spondylotic ridging.

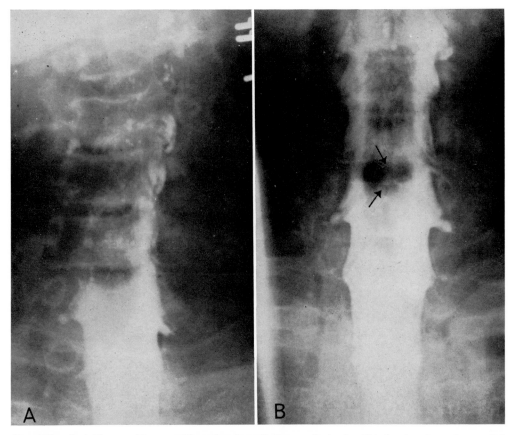

Fig. 405. *A*, A 58-year-old man with neck pain radiating to the back of his head and numbness of the left hand. Cervical myelogram showed a delay at the sixth interspace, the column assuming an L-shaped configuration. *B*, When the column filled the canal, a midline defect appears (arrows). At operation a midline cervical ridge was found together with a small discal herniation on the left side.

References

Allen, K. L.: Neuropathies Caused by Bony Spurs in the Cervical Spine with Special Reference to Surgical Treatment, J. Neurol., Neurosurg. & Psychiat., *15*, 20, 1952.

Bailey, R. W.: Observations of Cervical Intervertebral-Disc Lesions in Fractures and Dislocations, J. Bone & Joint Surg., *45-A*, 461, 1963.

Bradshaw, P.: Some Aspects of Cervical Spondylosis, Quart. J. Med., *26*, 177, 1957.

Browder, J. and Watson, R.: Lesions of the Cervical Intervertebral Disc. New York State J. Med., *45*, 730, 1945.

Bucy, P. C., Heimberger, R. F. and Oberhill, H. R.: Compression of the Cervical Spinal Cord by Herniated Intervertebral Discs, J. Neuorsurg., *5*, 471, 1948.

Bull, J. W. D.: Rupture of an Intervertebral Disc in the Cervical Region, Proc. Royal Soc. Med., *41*, 513, 1948.

Cloward, R. B.: Cervical Diskography, Ann. Surg., *150*, 1052, 1959.

Dandy, W. E.: Loose Cartilage from Intervertebral Disk Simulating Tumor of the Spinal Cord, Arch. Surg., *19*, 660, 1929.

Elliot, F. A. and Kremer, M.: Brachial Pain from Herniation of Cervical Intervertebral Disc, Lancet, *1*, 4, 1945.

Elvidge, A. R. and Li, C-L.: Central Protrusion of Cervical Intervertebral Disk Involving Descending Trigeminal Tract, Arch. Neurol. & Psychiat., *63*, 455, 1950.

Epstein, B. S. and Davidoff, L. M.: Iodized Oil Myelography of Cervical Spine, Am. J. Roentgenol., *52*, 253, 1944.

Frykholm, R.: Cervical Nerve Root Compression Resulting from Disc Degeneration and Rootsleeve Fibrosis, Acta chir. scandinav., Supp. 160, 1951.

Haley, J. C. and Perry, J. H.: Protrusion of Intervertebral Discs, Am. J. Surg., *80*, 394, 1950.

Hawk, W. A.: Spinal Compression Caused by Ecchondrosis of the Intervertebral Fibrocartilage, Brain, *59*, 204, 1936.

Höök, O., Lidvall, H. and Åström, K-E.: Cervical Disk Protrusions with Compression of the Spinal Cord, Neurology, *10*, 834, 1960.

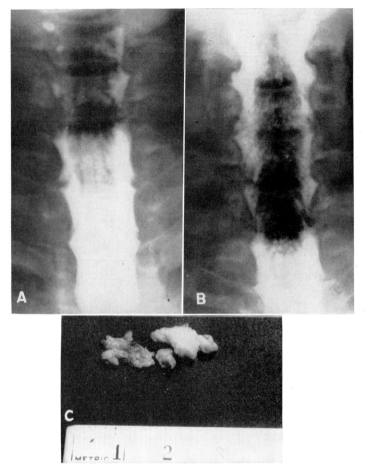

FIG. 406. Midline herniated disc at the sixth cervical interspace in a 50-year-old man with severe left chest pain, followed by numbness, weakness and diminished reflexes in the left upper arm after a sudden trauma. There was also pain in the right arm. On fluoroscopic inspection the Pantopaque met an almost transverse obstruction at the sixth interspace, *A*. When the patient was kept in the inverted position, Pantopaque flowed down the lateral gutters. The spinal cord is widened, *B*. At operation a herniated disc was found in the midline and removed, *C*.

Hussar, A. E. and Guller, E. J.: Correlation of Pain and the Roentgenographic Findings of Spondylosis of the Cervical and Lumbar Spine, Am. J. Med. Sci., *232*, 518, 1956.

Josey, A. I.: Headache Associated with Pathologic Changes in the Cervical Region, J.A.M.A., *140*, 944, 1949.

Kahn, E. A.: The Role of the Dentate Ligaments in Spinal Cord Compression and the Syndrome of Lateral Sclerosis, J. Neurosurg., *4*, 191, 1947.

Kristoff, F. V. and Odom, G. L.: Ruptured Intervertebral Disk in Cervical Region, Arch. Surg., *54*, 287, 1947.

Mair, W. G. P. and Druckman, R.: The Pathology of Spinal Cord Lesions and Their Relation to the Clinical Features in Protrusion of Cervical Intervertebral Discs, Brain, *76*, 70, 1953.

Michelsen, J. J. and Mixter, W. J.: Pain and Disability of Shoulder and Arm Due to Herniation of Nucleus Pulposus of Cervical Intervertebral Disks, New England J. Med., *231*, 279, 1944.

Morton, S. A.: Localized Hypertrophic Changes in Cervical Spine with Compression of Spinal Cord and its Roots, J. Bone & Joint Surg., *18*, 893, 1936.

Myers, A.: Degeneration of Cervical Intervertebral Disks Following Whip-Lash Injury, Bull. Hosp. Joint Dis., *14*, 74, 1953.

O'Connell, J. E. A.: Involvement of the Spinal Cord by Intervertebral Disk Protrusions, Brit. J. Surg., *43*, 216, 1955.

Oppenheimer, A. and Turner, E. L.: Discogenic Disease of the Cervical Spine with Segmental Neuritis, Am. J. Roentgenol., *37*, 484, 1937.

Pool, J. L.: Cervical Disc Syndrome, Bull. New York Acad. Med., *29*, 47, 1953.

Raney, A. A. and Raney, R. B.: Headache: Common Symptom of Cervical Disk Lesions, Arch. Neurol. & Psychiat., *59*, 603, 1948.

Schneider, R. C.: Acute Traumatic Posterior Dislocation of an Intervertebral Disc with Paralysis, J. Bone & Joint Surg., *31-A*, 566, 1949.

Scoville, W. B.: Types of Cervical Disk Lesions and Their Surgical Approaches, J.A.M.A., *186*, 479, 1966.

Semmes, R. and Murphey, F.: The Syndrome of Unilateral Rupture of the Sixth Cervical Intervertebral Disk, with Compression of the Seventh Cervical Nerve Root, J.A.M.A., *121*, 1209, 1943.

Spurling, R. G. and Segerberg, L. H.: Lateral Intervertebral Disk Lesions in Lower Cervical Region, J.A.M.A., *151*, 354, 1953.

Stern, W. E. and Rand, R. W.: Spinal Cord Dysfunction from Cervical Intervertebral Disk Disease, Neurology, *4*, 883, 1954.

Stookey, B.: Compression of Spinal Cord and Nerve Roots by Herniation of the Nucleus Pulposus in Cervical Region, Arch. Surg., *40*, 417, 1940.

Strully, K. J., Gross, S. W., Schwartzman, J. and von Storch, T. J. C.: Progressive Spinal Cord Disease. Syndromes Associated with Herniation of Cervical Intervertebral Disks, J.A.M.A., *146*, 10, 1951.

Taylor, A. R.: Mechanism and Treatment of Spinal Cord Disorders Associated with Cervical Spondylosis, Lancet, *1*, 717, 1953.

Teng, P.: Spondylosis of the Cervical Spine with Compression of the Spinal Cord and Nerve Roots, J. Bone & Joint Surg., *42-A*, 392, 1960.

Whiteleather, J. E., Semmes, R. E. and Murphey, F.: Herniation of Cervical Intervertebral Disk, Radiology, *46*, 213, 1946.

Yuhl, E. T., Hanna, D., Rasmussen, T. and Richter, R. B.: Diagnosis and Surgical Therapy of Chronic Midline Cervical Disk Protrusions, Neurology, *5*, 494, 1955.

ANTERIOR DISCAL PROTRUSIONS

In discussing herniations of the intervertebral discs, usually attention is directed towards symptom-producing posterior protrusions. There is also a group of discal malpositions associated with discogenic disease in which displacement of nuclear material occurs anteriorly.

Batts (1939) noted 3 anterior protrusions in 50 cadavers specimens with herniated discs. His Figure I depicted a thinned disc with the nucleus pulposus extruded anteriorly, where it was covered with bony bridging between the anterior portions of the vertebral bodies. The changes were considered secondary to the discal alterations. Schmorl and Junghanns also demonstrated on anatomic preparations that the so-called "persistent epiphyses" or "limbic bones" seen on the anterosuperior aspects of the vertebral bodies represented another form of discal

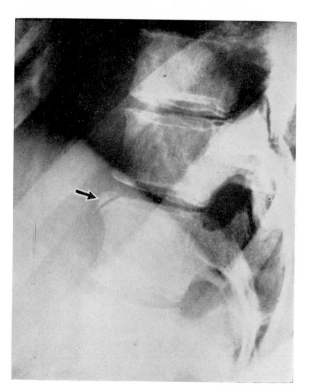

Fig. 407. Small, triangular bony fragment at anterosuperior aspect of the first lumbar vertebra (arrow), miscalled persistent epiphysis or limbic bone. This has been demonstrated as being due to anterior discogenic disease with forward nuclear protrusion.

extrusion separating a small fragment of bone from the body of the involved vertebra. Association of such changes with back pain in 8 cases was reported by Hellstadius (1947). These lesions are observed mainly in the lumbar vertebrae (Fig. 407).

By means of discography, Lindblom (1951) demonstrated on 3 anatomic preparations and 5 living patients that opaque medium entered the fissure lines separating the intervertebral discs from the marginal bony fragments, confirming the work of Schmorl and Junghanns *in vivo*. Anterior herniations of the nucleus pulposus revealed by discography was reported also by Cloward and Buzaid (1952). Cloward (1952) described a case in a 42-year-old man with chronic low-back pain in whom discograms showed anterior herniation of a large disc fragment.

Lindblom (1951) reported that extension of diodrast during discography into an anteriorly ruptured first lumbar disc caused severe abdominal pain. A similar reaction took place in 2 patients without bony separation from the vertebral body. He mentioned that Grill had directed attention to the possibility of abdominal pain arising from anterior discal herniations.

A rare example of anterior thoracic discal protrusion causing slight dysphagia and a defect of the esophagus because of extrinsic pressure was reported by LaSorte and Brown (1959). Occasionally anterior discal extrusions presenting marginal defects are seen in the cervical vertebrae (Fig. 378).

References

Batts, M., Jr.: Rupture of the Nucleus Pulposus, J. Bone & Joint Surg., *21*, 121, 1939.

Beggs, A. C.: Nuclear Herniations of the Intervertebral Disc, J. Bone & Joint Surg., *36-B*, 180, 1954.

Cloward, R. B.: Anterior Herniation of a Ruptured Lumbar Intervertebral Disk, Arch. Surg., *64*, 457, 1952.

Cloward, R. B. and Buzaid, L. L.: Discography, Am. J. Roentgenol., *68*, 552, 1952.

Hellstadius, A.: Paradiscal Defects in the Anterior Portion of the Vertebral Body, with Remarks on the Pathogenesis of the Lesions in Question, Acta orthop. scandinav., *17*, 50, 1947.

LaSorte, A. F. and Brown, N.: Ruptured Anterior Nucleus Pulposus Between T 1 and T 2 Causing a Discrete Esophageal Defect and Minimal Dysphagia, Am. J. Surg., *98*, 631, 1959.

Lindblom, K.: Discography of Dissecting Transosseous Ruptures of Intervertebral Discs in Lumbar Region, Acta radiol., *36*, 12, 1951.

POSTOPERATIVE COMPLICATIONS OF DISCAL SURGERY

Leavens and Bradford (1954) reported a case in which, after removal of a herniated disc, their rongeurs passed through a fissure in the anterior aspect of the annulus fibrosus. They believed this explained abdominal vascular accidents, and cited 2 cases from the literature in addition to 12 of which they had personal knowledge in which abdominal aortic injuries terminated fatally. I recall 1 case in which the patient died on the operating table because the abdominal aorta was torn by pituitary rongeurs during the operation. Smith, Hughes, Sapp, Joy and Mittingly (1957) reported 2 patients with high output circulatory failure due to arteriovenous fistulas following surgery for herniated discs. They noted that 9 cases had been reported, 5 of which had been recognized only after the fistulas had resulted in circulatory failure. A long time may elapse between the creation of an arteriovenous fistula and its radiologic or clinical diagnosis. Aortography is important in radiologic identification of this lesion. By 1963 Spittell and his co-workers collected 22 such cases and added 3 more. The arteriovenous fistulas involved the aorta or the iliac arteries and the inferior vena cava or the iliac veins. Stape and Friedenberg (1965) reported the angiographic demonstration of an ilio-iliac arteriovenous fistula diagnosed 9 years after operation. A continuous bruit was heard over the back, loudest at the fourth lumbar interspace. Bowel perforation following lumbar disc surgery was reported by Smith and Estridge (1964), who mentioned that only 3 out of 140 reported intraabdominal injuries were of this variety. Their patient, a 52-year-old woman, had a complete block at the lumbosacral interspace. Following operation the patient developed an ileus due to laceration of the ileum and peritonitis, with disc space infection.

Inflammatory intervertebral disc disease as a complication of discal surgery occurs occasionally (Fig. 242). This is associated with severe postoperative pain requiring prolonged treatment. A concomitant osteomyelitis of the adjacent vertebrae often is present, which on healing presents evidence of sclerosis and fusion (Stern and Crandall, 1959). Schultz (1958) observed that in some of these patients the process might be a type of aseptic necrosis.

With the advent of anterior body fusion of the cervical spine for the treatment of degenerative joint and discal disease, considerable discussion still takes place as to postoperative changes in these patients. In comments made by discussors of a paper presented by Robinson and his co-workers (1962) difficulties in interpretation of radiologic evaluation of fusion was emphasized. Jones (1962) made a cineradiographic study of patients with cervical spine fusion. In his group of 41 patients were 22 who had undergone anterior body fusion operations. Of these 5 were asymptomatic regardless of the degree of motion observed, 3 were definitely improved, and 13 had either persistence of complaints or recurrence of symptoms after a period of relief. He noted that 1 patient with an obvious failure of fusion had been completely relieved of symptoms.

Galera and Tovi (1968) reviewed 59 patients with cervical spondylosis who had been operated upon by them during the past 7 years by the technique developed by Cloward. They reported that 17 per cent showed a satisfactory response and 83 per cent showed a poor response to this procedure. They also noted that in 12 cases the anterior angulation of the cervical spine was found to have increased after surgery. It was stressed that even with operation at different levels it is not possible to enlarge effectively the congenitally narrow spinal

canal found in a great number of these cases. They suggested that this technique should be used only in those cases with a clinically and radiologically localized process without alterations of the lordotic cervical curvature and with a canal of normal width. In our own practice we have found the results of foramenotomy and laminectomy with removal of osteophytes to provide adequate relief without resorting to anterior spinal fusion and discal excision.

The implication that cineradiographic examination is decisive in examinations performed for determination of failure of fusion cannot be regarded as certain. I have reviewed cineradiographic examinations of the cervical spine made by others, and colleagues have reviewed mine with a definite lack of agreement on the observations, particularly when slight changes are present. Nevertheless, these are important records, and perhaps with additional experience we will arrive at more definite conclusions. Serial studies are especially important in those patients with persistent symptoms for identification of degenerative changes in the intervertebral discs and vertebrae above and below the fused area (Fig. 408). Other complications which have been encountered include rejection of the graft, osteomyelitis, protrusion of the graft anteriorly, and soft tissue infections.

References

Galera, R. and Tovi, D.: Anterior Disc Excision with Interbody Fusion in Cervical Spondylotic Myelopathy and Rhizopathy, J. Neurosurg., 28, 305, 1968.

Geiger, L. E.: Fusion of Vertebrae Following Resection of Intervertebral Disc, J. Neurosurg., 18, 79, 1961.

Horton, R. E.: Arteriovenous Fistula Following Operation for Prolapsed Intervertebral Disk, Brit. J. Surg., 49, 77, 1961.

Jones, M. D.: Cineroentgenographic Studies of Patients with Cervical Spine Fusion, Am. J. Roentgenol., 87, 1054, 1962.

Leavens, M. E. and Bradford, F. K.: Ruptured Intervertebral Disc, J. Neurosurg., 10, 544, 1953.

Robinson, R. A., Walker, A. E., Ferlic, D. C. and Wiecking, D. K.: The Results of Anterior Interbody Fusion of the Cervical Spine, J. Bone & Joint Surg., 44-A, 1569, 1962.

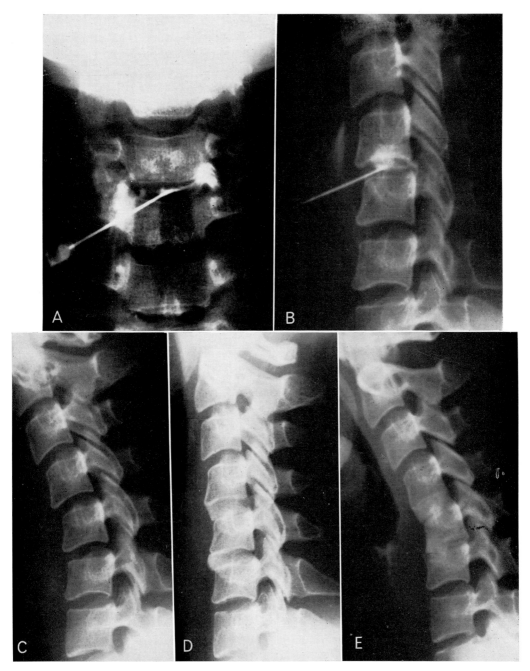

FIG. 408. *A*, This 37-year-old woman was in an automobile accident, and had difficulty in moving her neck thereafter. A cervical discogram showed extravasation of Hypaque laterally and towards the floor of the cervical canal, *B*. The normal cervical curve was reversed, *C*. Anterior spinal fusion was done, straightening the curve, *D*. Thereafter the patient developed neck pain which at times was severe. Re-examination of the cervical spine showed a breakdown of the fusion between C5 and 6, while the one above was well maintained. At this time, 8 months after operation, cineradiographic examination of the cervical spine was made. The difference of opinion as to which segment was unstable, and whether or not abnormal movement existed at the interspaces above and below the fused segments, was wide. However, there was little doubt that bony changes were present at the sixth cervical level.

Schultz, E. C.: Postoperative Bone Changes Following Lumbar Disc Removal, J. Neurosurg., *15*, 537, 1958.

Smith, R. A. and Estridge, M. N.: Bowel Perforation Following Lumbar Disc Surgery, J. Bone & Joint Surg., *46-A*, 826, 1964.

Smith, V. M., Hughes, C. W., Sapp, O., Joy, R. J. T. and Mittingly, T. W.: High-Output Circulatory Failure Due to Arteriovenous Fistula, Complication of Intervertebral Disc Surgery, Arch. Int. Med., *100*, 833, 1957.

Spittell, J. A., Jr., Palumbo, P. J., Love, J. G. and Ellis, F. H., Jr.: Arteriovenous Fistula Complicating Lumbar-Disk Surgery, New England J. Med., *268*, 1162, 1963.

Staple, T. W. and Friedenberg, M. J.: Ilio-Iliac Arteriovenous Fistula Following Intervertebral Disc Surgery, Clin. Radiol., *16*, 248, 1965.

Stern, W. E. and Crandall, P. H.: Inflammatory Intervertebral Disc Disease as a Complication of the Operative Treatment of Lumbar Herniations, J. Neurosurg., *16*, 261, 1959.

8

Diseases of the Spinal Cord and Its Coverings

Inflammatory Diseases

ARACHNOIDITIS

Arachnoiditis presents a variable clinical picture, primarily of pain referable to nerve patterns. When lumbar areas are affected, back pain and sciatica may be intermittent, and suggest the diagnosis of a herniated disc. In the cervical or thoracic spinal canal, symptoms may be relatively acute and simulate a tumor. Among the causes of arachnoiditis are the various inflammatory diseases such as meningitis (Mackay, 1939), pneumonia, typhoid fever, and virus diseases (Stookey, 1927). Tuberculosis and syphilis also may produce arachnoidal reactions. Parasitic infestations with meningeal involvement is infrequent in the United States, but is reported in South American, Asian and East European countries. Hydatid disease, cysticercosis and torulosis are among the more frequent offenders. These have been discussed in Chapter 4. Arachnoiditis may be associated with trauma, possibly incident to bleeding within the spinal canal. In this connection the experiments of Bagley (1928) are of interest. He injected the blood of dogs into the subarachnoid space by way of the cisterna magna, and produced frequent meningeal reactions in response to a few cubic centimeters of blood. In most cases this reached the state of proliferative meningitis, and he cited clinical cases of a similar nature. Nelson (1943) reported the case of a 50-year-old man with thrombopenic purpura with arachnoid-

itis, and postulated that meningeal bleeding occurring during convulsive episodes may have preceded sterile meningitis, which went on to fibrotic organization and cavitations. At necropsy, the inflammatory process began at the midthoracic region and extended down to the cauda equina. There was marked thickening of the dura with adherence of the nerve roots of the cauda equina. The cord above the lesion was normal, but below sections revealed numerous cavities in the dorsal and lumbar regions. The normal architecture of the cord appeared to be markedly distorted. In one of our patients with a bleeding aneurysm of the anterior communicating artery arachnoiditis appeared about 6 months after an acute episode, at which time bloody fluid had been obtained from the lumbar spinal canal The effect of blood in potentiating the production of arachnoiditis in the presence of Pantopaque was investigated by Howland and his co-workers (1963). They found that Pantopaque mixed with blood produced severe localized inflammation in dogs. Interestingly enough, they noted no reaction to blood alone. Seghal, Gardner and Dohn (1962) described acute meningeal reactions immediately after injection of Pantopaque and removal of 7 out of 8 ml injected. Their patients complained of pain in both hips and the lower back. Repeat lumbar punctures revealed 309 leukocytes in the cerebrospinal fluid. They also noted acute reactions which subsided to a chronic state. For relief they suggested adrenal corticosteroid

39

instillation into the subarachnoid space. I have not seen such an occurrence except in 1 adult female patient in whom myelographic examination was followed by a rather violent meningeal reaction. This patient had had a previous spinal fusion, and I suspect that it is more likely that infection was introduced by the lumbar puncture needle than by the presence of Pantopaque. There was no difficulty either in the instillation or the removal of the Pantopaque.

Progressive hypertrophic neuritis (Déjérine-Sottas disease) occurs as a rare heredofamiliar disorder in which the connective tissue and the sheaths of Schwann proliferate around the nerve fibers in multiple concentric layers. The fibers are gradually replaced by this proliferation, which also progresses around the fibers and increases their bulk. Radiologically this condition is identified by pronounced swelling of the thickened nerve roots displacing Pantopaque in thick, relatively parallel streaks. The passage of the opaque medium down the canal may be partly or completely blocked, presenting a dentate appearance of the caudad end of the column. Difficulty in obtaining an adequate flow of cerebrospinal fluid may be encountered if the tap is in the involved area. Removal likewise becomes difficult (Fig.

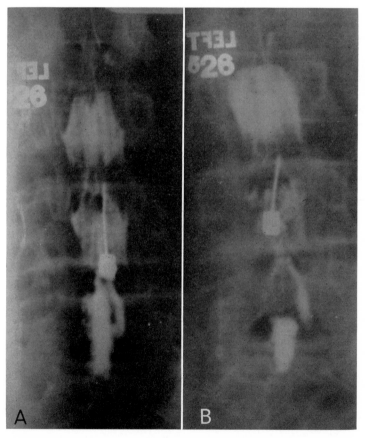

Fig. 409. *A,* Difficulty was encountered in performing lumbar puncture in this 70-year-old man who had inability to walk for about a month, and had been dragging his left leg for 18 months. Weakness in both legs present at the time of examination. A few drops of xanthochromic fluid were obtained at lumbar puncture. The CSF protein content was over 800 mg per cent. After injection of 1.5 ml of Pantopaque the nerve roots were visualized as thickened structures, and delay in passage at the third, fourth and fifth interspaces was present. In the erect position, *B,* an almost complete block is seen at L3, and the column assumes a "paint-brush" appearance. At operation the dura was opened and the roots were seen to be markedly inflamed and swollen. A biopsy was not performed.

409). The peripheral nerves also are affected, and nodular masses occasionally can be palpated. When the intraspinal nerves become massively involved, enlargement of intervertebral foramina may appear because of expanded nerve roots. Hypertrophic interstitial neuritis may involve peripheral nerves, spinal nerve roots and the cauda equina singly or together. When the cauda equina alone is diseased, the diagnosis can be made myelographically (Hinck and Sachdev, 1965). Infrequently a tumor growing on a nerve root extends sufficiently into the spinal canal to produce a block which

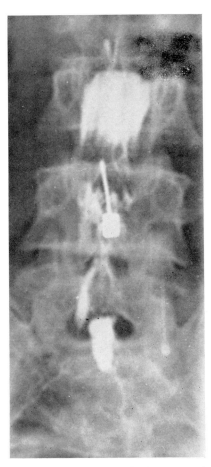

FIG. 410. Arachnoiditis following removal of a herniated fourth lumbar disc. Recurrent pain, with almost complete block at the third lumbar interspace. Irregular collections of Pantopaque below the obstruction were caught in thick, fibrinous exudate which had almost obliterated the spinal canal.

can easily be confused with that due to a neurofibroma (Symonds and Blackwood, 1962). Similar changes occasionally appear in the presence of a large obstructing lesion such as an extruded lumbar disc. Localized arachnoiditis following disc surgery, sometimes associated with a peridural inflammation, similarly can cause obstruction with a serrated caudal margin of the Pantopaque column (Fig. 410). Schut and Groff (1968) reported a patient with complete lumbar myelographic block caused by redundant nerve roots which produced serpentine shadows simulating dilated blood vessels.

Arachnoiditis with calcification is infrequent. It has been observed together with a vascular spinal anomaly and subarachnoid hemorrhage (Gatzke, Dodge and Dockerty, 1957). Calcifications of unknown origin producing multiple myelographic defects in the lumbar area were seen by Faeth (1958). At operation these stones were adherent to the roots and their tiny vessels, and apparently did not arise from the arachnoid. However, it is not infrequent to find thin calcific plaques a few millimeters in diameter in normal meninges at postmortem examination in elderly patients. Wise and Smith (1965) observed deposition of bone in inflammatory lesions, and suggested that previous trauma, subarachnoid hemorrhage and spinal anesthesia were predisposing causes. Calcifications appear in an asymptomatic form, but also can produce cord and nerve root compression in rare instances where progressive increase in size takes place. Most of the time there is no correlation with systemic disease or neurologic manifestations (Knoblich and Olsen, 1966).

Arachnoiditis has been associated with continuous caudal anesthesia. Peacher and Robinson (1944) described 2 cases, 1 of which had a secondary osteomyelitis, while the other had either an epidural or subdural abscess which responded to chemotherapy. Kennedy, Effron and Perry (1950) reported on the occurrence of inflamamtory lesions following spinal anesthesia. Rosenbaum, Long, Henchey and Trufant (1952) de-

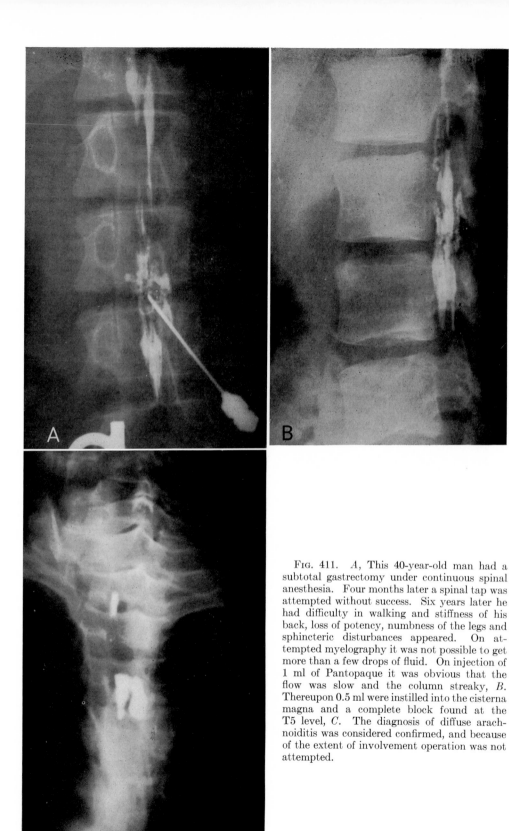

Fig. 411. *A*, This 40-year-old man had a subtotal gastrectomy under continuous spinal anesthesia. Four months later a spinal tap was attempted without success. Six years later he had difficulty in walking and stiffness of his back, loss of potency, numbness of the legs and sphincteric disturbances appeared. On attempted myelography it was not possible to get more than a few drops of fluid. On injection of 1 ml of Pantopaque it was obvious that the flow was slow and the column streaky, *B*. Thereupon 0.5 ml were instilled into the cisterna magna and a complete block found at the T5 level, *C*. The diagnosis of diffuse arachnoiditis was considered confirmed, and because of the extent of involvement operation was not attempted.

scribed several cases of paralysis following saddle block anesthesia in obstetrical patients. Schwarz and Bevilacqua (1964) reported necropsy observations on a patient who developed a flaccid paraplegia immediately after a continuous spinal anesthesia for a hysterectomy. Extensive meningeal, neural and vascular changes were found in the cord and meninges. A review of the literature disclosed 31 cases with necropsies. Progressive arachnoiditis appeared in a patient seen by us who had had spinal anesthesia for a subtotal gastrectomy 10 years before he came for help. The onset of symptoms had been gradual over a period of about 5 years (Fig. 411).

The irritative effects of lipiodol on the meninges with the production of a mild arachnoiditis was demonstrated experimentally in dogs by Craig (1942). Mention has been made of arachnoiditis following the use of Thorotrast and Pantopaque in the discussion of complications of myelography. Walker (1947) described 2 cases of arachnoiditis after the intrathecal administration of penicillin. He stated that such reactions occurred only with large amounts, but that when smaller doses were used this complication was rare. In his second case, cisternal and lumbar myelography showed changes characteristic of arachnoiditis, and this was confirmed at operation.

With the advent of frequent operations for herniated discs it was noted that occasionally these lesions were accompanied by inflammatory changes in the leptomeninges. French (1946) reviewed 200 such cases, and found 13 with arachnoiditis, 8 with concomitant herniated discs. The remaining 5 were early cases, and protrusions may have been overlooked. The association of arachnoiditis with spinal surgery was mentioned by Smolik and Nash (1951), who reported 4 cases as a complication of lumbar intervertebral disc operations. Davidoff, Gass and Grossman (1947) reported 5 cases of arachnoiditis following operation for benign spinal cord tumors. Their first case had arachnoiditis associated with recurrence of a meningi-

oma 14 years after the removal of the original tumor. In their fifth case, necropsy disclosed foci of meningiomatous tissue with dense arachnoidal proliferations 10 years after the original operation.

It was believed by earlier authors, notably Stookey (1927) and Elkington (1936), that spinal arachnoiditis was more common in the cervical and thoracic regions. However, French (1946) and Ramsey, French and Strain (1946) indicated that in their experience the occurrence of arachnoiditis in the lumbar region was more common, and this has been my experience. Six of the 7 cases reported by Seaman, Marder and Rosenbaum (1953) involved the lumbar spinal canal. Twenty-eight of the 41 cases reported by Lombardi, Passerini and Migliavacca (1962) were in the thoracic spinal canal. The lumbar region was involved in 7, and the cervical canal in 6.

Arachnoiditis is characterized by diffuse adhesions, which may be minimal and localized, or diffusely disseminated as thick, whitish fibrotic intermeshed bands which occur in all gradations of severity. Thin, stringy fibrous tissue containing large numbers of polymorphonuclear cells first appear, and as organization takes place, a thickened membranous fibrotic lesion is formed (Kulowski and Scott, 1934). The arachnoidal inflammation is recurrent, and may be widespread or locally circumscribed, and associated with the formation of cystic areas. The thickening may be moderate or extensive. It distorts the dural sac, and extends into the nerve root pouches, deforming and compressing the nerve roots themselves (Rexed, 1947). Intramedullary changes, notably atrophy and cavitation, have been described as a result of pressure and circulatory disturbances (Lubin, 1940) (Schwarz and Bevilacqua, 1964).

Examination of the cerebrospinal fluid may help. Manometric readings range from normal values to complete block. The cerebrospinal fluid protein content varies from normal to extremely high values with xanthochromic or thick yellowish fluid.

French (1947) mentioned that the protein content may exceed 400 mg per cent, and we have observed even higher values. Difficulty in performing a spinal tap, or slow return of thick fluid sometimes point to the diagnosis. If this occurs, only a few drops of Pantopaque should be instilled under image intensification fluoroscopic control. The appearance of a streaky pattern which flows slowly should alert the examiner to stop the injection.

We have seen 37 cases of arachnoiditis. Only 4 of these involved the dorsal spinal canal. The clinical picture suggested a spinal cord tumor, with complete block in the mid-dorsal area. The true nature of the lesion was disclosed at operation, and the postoperative results were poor. In 10 cases arachnoiditis involving the lumbar spinal canal was concomitant with large herniated discs. The dura was opened to gain access to the prolapsed discs, and the thickened nerve roots and arachnoidal inflammations were then identified. In some of these cases exploration of the spinal canal by the lateral approach failed to disclose the protruded discs, which were identified only after the dura had been opened. Almost all had complete or almost complete spinal canal block.

In 16 cases arachnoiditis was associated with previous surgery for herniated discs. In 6 of these a second operation disclosed in addition to the arachnoiditis, recurrences of the protruded discs. The time interval between the first operation and the need for subsequent operation was variable. In 1 case only 6 weeks elapsed, while in the others the intervals varied from 3 to 10 years. One patient had had intrathecal medication for meningitis about 10 years before, and another had had a briskly bleeding aneurysm of the circle of Willis 6 months before the appearance of spinal symptoms.

In 5 other cases there was no known reason

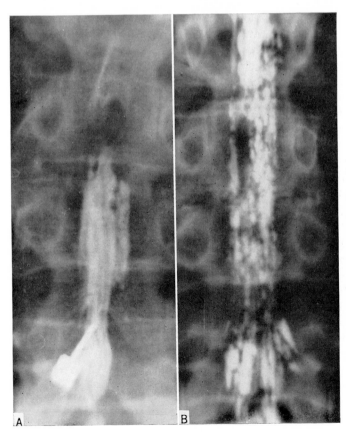

Fig. 412. Arachnoiditis in a 38-year-old man who had had staphylococcic meningitis 20 years before, treated with multiple lumbar punctures and intrathecal medication including Prontosil, sulfapyridine and bacteriophage. The flow of cerebrospinal fluid was slow, and 3 ml of Pantopaque was instilled, A. Under fluoroscopic inspection the flow was very slow, and the column broke up into many droplets which did not reunite, B.

for the arachnoiditis, and in each case the clinical diagnosis was either spinal cord tumor or herniated disc.

Plain roentgenograms of the spine usually are normal, except when opaque media such as Thorotrast or Pantopaque had been used previously. The demonstration of a previous laminectomy may be a helpful hint. The diagnosis of arachnoiditis is best made by means of myelography, but the picture is indeed a variable one. In its most characteristic form myelograms reveal a spotty irregular, loculated pattern which may extend over several segments (Fig. 412). When this exists, the passage of Pantopaque through the area is slow and irregular, but no single point of abrupt obstruction is observed. In a simpler form, and particularly when associated with large herniated discs, radiolucent streaks parallel to the long axis of the canal may be observed. These terminate in a dentate pattern at the line of the block and correspond to the thickened roots of the cauda equina. Serpentine shadows also may become visible, an indication of dilated venous channels. Associated with this may be irregular defects in the Pantopaque column caused by patches of agglutinated tissue (Fig. 410). A recurrent herniated disc can produce a confusing myelographic defect. Nevertheless, such a lesion may require operation for relief of symptoms (Fig. 413).

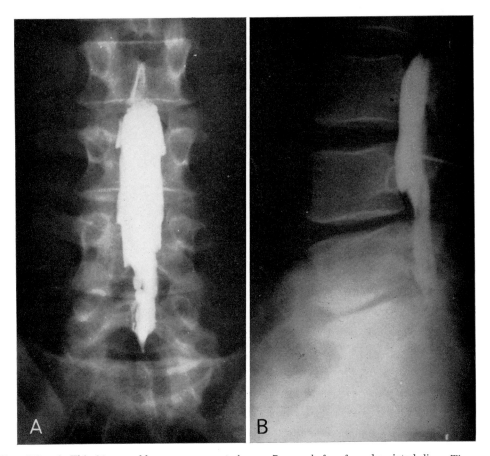

Fig. 413. A, This 36-year-old man was operated upon 7 years before for a herniated disc. There was recurrence of pain in the right lower leg. On lumbar tap a good return of fluid was obtained. On instilling the Pantopaque an irregular narrowing of the column was seen at the L4 interspace, and the sac terminated at the level of the L5 neural arch. B, On lateral examination an indentation is present in the anterior aspect of the column at L4. At operation a recurrent herniated disc was found at L4. The dural sac was enveloped in multiple adhesions attributed to periduritis, probably with concomitant localized arachnoiditis.

The most variable myelographic patterns are encountered in the lumbar or lower thoracic areas. French (1947) mentioned that recurrent arachnoiditis of the dorsal spinal canal discloses an irregular appearance of the oil column with partial or complete block. Lubin (1940), in a report of adhesive cervical arachnoiditis, included a 36-year-old man in whom combined cisternal and lumbar punctures revealed a complete block. At necropsy this patient had intradural adhesions extending from the third to the sixth cervical segments. The arachnoid was markedly hyperplastic and adherent to the cord. Cavitations within the cord were attributed to interference with its blood supply. Blumstein and Baker (1943) regarded arrest of iodized oil at multiple levels as an important indication of arachnoiditis. Of interest in their report is a case of arachnoiditis with necropsy in a 17-month-old infant.

In our cases of lumbar arachnoiditis, particularly those with previous surgery, an interesting change was an irregular tapered thinning of the caudal sac (Figs. 413 and 414). In some, irregular, small scallops were seen in the lateral margins of the distal thecal sac. The area of narrowing extended for as much as three spinal segments. In these cases sometimes recurrent herniated discs could be identified myelographically

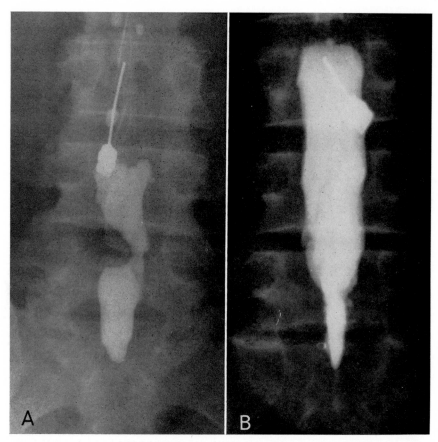

Fig. 414. *A*, A 41-year-old man who had been operated on for a herniated disc at L4. The caudal sac at that time was normal. Three years later he returned with recurrent pain much the same as noted prior to operation. A narrowed, tapered caudal sac was seen, *B*. At operation a recurrent herniated L4 disc was found, and there was degenerated discal tissue at L5 on the left side. Periduritis was present. The dura was opened and it was apparent that the arachnoid was markedly thickened, milky white in color, with adhesions between the nerve roots at the terminal end of the sac. Two small bits of thickened arachnoid were taken for biopsy.

(Fig. 413). At operation the subarachnoid space in these patients was practically obliterated, but sufficient space remained to permit seepage of the Pantopaque downwards. In others a complete block was encountered, and the distal end of the Pantopaque column assumed a variable appearance, of which the dentate-impressions of the swollen nerve roots was the most frequent. Care should be taken not to misinterpret subdural and epidural Pantopaque as evidences of arachnoiditis.

EPIDURAL ADHESIONS

We have observed several cases in which the dura at the level of the fourth and fifth lumbar intervertebral spaces was sharply kinked and adherent to the overlying ligamentum flavum. The adhesions also extended under the neural arches. In 1 of the patients, a 28-year-old woman, the clinical diagnosis was herniated disc, and myelographic examination disclosed a semicircular filling defect on the left side of the canal at the fourth lumbar interspace, which was considerably narrowed. At operation no disc protrusion was encountered and only kinking of the dural sac was observed (Fig. 415B). Before the adhesions were separated no pulsations were observed in the spinal epidural vessels below the area of adhesions. However, when the adhesions were separated pulsations returned. No reason for the presence of this lesion could be ascertained.

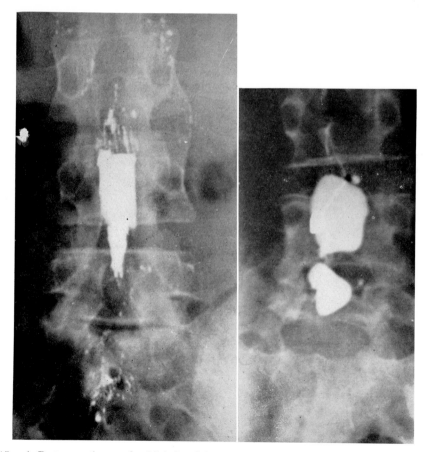

FIG. 415. *A*, Post-operative arachnoiditis involving lower lumbar spinal canal, erect myelogram. Note the tapering of the caudal end of the Pantopaque column and block at the level of the laminectomy. Operative verification. *B*, Another patient, with a myelographic defect at the fourth lumbar interspace due to inflammatory adhesions kinking the dural sac against the neural arch and ligamentum flavum.

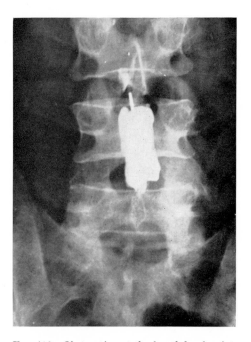

Fig. 416. Obstruction at the fourth lumbar interspace due to epidural scarring following removal of herniated disc 3 years before recurrence of back and sciatic pain. At operation the dural sac was opened and arachnoiditis involving the cauda equina also was present.

In another case, the patient had had a large protruded disc removed from the fourth lumbar interspace and a smaller one from the lumbosacral interspace. Another myelogram 3 years later revealed an obstructive defect at the fourth lumber interspace and it was believed that a recurrent herniated disc existed. There was a free flow of Pantopaque through the entire spinal canal above this level. At operation, adhesions were encountered between the dura, the ligamentum flavum and the adjacent bone, causing the defect noted on the myelograms (Fig. 416). The herniated disc had not recurred.

The latter case is much the same as described by Knuttson (1949), who mentioned that deformity may be due to postoperative hemorrhage with thickened scar formation and adhesions. In such cases the impression of a recurrent disc may be difficult to refute, and he reported 3 in which a second opera-

tion showed no recurrence of a herniated disc but only scar formation. He concluded that the deformity followed extirpation of the ligamentum flavum followed by adhesions, together with a local hernia-like protrusion of the posterolateral aspect of the dura. The coexistence of peridural scarring and arachnoiditis is not uncommon, particularly when previous discal surgery has been performed. Trauma also may be followed by localized dural thickening and adhesions unassociated with arachnoiditis (Fig. 417).

Epidural and Subdural Infections

Epidural infections usually are situated in the dorsal aspect of the spinal canal, and may extend laterally. The reason for this is that the space between the dura and the periosteum is widest in this area. The dura is so situated that its ventral aspect is close to the vertebral bodies and the intervertebral discs, so that the epidural space is narrow anteriorly. The epidural space is widest in the thoracic and lumbar regions, and is minimal in the cervical area. Below the seventh cervical segment the epidural space may reach a depth of 0.5 to 0.7 cm. Below the fourth to eighth thoracic vertebrae it again tapers and becomes shallow below the eleventh thoracic to the second lumbar vertebra. Over the remaining lumbar vertebrae the epidural space attains its greatest depth. Within the epidural space is a layer of fat, connective tissue and arterial and venous plexuses (Reeves, 1940). It is within the fatty and loose areolar tissue that infection may take place. The most common cause is metastatic abscess formation secondary to a staphylococcic infection. Other infections such as pneumococcus, B. pyocyaneus and aerobactor aerogenes have been reported, as have been mycotic infections (Miller and Hesch, 1962). Spinal epidural abscesses associated with streptococcal infections, actinomycosis, typhoid and pyocyaneus infections have also been reported in isolated cases. Heusner (1948) collected 200 cases of spinal epidural sepsis. Free

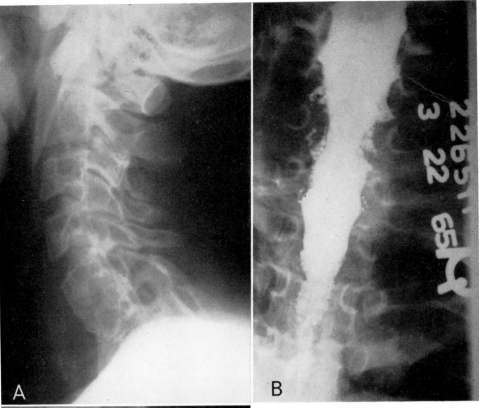

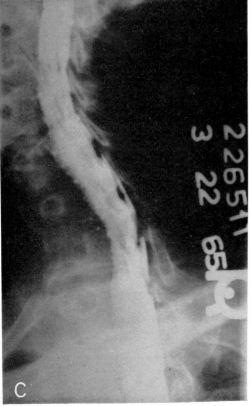

Fig. 417. A, This 47-year-old man suffered a fracture of his lower cervical spine, followed by fusion of the fifth, sixth and seventh cervical vertebrae. Three years later he complained of pain in both arms and weakness of both shoulders. Myelography revealed a waist-like broad defect, B, in the lower cervical region. The AP configuration of the thecal sac also was narrowed and humped at the level of the old fracture, C. At operation the lower cervical dura was wrapped in peridural adhesions. The laminae between C5, 6 and 7 were very thick and the ligamenta flava were obliterated. Proliferation of bone compressed the nerve roots emerging from both foramina at the fifth cervical interspace.

pus in the epidural space without granulation tissue on the dura constitutes the acute phase of an epidural abscess. If both free pus and dural granulations are found, the condition is considered subacute, and if a solid epidural fibrous mass without definite macroscopic evidence of infection is discovered, the abscess is considered chronic. In neglected lesions the pus may track into the paravertebral muscles as well as the epidural space (Echols, 1941). Browder and Meyers (1937, 1941) considered that such infections were preceded by vertebral osteomyelitis, and that the extension of the infection was from the bony structures to the epidural space. Rankin and Flotow (1946) commented that epidural infections almost never resulted from leptomeningitis perforating the dura. Raney (1939) reported 3 cases of pneumococcic epidural abscess associated with pneumonia. Rangell and Glassman (1945) described a case which they believed to be the first of this variety in which an acute spinal epidural abscess followed a diagnostic lumbar puncture within 3 days. Negrin and Clark (1952) also reported that pyogenic infections may take place by direct contaminations of the subdural space by a spinal or caudal needle puncture. They differentiated this from metastatic epidural infections by the fact that the latter overlay the cord, at least in part, while subdural extension involves particularly the region of the cauda equina. In either event surgical intervention is required practically as an emergency procedure.

Another route for epidural infections is by way of congenital dermal sinuses (Walker and Bucy, 1934). Stammers (1938) reported 2 cases of interest in children, one a 2-year-old child with a low grade meningitis due to a dermal sinus which extended from the surface of the upper sacral region through a bifid fifth lumbar vertebra to communicate with a dermoid cyst within the spinal canal. The second, a 4-year-old boy, had meningitis incident to a discharging sacrococcygeal sinus attached to the dura. Waring and Pratt-Thomas (1945) reported 2 cases in which a congenital dermal sinus was the source of meningeal infection. Mount (1949) mentioned a case of congenital dermal sinus in the upper thoracic region which led to an abscess within the spinal cord in a 10-year-old girl.

Epidural granulomas form either from chronic pyogenic infections, or with tuberculosis, syphilis, actinomycosis, or coccidioidal infections. They may also be non-infectious in nature, such as incident to foreign bodies (Bucy and Oberhill, 1950). These are mass lesions and are considered with tumors. Spinal epidural hematomas result in similar changes and are considered later in this chapter.

The clinical picture of spinal epidural infections varies with the extent of spinal cord compression and the toxicity produced by the process. In acute cases a rapid progression of pain and paralysis below the level of involvement takes place, together with local tenderness and fever. Sphincteric disturbances and motor weakness occur within a week after the onset of pain. The pain may be accentuated by bending or other movement, and associated with nuchal rigidity, a positive Kernig sign and muscular spasm. In subacute and chronic cases symptoms are slower in progression, and the total effect may simulate an intraspinal tumor.

As a rule plain film roentgenograms of the spine are not helpful. However, in suspected epidural infections, a careful study of the vertebrae for breakdown of bone pointing towards osteomyelitis should be undertaken. Stereoroentgenograms are helpful, and in doubtful instances body section radiography for detailed inspection of the vertebral bodies and the neural arches provides diagnostic information. One should not hesitate to employ myelography in patients suspected of an epidural abscess, particularly of the acute variety. In such cases the myelogram may disclose a complete block at the level of the lesion, and if this or any other filling defect is noted, immediate surgical intervention is indicated. In some instances it is advisable to instill

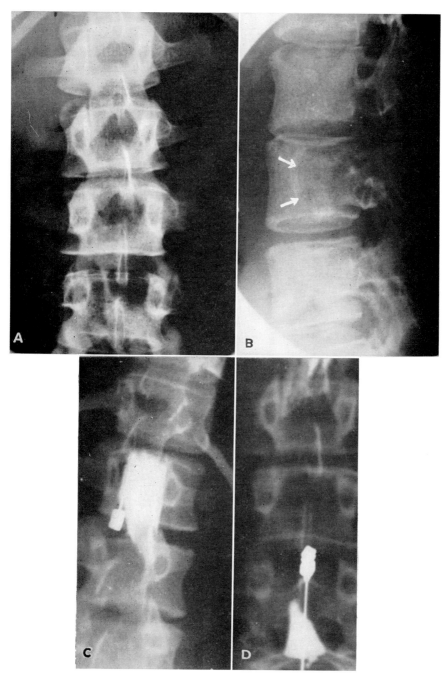

Fig. 418. *A,* Anteroposterior view of lumbar spine of 18-year-old male patient with rapidly progressing weakness and paraplegia of lower extremities. No osseous changes visible in this projection. *B,* Same case, lateral view. Note the destruction of bone in the posterior aspect of the body of the second lumbar vertebra (arrows). *C,* Pantopaque instilled at the first lumbar interspace. Note the block at the second lumbar interspace. *D,* Same case. Pantopaque instilled at lumbosacral interspace, with block at the fourth lumbar interspace. At necropsy the epidural space between the upper and lower obstructions was obliterated by an abscess emanating from the second lumbar vertebra. It could not be ascertained whether this was purely osteomyelitis, or if there was concomitantly a degeneravted neoplasm.

the Pantopaque both by the lumbar and the cisternal routes, particularly when a complete block is present and symptoms are referable to a wide area of the spinal cord. In 1 case seen by us the epidural infection extended from the fifth to the second lumber vertebrae (Fig. 418).

Freedman and Alpers (1948) observed that spinal subdural abscesses received little attention in the literature. They reported 2 such cases, with signs and symptoms characteristic of an intraspinal abscess, namely, back pain which occurred with an acute inflammatory disease, followed by signs of progressive involvement of the spinal cord, and accompanied by subarachnoid block. There was no evidence of extradural inflammation or deformity of the cord. The dura was thickened and infiltrated with inflammatory cells, with the formation of subdural abscesses. In 1 case the inflammation extended from the cervical region to the cauda equina. The authors noted that the preoperative differentiation of extradural and subdural spinal abscess is probably impossible, an observation reiterated by Negrin and Clark (1952).

Hypertrophic spinal meningitis is a disease of unknown etiology which results in thickening of the dura with a proliferation of collagenous fibers arranged in parallel rows and infiltrated with cells characteristic of a chronic inflammatory reaction (Bucy and Freeman, 1952). This occurs most frequently in the cervical and the cervicothoracic region, but may appear anywhere in the spinal canal. The lesion sometimes is localized to a single level, or extends for variable distances over the cord. In extreme instances the entire cord is involved. Because of the marked hypertrophy of the dura mater, which at times reaches over 1 cm in depth, the cord is compressed and softening and cavitation within it appears. The clinical picture varies with the location and extent of the inflammation. Plain film roentgenographic examination of the spine is normal. Myelographic examination discloses a block. Guidetti and La Torre

(1967) observed that because of the posterior position of the inflammatory process the cord and the subarachnoid space is displaced forward, permitting the Pantopaque to accumulate in a characteristic beak-shaped pattern which they regard as diagnostic.

References

Bagley, C. Jr.: Blood in Cerebrospinal Fluid, Arch. Surg., *17*, 18 and 30, 1928.

Blumstein, A. and Baker, A. B.: Arachnoiditis (Diffuse Proliferative Leptomeningitis), Ann. Int. Med., *18*, 809, 1943.

Browder, J. and Meyers, R.: Infections of Spinal Epidural Space, Am. J. Surg., *37*, 4, 1937.

————: Pyogenic Infections of the Spinal Epidural Space, Surgery, *10*, 296, 1941.

Bucy, P. C. and Freeman, L. W.: Hypertrophic Spinal Pachymeningitis, J. Neurosurg., *9*, 564, 1952.

Bucy, P. C. and Oberhill, H. R.: Intradural Spinal Granulomas, J. Neurosurg., *7*, 1, 1950.

Craig, R. L.: Effect of Iodized Poppyseed Oil on the Spinal Cord and Meninges, Arch. Neurol. & Psychiat., *48*, 799, 1942.

Davidoff, L. M., Gass, H. and Grossman, J.: Postoperative Spinal Adhesive Arachnoiditis and Recurrent Spinal Cord Tumor, J. Neurosurg., *4*, 451, 1947.

Dus, V.: Spinal Peripachymeningitis (Epidural Abscess), J. Neurosurg., *17*, 972, 1960.

Echols, D. H.: Emergency Laminectomy for Acute Epidural Abscess of Spinal Canal, Surgery, *10*, 287, 1941.

Elkington, J., St. C.: Meningitis Serosa Circumscripta (Spinal Arachnoiditis), Brain, *59*, 181, 1936.

Epstein, B. S. and Govoni, A. F.: Aspetti Mielografici della Aracnoiditis, La Radiologia Medica, *45*, 113, 1959.

Faeth, W. H.: Spinal Lithiasis, J. Neurosurg., *15*, 116, 1958.

Feder, B. H. and Smith, J. L.: Roentgen Therapy in Chronic Spinal Arachnoiditis, Radiology, *78*, 192, 1962.

Freedman, H. and Alpers, B.: Spinal Subdural Abscess, Arch. Neurol. & Psychiat., *60*, 49, 1948.

French, J. D.: Clinical Manifestations of Lumbar Spinal Arachnoiditis, Surgery, *20*, 718, 1946.

————: Recurrent Arachnoiditis in Dorsal Spinal Region, Arch. Neurol. & Psychiat., *58*, 200, 1947.

Frey, E. and Zimmerli, B.: Pantopaque Myelography in Tuberculous Arachnoiditis, Radiol. Clin., *31*, 178, 1962.

Gatzke, L. D., Dodge, H. W. and Dockerty, M. B.: Arachnoiditis Ossificans, Proc. Staff Meet., Mayo Clin., *32*, 698, 1957.

Grant, F. C.: Epidural Spinal Abscess, J.A.M.A., *128*, 509, 1945.

Guidetti, B. and La Torre, E.: Hypertrophic Spinal Pachymeningitis, J. Neurosurg., 26, 496, 1967.

Heusner, A. P.: Nontuberculous Spinal Epidural Infections, New England J. Med., 239, 845, 1948.

Hinck, V. C. and Sachdev, N. S.: Myelographic Findings in Hypertrophic Interstitial Neuritis, Am. J. Roentgenol., 95, 947, 1965.

Howland, W. J., Curry, J. L. and Butler, A. K.: Pantopaque Arachnoiditis. Experimental Study of Blood as a Potentiating Agent, Radiology, 80, 489, 1963.

Hurteau, E. F., Baird, W. C. and Sinclair, E.: Arachnoiditis Following the Use of Iodized Oil, J. Bone & Joint Surg., 36-A, 393, 1954.

Kennedy, F., Effron, A. S. and Perry, G.: The Grave Spinal Cord Paralyses Caused by Spinal Anesthesia, Surg., Gynec. & Obst., 91, 385, 1950.

Kennedy, F., Elsberg, C. A. and Lambert, C. I.: Radiculitis of the Cauda Equina, Am. J. Med. Sci., 147, 645, 1924.

Knoblich, R. and Olsen, B. S.: Calcified and Ossified Plaques of the Spinal Arachnoid Membranes, J. Neurosurg., 25, 275, 1966.

Knuttson, F.: Myelogram Following Operation for Herniated Disk, Acta radiol., 32, 60, 1949.

Krumdieck, N. and Stevenson, L.: Spinal Epidural Abscess Associated with Actinomycosis, Arch. Path., 30, 1223, 1940.

Kulowski, J. and Scott, W.: Localized Adhesive Spinal Arachnoiditis, J. Bone & Joint Surg., 16, 699, 1934.

Lewtas, N. A. and Dimant, S.: The Diagnosis of Hypertrophic Interstitial Polyneuritis by Myelography, J. Fac. Radiologists, 8, 276, 1957.

Lombardi, G., Passerini, A. and Migliavacca, F.: Spinal Arachnoiditis, Brit. J. Radiol., 35, 314, 1962.

Lubin, A. J.: Adhesive Spinal Arachnoiditis as a Cause of Intramedullary Cavitation, Arch. Neurol. & Psychiat., 44, 409, 1940.

Mackay, R. P.: Chronic Adhesive Spinal Arachnoiditis, J.A.M.A., 112, 802, 1939.

Miller, W. H. and Hesch, J. A.: Nontuberculous Spinal Epidural Abscess. Report of a Case in a 5-week-old Infant, Am. J. Dis. Child., 104, 269, 1962.

Mount, L. A.: Congenital Dermal Sinuses, J A.M.A., 139, 1253, 1949.

Mulvey, R. B.: An Unusual Myelographic Pattern of Arachnoiditis, Radiology, 75, 778, 1960.

Negrin, J. and Clark, R. A., Jr.: Pyogenic Subdural Abscess of the Spinal Meninges, J. Neurosurg., 9, 95, 1952.

Nelson, J.: Intramedullary Cavitation Resulting from Adhesive Spinal Arachnoiditis, Arch. Neurol. & Psychiat., 50, 1, 1943.

Parker, J. J. and Anderson, W. B.: Myelitis Simulating Spinal Cord Tumor, Am. J. Roentgenol., 95, 942, 1965.

Peacher, W. G. and Robertson, C. L.: Neurologic Complications Following Use of Continuous Caudal Anesthesia, Arch. Neurol. & Psychiat., 52, 531, 1944.

Ramsey, G. H., French, J. D. and Strain, W. H.: Lesions of Intervertebral Discs and Spinal Cord. In Clinical Radiology, G. U. Pillmore, editor, Philadelphia, F. A. Davis Co., 1946.

Raney, R. B.: Acute (Pneumococcic) Metastatic Spinal Epidural Abscess, Bull. Los Angeles Neurol. Soc., 4, 31, 1939.

Rangell, L. and Glassman, F.: Acute Spinal Epidural Abscess as a Complication of Lumbar Puncture, J. Nerv. & Ment. Dis., 102, 8, 1945.

Rankin, R. M. and Flothow, P. G.: Pyogenic Infection of Spinal Epidural Space, West. J. Surg., 54, 320, 1946.

Reeves, D. L.: Acute Metastatic Spinal Epidural Abscess, Arch. Surg., 41, 994, 1940.

Rexed, B.: Arachnoidal Proliferations with Cyst Formation in Human Spinal Nerve Roots at their Entry into the Intervertebral Foramina, J. Neurosurg., 4, 414, 1947.

Rosenbaum, H. E., Long, F. B., Jr., Hinchey, T. R. and Trufant, S. A.: Paralysis with Saddle Block Anesthesia in Obstetrics, Arch. Neurol. & Psychiat., 68, 783, 1952.

Schut, L. and Groff, R. A.: Redundant Nerve Roots as a Cause of Complete Myelographic Block, J. Neurosurg., 28, 394, 1968.

Schwarz, G. A. and Bevilacqua, J. E.: Paraplegia Following Spinal Anesthesia, Arch. Neurol., 10, 308, 1964.

Seaman, W. B., Marder, S. N. and Rosenbaum, H. E.: Myelographic Appearance of Adhesive Spinal Arachnoiditis, J. Neurosurg., 10, 145, 1953.

Sehgal, A. D., Gardner, W. J. and Dohn, D. F.: Pantopaque "Arachnoiditis." Treatment with Subarachnoid Injection of Corticosteroids. Cleveland Clin. Quart., 29, 177, 1962.

Slager, U. T.: Arachnoiditis Ossificans: Report of a Case and Review of the Subject, Arch. Path., 70, 322, 1960.

Smolik, A. E. and Nash, F. P.: Lumbar Spinal Arachnoiditis, Ann. Surg., 133, 490, 1951.

Stammers, F. A.: Spinal Epidural Suppuration with Special Reference to Osteomyelitis of the Vertebrae, Brit. J. Surg., 26, 366, 1938.

Stookey, B.: Adhesive Spinal Arachnoiditis Simulating Spinal Cord Tumor, Arch. Neurol. & Psychiat., 17, 151, 1927.

Symonds, C. P. and Blackwood, W.: Spinal Cord Compression in Hypertrophic Neuritis, Brain, 85, 251, 1962.

Walker, A. E. and Bucy, P. C.: Congenital Dermal Sinuses; Source of Spinal Meningeal Infection and Subdural Abscess, Brain, 57, 401, 1934.

Walker, A. E.: Toxic Effects of Intrathecal Administration of Penicillin, Arch. Neurol. & Psychiat., 58, 39, 1947.

Waring, J. I. and Pratt-Thomas, H. R.: Congenital Dermal Sinus as a Source of Meningeal Infection, J. Pediat., 27, 79, 1945.

Winkelman, N. W., Gotten, N. and Scheibert, D.: Localized Adhesive Spinal Arachnoiditis. A Study of Twenty-five Cases with Reference to Etiology, Trans. Amer. Neurol. Assn., 15, 1953.

Wise, B. L. and Smith, M.: Spinal Arachnoiditis Ossificans, Arch. Neurol., 13, 391, 1965.

Intraspinal Dermoids and Epidermoids, and Dermal Sinuses

Hamartomas are heterotopic formations composed of elements of the skin. These are dysembryonic malformations rather than true neoplasms, but are regarded as tumors because of their expanding nature. Epidermoids consist of tissues derived from the superficial layers of the skin. Dermoids originate from all layers of the skin, both epithelial and mesenchymal, with accessory cutaneous organs such as sebaceous glands, sweat glands and hair follicles. Dermal sinuses are tubular formations which have the histologic characteristics of epidermoids, dermoids or both, but which are always in direct communication with the skin. In all three conditions the viable cells form a thin capsule, and the interior is composed of cheesy amorphous masses of cornified epithelial cells. With dermoids, sebaceous matter and hair are encountered. List (1941) classified hair-containing tumors as dermoids in his study, even though microscopic examination of the cyst wall showed no cutaneous structures.

Epidermoids occur in a fairly uniform distribution over the thoracic and lumbosacral cord, and are most frequent in the region of the cauda equina. Dermoids appear to have an affinity for the lumbosacral portion of the cord. Dermal sinuses occur chiefly in the lowermost portion of the spine or in the upper thoracic region. They are seldom encountered in the cervical region. As a rule, these lesions are single, but instances of multiple epidermoids or dermoids, either due primarily to multiple origin or to implantation metastases in the subarachnoid space from rupture of the main nodule have been recorded. Intraspinal epidermoids have been reported following lumbar puncture with implantation of skin elements into the spinal canal (Manno, Eihlein and Kernohan, 1962) (Boyd, 1966).

Communications between pilonidal sinuses and intraspinal dermoids were described by Sachs and Horrax (1949), who collected 14 such cases from the literature, and considered them as congenital mechanical defects in fusion. They assembled 59 dermoid and epidermoid tumors of the spinal cord from the literature, and added 2. There were 25 teratomas of the spinal cord and of this group the dural or intradural tumor was associated with a congenital dermal sinus in 22 cases. They reported an adult male with slowly progressive neurologic symptoms who had a cervical congenital dermal sinus which communicated with the dura and an intraspinal dermoid.

Sacrococcygeal teratomas in infants and children were reviewed by Ravich and Smith (1951), who described 9 verified cases of their own. Large tumors which presented externally usually were present at birth, but sometimes remained inconspicuous until rapid growth and malignant changes appeared. Ulceration and infection may lead to death while the tumors are benign. Obstructive symptoms referable to the rectum, the ureters or urethra appear because of extrinsic pressure. Malignant transformation is relatively common, the usual type being papillary adenocarcinoma. In 3 of the cases reported by Ravich and Smith death occurred because of metastases, and in 1 there was massive local recurrence after incomplete removal of a benign teratoma.

Intraspinal epidermoid tumors occur both in children and in adults. Moore and Walker (1951) reported a 52-year-old man who had had symptoms over 20 years. Malignant degeneration in an intramedullary teratoma was reported by Lemmen and Wilson (1951) in an 11-year-old girl. Intraspinal epidermoids may be either intradural or extradural. According to Craig (1943), who gathered 43 such cases, half of the 20 cases of epidermoids were intramedullary. Of the 23 dermoids, an extramedullary situation was more frequent, and these were occasionally extradural. He reported a subpial epidermoid associated with spina bifida of the first sacral segment. Occasionally a teratoma arises within the spinal cord and extends to the extramedullary region. Such

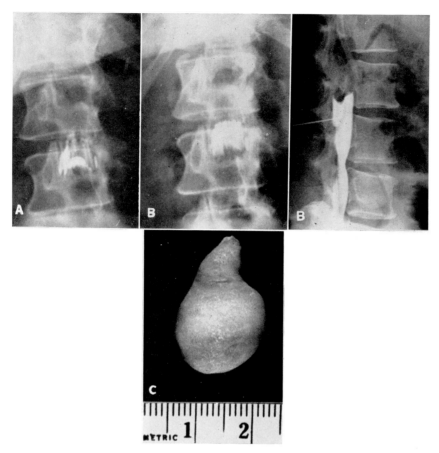

Fig. 419. *A*, Block at the level of the second lumbar vertebra, superior aspect. Cisternal instillation of Pantopaque. *B*, Pantopaque instilled from below reveals an arcuate block at the level of the second lumbar vertebra. *C*, Operative specimen, epidural epidermoid. This patient, a 22-year-old woman, had been considered hysterical for about a year.

a case was reported by Black and German (1950) in which the tumor practically filled the entire spinal canal. Mosberg (1951) commented on the high association of intraspinal tumors with other congenital anomalies during the first year of life. A rare complication of an intraspinal teratomatous tumor is arachnoiditis following a rupture of the tumor and spread of its contents in the subarachnoid space.

Plain film roentgenotrams with congenital large tumors reveal widening of the antero-posterior and lateral diameters of the spinal canal, with erosion of the pedicles and some-times arcuate indentations in the dorsal aspects of the adjacent vertebrae. Spina bifida is frequently present. These changes some-times are sufficient for diagnosis. If the plain films are normal, as is more frequent in older patients, there should be no hesitation to employ myelography, particularly if a midline dimple is present. As a rule myelo-grams in such cases will show only block rather than any characteristic defect, except perhaps for the existence of diastematomy-elia (Naffziger and Jones, 1935; Ingraham and Bailey, 1946; Hannan and Geist, 1950). In occasional cases the head of the Panto-paque column assumes a rounded or some-what scalloped configuration (Fig. 419). Occasionally the block is almost transverse in configuration (Fig. 420). At operation some tumors are well encapsulated, while others are interspersed in the roots of the cauda equina, making complete removal im-possible.

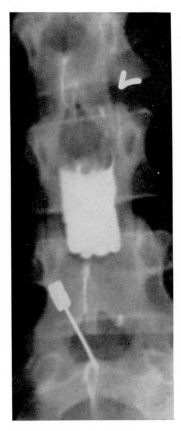

FIG. 420. Complete block due to extradural dermoid at the level of the third lumbar vertebra in a 19-year-old girl, who had been considered "neurotic" for 2 years.

Teratomas in the presacral region are fairly frequent. Mayo, Baker and Smith (1953) reported that congenital tumors accounted for 62 per cent of 161 presacral tumors gathered from the literature. Inflammatory lesions constituted 11 per cent, 11 per cent neurogenic growths, bony neoplasms constituted 9 per cent and miscellaneous growths occurred in 7 per cent. Roentgenologically these tumors manifested themselves by bone erosion and displacement of adjacent viscera. Operation and pathologic examination are usually required for definite identification. McCarty (1950) observed that the most frequent congenital presacral tumors were dermoids and teratomas, usually attached to the anterior sacral wall and the coccyx.

In a report of 40 cases of sacrococcygeal teratomas in infants and children Gross, Clatworthy and Meeker (1951) noted that the growths were more common in females. Plain roentgenograms in 37 cases showed soft tissue masses at the coccyx in 35. Calcifications were seen in 16 and distant metastases to the lungs and bones occurred in 6.

The presence of a cutaneous dimple or of a discharging sinus in the middle of the back indicates the existence of a pilonidal sinus. This in turn may indicate a coexistent intraspinal mass lesion (Fig. 146). Of equal importance is extension of infection into the spinal canal by way of a dermal sinus. As a rule these extend to the epidural space and the meninges, but rarely they enter the spinal cord. Such a case was reported by Kooistra (1942) in a 19-year-old girl with a sinus over the third thoracic vertebra. Myelograms showed a block at the third thoracic vertebra. The inner aspects of the left pedicles at this level were thinned. The clinical picture was that of a spinal cord tumor, and operation disclosed a mass extending from the seventh cervical to the fourth thoracic vertebra.

Meningitis or myelitis of an acute or chronic nature may follow infection extending along a pilonidal sinus. Craig (1943) suggested that a sterile form of meningitis may be caused by liberation of fatty acids from a cyst within the subarachnoid space. Shenkin, Hunt and Horn (1944) reported a 2-year-old infant with transverse myelitis and widespread leptomeningitis caused by infection along a pilondal sinus in direct continuity with a patent filum terminale continuous with the central canal of the spinal cord. When this is suspected, it is better to attempt gas myelography before resorting to the instillation of Pantopaque, because the injection of foreign material into an infected subarachnoid space should be avoided.

References

Black, S. P. W. and German, W. J.: Four Congenital Tumors Found at Operation within the Vertebral Canal. J. Neurosurg., 7, 49, 1950.

Boyd, H. R.: Iatrogenic Intraspinal Epidermoid, J. Neurosurg., *24*, 105, 1966.

Craig, R. L.: Epidermoid Tumor of the Spinal Cord, Surgery, *13*, 354, 1943.

French, L. A. and Peyton, W. T.: Mixed Tumors of the Spinal Canal, Arch. Neurol. & Psychiat., *47*, 737, 1942.

Gross, R. E., Clatworthy, H. W., Jr. and Meeker, I. A., Jr.: Sacrococcygeal Teratomas in Infants and Children, Surg., Gynec. & Obst., *92*, 341, 1951.

Hannan, J. R. and Geist, R. M., Jr.: Teratomatous Tumors of Spinal Canal, Am. J. Roentgenol., *63*, 875, 1950.

Hansebout, R. R. and Bertrand, G.: Intraspinal Teratoma Simulating Protruded Intervertebral Disc., J. Neurosurg., *22*, 374, 1965.

Higazi, I.: Intraspinal Epidermoids, J. Neurosurg., *20*, 805, 1963.

Ingraham, F. D. and Bailey, O. T.: Cystic Teratomas and Teratoid Tumors of the Central Nervous System in Infancy and Childhood, J. Neurosurg., *3*, 511, 1946.

Kooistra, H. P.: Pilonidal Sinuses Occurring Over Higher Spinal Segments, Surgery, *11*, 63, 1942.

Lemmen, L. J. and Wilson, C. M.: Intramedullary Malignant Teratoma of Spinal Cord, Arch. Neurol. & Psychiat., *66*, 61, 1951.

List, C. F.: Intraspinal Epidermoids, Dermoids and Dermal Sinuses, Surg., Gynec. & Obst., *73*, 525, 1941.

Manno, N. J., Eihlein, A. and Kernohan, J. W.: Intraspinal Epidermoids, J. Neurosurg., *19*, 754, 1962.

Mayo, C. W., Baker, G. S. and Smith, L. R.: Presacral Tumors, Proc. Staff Meet., Mayo Clin., *28*, 623, 1953.

McCarty, R. B.: Presacral Tumors, Ann. Surg., *131*, 424, 1950.

Moore, W. W. and Walker, E.: Intraspinal Epidermoid Tumor, J. Neurosurg., *8*, 343, 1951.

Naffziger, H. C. and Jones, O. W., Jr.: Dermoid Tumors of Spina Cord, Arch. Neurol. & Psychiat., *33*, 941, 1935.

Ravich, M. M. and Smith, E. I.: Sacrococcygeal Teratoma in Infants and Children, Surgery, *30*, 733, 1951.

Reeves, D. L.: Epidermoid (Mixed) Tumors of the Central Nervous System, J. Neurosurg., *26*, 21, 1967.

Sachs, E. and Horrax, G.: Cervical and Lumbar Pilonidal Sinus Communicating with Intraspinal Dermoids, J. Neurosurg., *6*, 97, 1949.

Shenkin, H. A., Hunt, A. D., Jr. and Horn, R. C., Jr.: Sacrococcygeal (Pilonidal) Sinus in Direct Continuity with the Central Canal of the Spinal Cord, Arch. Neurol. & Psychiat., *52*, 423, 1944.

Intraspinal Neoplasms

Aside from extradural lesions, tumors within the spinal canal occur as intramedullary growths, as extramedullary tumors, or tumors which perforate the dura and are both intradural and extradural but extramedullary. Extradural tumors arising from outside the spinal canal, such as metastatic tumors, dermoids, melanomas, sarcomas, chordomas and lymphomas behave like primary intraspinal tumors at times. While many present evidence of their existence on plain film roentgenograms, others are deceptive in that preliminary studies are regarded as within normal limits. Radioactive bone scans can be helpful when this occurs. In a review of 557 intraspinal tumors by Rasmussen, Kernohan and Adson (1940) intramedullary tumors constituted 11 per cent of the series. Extradural growths were present in 28 per cent, and combined intradural and extradural growths were present in 8 per cent. Intradural extramedullary growths made up 53 per cent of this series. Eleven years later Woltman, Kernohan, Adson and Craig (1951) reported on 979 intraspinal tumors, and in this group there were 220 intramedullary gliomas, constituting 22.5 per cent of the series. Elsberg (1941) reported that of 275 spinal cord tumors 92 were intramedullary, 175 were extramedullary and 81 were extradural. Of the extramedullary tumors perineurial fibroblastomas were the most common, and meningiomas were almost equally frequent. Both groups together composed approximately 60 per cent of the reported intraspinal neoplasms. These growths occurred either entirely within or without the dura, but the intradural situation was more frequent. Of the 59 perineurial fibroblastomas reported by Elsberg, 34 were intradural and 25 were extradural. Of his 73 meningiomas, 69 were intradural and 4 extradural. Tucker, Aramsri and Gardner (1962) collected 167 cases, including 57 neurofibromas, 47 meningiomas, 15 ependymomas and 16 gliomas. There were scattered instances of teratomas, lipomas, chordomas, lymphomas, giant cell tumors, aneurysmal bone cysts, sarcomas and cysts. Epstein (1966) reviewed 187 patients with intraspinal masses, including sporadic cases of rarities such as lymphangiomas, and malignant peritheliomas, intraspinal metastatic tumors from intracranial tumors such as those of the cerebellum and the pituitary among others. Trachdjiam and Matson (1965) reported on a 30-year experience with intraspinal tumors in infants and children encompassing 115 neoplasms, of which 63 were benign and 52 malignant. Intramedullary gliomas were most frequent, and in company with extradural sarcomas arising in paraspinal lymphoid tissue, were seen in children of all ages.

Rasmussen, Kernohan and Adson (1940) reported that 67 per cent of 163 neurofibromas were intradural and 15 per cent extradural. The remainder were both intradural and extradural. These figures indicate that the two most frequent growths within the spinal canal are usually intradural, but extradural or both extra- and intradural positions are not uncommon.

Occasionally one encounters multiple tumors within the spinal canal (Lichtenstein, 1941). This is relatively frequent in neurofibromatosis and will be mentioned again under that heading. Occasionally meningiomas may be present together with perineurial fibroblastomas. Such a case was reported by Svien, Camp and Adson (1949) in a 29-year-old woman who had three primary intraspinal tumors. Two of these were intradural meningiomas in the upper thoracic spinal canal, and a neurofibroma was removed from the cervical canal later. Twelve years thereafter the patient had symptoms referable to the cerebellopontine angle and the cervical cord. Myelography revealed a complete block at the fourth thoracic vertebra and a partial block at the first lumbar interspace. Operation disclosed an intradural extramedullary neurofibroma arising from the anterior root of the fifth cervical nerve and another from the posterior root of the right fourth lumbar nerve.

Tumors within the spinal canal, especially meningiomas, are most frequent in the thoracic region, and occur with about equal frequency in the cervical and lumbar areas. Of the 557 cases reported by Rasmussen, Kernohan and Adson (1940) 18 per cent

were in the cervical region, 54 per cent in the thoracic region and 21 per cent in the lumbar region. Seven per cent were in the sacral area. Of the 296 cases reported by Elsberg (1941) approximately the same distribution was noted. In the later report by Waltman, Kernohan, Adson and Craig (1951) it was mentioned that of 220 intramedullary gliomas 19 per cent were in the cervical region, 31 per cent in the thoracic region, 48 per cent in the lumbar region, and 2 per cent in the sacral region. This reflected the considerable number of ependymomas, which occur most frequently in the lumbar spinal canal.

The clinical picture associated with spinal cord tumors requires no elaboration here. It should be recalled that the classical picture of spinal cord impairment is not constant with tumors, and the symptoms and signs may simulate other diseases such as herniated discs (Toumey, Poppen and Hurley, 1950). The coexistence of spinal cord tumors with herniated discs is not unknown, and care in diagnosis is required to avoid overlooking such a combination of lesions. Atypical syndromes produced by extramedullary spinal cord tumors in the cervical region simulate degenerative conditions of the spinal cord. Symptoms referable to the posterior cranial fossa are produced by high cervical tumors projecting into the foramen magnum. A clinical picture simulating acute anterior poliomyelitis with intraspinal tumors in children was described by Chambers (1952). These patients suddenly became paralyzed and had stiff necks, fever and high spinal fluid cell counts. In 1 such case myelography revealed a block, and 2 others had destructive bony changes. One case was verified as an angioma.

Exaggeration of the usual lumbar lordotic curve in children sometimes is a sign of a tumor of the cauda equina (Furlow, 1950). Progressive scoliosis is observed in children with progressive neurologic disorders such as Friedreich's ataxia, syringomyelia, poliomyelitis, neurofibromatosis or various intraspinal tumors. Progressive scoliosis in patients with an already established scoliosis has been associated with paraplegia attributed to unequal growth of the dura and the spine, tight dural bands, bone spurs, and angulation of the cord. However, spinal cord tumors can occur in these children, and myelographic evidence of block is important in establishing this possibility (Curtiss and Collins, 1961).

References

Arseni, C. and Samitca, D. C.: Primary Intraspinal Tumors in Children, J. Neurosurg., *18*, 135, 1961.

Black, B. K. and Kernohan, J. W.: Primary Diffuse Tumors of the Meninges (So-called Meningeal Meningiomatosis), Cancer, *3*, 805, 1950.

Bull, J. W. D.: Spinal Meningiomas and Neurofibromas, Acta radiol., *40*, 283, 1953.

Chambers, W. R.: Intraspinal Tumors in Children Resembling Anterior Poliomyelitis, J. Pediat., *41*, 288, 1952.

Craig, W. McK., Svien, H. J., Dodge, H. W., Jr. and Camp, J. D.: Intraspinal Lesions Masquerading as Protruded Lumbar Intervertebral Disks, J.A.M.A., *149*, 250, 1952.

Cramer, F. and Hudson, F.: Myelographically Demonstrated Lesions of the Cervical Intervertebral Discs, Co-existing with Tumors and Other Causes of Myelopathy, Acta radiol., *46*, 31, 1956.

Curtiss, P. H., Jr. and Collins, W. F.: Spinal Cord Tumor—A Cause of Progressive Neurological Changes in Children with Scoliosis, J. Bone & Joint Surg., *43-A*, 517, 1961.

Dodge, H. W., Jr., Svien, H. J., Campt, J. D. and Craig, W. McK.: Tumors of the Spinal Cord Without Neurological Manifestations, Producing Low Back and Sciatic Pain, Proc. Staff Meet., Mayo Clin., *26*, 88, 1951.

Elsberg, C. A.: *Tumors of the Spinal Cord*, New York, Paul B. Hoeber, Inc., 1925.

————: *Surgical Diseases of the Spinal Cord, Membranes and Nerve Roots*, New York, Paul B. Hoeber, Inc. 1941.

Epstein, B. S.: Spinal Canal Mass Lesions, Radiol. Clin. North America, *4*, 185, 1966.

Furlow, L. T.: Lumbar Lordosis as a Sign of Cauda Equina Tumors in Children, Southern Surg., *16*, 1065, 1950.

Grant, F. C. and Austin, G. M.: The Diagnosis, Treatment and Prognosis of Tumors Affecting the Spinal Cord in Children, J. Neurosurg., *13*, 535, 1956.

Lichtenstein, B. W.: Multiple Primary Tumors of Spinal Cord, Arch. Neurol. & Psychiat., *46*, 59, 1941.

Love, J. G., Wagener, H. P. and Woltman, H. W.: Tumors of Spinal Cord Associated with Choking of Optic Disks, Arch. Neurol. & Psychiat., *66*, 171, 1951.

Meyer, B. C. and Fine, B. D.: Atypical Syndromes Produced by Extramedullary Tumor of Cervical Portion of Spinal Cord, Arch. Neurol. & Psychiat., *61*, 262, 1949.

Oberhill, H. R., Smith, R. A. and Bucy, P. C.: Neoplasms of Central Nervous System Simulating Degenerative Disease of Spinal Cord, J.A.M.A., *151*, 612, 1953.

Rand, R. W. and Rand, C. W.: *Intraspinal Tumors of Childhood*, Springfield, Charles C Thomas, 1960.

Rasmussen, T. B., Kernohan, J. W. and Adson, A. W.: Pathological Classification, with Surgical Consideration of Intraspinal Tumors, Ann. Surg., *111*, 513, 1940.

Richardson, F. L.: A Report of 16 Tumors of the Spinal Cord in Children, J. Pediat., *57*, 42, 1960.

Svien, H. J., Camp, J. D. and Adson, A. W.: Multiple Primary Tumors of the Spinal Cord, Surg. Clin. North America, *29*, 1223, 1949.

Tachdjian, M. O. and Matson, D. D.: Orthopedic Aspects of Intraspinal Tumors in Infants and Children, J. Bone & Joint Surg., *47-A*, 223, 1965.

Toumey, J. W., Poppen, J. L. and Hurley, M. T.: Cauda Equina Tumors as a Cause of the Low-Back Syndrome, J. Bone & Joint Surg., *32-A*, 249, 1950.

Tucker, A. S., Aramsri, B. and Gardner, W. J.: Primary Spinal Tumors, Am. J. Roentgenol., *87*, 371, 1962.

Weinberg, M. H.: Tumor of Spinal Cord at Foramen Magnum, Confinia Neurol., *2*, 292, 1939.

Woltman, H. W., Kernohan, J. W., Adson, A. W. and Craig, W. McK.: Intramedullary Tumors of Spinal Cord and Glimoas of Intradural Portion of Filum Terminale, Arch. Neurol. & Psychiat., *65*, 378, 1951.

INTRAMEDULLARY TUMORS

These tumors are predominantly gliomas. In a series of 35 cases reported by Woods and Pimenta (1944), 12 were ependymomas, 7 astrocytomas, 4 spongioblastomas, 2 glioblastomas, 2 mixed gliomas and 1 was an oligodendroglioma. Of the others, 2 were unclassifiable, 1 was a melanoblastoma, 3 were dermoid cysts and 1 patient had an intraspinal blood clot. They mentioned that they found references in the literature to 7 cases diagnosed as intramedullary tumors, and which at operation were intramedullary tuberculomas. Intramedullary metastatic tumors are rare.

Because of their intramedullary position, these tumors do not produce changes in the bony walls of the spinal canal unless they become large enough to compress the adjacent

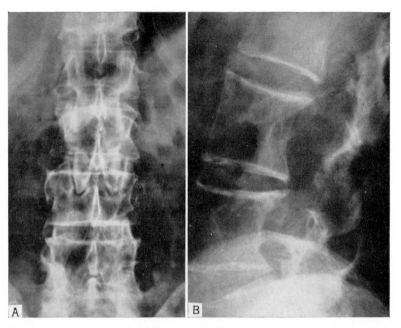

Fig. 421.   Ependymoma of lumbar spinal canal in a 62-year-old man with low back pain radiating down right leg, weakness of right leg, foot drop, and diminished sensation.   The pedicles on the left side are destroyed, and the neural arches of the midlumbar vertebrae are thinned, *A*.   The lateral projection, *B*, shows the destruction of the pedicles and of the posterior aspects of the second and third lumbar vertebrae.

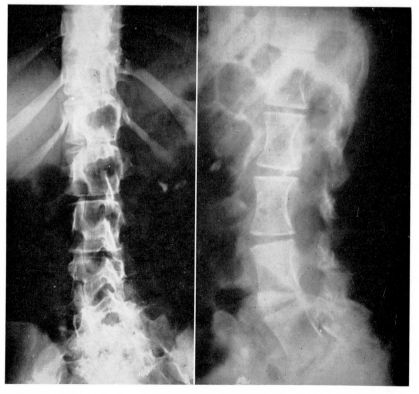

Fig. 422.   Ependymoma of the lumbar spinal canal.   This was a huge tumor which originated from the filum terminale and filled the canal, producing marked compressive changes in the dorsal aspects of the lumbar vertebrae.   This configuration is sometimes referred to as a "dog spine."

bony walls, as for example with the large ependymomas involving the cauda equina (Figs. 421 and 422). In some instances ependymomas affect the pedicles, laminae or the anterior confines of the spinal canal for one or two segments, but with more bulky tumors almost the entire lumbar spinal canal may be involved. These lesions sometimes atrophy the neural arches, spread and thin out the pedicles so that they are almost invisible, and indent the dorsal aspects of the vertebrae producing multiple scallops in this region. Ependymomas originate most often in the filum terminale, and occasionally extend up into the lower thoracic spinal canal. Horrax and Henderson (1939) mentioned an ependymoma extending from the foramen magnum to the third lumbar vertebra, the tumor measuring 38.5 cm in length. Other ependymomas are more localized, and produce an obstructive picture without bone involvement. These are more likely to appear in the thoracic region (Fig. 423). Rarely an ependymoma invades the adjacent muscles or metastasizes widely (Patterson, Campbell and Parsons, 1961). Extensive vertebral invasion by an adjacent ependymoma also has been observed. Subarachnoid hemorrhage is associated with intraspinal tumors, and filar ependymomas were reported as the cause of such bleeding in 8 out of 15 tumors (Nassar and Correll, 1968).

In the differential diagnosis of ependymomas, especially those with indentations into the dorsal aspects of the vertebral bodies, consideration must be given to those conditions which are accompanied by scalloping of the vertebrae. Among these conditions are syringomyelia and hydromyelia, extradural arachnoidal cysts, and tumors such as lipomas and dermoids. The widened spinal canal observed with arachnodactyly (Marfan's syndrome) also should be kept in mind (Nelson, 1955). The Ehler-Danlos syndrome similarly rarely produces this change. The only report of this occurrence is that of Mitchell, Lourie and Berne (1967). Neurofibromatosis not infrequently is associ-

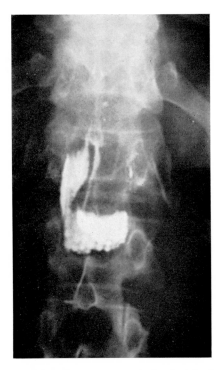

Fig. 423. Ependymoma at the level of the interspace between the twelfth thoracic and first lumbar vertebrae, with complete obstruction.

ated with scalloping, which tends to be irregular in distribution and extent, often associated with kyphoscoliosis. Among the congenital disorders with scalloping are Hurler's syndrome, Morquio's disease and achondroplasia. These are easily differentiated from the scalloping of ependymomas. Idiopathic widening of the spinal canal occasionally causes difficulty in diagnosis (Jefferson, 1958), and myelography is useful in identifying this condition, as well as many of the others mentioned. Inasmuch as ependymomas large enough to produce pronounced scalloping usually cause thinning and spreading of the pedicles and erosive changes in the neural arches, they should be readily recognized. However, those which cause only minor changes require additional investigation. Myelography in these instances can be accomplished adequately, but in the presence of really bulky tumors cautious instillation of Pantopaque is recommended.

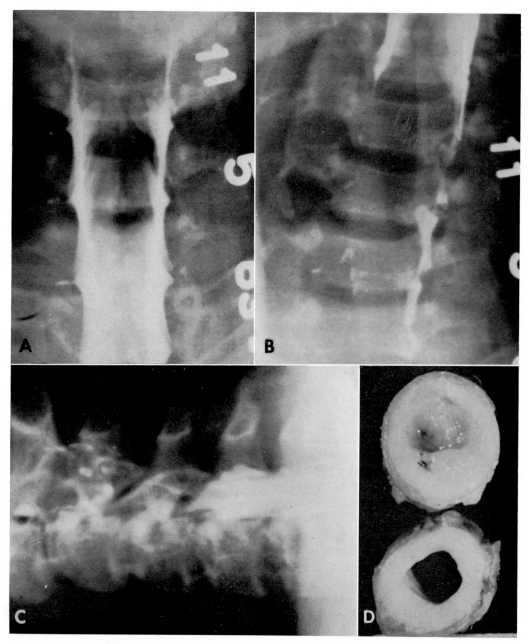

Fig. 424. *A*, Intramedullary glioma in a 13-year-old girl with pain in both arms, loss of dexterity and a stiff neck for 1 month, attributed to a fall from a bicycle. This was followed by loss of sensation of both hands and weakness of both hands and forearms. Plain spine films were normal. Myelography revealed spreading of the column in the cervical region with delay in the descent of Pantopaque, *B*. A transcervical study reveals an irregular partial block, *C*. At necropsy about 9 months after operation and intensive x-ray therapy, it was found that the tumor entered the medulla oblongata and the upper segment of the cord. A wide hydromyelia had formed in the tumefied area, *D*. This was filled with a rather gelatinous fluid. (From Epstein, B. S.: Spinal Canal Mass Lesions, Radiol. Clin. North America, *4*, 185, 1966.)

Myelography is important in the diagnosis of intramedullary tumors other than large ependymomas. The typical picture produced by gliomas is spinal canal block. The head of the column assumes a cap-like configuration on lumbar myelography, and extending cephalad from this rather shallow deformity are streaks of contrast medium to either side of the swollen spinal cord which are thin and arcuate, with flattened axillary pouches (Fig. 424). If the tumor is sufficiently large, none of the Pantopaque passes beyond the lesion. While the picture of a concave filling defect with upward extending streaks embracing a swollen area within the spinal cord is the customary picture of an intramedullary growth, it is not infrequent to observe a block as the sole myelographic indication. Atypical configurations of the Pantopaque column with irregular margins of the lateral aspects or transverse defects also occur (Fig. 425). If it is necessary to identify the superior aspect of the tumor in the presence of complete block, Pantopaque is instilled cisternally and the examination continued with the patient erect. No more than 0.5 to 1.0 ml of Pantopaque is instilled if block is suspected even if the flow of fluid is free and manometric determinations are normal or equivocal. If block is present, it is preferable not to remove excessive quantities of cerebrospinal fluid, and only that Pantopaque which can be withdrawn easily is evacuated.

Not all intramedullary gliomas produce the spindle-shaped widening of the cord considered typical of the lesion. Some are sharply localized to one level, others taper off and invade the cord at several levels, and some cystic gliomas involve a major portion of the cord (Fig. 426).

Other spinal cord lesions may be associated with bulging of the cord or obstructions within the spinal canal, and produce a similar myelographic picture. Among these are large herniated cervical discs or ridges and syringomyelia. Syringomyelia as a rule is associated with widening of the spinal cord, usually in the cervical area. This produces a widening of the radiolucent space corresponding to the spinal cord, with relatively narrow lateral channels of Pantopaque. Tuberculomas, lipomas, intramedullary blood clots, intramedullary cysts of diverse origin, and an occasional case of sarcoid present similar changes. The demonstration of a "collapsing cord" by means of gas myelography is diagnostic of syringomyelia (Westberg, 1966).

Cooper, Craig and Kernohan (1951) commented on primary extramedullary gliomas. They reported 15 such tumors along the spinal axis which apparently had no attachment to and had not arisen from seeding from a primary intramedullary or intracerebral neoplasm. Included in this series

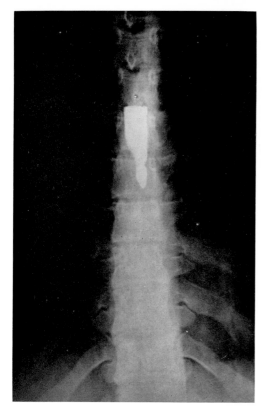

Fig. 425. Complete block with an atypical configuration in the midthoracic spine. cisternal injection of Pantopaque. Intramedullary glioma found at operation.

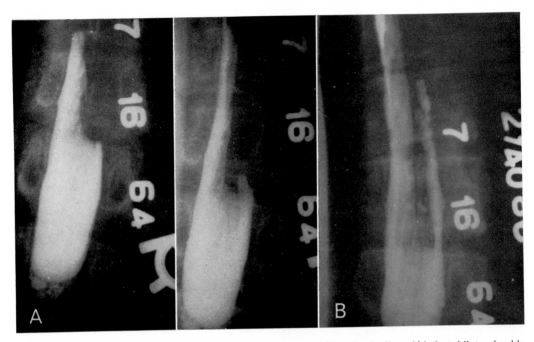

FIG. 426. *A*, This 16-year-old boy was first seen because of a stiff neck, tingling of his feet, bilateral ankle clonus and a curvature of his spine. Myelography revealed a holdup of the column at L1, with slow passage on either side of a swollen cord. The thoracic canal, *B*, filled slowly, so much so that it was felt that the Pantopaque might be subdural. The examination was repeated 2 days later with exactly the same findings. The cinemyelographic record of the myelogram was particularly striking. At operation a large tumor involving the entire thoracic cord was found. Needling disclosed cystic changes. A dorsal split of the cord was made, and a hard nodule was removed. A diagnosis of cystic diffuse glioma was made.

were 9 cases in which the growths were intra- and extradural. These authors believed that heterotopic gliomas arose from glial tissues which had been pinched off from the neuraxis in the course of its development. These unusual growths may be associated with other anomalies, such as spina bifida, club feet, undescended testes and spondylolisthesis. Prior to this communication Bailey (1936) had reported a case of astrocytoma of the leptomeninges. He too noted that glial heterotopias were accompanied by other anomalies. While it is usual to find that intramedullary growths are inoperable, not every one is hopeless. Grant (1944) reported the successful removal of a large intramedullary encapsulated astrocytoma from the upper thoracic region of an 18-year-old male. Love and Rivers (1962) reported a 31-year cure following removal of a cervical intramedullary glioma.

References

Bailey, O. T.: Relation of Glioma of the Leptomeninges to Neuroglia Nests, Arch. Path., *21*, 584, 1936.

Boijsen, E.: The Cervical Spinal Canal in Intraspinal Expansive Processes, Acta radiol., *42*, 101, 1954.

Cooper, I. S., Craig, W. McK. and Kernohan, J. W.: Tumors of Spinal Cord, Surg., Gynec. & Obst., *92*, 183, 1951.

Cuneo, H. M.: Invasion of the Spinal Cord by Malignant Schwannoma, J. Neurosurg., *14*, 242, 1957.

Grant, F. C.: Successful Removal of a Large Intramedullary Tumor of the Spinal Cord, Arch. Neurol. & Psychiat., *52*, 157, 1944.

Haft, H., Ransohoff, J. and Carter, S.: Spinal Cord Tumors in Children, Pediatrics, *23*, 1152, 1959.

Horrax, G. and Henderson, D. G.: Encapsulated Intramedullary Tumor Involving Whole Spinal Cord from Medulla to Conus, Surg., Gynec. & Obst., *68*, 814, 1939.

Jefferson, A.: Localized Enlargement of Spinal Canal in Absence of Tumour, Congenital Abnormality, J. Neurol., Neurosurg. & Psychiat., *18*, 305, 1955.

King, A. B.: Intramedullary Epidermoid Tumor of the Spinal Cord, J. Neurosurg., *14*, 353, 1957.

Love, J. G. and Rivers, M. H.: Thirty-one-year Cure Following Removal of Intramedullary Glioma of Cervical Portion of Spinal Cord, J. Neurosurg., *19*, 906, 1962.

Mitchell, G. E., Lourie, H. and Berne, A. S.: The Various Causes of Scalloped Vertebrae With Notes on Their Pathogenesis, Radiology, *89*, 67, 1967.

Moll, M. H.: Diagnosis of Spinal Block by Means of Lipiodol, J. Neurol. & Psychopath., *13*, 14, 1932.

Nassar, S. I. and Correll, J. W.: Subarachnoid Hemorrhage Due to Spinal Cord Tumors, Neurology, *18*, 87, 1968.

Nelson, T. D.: Marfan Syndrome with Special Reference to Congenital Enlargement of the Spinal Canal, Brit. J. Radiol., *31*, 561, 1958.

Patterson, R. H., Campbell, W. G., Jr. and Parsons, H.: Ependymoma of the Cauda Equina with Multiple Visceral Metastases, J. Neurosurg., *18*, 145, 1961.

Shenkin, H. A. and Alpers, B. J.: Gliomas of Spinal Cord, Arch. Neurol. & Psychiat., *52*, 87, 1944.

Walker, E. A., Jessica, C. M. and Marcovich, A. W.: Myelographic Diagnosis of Intramedullary Spinal Cord Tumors, Am. J. Roentgenol., *45*, 321, 1941.

Wells, C. E. C., Spillane, J. D. and Bligh, A. S.: The Cervical Spinal Canal in Syringomyelia, Brain, *82*, 3, 1959.

Westberg, G.: Gas Myelography and Percutaneous Puncture in the Diagnosis of Spinal Cord Cysts, Acta radiol. Supp., *252*, Stockholm, 1966.

Woods, W. W. and Pimenta, A. M.: Intramedullary Lesions of Spinal Cord, Arch. Neurol. & Psychiat., *52*, 383, 1944.

Wortzman, G. and Botterell, E. H.: A Mobile Ependymoma of the Filum Terminale, J. Neurosurg., *20*, 164, 1963.

INTRASPINAL LIPOMAS

These tumors constitute approximately 1 per cent of all intraspinal growths, and appear either as intradural or extradural masses. Frequently they attain considerable size and manifest themselves by compression of the spinal cord and cauda equina during infancy, puberty or during the third to fifth decades (Taniguchi and Mufson, 1950). As a rule symptoms are slowly progressive. Ehni and Love (1945) reviewed 29 cases of intradural lipomas and found that they occurred chiefly in the cervical and thoracic regions, most often on the dorsal aspect of the cord. These growths are composed of adult adipose tissue which may be accompanied by an excessive amount of fibrous stroma and vascular and other elements. There is a tendency, particularly in lumbar lesions in infancy, for such tumors to be accompanied by congenital deformities, such as sacral malformations and meningoceles. Wycis (1953) reported a 48-year-old woman who also had a Klippel-Feil deformity. The lipoma was of considerable size and had practically replaced the spinal cord tissue. Wycis postulated that the Klippel-Feil deformity might be one which involved both the skeletal and neurogenic tissues, and that the intramedullary lipoma might have arisen from misplaced cell rests accompanying a myelodysraphia. Of particular interest is that there was a paucity of symptoms even though the tumor was so large that it practically obliterated the spinal cord tissue.

Crosby, Wagner and Nichols (1953) reported a lipoma situated in an extramedullary subpial location. When this patient was first operated upon it was believed that the tumor was intramedullary, but close inspection and a second operation disclosed that it was actually extramedullary. The tumor was so enveloped in the spinal cord that its exact location was determined only after the most careful scrutiny. They postulated an extramedullary origin for this growth, and that lipomas may be operable even though at first inspection this seems improbable. Wilson, Bartle and Dean (1940) reported a 21-year-old woman with an intradural spinal lipoma and mentioned that the tumor probably arose beneath the pia arachnoid. The suggestion that these tumors are actually extramedullary but intrude into the substance of the cord because of close apposition has considerable clinical importance. However those lipomas which are enmeshed in the roots of the cauda equina, particularly when associated with myelomeningoceles or meningoceles, have an ominous prognosis and may actually be harmed by surgical intervention.

Lassman and James (1967) reported their operative findings in 26 patients with lumbosacral lipomas. In all there was a superficial fatty tumor over the lumbosacral spine in or near the midline. The larger masses were found in children, while smaller tumors were present in adults. There were 15 children and 4 adults in their group, and all showed evidence of defects in the lumbosacral spine including widening of the interpedicular distances and some dysgenesis of the sacrum. On myelographic examination various abnormalities such as diastematomyelia, a low-placed conus or filling defects were noted. Every case presented some myelographic abnormality. At operation the subcutaneous lipoma was found in continuity with the conus, the filum terminale or the cauda equina in 18 patients. The other 8 had abnormalities affecting the neural tissue and were amenable to surgical alleviation. They found no correlation between the clinical state and the type of anomaly found at operation to serve as a guide for operation, and favored surgical removal of the lipoma and deep exploration of the thecal sac as a preventive measure.

Spinal lipomas also occur extradurally, and as a rule these present a more acute clinical picture. Extradural lipomas are sometimes seen in the thoracic region, but appear in the lumbar region as well, particularly involving the cauda equina. These are often accompanied by other congenital malformations such as deformities of the sacrum, myelomeningoceles and subcutaneous deposits of fat overlying the lumbosacral region which may extend into the spinal canal. These form lipomeningoceles which enter the dura and entwine about the cauda equina. Lipomas of the lumbar canal can tether the conus, so that it is low in the spinal canal. This can be identified myelographically by demonstrating the low position of the conus or identifying the anterior spinal artery in an abnormally caudad location. The nerve roots are directed upwards because of the caudal displacement of the conus and the abnormally shortened cauda equina. Symptoms attributable to tethering of the conus

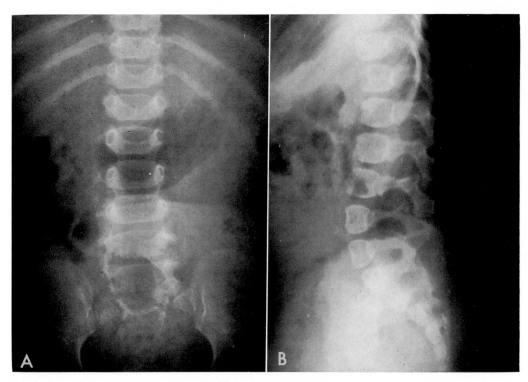

FIG. 427. *A*, A 2-month-old infant with a large lipomeningocele involving the lumbar canal. A subcutaneous lipoma was present over the lumbar area. The neural arches of L5 and S1 are deformed and the pedicles are spread. On the lateral view, *B*, a marked widening of the canal is present and the fourth and fifth lumber vertebrae are hypoplastic. Verified at operation.

together with cauda equina and conus deficits include progressive neurologic deficiencies of the legs and sphincter disturbances. These tumors sometimes produce symptoms slowly, so that they attain large size before the mild neurologic deficit becomes apparent.

Plain film roentgenograms sometimes are helpful in the identification of intraspinal lipomas, particularly large ones in the lumbosacral region. Because of the bulk of the lesion indentations appear in the dorsal aspects of the vertebral bodies and the spinal canal becomes widened, with increased interpedicular distances and thinning of the neural arches. Concomitant sacral malformations and congenital defects of the lumbar spine are relatively frequent in infants. Rarely the fatty content of the tumor results in a radiolucency which can be seen on plain films (Roller and Pribram, 1965). Extension of a lipoma into the thoracic cavity was reported by Maier (1962) who described a 17-month-old girl with a block at the T7 level together with an opacity in the left upper chest and erosion of the posterior portions of the left fourth and fifth ribs due to extension of the lipoma into the chest in dumbbell fashion.

The variability in the size of intraspinal lipomas is wide. Some are small, so much so that they resemble herniated discs myelographically (Fig. 428). Others are relatively localized, and present a myelographic picture of an intramedullary tumor (Fig. 429). Those which extend over many segments can cause considerable difficulty in diagnosis because of their tendency to cause obstruction. It may become necessary in these patients to resort to cisternal instillation of Pantopaque. Halaby, Peterson and Leaver (1964) suggested that a combination of a large cord mass and block in the absence of neurologic deficits of comparative severity might be considered characteristic of lipoma.

In differential diagnosis consideration must be given to slow-growing gliomas, syringomyelia, subarachnoid and intraspinal cysts, degenerative diseases of the spinal cord and other neoplastic or congenital lesions.

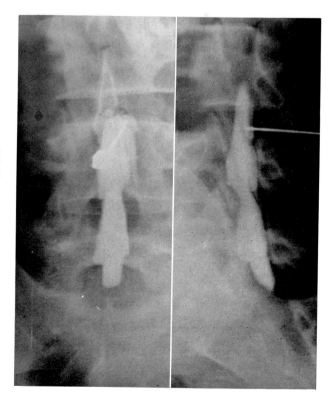

FIG. 428. Myelographic defect at the fourth lumbar interspace on the left side, anteroposterior and lateral myelograms. The clinical picture in this 45-year-old male was characteristic of a herniated disc. At operation an extradural lipofibroma was encountered. Complete relief of symptoms followed removal of the tumor.

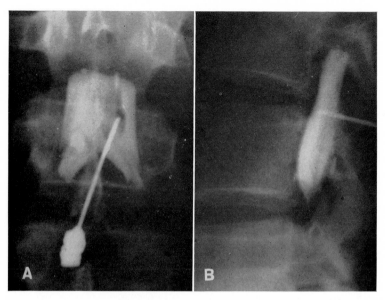

Fig. 429. Intradural lipoma involving the conus in the upper lumbar region in a 41-year-old man with a subcutaneous lipoma over the midline lumbosacral area. No pain or motor loss. Diminished sensation in sacrococcygeal region, penis and scrotum. The patient had difficulty in voiding and catheterized himself for relief. No loss of potency. Lumbar taps in the lower lumbar interspaces were not productive of a good flow of fluid. At the first interspace a good flow was obtained, and 1.5 ml of Pantopaque was instilled. Note the complete block, and the spreading of the Pantopaque column.

References

Bassett, R. C.: Neurologic Deficit Associated with Lipomas of the Cauda Equina, Ann. Surg., *131*, 109, 1950.

Bucy, P. C. and Ritchey, H.: Klippel-Feil's Syndrome Associated with Compression of the Spinal Cord by an Extradural Hemangiolipoma, J. Neurosurg., *4*, 476, 1947.

Caram, P. C., Scarcella, G. and Carton, C. A.: Intradural Lipomas of the Spinal Cord, J. Neurosurg., *14*, 28, 1957.

Crosby, R. N., Wagner, J. A. and Nichols, P., Jr.: Intradural Lipoma of Spinal Cord, J. Neurosurg., *10*, 81, 1953.

Dubowitz, V., Lorber, J. and Zachary, R. B.: Lipoma of the Cauda Equina, Arch. Dis. Childhood, *40*, 207, 1965.

Ehni, G. and Love, J. G.: Intraspinal Lipomas, Arch. Neurol. & Psychiat., *53*, 1, 1945.

Halaby, F. A., Peterson, R. B. and Leaver, R. C.: Spinal Lipoma, Am. J. Roentgenol., *92*, 1293, 1964.

Lassman, L. P. and James, C. C.M.: Lumbosacral Lipomas, J. Neurol. Neurosurg. & Psychiat., *30*, 174, 1967.

Maier, H. C.: Extradural and Intrathoracic Lipoma Causing Spinal Cord Compression, J.A.M.A., *181*, 610, 1962.

Roller, G. J. and Pribram, H. F. W.: Lumbosacral Intradural Lipoma and Sacral Agenesis, Radiology, *84*, 507, 1965.

Slade, H. W. and Vinas, F. J.: Intramedullary Lipoma of the Spinal Cord, Neurology, *6*, 449, 1956.

Talbert O. R. and Simmons, C. N.: Spinal Leptomeningeal ("Pial") Lipoma, Neurology, *11*, 645, 1961.

Taniguchi, T. and Mufson, J.: Intradural Lipoma of Spinal Cord, J. Neurosurg., *7*, 584, 1950.

Wycis, H. T.: Lipoma of Spinal Cord Associated with Klippel-Feil Syndrome, J. Neurosurg., *10*, 675, 1953.

Yashon, D. and Beatty, R. A.: Tethering of the Conus Medullaris Within the Sacrum. J. Neurol., Neurosurg. & Psychiat., *29*, 244, 1966.

Intradural Extramedullary Tumors

These constitute about 60 per cent of all spinal tumors, and are principally perineurial fibroblastomas or meningiomas. In 275 such cases reported by Elsberg (1941), 159 were intradural, mostly in the cervical and thoracic regions. In a review of 179 cervical intraspinal neoplasms, Webb, Craig and Kernohan (1953) found 68 intradural extramedullary growths. Neurofibromas constituted 38.5 per cent and meningiomas

29.9 per cent. Vascular tumors accounted for 8.4 per cent of their cases. Extradural meningiomas and neurofibromas also were observed. Of the 73 meningiomas reported by Elsberg (1941) 69 were intradural and 4 were extradural. Five of the 59 perineurial fibroblastomas were extradural. Recent surveys of spinal cord tumors including those of the meninges report about the same incidence (Lombardi and Passirini, 1961, 1964) (Epstein, 1966).

Meningiomas. These tumors arise from cells of the spinal arachnoid, usually in the villi which lie close to the crossing nerve roots (Fig. 430). The arachnoidal attachment of these neoplasms may be minute. Infrequently a meningioma penetrates the dura and becomes extradural, with disappearance of its arachnoidal pedicle. The pia arachnoid may be incorporated in the tumor, and occasionally malignant varieties may cross the pial barrier and actually invade the cord. Combined intra- and extradural meningiomas have been observed. Rarely a meningioma actually invades adjacent bone (Hannan, Hughes and Mulvey, 1949). Of 130 cases of intraspinal meningiomas reported by Brown (1942), 78 per cent were in the thoracic region, 18 per cent in the cervical region, and 4 per cent in the lumbar and lumbosacral regions. There were 8 varieties distributed as follows: meningothelial, 56 per cent; fibroblastic, 28 per cent; psammomatous, 15 per cent; osteoblastic, 4 per cent; lipomatous, 2 per cent; chondromatous and melanomatous each 1 per cent; and malignant, 6 per cent.

Meningiomas occur more often in middle-aged females, the incidence varying from 66 to 80 per cent in different series.

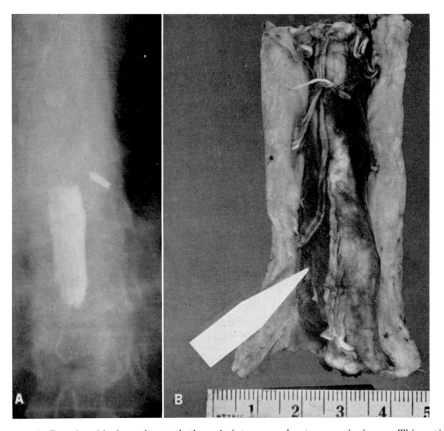

FIG. 430. *A*, Complete block at the tenth thoracic interspace due to a meningioma. This patient had complained of back pain for 2 years, and had been paralyzed for several months before myelography was performed. *B*, Photograph of tumor *in situ*, necropsy specimen. The cord is deviated to the left.

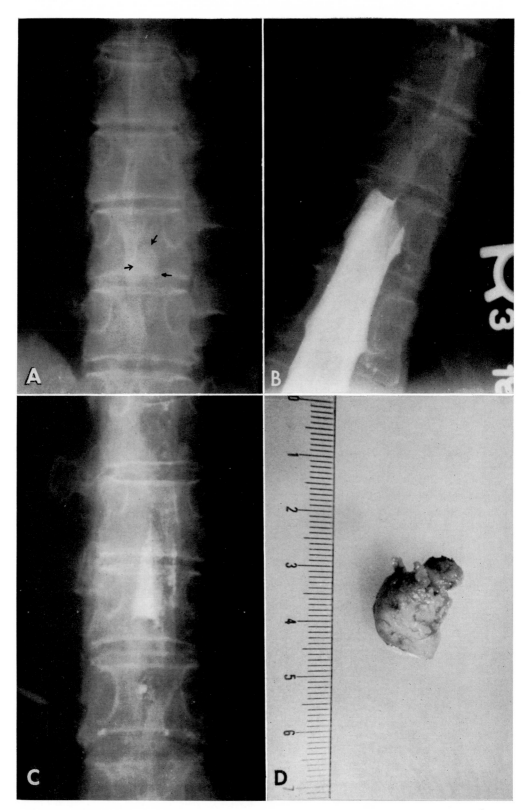

FIG. 431. *A*, This patient, a 57-year-old woman, had numbness of both legs for 5 years, considered to be due to degenerative disease. Manometric examinations were normal, and the CSF protein content was 50 mg per cent. On plain film examination a calcareous deposit is seen overlying the inferior margin of T10 (arrows). Myelography revealed a block with a cup-shaped defect at this level, *B*. A small quantity of Pantopaque got past the lesion, and on return flow the upper level of the tumor is visible, *C*. At operation a psammomatous meningioma situated laterally in an intradural position was removed.

A typical intraspinal meningoma occurs as a well-demarcated, spherical or ovoid smooth or lobulated encapsulated tumor. Its capsule is quite tough and broadly attached to the dura. Sometimes it is fixed to the dentate ligament and adjacent arachnoid. with the nerve roots drawn tautly across the tumor (Fig. 430). Occasionally no dural attachment can be identified. It occurs as a single lesion, although occasionally multiple meningiomas do occur (List, 1943) (Rand, 1952). The tumor seldom invades the extradural fat or adjacent bone, and dumbbell configurations are observed only rarely. Meningiomas extend over one, two or sometimes three interspaces, and are usually dorsolateral in position. Occasionally they occur ventrolaterally or encircle the spinal cord. On cut section they are fleshy, firm and relatively avascular, although the surrounding tissues may become highly vascularized. Fine, gritty calcareous particles and sometimes larger spicules of bone or calcium are occasionally present, the calcifications occurring as a rule as small, concentrically laminated psammoma bodies (Fig. 431).

High cervical meningiomas may intrude into the foramen magnum and cause increased intracranial pressure by obstructing the cerebrospinal fluid circulation. Smolik and Sachs (1954) reported 6 such cases out of 234 verified spinal cord tumors. Meningiomas in the cervical spinal canal at the first or second cervical segments are difficult to localize on the basis of the clinical picture along. Grant (1940) mentioned that they might simulate degenerative diseases of the spinal cord. Epstein and Davidoff (1946) noted the presence of low cervical and shoulder pain as well as symptoms referable to the lower limbs in patients with high cervical meningiomas. Cervico-occipital pain, weakness of the ipsilateral arm, atrophy of the small hand muscles, spastic paresis, altered position sense in the arms also are present. Stein, Leeds, Taveras and Pool (1963) distinguished between meningiomas arising above the foramen magnum extending into the upper cervical spinal canal as craniospinal in location (Fig. 432), and those extending into the posterior fossa from the upper cervical spinal canal as spinocranial in position. If sufficient pressure is exerted in the posterior cranial fossa, the symptom pattern can be confusing in the event of a high cervical tumor. However, spinocranial lesions usually extend relatively slightly craniad. The outline of high cervical spinal canal tumors occasionally can be made out on a plain film roentgenogram (Fig. 442). Protrusions into the upper cervical canal frequently can be discerned during pneumoencephalography or cervical air myelography (Fig. 433).

The clinical picture encountered with meningiomas in the thoracic spinal canal is predicated on cord pressure, and as a rule the approximate level of the lesion can be identified clinically. Tumors in the lower lumbar area cause confusing neurologic pictures, often indistinguishable from herniated discs.

Dyke (1941) estimated that 25 per cent of extramedullary intradural tumors might be localized by changes in the contiguous vertebrae. Buchstein (1941) observed that plain film changes with meningiomas was considerably less than seen with perineurial fibroblastomas, only 10 per cent of the meningiomas producing visible changes as compared with 45 per cent of perineurial fibroblastomas. In our experience meningiomas rarely produced bony alterations. Psammomatous meningiomas may contain sufficient calcification to indicate their presence radiologically (Fig. 431). In a series of 130 cases reported by Brown (1942), 15 per cent were either of this variety or osteoplastic in type, and 4 per cent of these were visible on plain roentgenograms. Bray (1942) suggested that body section roentgenograms might help to identify such calcifications, which he found in about 10 per cent of meningiomas. He reported 3, including 2 meningiomas, 1 psammomatous and the other osteoplastic. The third case was a hemangioblastoma containing calcium. The calcifications appeared as olive-shaped

41

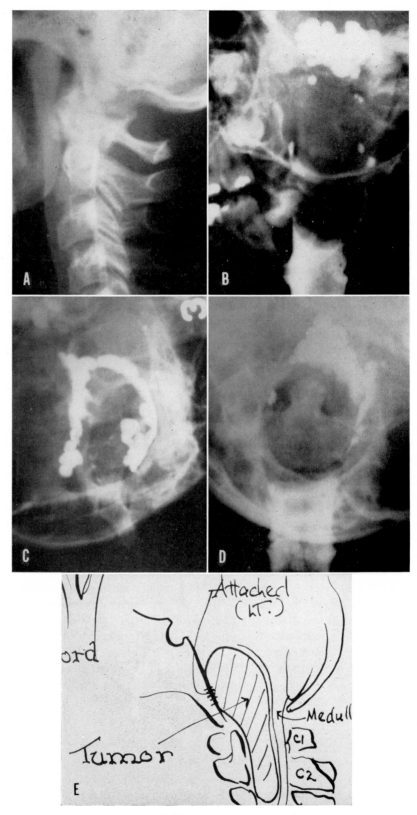

Fig. 432   (*Legend on opposite page.*)

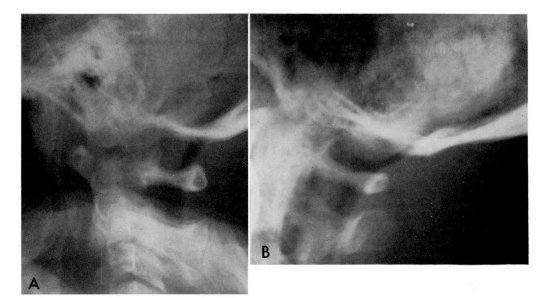

FIG. 433. *A*, Lateral neck film taken during lumbar pneumoencephalography in a 7-year-old boy with a posterior fossa astrocytoma. Herniation of the cerebellar tonsil to the level of the neural arch of C1 is present. *B*, Air myelogram showing cervical tonsillar herniation in a 16-year-old girl with aqueductal stenosis.

opacities within the spinal canal. No associated pedicle thinning or foraminal enlargement was observed. In a case of a cervicothoracic meningioma reported by Osgood, Arnett and Lewy (1944), calcification measured 4 cm in length and 2 to 5 mm in thickness. Culver, Concannon and Koenig (1949) presented 5 cases out of a series of 15 meningiomas in which homogeneous increased density indicative of tumoral calcification was present, and was best seen on the lateral roentgenograms.

Myelography is most important in the diagnosis of intraspinal meningiomas. If a block is suspected, lumbar instillation of about 1 ml of Pantopaque is sufficient. Tumors situated anterolaterally or postero-laterally can be identified by indentation of the column and contralateral shifting of the spinal cord on the corresponding side. Anteroposterior localization is made on the lateral projections. Since many meningiomas are situated in the thoracic area, one must obtain an adequate flow to the upper thoracic and cervical levels. This may be rather difficult in patients with exaggerated thoracic curvatures, but this usually can be overcome by placing the patient in a lateral or if necessary, in the supine position. Meningiomas often produce complete or almost complete block, so that the diagnosis usually is established easily. If the uppermost extent of the lesion is to be determined in the presence of com-

---

FIG. 432. Cervico-occipital meningioma in a 14-year-old boy who complained of a stiff neck, pain in the left side of his neck, weakness of all limbs, and altered gait for 8 months. Plain film examination (*A*) shows the usual cervical curve to be maintained. Of particular interest is an indentation into the anterior aspect of the occipital bone just behind the foramen magnum and an elongation of the superior notch of the lamina of C1. Myelography (*C*) reveals block at the interspace between C2 and 3. Pantopaque enters the posterior fossa, and the upper aspect of the tumor is identified on caudad flow (*C* and *D*). The tumor (*E*) extends high into the posterior fossa in an antero-lateral position.

plete obstruction, cisternal instillation of Pantopaque sometimes is required. This becomes quite important if multiple tumors are suspected. Usually it is possible to get a few droplets of Pantopaque above the lesion, so that its cephalad border is identified on placing the patient erect (Fig. 431).

If the tumor is only partially obstructive, the examiner must be alert to identify small arcuate defects in the head of the Pantopaque column which may be quite transient. The entire canal should be checked, up to and including the foramen magnum. The upper and lower limits of the tumor can be determined readily when partly obstructive lesions are present by observing the downward flow of Pantopaque. Cinemyelograms are helpful.

In a review of 26 spinal canal meningiomas, complete block was observed in 12 of 19 patients with thoracic lesions. The Pantopaque column assumed a varying cap-

like configuration of its cephalad end, and it was often possible to get a few drops past the tumor. Displacement of the cord was identifiable by filling of the space between the dura and the cord resulting in a wedge-shaped accumulation of contrast material (Fig. 431*B*). Centrally placed meningiomas, especially if large, cause a divergence of the lateral margins of the column somewhat like that seen with intramedullary tumors, other extramedullary tumors and occasionally with large compressive lesions such as spondylosis or tumors. Lumbar canal meningiomas usually did not produce block. In the lower cervical canal block was again the most common manifestation. Tumors high in the cervical region displaced the column dorsad from the dens and indented its lateral aspect.

In differential diagnosis the possibility of a neurofibroma is usually considered first. If the neurofibroma is of about the same

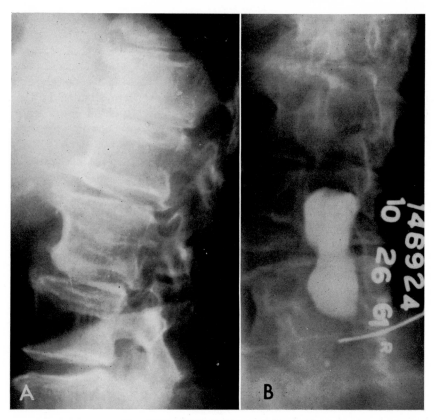

Fig. 434. (*Continued on opposite page.*)

size as one would expect a meningioma to be, the differential diagnosis is difficult. However, small neurofibromas, especially those seen with multiple lesions, often are small and are completely enveloped in the contrast material. This produces a round defect, often multiple, and can be distinguished with considerable accuracy (Fig. 437). Other lesions, depending on the location of the tumor, include a wide variety of lesions within the cord, extradural lesions such as vertebral metastatic tumors, epidural metas-

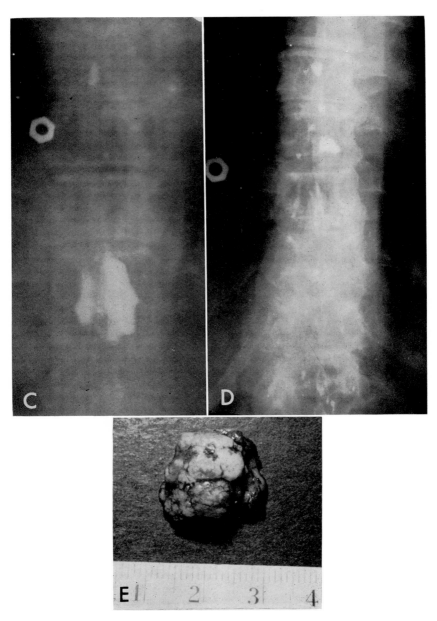

FIG. 434. *A*, A 65-year-old woman with low back pain for 2 weeks, with paresis of the left leg. A sensory level was found at about T9. The lumbosacral spine reveals marked spondylotic change. Difficulty in spinal tap was encountered, and only 3 ml of Pantopaque were instilled. A block was encountered at L2, *B*. However, a small amount got above this region, and an extramedullary lesion was found at T8 on cephalad and caudad flow, *C* and *D*. At operation a meningioma was removed from this site, *E*.

tases, or herniated thoracic discs, cranio-spinal tumors, Arnold-Chiari malformation, pronounced cervical spondylosis, or other lesions producing downward displacement of the cerebellar tonsils, clivus tumors, and degenerative diseases.

The benefits of surgical removal of menin-giomas are obvious. It is less well known, however, that meningiomas may recur. Three such cases were reported by Cushing and Eisenhardt (1938), recurring 2 years in 2 cases and 9 years after removal in the third. Davidoff, Gass and Grossman (1947) reported the recurrence of a meningioma 14 years after the removal of a lesion from the lower thoracic region. One should also recognize the possibility of other coexistent lesions. Freedman, Feiring and Davidoff (1949) reported metastases from carcinoma of the breast together with intraspinal

meningiomas in three cases. The coexistence of spondylosis and intraspinal tumors can be overlooked unless the clinical and radiologic pictures are correlated. In several elderly patients we have encountered marked mye-lographic defects in the lumbar canal, in some approaching complete block, with a clinical picture of a thoracic canal lesion. In these patients Pantopaque must be intro-duced above the block to outline the cervical and thoracic canal. Unless this is done one may easily overlook an intraspinal tumor (Fig. 434).

Neurofibromatosis and Perineurial Fibro-blastomas. This hereditary condition occurs in both sexes about equally, and is manifest either from infancy or becomes apparent later in life. Many patients are unaware of their affliction until the appearance of char-acteristic tumors about the time of puberty.

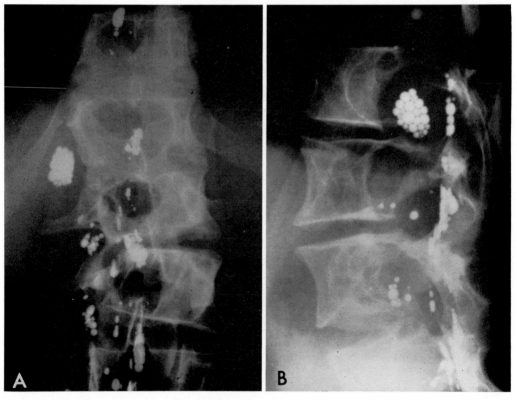

FIG. 435. A 32-year-old man with generalized neurofibromatosis. Progressive weakness for 1 year had been followed by inability to wal. The plain films disclosed multiple excavations in the lumbar vertebrae. Myelography revealed that these were caused by cysts communicating with the subarachnoid space, with Pantopaque extending from the thecal sac into the paravertebral cysts in both the frontal, *A*, and the lateral projections, *B*.

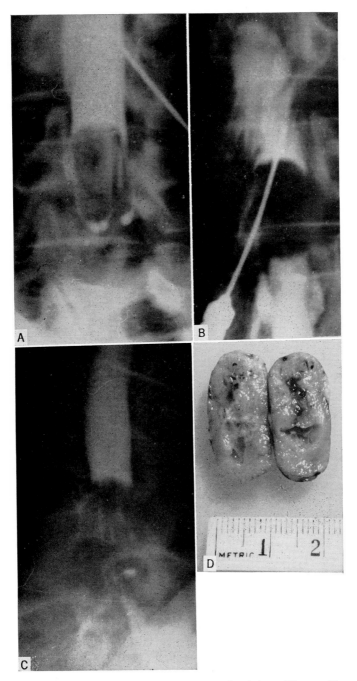

Fig. 436. Intradural neurofibroma at the fourth lumbar level in a 58-year-old woman considered "neurotic" for several years. Bizarre reflex changes and intermittent pain initiated the myelographic examination. A partial block was found at the level of the superior aspect of the fourth lumbar vertebra, A, and a cap-like deformity was demonstrated at its upper and lower levels, B and C. The tumor, D, was attached by several filaments to one of the roots of the cauda equina.

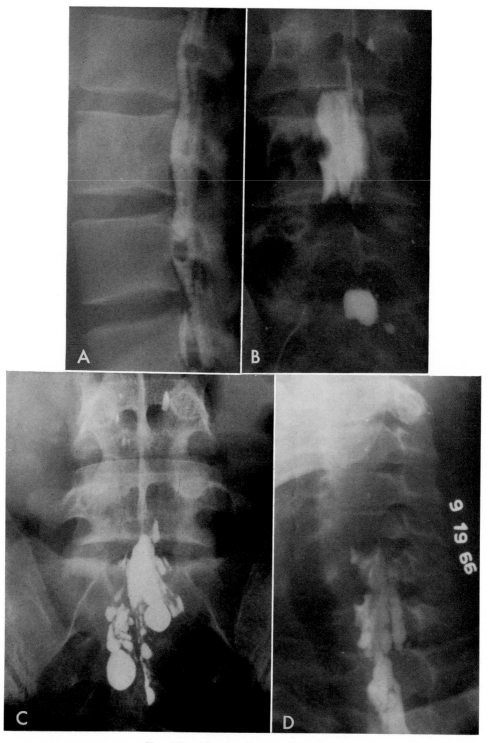

FIG. 437.   (Continued on opposite page.)

Neurofibromatosis is included among the neurocutaneous syndromes such as tuberous sclerosis, Sturge-Weber syndrome and von Hippel-Lindau disease. It is recognized readily in its completely developed form by the presence of multiple tumors along the peripheral nerves, skin pigmentation and a variety of concomitant congenital malformations, among which are meningoceles, glaucoma, spina bifida and mental defects (Uhlmann and Grossman, 1940). A great variety of skeletal changes appear, including abnormalities in growth and irregular lytic defects in the appendicular and axial skele-ton. Noteworthy among these are defects in the orbital walls and the sphenoid, irregularities in growth of the tibia and fibula producing bowing, unequal lengths and pseudarthrosis of the lower limbs, soft tissue swellings and asymmetry of the face and limbs. Pronounced changes may appear in the vertebral column (Fig. 435). Bony changes are present in about 7 per cent of cases (Friedman, 1944; Mackenzie, 1950). A variation of this condition occurs with only skin pigmentation and minor skeletal anomalies.

Intraspinal neurofibromas without skeletal

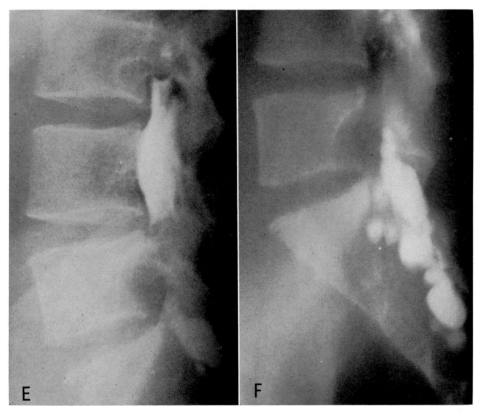

Fig. 437. *A*, A 36-year-old man with generalized neurofibromatosis. A stumbling gait, and weakness of both arms had been present for a year. Multiple neurofibromas are present in the lumbar canal, well seen on the transabdominal view. *B*, A block is present at L4, and a small neurofibroma is seen above this on the right side. *C*, When the patient was permitted to remain erect for about 10 minutes, the caudal sac filled, and multiple large arachnoidal cysts appeared. On passing the Pantopaque into the cervical canal, *D*, a block was encountered at the C6 level, and small defects indicative of multiple neurofibromas could be seen. At operation the cervical spinal canal was opened and numerous neurofibromas were found on many of the nerve roots. These extended through the intervertebral foramina, forming multiple dumbbell tumors. Note the change on the inferior margin of the left transverse process of L5, *C*, representing a neurotrophic disturbance inasmuch as no tumor is known to be there, although one cannot be sure of this. *E*, A large indentation is present on the dorsal aspect of L5, and cystic changes are seen in the sacral canal, *F*.

deformities, referred to as perineurial fibro-blastomas, schwannomas, neurinomas or neurilemmomas, originate in the sheaths of the spinal nerve roots and occur as smooth, sometimes nodular or irregularly lobulated growths surrounded by firm, fibrous cap-sules. The tumors are the next most fre-quent ones encountered within the spinal canal, and are usually intradural but extra-medullary in location. However, some-times they are entirely extradural in position, and occasionally occur both intradurally and extradurally. In rare instances they arise within the spinal cord (Walthard, 1927). They manifest themselves clinically by com-pression of the cord and the nerve roots. The clinical picture sometimes is complicated because of multiple intraspinal neurofibromas which can vary in size from a millimeter or two to over 2.5 cm (Fig. 436).

Perineurial fibroblastomas occur most fre-quently in the cervical and the thoracic spinal canal, but are not uncommon in the lumbar region. Instances of these growths within the sacral canal also have been re-corded. Rasmussen, Kernohan and Adson (1940) reported that among 167 intraspinal neurofibromas, 30 were in the cervical spinal canal, 70 in the thoracic, 55 in the lumbar and 2 in the sacral spinal canal. Wolf's (1941) distribution of 67 such tumors included 25 in the cervical canal, 31 in the thoracic, 10 in the lumbar and 1 in the sacral canal. The incidence of central nervous system involve-ment in neurofibromatosis was reported by Holt and Wright (1948). Neurofibromatosis was present in 127 cases out of a total of 245, 219 admissions. Approximately 10 per cent presented evidences of intracranial growths, a manifestation of the predilection of neurofibromatosis for localizing in the eighth cranial nerve. Hypoglossal neuro-fibromas are infrequent. They can be identi-fied radiologically by demonstration of widening of the hypoglossal canal (Valvas-sori and Kirdani, 1967). Ignelzi and Bucy (1967) reported this tumor without bone in-volvement but with angiographic evidence

of a small left vertebral artery which did not fill above the foramen magnum. With the increasing use of positive contrast examina-tions of the posterior fossa it can be expected that these tumors will be identified more often than up to now.

Neurofibromatosis often produces scoliosis or kyphoscoliosis when erosive changes are present in the bones. These result from multiple intraspinal tumors with compres-sive changes incident to the adaptive neces-sities created by the presence of these masses in the spinal canal and the intervertebral foramina. In addition, and perhaps more often, saccular dilatations of the meninges produce changes in bone because of pulsatile activity (Fig. 435). Dysplastic changes also occur in the bones which are difficult to ex-plain, but are much the same as those due to either masses or saccular lesions. Widen-ing of the spinal canal, indentation into the dorsal aspect of the vertebral bodies and widening of one or many intervertebral foramina appear with these diverse lesions. If saccular lesions are suspected, myelo-graphic confirmation might better be ob-tained from air myelograms inasmuch as it avoids the introduction of positive contrast material (Loop, Akeson and Clawson, (1965). If intraspinal mass lesions are responsible for the bony alterations, positive contrast exam-inations provide more reliable information. Prominence of the axillary sleeves is a fairly common change, and in some instances these protrude well beyond the bony margins of the intervertebral foramina, much like a dumbbell tumor (Fig. 443). Occasionally multiple tumors are accompanied by large pouch-like axillary sleeves (Fig. 437).

The advanced bone changes just described are not seen with the more frequent single neurofibromas. These lesions infrequently attain sufficient size to erode adjacent bone grossly. However, often enough they pro-duce less conspicuous changes in the adja-cent vertebral body, laminae or pedicles (Fig. 438), so that identification of these changes permits diagnosis of an intraspinal

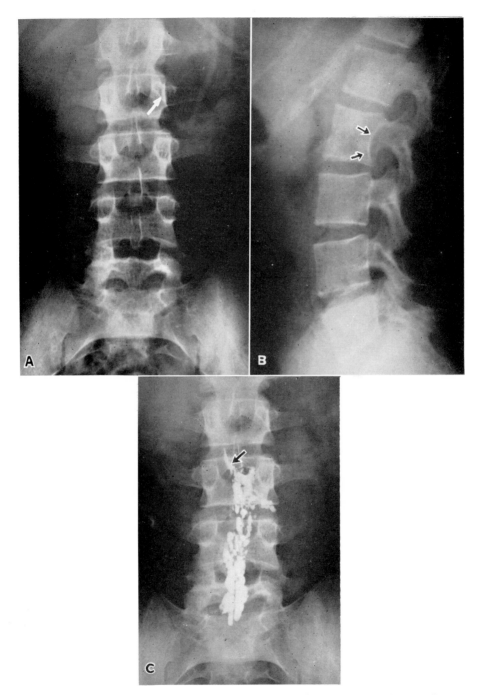

Fig. 438. *A*, Perineurial fibroblastoma in a 16-year-old boy with progressive weakness and pain in both legs. The cerebrospinal fluid protein content was over 650 mg per cent. Anteroposterior roentgenogram showing thinning of the left pedicle of the second lumbar vertebra (arrow). *B*, Lateral lumbar spine. Note the arcuate indentation of the dorsal aspect of the second lumbar vertebra (arrows). *C*, The flow of Pantopaque was slow, and multiple irregular defects are present in the column. A curvilinear defect is present extending to the right of the midline at the upper aspect of the second lumbar vertebra (arrows). At operation a large perineurial fibroblastoma was found, and there was marked tortuosity and dilatation of the veins below the obstruction.

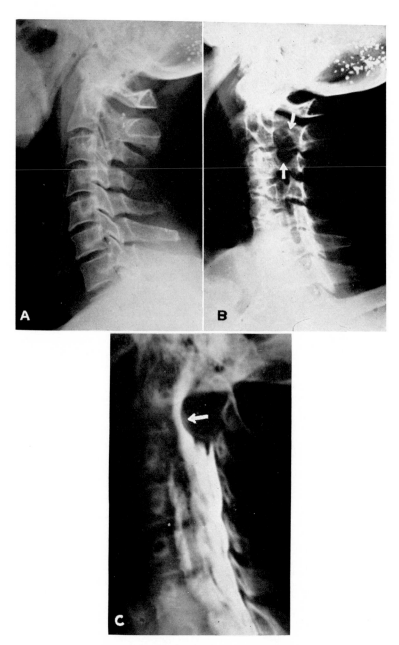

Fig. 439. *A*, Lateral cervical spine roentgenogram in a 56-year-old male with pain radiating to the occiput from the neck, and headache. No changes seen on this film. Pantopaque droplets from a myelogram done 10 years before are present in the cisterna magna. The patient's complaints had been attributed to this. *B*, Oblique view. Note the widening of the second intervertebral foramen (arrows). *C*, Myelographic defect due to large perineurial fibroblastoma.

mass. Widening of the intervertebral foramina constitutes another important diagnostic sign (Fig. 439).

Eden (1941) reported that in a series of 234 spinal tumors, 32 were of the dumbbell variety. Of these 25 were solitary or multiple neurofibromas, 3 were meningiomas, 2 were hemangioendotheliomas, 1 a ganglioneuroma and 1 an endothelial cell sarcoma.

It is possible for the intraspinal component of such growths to be small, while the extraspinal portions reach considerable size. Friedl (1946) noted that the extraspinal component may attain the size of a child's head. It is not uncommon to observe a smoothly circumscribed solid mass in the paravertebral area of the chest, usually in its upper aspect, which at first glance looks like an encapsulated growth or collection of fluid. Associated with this may be pressure changes in the posterior aspect of the ribs. In such cases the thoracic spine must be examined to ascertain changes in the intervertebral foramina and the neural arches to avoid overlooking a dumbbell tumor. In doubtful cases myelography may disclose the nature of the lesion if an intrathoracic meningocele communicating with the cerebrospinal fluid spaces is present. Gas myelography is preferable for this purpose. Svien (1950) noted the occurrence of 5 dumbbell tumors in 37 spinal cord neoplasms in children. One of these was a $5\frac{1}{2}$-year-old child with progressive difficulty in walking,

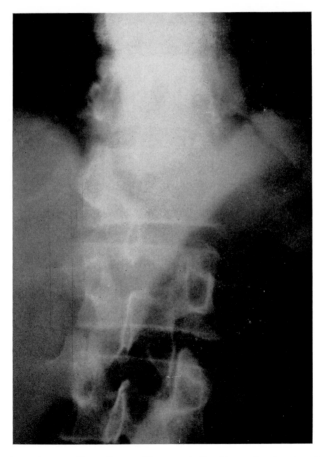

Fig. 440. Sarcomatous degeneration of neurofibroma at the thoracolumbar junction in a 35-year-old man with generalized neurofibromatosis. At operation the growth could be traced down to the spine, where it entered the spinal canal. Note the destruction of bone at the left lateral aspect of the twelfth thoracic vertebra, and the adjacent rib.

followed by paralysis of the lower extremities and bowel and bladder incontinence. A paravertebral mass was present extending from the seventh to the eleventh thoracic vertebrae. Bilateral thoracic laminectomy exposed a large encapsulated extradural tumor entering the spinal canal from the chest through the enlarged foramen between the ninth and tenth thoracic vertebrae. The intraspinal portion of the tumor was found to be a ganglioneuroma. A similar case in a 3-year-old girl with calcification inside the tumor was reported by Sames (1950). Grafton and Dodge (1952) reported on 60 cases of dumbbell neurofibromas affecting the spinal canal, occurring in approximately 1000 operated cases of spinal canal tumors. Spinal cord compression is most frequent with thoracic spinal canal neurofibromas. In the cervical region the predominating symptoms are those of both cord and nerve root compression. Those in the lumbar spinal canal are more likely to produce symptoms of nerve root compression. The possibility of multiple neurofibromas may be suggested by a bizarre symptom pattern (Fig. 441).

While neurofibromas are benign tumors, neoplastic degeneration can take place. Herrman (1950) reported 4 cases of neurofibromatosis, of which 3 developed sciatic nerve sarcomas and the fourth a retroperitoneal sarcoma. We had a case in which a large intrathoracic neurofibroma underwent sarcomatous degeneration, and another in which sarcomatous degeneration produced extensive destruction of the adjacent vertebrae (Fig. 440). Cuneo (1957) reported invasion of the spinal cord by a malignant schwannoma.

Myelographic examination is required for diagnosing intraspinal neurofibromas. In the case of an evident tumor, myelography serves to exclude multiple tumors (Fig. 441) or other masses which produce no visible or even clinical changes at the moment. The myelographic deformity varies from a complete obstruction to the passage of contrast material around single or multiple sharply circumscribed circular or oval masses without obstruction (Fig. 437). Spinocranial tumors of neurofibromatous origin likewise require careful observation of the upper cervical canal, and on occasion, can be seen on plain film ex-

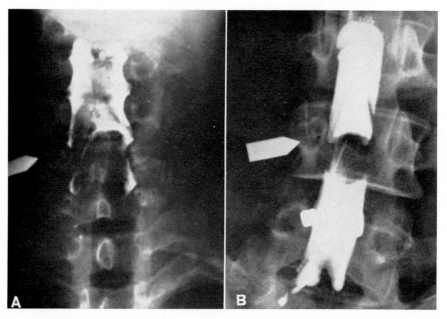

Fig. 441.   A, Neurofibroma in the lower cervical spinal canal.   B, Same case.   Another neurofibroma is present in the lower lumbar spinal canal.   Symptoms were referable to the upper and lower limbs, presumably due to a "demyelinizing disease."

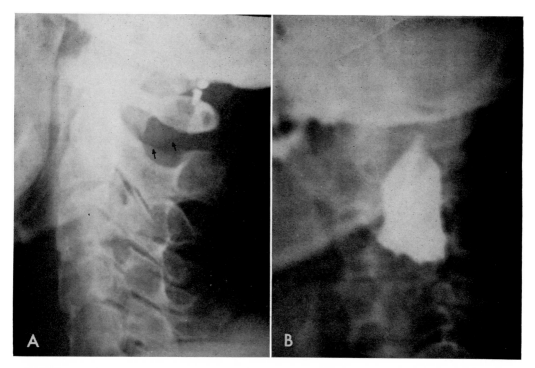

Fig. 442. *A*, A 37-year-old woman with sensory changes referable to the upper cervical cord and pain in the left leg for about 15 months. On plain film examination a soft tissue density projects downwards in the upper cervical canal (arrows). A block in this area is demonstrable on myelography, *B*. At operation an extramedullary extradural neurofibroma was found situated anterior and to the left of the cord at the level of C1, 2 and 3.

aminations (Fig. 442). Cineradiographic observations serve to confirm, or even to demonstrate small lesions, particularly those which are quickly enveloped in Pantopaque. It must also be kept in mind that other lesions may be responsible for symptoms, much in the same way as observed with meningiomas. Differentiation of widening of the spinal canal as an isolated lesion or concomitant with neurofibromatosis sometimes makes it necessary to continue investigations with myelography (Fig. 443). Differential diagnosis in the presence of a single neurofibroma is much the same as with meningiomas. With multiple neurofibromas it is possible that two or more may be present in the absence of systemic or skeletal changes. However, with many scattered lesions it is more likely that bony changes will be present. The question whether these are due to the pressure effect of tumors, to pulsatile effects incident to dilatation of cerebrospinal fluid containing structures, or just to dysplastic changes without other lesions is best settled by means of myelography.

References

Barson, A. J. and Cole, F. M.: Neurofibromatosis with Congenital Malformation of the Spinal Cord, J. Neurol., Neurosurg. & Psychiat., *30*, 71, 1967.

Bray, E. D.: Calcification and Ossification of Spinal Tumors, Brit. J. Radiol., *15*, 365, 1942.

Brown, M. H.: Intraspinal Meningiomas, Arch. Neurol. & Psychiat., *47*, 271, 1942.

Buchstein, H. F.: Meningiomas of Spinal Cord, Minnesota Med., *24*, 539, 1941.

Chandler, A. and Herzberger, E. E.: Lateral Intra-thoracic Meningocele, Am. J. Roentgenol., *90*, 1216, 1963.

Cloward, R. B.: Destruction of Cervical Vertebra by Solitary Neurofibroma. Report of a Case with Quadriplegia, J. Neurosurg., *17*, 510, 1960.

Craig, W. McK., Brown, J. R. and Osborn, J. E.: Tumors of the Foramen Magnum, Neurology, *6*, 73, 1956.

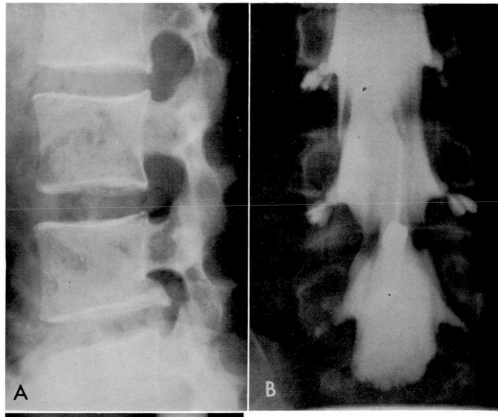

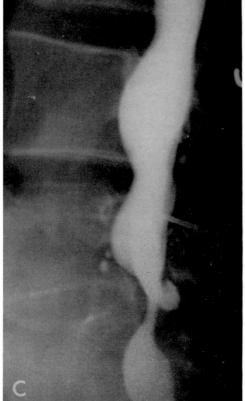

Fig. 443. *A*, The patient was a 26-year-old man with generalized neurofibromatosis. Symptoms were referable to the lower lumbar spine. Plain film examination disclosed a large spur projecting from the posteroinferior margin of L4 (*A*). An increased concavity is seen in the dorsal aspect of the bodies of L2, 3, 4 and 5. On myelographic examination, *B* and *C*, a large indentation is noted into the lateral and anterior aspects of the Pantopaque column. The canal is wide, requiring 30 ml to fill it adequately. The axillary pouches are unusually prominent and bulge beyond the intervertebral foramina. At operation the spur was found to compress the cauda equina and emerging nerve roots. Symptoms were relieved after operation.

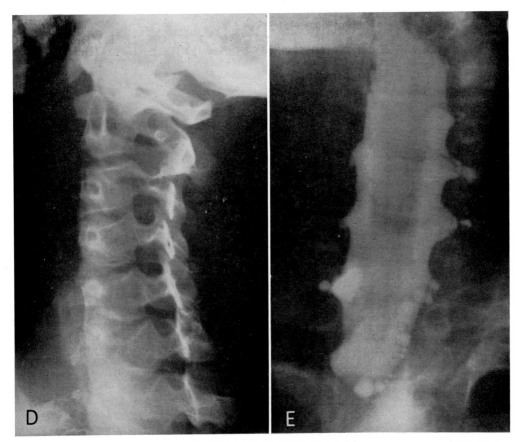

Fig. 443. (*Continued.*) On passing the Pantopaque into the cervical canal, which has large intervertebral foramina, *D*, large arachnoidal sacs project beyond the intervertebral foramina, part of the picture of neurofibromatosis affecting the bones without intraspinal tumors, *E*.

Culver, G. J., Concannon, J. P. and Koenig, E. C.: Calcification in Intraspinal Meningiomas, Am. J. Roentgenol., *62*, 237, 1949.

Cuneo, H. M.: Invasion of the Spinal Cord by Malignant Schwannoma, J. Neurosurg., *14*, 242, 1957.

Cushing, H. and Eisenhardt, L.: *Meningiomas*, Springfield, Charles C Thomas, 1938.

Davidoff, L. M., Gass, H. and Grossman, J.: Postoperative Spinal Adhesive Arachnoiditis and Recurrent Spinal Cord Tumor, J. Neurosurg., *4*, 451, 1947.

Dodge, H. W., Jr., Love, J. G. and Gottlieb, C. M.: Benign Tumors at the Foramen Magnum, J. Neurosurg., *13*, 603, 1956.

Dyke, C. G.: Roentgen Ray Diagnosis of the Spinal Cord, Meninges and Vertebrae. In *Surgical Diseases of the Spinal Cord, Membranes and Nerve Roots*, C. A. Elsberg, New York, Paul B. Hoeber, Inc., 1941.

Early, C. B. and Sayers, M. P.: Spinal Epidural Meningioma, J. Neurosurg., *25*, 571, 1966.

Eden, K.: Dumb-bell Tumours of the Spine, Brit. J. Surg., *28*, 549, 1941.

Elsberg, C. A.: *Surgical Diseases of the Spinal Cord,*

Membranes and Nerve Roots, New York, Paul B. Hoeber, Inc., 1941.

Epstein, B. S. and Davidoff, L. M.: Myelographic Diagnosis of Extramedullary Cervical Spinal Cord Tumors, Am. J. Roentgenol., *55*, 413, 1946.

Feiring, E. H. and Barron, K.: Late Recurrence of Spinal Cord Meningiomas, J. Neurosurg., *19*, 652, 1962.

Freedman, D. A., Feiring, E. H. and Davidoff, L. M.: Carcinoma of the Breast and Intraspinal Meningioma, J. Neuropath. & Exper. Neurol., *8*, 85, 1949.

Friedl, E.: Erweiterung des Wirbelkanales bei Geschwülsten des Rückenmarkes, der Nervenwurzeln unter der Rückenmarkshaute, Radiol. clin., *15*, 275, 1946.

Friedman, M. M.: Neurofibromatosis of Bone, Am. J. Roentgenol., *51*, 623, 1944.

Grafton, J. G. and Dodge, H. W., Jr.: Dumbbell (Hourglass) Neurofibromas Affecting the Spinal Cord, Surg., Gynec. & Obst., *94*, 161, 1952.

Graumann, W. and Braband, H.: Die Kombination Intrathorakaler Meningozelen mit der Neurofibromatosis Generalisata Recklinghausen, Fortschr. Röntgenstr., *97*, 484, 1962.

Haft, G. H. and Shenkin, H. A.: Spinal Epidural Meningioma, J. Neurosurg., *20*, 801, 1963.

Hannan, J. R., Hughes, C. R. and Mulvey, B. E.: Spinal Cord Tumors, Radiology, *53*, 711, 1949.

Heard, G., Holt, J. F. and Naylor, B.: Cervical Vertebral Deformity in von Recklinghausen's Disease of the Nervous System. A Review with Necropsy Findings, J. Bone & Joint Surg., *44-B*, 880, 1962.

Heard, G. and Payne, E. E.: Scalloping of the Vertebral Bodies in von Recklinghausen's Disease of the Nervous System (Neurofibromatosis), J. Neurol., Neurosurg. & Psychiat., *25*, 345, 1962.

Herrman, N. J.: Sarcomatous Transformation in Multiple Neurofibromatosis, Ann. Surg., *131*, 206, 1950.

Hirano, A. and Carton, C. A.: Primary Malignant Melanoma of the Spinal Cord, J. Neurosurg., *17*, 935, 1960.

Holt, J. F. and Wright, E. M.: Neurofibromatosis, Radiology, *51*, 647, 1948.

Ignelzi, R. J. and Bucy, P. C.: Intracranial Hypoglossal Neurofibroma, J. Neurosurg., *26*, 352, 1967.

Laws, J. W. and Pallis, C.: Spinal Deformities in Neurofibromatosis, J. Bone & Joint Surg., *45-B*, 674, 1963.

List, C. F.: Multiple Meningiomas, Arch. Neurol. & Psychiat., *50*, 335, 1943.

Lombardi, G. and Passerini, A.: Spinal Cord Tumors, Radiology, *56*, 381, 1961.

————: Multiple Lesions of the Spinal Cord, Am. J. Roentgenol., *92*, 1298, 1964.

Loop, J. W., Akeson, W. H. and Clawson, D. K.: Acquired Thoracic Abnormalities in Neurofibromatosis, Am. J. Roentgenol., *93*, 416, 1965.

Mackenzie, J.: Neurofibromatosis (von Recklinghausen's Disease), Brit. J. Radiol., *23*, 667, 1950.

Miller, A.: Neurofibromatosis with Reference to Skeletal Changes, Compression Myelitis and Malignant Degeneration, Arch. Surg., *32*, 109, 1936.

Osgood, E. C., Arnett, J. H. and Lewy, F. H.: Calcified Spinal Meningioma, Radiology, *43*, 62, 1944.

Preiser, S. A. and Davenport, C. B.: Multiple Neurofibromatosis (von Recklinghausen's Disease) and its Inheritance, Am. J. Med. Sci., *156*, 507, 1918.

Rand, R. W.: Multiple Spinal Cord Meningiomas, J. Neurosurg., *9*, 310, 1952.

Rasmussen, T. B., Kernohan, J. W. and Adson, A. W.: Pathologic Classification, with Surgical Consideration of Intraspinal Tumors, Ann. Surg., *111*, 513, 1940.

Raynor, R. B. and Mount, L. A.: Bilateral Cervical Neurofibromata Presenting as Cervical Spondylosis, J. Neurosurg., *19*, 1074, 1962.

Russell, J. Y. W.: Neurofibromatosis: A Bizarre Disease, Brit. J. Surg., *52*, 251, 1965.

Sames, C. P.: Dumb-bell Ganglioneuromata, Brit. J. Surg., *37*, 467, 1950.

Sammons, B. P. and Thomas, D. F.: Extensive Lumbar Meningocele Associated with Neurofibromatosis, Am. J. Roentgenol., *81*, 1021, 1959.

Scott, J. C.: Scoliosis and Neurofibromatosis, J. Bone & Joint Surg., *47-B*, 240, 1965.

Shapiro, J. H., Och, M. and Jacobson, H. G.: Differential Diagnosis of Intradural (Extramedullary) and Extradural Spinal Canal Tumors, Radiology, *76*, 718, 1961.

Shealy, C. N. and Le May, M.: Intrathoracic Meningocele, Two Additional Cases of This Rare Entity, J. Neurosurg., *21*, 880, 1964.

Shephard, R. H. and Sutton, D: Dumb-bell Ganglioneuromata of the Spine with a Report of Four Cases, Brit. J. Surg., *45*, 305, 1958.

Sinclair, J. E. and Yang, Y. H.: Ganglioneuromata of the Spine Associated with Von Recklinghausen's Disease, J. Neurosurg., *18*, 115, 1961.

Smolik, E. A. and Sachs, E.: Tumors of Foramen Magnum of Spinal Origin, J. Neurosurg., *11*, 161, 1954.

Stein, B. M., Leeds, N. E., Taveras, J. M. and Pool, J. L.: Meningiomas of the Foramen Magnum, J. Neurosurg., *20*, 740, 1963.

Svien, H. J.: Intraspinal and Intrathoracic Tumor with Paraplegia in a Child, Proc. Staff Meet., Mayo Clin., *25*, 715, 1950.

Uhlmann, E. and Grossman, A.: von Recklinghausen's Neurofibromatosis with Bone Manifestations, Ann. Int. Med., *14*, 225, 1940.

Valvassori, G. E. and Kirdani, M.: The Abnormal Hypoglossal Canal, Am. J. Roentgenol., *99*, 705, 1967.

Walthard, K. M.: Morbus Recklinghausen mit teilweiser intramedullaren Localization und mit nervosbedingten Hyperthermie im postoperative Verlauf, Deutsch. Ztschr. f. Nervenh., *99*, 125, 1927.

Webb, H. J., Craig, W. McK. and Kernohan, J. W.: Intraspinal Neoplasms in Cervical Region, J. Neurosurg., *10*, 360, 1953.

Weimann, R. B., Hallman, G. L. and Greenberg, S. D.: Intrathoracic Meningocele, J. Thor. & Cardiovasc. Surg., *46*, 40, 1963.

Wood, E. H., Jr.: Diagnosis of Spinal Meningiomas and Schwannomas by Myelography, Am. J. Roentgenol., *61*, 683, 1949.

SPINAL CORD AND INTRASPINAL MENINGEAL
TUMOR IMPLANTS

It has long been recognized that brain tumors can spread to the spinal meninges by way of the cerebrospinal fluid circulation. Spiller (1907) described the extension of an ependymoma of the fourth ventricle to the lower thoracic region of the cord. Cairns and Russell (1931) observed spinal metastases in more than one-third of the 22 cases of cerebral glioma studied. Included in the various brain tumors were medulloblastomas, glioblastomas multiforme, astrocytomas, ependymomas and neuroepitheliomas. Half of these growths originated above and half below the tentorium. Wolf (1941) mentioned that spinal metastases from brain tumors occurred in approximately 4 per cent of all spinal cord neoplasms encountered in routine examinations of the cord at necropsy. The fact that these extensions were by means of the cerebrospinal fluid was highlighted by the report of Halpern (1942), who observed silver clips used in a posterior fossa craniotomy in the spinal canal (Fig. 445). Three additional cases of subarachnoid and ventricular implants were reported by Tarlov and Davidoff (1946). Svien, Gates and Kernohan (1949) reported 19 cases of ependymomas of the fourth ventricle with an incidence of 31.6 per cent of spinal subarachnoid implantations. In none of these

6 patients did the history suggest the presence of implants in the canal.

Symptomatic implants in the subarachnoid space are not uncommon. These appear anywhere in the spinal canal, most often in the lumbar region. With large deposits spinal canal block can be prominent. More often several defects are apparent in the Pantopaque column, inasmuch as multiple deposits are the rule (Fig. 445). Seeding of the subarachnoid space may be accompanied by dissemination in the ventricles of the brain and intramedullary lesions (Perese, Slepian and Nigogosyan, 1959). Massive involvement of the cauda equina and the conus was described by Strang and Nordenstam (1961) 2 years after craniotomy for an intracerebral oligodendroglioma in a 30-year-old man.

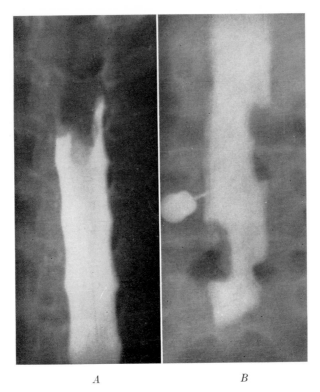

A   *B*

Fig. 444. *A*, Intraspinal metastases in the upper thoracic spinal canal in a 6-year-old girl operated upon 2 years before for a cerebellar spongioblastoma. Progressive pain in the lower thoracic and high epigastric areas. Manometrics normal. Relief with intrathecal methotrexate followed by x-ray therapy (courtesy of Dr. Leo M. Davidoff). *B*, Intradural metastases from a cerebellar astrocystoma in a 32-year-old man operated upon 5 years before present examination. The clinical diagnosis had been a herniated disc. (Courtesy of Dr. Joseph A. Epstein.)

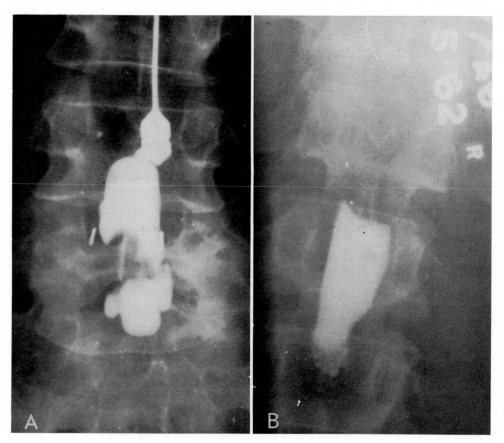

Fig. 445. Two silver clips are seen in the lower lumbar spinal canal. This patient, a 37-year-old man, had been operated upon for a pituitary adenoma and had received x-ray therapy for this condition. He did well for about 6 years, when he returned because of pain radiating down the left leg for 2 months and symptoms attributed to recurrence of the pituitary tumor. No bone changes visible in the spine. The silver clips had gravitated into the caudal sac. Myelography revealed multiple rounded filling defects in the entire lumbar canal, with a block at L1. Laminectomy performed at two levels revealed tumorous implants at T12 and at L4 and 5. The tumors were intradural and completely caught up the conus and the cauda equina above, while below this multiple tumor nodules involved the distal cauda equina fila. The patient was relieved symptomatically after operation followed by x-ray therapy, but expired because of progressive invasion of the base of the brain by pituitary carcinoma. (From Epstein, J. A., Epstein, B. S., Molho, L. and Zimmerman, H. M., Carcinoma of the Pituitary Gland with Metastasses to the Spinal Cord and Roots of the Cauda Equina, J. Neurosurg., *21*, 846, 1964.)

Seeding of the roots of the cauda equina presents a bizarre clinical picture. Lymphosarcoma, with spread to the cauda equina resulting in partial block, was reported by Van Allen and Rahme (1962). Longitudinal parallel striations of varying density and width was found at operation to be due to a mass of swollen roots with extensive tumor infiltration. Myelography in this patient had been suggestive of arachnoiditis or angiomatous malformation. Daniel (1964) observed secondary deposits along the roots of the cauda equina in a patient who had a lung carcinoma. We observed a woman who had a breast carcinoma and seeding of all of the roots of the cauda equina. Myelography disclosed only thickened nerve roots. At necropsy it was found that the nerve roots were encased in sheaths of tumor which were of varying depths, resulting in the beaded appearance along the length of each root (Fig. 446).

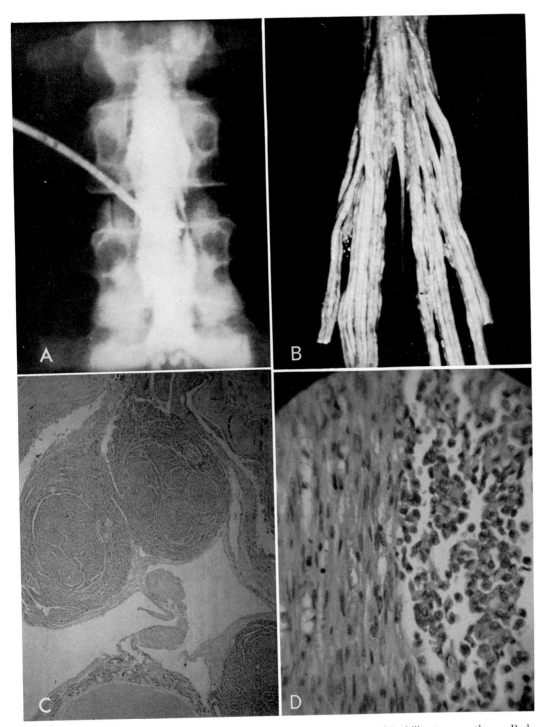

FIG. 446. *A*, A 49-year-old woman with pain and stiffness of the legs, and inability to move them. Radical mastectomy had been done 7 months before. CSF proteins were 114 mg per cent. Plain film examination of the spine was normal. Myelography showed no evidence of block, but the nerve roots of the cauda equina appeared to be thickened. In view of the clinical picture it was presumed that she had a cauda equina syndrome and x-ray therapy was started. She expired a week later after developing bladder and fecal retention, diplopia and bilateral aspiration pneumonia. At necropsy metastases to the leptomeninges of the lower half of the spinal cord, the cauda equina and the brain were found. The roots of the cauda equina were thickened and beaded, *B*. On microscopic study each root of the cauda equina was enveloped in a ring of tumor tissue which infiltrated into the spaces between the individual rootlets, *C* and *D*. The filum terminale was involved.

Metastases to the spinal cord also occur, sometimes together with implants in the subarachnoid space. Invasion of the roots of the cauda equina together with multiple subarachnoid deposits and two silver clips which had migrated to the caudal sac were reported by Epstein, Epstein, Molho and Zimmerman (1964) in a 34-year-old man with a pituitary carcinoma (Fig. 445). Belmusto, Owens and la Pava (1966) reported on the occurrence of intramedullary spinal cord metastases. These manifest themselves in the same way as intramedullary primary tumors, but can be slow growing and clinically deceptive. When small, no symptoms are evident. Later, as the tumor increases in size, degenerative and hemorrhagic changes can injure the cord so that symptoms appear rapidly. With large tumors myelography indicates the swelling of the cord associated with intramedullary tumor, but with small lesions examination may be unremarkable.

While the most common site of origin for intraspinal meningeal tumor implants is from the brain, occasional cases of carcinomatosis from more distant areas occur. Meissner (1953) reported on the incidence of meningeal carcinosis in 4 cases of carcinoma of the stomach. We have seen small implants with no clinical evidence to suggest their presence in cases of leukemia, malignant lymphoma, melanoma, and breast, lung, kidney and gastric neoplasms. In a report of primary malignant melanoma of the spinal cord, King, Chambers and Garey (1952) mentioned that in their second case the cerebrospinal fluid was black, indicating the presence of free melanin. This was believed to have produced a chemical arachnoiditis which caused hydrocephalus by obstruction of the foramina of Magendie and Luschka. Spinal canal block was encountered at the level of the first lumbar vertebra, and at operation an intradural tumor was found enmeshing the cauda equina, filling the intramedullary region of the conus and penetrating the spinal cord on its anterior surface. At necropsy seeding of

cells by way of the cerebrospinal fluid to the brain was found. Hirano and Carton (1960) discussed primary malignant melanomas of the cord. In a review of 26 patients they found that 8 tumors were intramedullary, 3 were both intra- and extramedullary, 10 were extramedullary but intradural in position, and 2 intradural lesions involved the dura mater and 2 extradural tumors affected the cord and the meninges. Primary melanoma of the cord was reported by Kiel, Starr and Hansen (1961). Tolnai and co-workers (1966) reported on primary malignant melanomatosis of the leptomeninges.

Unless spinal meningeal implants attain sufficient size to cause symptoms, their presence usually is detected only at necropsy. There is a practical point in recognizing these lesions which finds application in the use of x-ray therapy. In children with leukemia the meninges may become seeded with tiny implants. Leukemia and more often lymphoma are occasionally associated with tumorous masses which cause rapid spinal cord or cauda equina compression and which require prompt and adequate treatment by decompression and x-ray therapy or x-ray therapy alone, as indicated clinically.

Meningeal implants on the cord are more frequent on its dorsal aspect. They are usually gray, white and firm, and most of the time are tiny. Compression and distortion of the cord and thickening of the leptomeninges may be observed when the implants are sufficiently large. Another form of meningeal involvement may be tumorous thickening in which the neoplastic layer reaches a thickness of more than a millimeter (Fig. 446).

References

Belmusto, L., Owens, G. and la Pava, S.: Aspects of Intramedullary Spinal Cord Metastases, N. Y. State J. Med., 66, 2273, 1966.
Cairns, H. and Russell, D. S.: Intracranial and and Spinal Metastases in Glioma of Brain, Brain, 54, 377, 1931.

Daniel, P. M.: Observations on the Pathology of Metastatic Tumours in the Nervous System, Proc. Royal Soc. Med., *57*, 1151, 1964.

Epstein, J. A., Epstein, B. S., Molho, L. and Zimmerman, H. M.: Carcinoma of the Pituitary Gland with Metastases to the Spinal Cord and Roots of the Cauda Equina, J. Neurosurg., *21*, 846, 1964.

Fowler, F. D., Alexander, E., Jr. and Davis, C. H., Jr.: Pinealoma with Metastases in the Central Nervous System, J. Neurosurg., *13*, 271, 1956.

Halpern, L.: Spinal Metastases in Cerebellar Medulloblastoma, J.A.M.A., *118*, 803, 1942.

Hirano, A. and Carton, C. A.: Primary Malignant Melanoma of the Spinal Cord, J. Neurosurg., *17*, 935, 1960.

Kiel, F. W., Starr, L. B. and Hansen, J. L.: Primary Melanoma of the Spinal Cord, J. Neurosurg., *18*, 616, 1961.

King, A. B., Chambers, J. W. and Garey, J.: Primary Malignant Melanoma of the Spinal Cord, Arch. Neurol. & Psychiat., *68*, 266, 1952.

Meissner, G. F.: Carcinoma of the Stomach with Meningeal Carcinosis, Cancer, *6*, 313, 1953.

Perese, D. M., Slepian, A. and Nigogosyan, G.: Postoperative Dissemination of Astrocytoma of the Spinal Cord Along the Ventricles of the Brain, J. Neurosurg., *16*, 114, 1959.

Strang, R. R. and Nordenstam, H.: Intracerebral Oligodendroglioma with Metastatic Involvement of the Cauda Equina, J. Neurosurg., *18*, 683, 1961.

Tarlov, I. M. and Davidoff, L. M.: Subarachnoid and Ventricular Implants in Ependymal and Other Glimoas, J. Neuropath, & Exper. Neurol., *5*, 213, 1946.

Tolnai, G., Campbell, J. S., Hill, D. P., Peterson, E. W., Hudson, E. W., Hudson, A. J. and Luney, F. W.: Primary Malignant Melanomatosis of Leptomeninges, Arch. Neurol., *15*, 404, 1966.

Svien, H. J., Gates, E. M. and Kernohan, J. W.: Spinal Subarachnoid Implantation Associated with Ependymoma, Arch. Neurol. & Psychiat., *62*, 847, 1949.

Van Allen, M. W. and Rahme, E. S.: Lymphosarcomatous Infiltration of the Cauda Equina, Arch. Neurol., *7*, 476, 1962.

Wolf, A.: Tumors of Spinal Cord, Nerve Roots and Membranes. In *Surgical Diseases of the Spinal Cord, Membranes and Nerve Roots*, C. A. Elsberg, New York, Paul B. Hoeber, Inc., 1941.

Wood, E. H., Taveras, J. M. and Pool, J. L.: Myelographic Demonstration of Spinal Cord Metastases from Primary Brain Tumors, Am. J. Roentgenol., *69*, 231, 1953.

EXTRADURAL TUMORS

These neoplasms originate from the dura, its surrounding tissues, or from the nerve sheaths outside the dural reflection. They also arise from metastatic tumor implants either in the epidural space or in the adjacent bone with extension into the spinal canal. Such growths are principally from the lungs and breast, but spine metastases occur from practically anywhere in the body. While frequently associated with visible changes on roentgenograms of the spine, the probability of neoplastic extension is not excluded by a negative x-ray examination. In these questionable instances scanning with radioactive strontium is useful. Myelography may prove helpful in the diagnosis of the patient's complaints.

Primary tumors arise in the adjacent bony, periosteal and vascular structures, particularly sarcomas which extend into the canal and produce compressive symptoms (Figs. 447 and 448). Another tumor frequently associated with spinal cord compression is multiple myeloma. Lymphosarcoma and Hodgkin's disease occur within the spinal canal, often without concomitant bony changes. These lesions also may extend into the canal from the posterior mediastium or the retroperitoneal region by way of the intervertebral foramina without visible bony change.

Inflammatory and granulomatous lesions such as epidural abscesses, tuberculomas, gummas and mycotic infections have been mentioned previously. These, too, may intrude into the epidural space. By far the most frequent condition producing epidural compression is herniation of the intervertebral disc. This, and intraspinal protrusion of osteophytes, have been discussed in previous chapters.

Hemangiomas of the posterior mediastinum invading the adjacent thoracic extradural region causing cord compression was reported by Toch, Hagstrom and Steinberg (1965). Spinal cord compression from extramedullary masses of hematopoietic tissue has been seen in patients with myelosclerosis (Lowman, Bloor and Newcomb, 1963) (Appleby and co-workers, 1964) (Sorsdahl, Taylor and Noyes, 1964). Acute spinal cord compression secondary to epidural hemato-

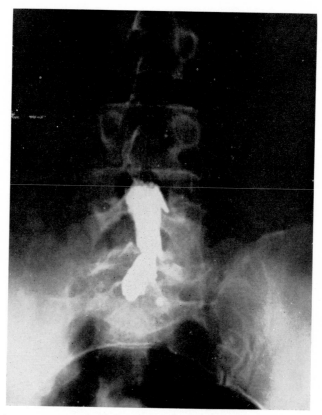

FIG. 447. Extradural fibrosarcoma at the lumbosacral interspace in a 44-year-old woman with low-back pain for 6 weeks before myelography. No bony involvement noted at operation or at post-mortem examination. Patient died in congestive heart failure due to long-standing mitral valve disease.

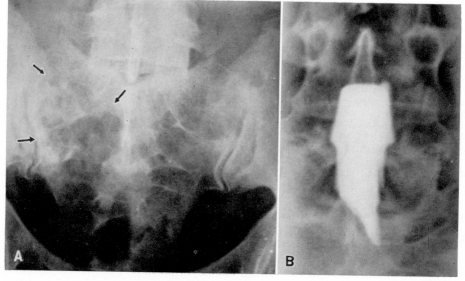

FIG. 448. A, Fibrosarcoma of the upper right sacrum in a 56-year-old woman with low back pain and sciatica. Mottled lytic and sclerotic areas are present adjacent to the right sacro-iliac joint (arrows). B, Same case, myelogram shows deflection of caudal sac due to epidural extension of the tumor.

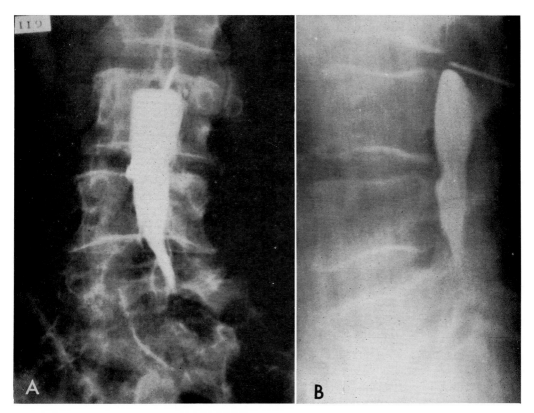

Fig. 449. *A*, A 70-year-old man with left sciatic pain and leg atrophy. Plain film examination of the spine was normal. He was known to have a bronchogenic carcinoma. Myelography revealed a tapered caudal sac displaced to the left. The pointed end of the sac is elevated from the floor of the canal, *B*. At operation extensive epidural tumor was found, and the left pedicle of L5 and its lamina were softened and tumorous.

poiesis which apparently did not extend through the intervertebral foramina has been reported.

Myelographic examination is important in identifying the site and extent of epidural lesions. Those low in the lumbar spinal canal produce a variety of changes in the caudal end of the Pantopaque column. In some a tapered blunt configuration is seen, sometimes with a high termination indicative of a complete block (Fig. 449). In others the caudal sac is tapered and deviated to one side by a laterally placed mass. Higher lesions produce extradural defects varying from complete block to a slight lateral displacement of the Pantopaque column. A good correlation exists between visible bone destruction and the level of block in symptomatic patients. However, whenever possible myelographic confirmation is desirable not only to localize the lesion more precisely, but to study the rest of the canal as well.

References

Appleby, A., Batson, G. A., Lassman, L. P. and Simpson, C. A.: Spinal Cord Compression by Extramedullary Haematopoiesis in Myelosclerosis, J. Neurol., Neurosurg. & Psychiat., *27*, 313, 1964.

Close, A. S., Taira, Y. and Cleveland, D. A.: Spinal Cord Compression Due to Extramedullary Hematopoiesis, Ann. Int. Med., *48*, 421, 1958.

Condon, W. B., Safarik, L. R. and Elzi, E. P.: Extramedullary Hematopoiesis Simulating Intrathoracic Tumor, Arch. Surg., *90*, 643, 1965.

Epstein, B. S.: The Myelographic Diagnosis of Epidural Metastases in the Lumbosacral Spinal Canal, Am. J. Roentgenol., *68*, 730, 1952.

Friedman, M. and Di Rienzo, A. J.: Treatment of Trophocarcinoma (Embryonal Carcinoma) of the Testis, Radiology, *80*, 550, 1963.

Heiser, S. and Swyer, A. J.: Myelography in Spinal Metastases, Radiology, *62*, 695, 1954.

Lowman, R. M., Bloor, C. M. and Newcomb, A. W.: Roentgen Manifestations of Thoracic Extramedullary Hematopoiesis, Dis. Chest. *44*, 154, 1963.

Melot, G. J., Potvliege, R., Martin, Ph. et Brihaye, J.: Myélographie dans les Infiltrations Néoplastiques de l'espace Épidural, Acta radiol., *1*, 736, 1963.

Sorsdahl, O. S., Taylor, P. E. and Noyes, W. D.: Extramedullary Hematopoiesis, Mediastinal Masses, and Spinal Cord Compression, J.A.M.A., *189*, 343, 1964.

Toch, H., Hagstrom, J. W. C. and Steinberg, I.: Hemangioma of the Mediastinum. Report of a Case with Compression of the Spinal Cord, Am. J. Roentgenol., *94*, 580, 1965.

Wright, R. L.: Malignant Tumors in the Spinal Extradural Space, Ann. Surg., *157*, 227, 1963.

Arachnoidal Cysts

These arise as congenital diverticula of the dura or as arachnoidal herniations through a dural defect which may follow trauma or surgery (Rosenblum and Derow, 1963) (Shahinfar and Schecter, 1966). The cysts communicate with the subarachnoid space through a pedicle. Hyndman and Gerber (1946) reported an instance of acquired extradural cysts in the cervical region in one patient and in the lumbar region of another after surgery. In both small persistent fistulas in the line of dural incision permitted herniation of the arachnoid. Occasionally an arachnoidal cyst remains with the dura. Primary arachnoidal cysts also arise from or within the septum posticum, a thin membranous partition which divides the posterior spinal subarachnoid space longitudinally from the cervical to the lower thoracic region. Cysts originating within the septum itself are rare (Perret, Green and Keller, 1962).

Extradural cysts are most frequent in the thoracic spinal canal, and occur occasionally in the cervical and lumbar regions as well. The walls are composed of avascular fibrous tissue lined with epithelial cells and contain fluid similar in consistency and chemical characteristics to cerebrospinal fluid. In some reported cases the fluid within the cysts was somewhat gelatinous.

According to DuToit and Fainsinger (1948) lumbar extradural cysts manifest themselves later than those in the thoracic region. This is ascribed to the greater capacity of the lumbar spinal canal and the ease of displacement of the cauda equina.

Congenital extradural cysts compress the spinal cord, producing progressive paraplegia with relatively little pain. Motor weakness of the legs, hyperactive deep reflexes, varying degrees of impairment of touch, pain, temperature and position sense as well as bowel and bladder disturbances may be encountered. Adams and Wegner (1947) reported intermittent compression of the cord with symptoms which were subacute and progressive up to a certain point, and then regressed so that the patient was relieved between attacks. The authors postulated that when the fluid pressure within the cyst reached a certain height its walls ruptured, relieving the compression. Another possibility was absorption of the cyst contents followed by reaccumulation.

Swanson and Fincher (1947) reported 4 acquired extradural arachnoidal cysts complicating 1,700 laminectomies. Three of these had had previous lumbar laminectomies for herniated discs. The fourth was related to a nonpenetrating injury of the lumbar spine. The predisposing cause was a dural tear in which a water-tight closure could not be made. The clinical aspects of their cases suggested recurrent intervertebral disc prolapse. Multiple inept punctures with a large spinal needle also may be a cause of extradural arachnoidal cysts. The case reported by Turner (1947) showed herniation of the arachnoid with a characteristic pedicle passing through a sharply delimited dural defect.

The plain film changes seen with arachnoidal cysts reflect the gradual increase in the size of the fluid-containing sac and its pressure against the adjacent bone. The earliest change is slight loss of bone in the inner aspects of the adjacent pedicles. This affects a single vertebra when a small cyst exists, while with larger sacs the pedicles of several segments become thinned and widened. Usually the pedicles at the upper and lower limits of the lesion are less altered than those in the middle where the bulk of the cyst is largest. As the cyst increases in size indentations appear against the posterior aspects of the vertebral bodies resulting in scalloped vertebrae. The neural arches likewise may become thinned (Fig. 450). Usually these changes can be differentiated from ependymomas easily when they appear in the cervical or thoracic spinal canal on the basis of localization alone. In the lumbar region the changes sometimes are difficult to distinguish from any bulky tumor.

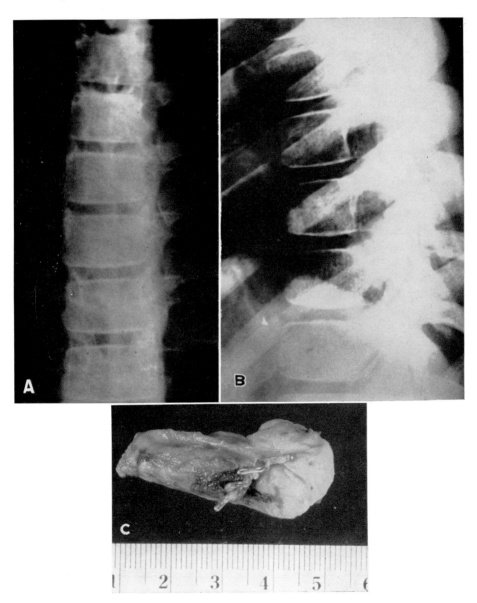

FIG. 450. *A*, Extradural cyst in the middorsal spine of an 11-year-old boy with progressive loss of function of both legs for 5 months. The interpedicular spaces are widened and the pedicle are thinned out. *B*, Lateral dorsal spine. A slight concavity is seen in the dorsal aspects of the sixth and seventh thoracic vertebrae, and the canal is widened. *C*, Operative specimen.

Myelography is helpful in differential diagnosis, and provides an almost pathognomonic sign when some of the contrast material, be it Pantopaque or air, enters the cyst. In some instances the neck of the cyst permits such communication, but in others this does not occur. It is sometimes helpful to repeat the films after a few hours to see if air or Pantopaque enters the sac. When Pantopaque envelops the lesion, it produces a partial block at each level where the cyst impinges against bone, and in some a complete block is produced. A localized small cyst, such as may be seen with a circumscribed area of arachnoiditis, may produce only a slight lateral filling defect simulating a herniated disc. Hart (1958) suggested that if operation did not disclose a discal lesion to explain the myelographic defect it might be necessary to open the dura.

Entrance of the lumbar puncture needle tip into lumbar extradural cysts was mentioned by Shahinfar and Schechter (1966). Calcification of cyst walls also has been observed occasionally (Rosenblum and Derow, 1963). Rounded paravertebral shadows caused by lateral extensions of extradural arachnoidal cysts which filled with Pantopaque on myelography were observed by Dastur (1963). Some eburnation and hollowing of the adjacent rib neck was present.

Plain film roentgenograms in children and adolescents may show concomitant changes of Scheuermann's disease (Cloward and Bucy, 1937). Adelstein (1941) observed that the association of Scheuermann's disease with progressive paraplegia indicated a spinal extradural cyst. None of the cases of Scheuermann's disease seen by us had extradural cysts.

References

Adams, R. D. and Wegner, W.: Congenital Cyst of the Spinal Meninges as Cause of Intermittent Compression of the Spinal Cord, Arch. Neurol. & Psychiat., 58, 57, 1947.

Adelstein, L. J.: Spinal Extradural Cyst Associated with Kyphosis Dorsalis Juvenalis, J. Bone & Joint Surg., 23, 94, 1941.

Cloward, R. B. and Bucy, P. C.: Spinal Extradural Cyst and Kyphosis Dorsalis Juvenalis, Am. J. Roentgenol., 38, 681, 1937.

Cuneo, H. M.: Spinal Extradural Cysts, J. Neurosurg., 12, 176, 1955.

Dastur, H. M.: The Radiological Appearance of Spinal Extradural Arachnoid Cysts, J. Neurol., Neurosurg. & Psychiat., 26, 231, 1963.

Decker, H. G. and Livingston, K. E.: Spinal Extradural Cyst, J. Neurosurg., 6, 248, 1949.

DuToit, J. G. and Fainsinger, M. H.: Spinal Extradural Cysts, J. Bone & Joint Surg., 30-B, 613, 1948.

Elsberg, C. A., Dyke, C. G. and Brewer, E. D.: Symptoms and Diagnosis of Extradural Cysts, Bull. Neurol. Inst. New York, 3, 395, 1934.

Good, C. A., Adson, A. W. and Abbott, K. H.: Spinal Extradural Cyst (Diverticulum of Spinal Arachnoid), Am. J. Roentgenol., 52, 53, 1944.

Hart, G. M.: Circumscribed Serous Spinal Arachnoiditis Simulating Protruded Lumbar Intervertebral Disc, Ann. Surg., 148, 266, 1958.

Hoffman, G. T.: Cervical Arachnoidal Cyst, J. Neurosurg., 17, 327, 1960.

Hyndman, O. R. and Gerber, W. F.: Spinal Extradural Cysts, Congenital and Acquired, J. Neurosurg., 3, 474, 1946.

Lehman, E. P.: Spinal Extradural Cysts, Am. J. Surg., 28, 307, 1935.

Mayfield, F. H. and Grantham, E. G.: Spinal Extradural Cysts, Surgery, 11, 589, 1942.

Murray, R. O.: Intradural Arachnoid Cyst of the Lumbar Spinal Canal, Brit. J. Radiol., 32, 689, 1959.

Nugent, C. R., Odon, G. L. and Woodhall, B.: Spinal Extradural Cysts, Neurology, 9, 397, 1959.

Perret, G., Green, D. and Keller, J.: Diagnosis and Treatment of Intradural Arachnoid Cysts of the Thoracic Spine, Radiology, 79, 425, 1962.

Rosenblum, D. J. and Derow, J. R.: Spinal Extradural Cysts: With Report of an Ossified Spinal Extradural Cyst, Am. J. Roentgenol., 90, 1227, 1963.

Schreiber, F. and Nielsen, A.: Lumbar Spinal Extradural Cyst, Am. J. Surg., 80, 124, 1950.

Schurr, P. H.: Sacral Extradural Cyst: an Uncommon Cause of Low Back Pain, J. Bone & Joint Surg., 37-B, 601, 1955.

Shahinfar, A. H. and Schechter, M. M.: Traumatic Extradural Cysts of the Spine, Am. J. Roentgenol., 98, 713, 1966.

Smith, G. W. and Chavez, M.: Lumbar Extradural Cysts—Congenital: Their Proper Classification, Arch. Neurol. & Psychiat., 80, 436, 1958.

Swanson, H. S. and Fincher, E. F.: Extradural Arachnoidal Cysts of Traumatic Origin, J. Neurosurg., 4, 530, 1947.

Turner, O. A.: Spinal Extradural Cyst, Arch. Neurol. & Psychiat., 58, 593, 1947.

SYRINGOMYELIA

The term "syringomyelia" indicates the presence of a tubular cavitation of the spinal cord which extends over distances varying from 2 or 3 segments to a lesion which involves practically the entire cord. Congenital dilatation of the central canal alone is referred to as hydromyelia.

As a rule, the first cervical segment of the cord is intact. In classical cases, the dilatation extends from the upper cervical spinal canal to the lower thoracic region. The lumbosacral enlargement as a rule is not affected. The syrinx usually extends horizontally across the cord in an irregular manner, sometimes assuming a U or an H shaped configuration. The distribution of the tubular syrinx varies, so that it may be prominent in the cervical region and relatively small in the thoracic cord. At times the lesion extends to both the right and left sides of the cord, and at others it is limited to a single side. The cavity may communicate with the central canal, particularly in the cervical region. When this takes place, the wall of the cavity is lined with ependymal cells, but in other areas no such ependymal lining is present. The fluid within the dilated spinal cord or canal is clear, slightly yellow sometimes, and resembles cerebrospinal fluid. The cavity usually is largest in the cervical region.

The clinical picture associated with syringomyelia is related to the destruction of the nerve cells and fibers in the region of the cavitation. Wasting of the muscles of the hands and forearms, with anesthesia and loss of appreciation of position and vibration, are all part of the symptom complex. The cavitation may involve the pons and the medulla oblongata, sometimes communicating with the floor of the fourth ventricle. If this is present, changes referable to the pons and cranial nerves emerging from the brain stem and the fibers of the medulla oblongata may appear. Scoliosis and peripheral neuropathic joint changes also may appear (Karck, 1963).

The appearance of the cord with syringomyelia varies. In the presence of small cavitations, the cord may show no visible change. With larger or multiple cavities, the cord becomes enlarged, particularly in those areas where there is considerable cavitation and fluid under pressure.

Syringomyelia and hydromyelic dilatation of the central canal of the cord not infrequently is found together with other congenital malformations, notably the Arnold-Chiari malformation, platybasia, hemivertebrae, myelomeningoceles, malformations of the cranio-occipital junction and the Klippel-Feil malformation.

The connection between the fourth ventricle and the central canal of the neural tube sometimes persist. This varies from a small dilatation of the central canal of no clinical importance to a long thin-walled tube filled with clear fluid.

Secondary syringomyelia occurs secondary to trauma, arachnoiditis, tumor, or following the absorption of blood from a hematomyelia. This, too, is associated with cavitation which varies in size and distribution, but usually is limited to a few segments. Cavitation of the spinal cord also may take place following x-ray therapy for spinal cord tumors (Fig. 424). Infarction of the cord secondary to embolization or to thrombosis of an angioma also may result in destruction of medullary tissue and secondary dilatation or cavitation.

Plain film examination of the spine in the presence of syringomyelia usually is not informatory in most cases. However, increase in the sagittal measurement of the spinal canal was reported in 15 out of 32 cases by Wells, Spillane and Bligh (1959). In two of these, scalloping of the posterior aspect of the vertebral bodies was present. These changes were attributed to adaptation of the bony canal to the unusual width of the syringomyelic cord.

Myelography reveals changes usually associated with an intramedullary growth, resulting in a spindle-shaped deformity of the cervical Pantopaque column with narrowing of the lateral margins. However, extensive syringomyelia may exist in the presence of a normal myelogram (McIlray and Richardson (1965). Of particular interest in the

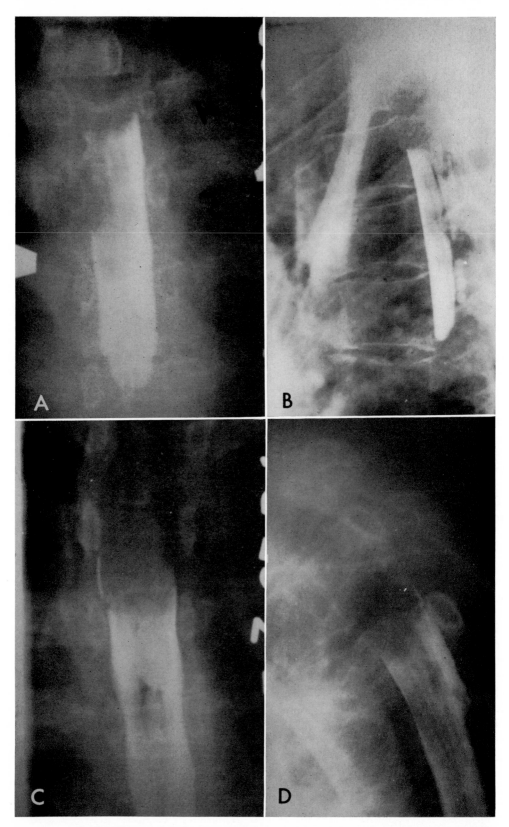

Fig. 451. *A*, Intramedullary mucoid cyst in a 14-year-old boy with a complete block at T4. The head of the column is slightly concave. In the lateral view, *B*, a complete block extends from the ventral to the dorsal aspect of the canal. Symptoms were relieved after aspiration of the cyst. About 2 years later symptoms recurred, and re-examination, *C* and *D*, again revealed a block at the same level. Reaspiration again produced a cloudy, yellowish mucoid material, with relief of symptoms.

diagnosis of syringomyelia is the use of gas myelography (Klefenberg and Saltzman, 1959). Removal of the cerebrospinal fluid results in a change in the configuration of the spinal cord when the patient is placed in the erect posture. This is revealed as a collapse of the cord as the fluid within it gravitates down to the lower lumbar area. If the dilatation of the cord in the cervical area persists, it is considered presumable evidence of an intramedullary tumor. The collapsing cord sign is important in the differential diagnosis of a solid versus a cystic lesion of the cord (Heinz, Schlesinger and Potts, 1966).

Pantopaque may be introduced into the fourth ventricle by examining the patient in the recumbent position. When the patient is placed in the erect posture, contrast material can be introduced into a dilated central canal, as occurred in one of the cases reported by Heinz and his co-workers.

Gas myelography also is useful in identifying the position of a bulge in the spinal cord. Westberg (1966) utilized the demonstration of large flaccid intramedullary cysts by gas myelography in the treatment of spinal cord cysts by percutaneous punctures. These cysts were found to extend throughout the cord in almost all of his patients. The fluid obtained from these cysts was similar to normal cerebrospinal fluid on chemical examination. These patients had clinical symptoms typical of syringomyelia.

Localized collections of mucoid fluid in the intramedullary substance of the cord also are encountered occasionally (Fig. 451) (Johnson, 1959). These present as tumors, and the thick, yellowish fluid encountered on needling the cord establishes the diagnosis of a colloid cyst. Recurrences of symptoms may follow reaccumulation of fluid.

References

Heinz, E. R., Schlesinger, E. B. and Potts, D. G.: Radiologic Signs of Hydromyelia, Radiology, *86*, 311, 1966.

Johnson, R. T.: Colloid Cysts of the Cervical Canal, J. Neurol, Neurosurg. & Psychiat., *22*, 342, 1959.

Karck, G.: Auffallende Skelettveränderungen bei Syringomyelie, Fortschr. Röntgenstr., *98*, 27, 1963.

Klefenberg, G. and Saltzman, F. F.: Gas Myelographic Studies in Syringomyelia, Acta radiol., *52*, 129, 1959.

McIlroy, W. J. and Richardson, J. C.: Syringomyelia. A Clinical Review of 75 Cases, Canadian M.A.J., *93*, 731, 1965.

McRae, D. L. and Standen, J.: Roentgenologic Findings in Syringomyelia and Hydromyelia, Am. J. Roentgenol., *98*, 695, 1966.

Wells, C. E., Spillane, J. D. and Bligh, A. S.: The Cervical Spinal Canal in Syringomyelia, Brain, *82*, 23, 1959.

Westberg, G.: Gas Myelography and Percutaneous Puncture in the Diagnosis of Spinal Cord Cysts, Acta radiol. Supp., 252, Stockholm, 1966.

INTRASPINAL VASCULAR MALFORMATIONS

Vascular malformations within the spinal canal are mainly arteriovenous, but either venous or arterial lesions have been observed. They involve principally the leptomeninges, and vary from single convoluted dilated vessels to huge intertwined varicosities. Occasionally a bruit can be heard over the involved area (Fig. 454). Vascular neoplasms such as capillary hemangiomas, hemangioendotheliomas, hemangioblastomas and hemangiomas associated with vertebral angiomas also project into the spinal canal, but are not considered true vascular malformations. Dilatation of the venous structures may result from intraspinal lesions causing obstruction to the return flow of blood (Fig. 452D). The effects of vascular dilatations within the spinal canal depends on their extent. Minute dilatations frequently exist without producing symptoms (Kaydi, 1929).

Local dilatations of epidural veins, particularly in the lumbosacral region, may compress adjacent nerve roots and produce a clinical and radiological picture indistinguishable from herniated discs (Fig. 452) (Cohen, 1941). Epstein (1947) reported 3 such cases, and others have been mentioned in the course of reports on intervertebral disc herniations (Johnson, 1940; Maltby and Pendergrass, 1946).

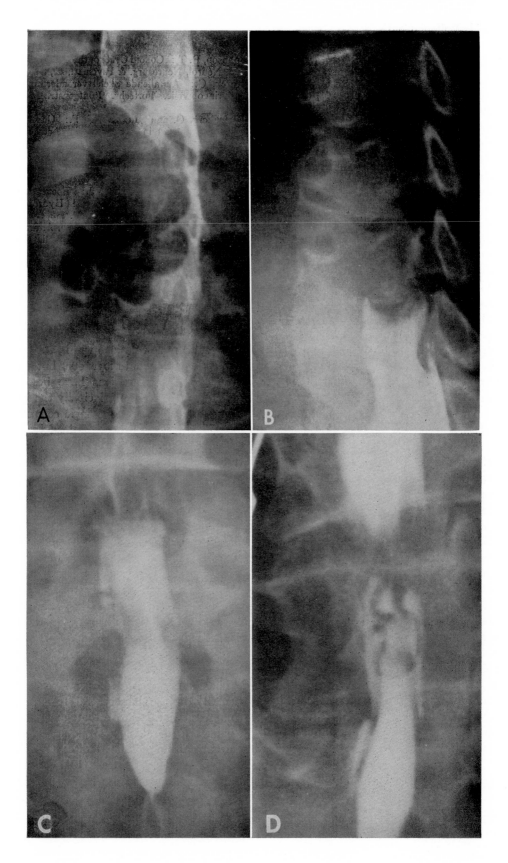

The association of subarachnoid angiomas with subcutaneous hemangiomas of a corresponding metamere was originally described by Berenbruch (1895), who demonstrated an actual vascular connection through the intervertebral foramen between an angioma of the cervicothoracic portion of the cord and multiple angiolipomas of the skin of the upper part of the trunk. Turner and Kernohan (1941) mentioned that instances of vascular tumors of the cord associated with nevi of the corresponding cutaneous metamere was reported only four times prior to 1941. In their study of 45 cases of vascular tumors of the spinal cord there were 18 angiomas, in none of which was there a vascular or pigmented nevus. Cross (1948) described a case of cutaneous and intraspinal angioma in the cervical region of a 19-year-old male. Trupp and Sachs (1948) also had a patient with a large skin telangiectasis who suddenly became paraplegic at a level corresponding with the skin lesion. It is probable that this group falls into the classification of Lindau's disease, consisting of familial hemangiomatous cysts, tumors of the central nervous system, associated angiomatosis of the retina and cysts of other parenchymatous organs. As brought out by Craig and Horrax (1949), these angiomatous lesions may extend the entire length of the cord.

Vascular malformations within the spinal canal may produce obstruction and cord compression simulating a spinal cord tumor or a herniated disc (Figs. 452 and 454). Elsberg (1925) cautioned against accepting varices as a sole cause for such a syndrome without searching for a tumor or other obstruction at a higher level which might cause venous obstruction and dilatation. However, epidural varices, while infrequent, are not associated with such lesions.

When an intraspinal angioma bleeds, there may be intense sudden pain in the back with radicular extension along the involved nerve roots. Symptoms may be intermittent and residual discomfort follows scar formation with nerve root pressure. Bassett, Peet and Holt (1949) stressed that at this stage the objective signs may be bizarre and segmentally incompatible with a single lesion because of the multiple foci of irritation. Consequently, the clinical picture may simulate multiple sclerosis, poliomyelitis or other inflammatory or degenerative diseases. Epstein and Davidoff (1943) pointed out that these symptoms of exacerbation and remission may indicate variations in vascular dilatation at a particular moment.

Intraspinal angiomas are localized according to their positions in the spinal canal. They are no respectors of anatomic position, and can be either localized (Fig. 454) or extend over practically the entire cord from the midcervical region to the lumbar enlargement and even over the cauda equina (Fig. 453). Venous angiomas appear as thin, blue-tinged vessels, while arterial anomalies present as thin, tortuous vessels which although arterial do not pulsate. They are differentiated from venous angiomas by the color of the blood, which is bright red. It is not possible to differentiate these one from the other on the basis of myelographic studies. Teng and Papatheodorou (1964) held that arteriovenous malformations were rare, occurring at the lower end of the cord and in the cauda equina. These differ in structure and color of vessels in that they are heavier and pul-

---

Fig. 452. *A*, This 42-year-old man had difficulty in walking and instability while standing for 3 months. Numbness of the right forearm, pain in both arms, and numbness of the left arm were noted for about a year. A large lobulated defect is seen in the lower spinal canal on the left side. On extension of the head a block is produced, *B*. At operation a large extradural intraspinal venous angioma with enormous varicosities was present. *C*, Myelographic defect on the left side of the lumbosacral interspace produced by a localized epidural varix. The clinical picture was that of a herniated disc in a 52-year-old man. *D*, Serpentine diluted veins below an extruded L3 disc in a 61-year-old man.

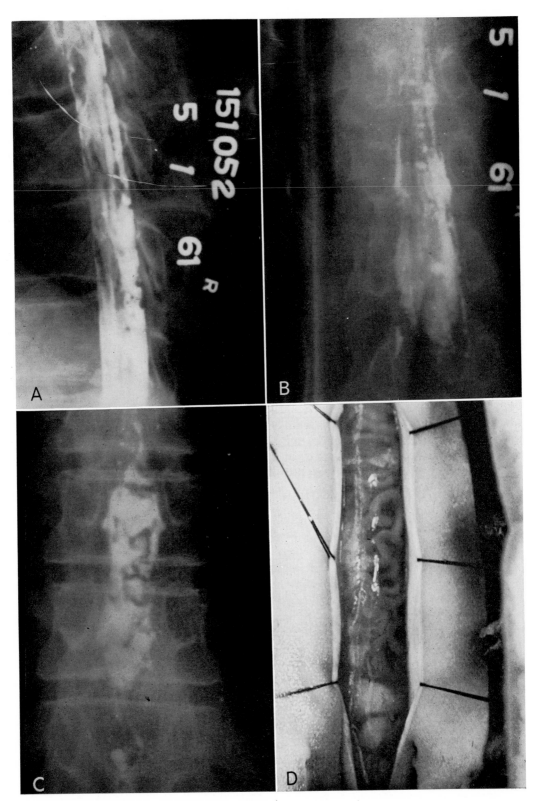

FIG. 452. (*Legend on opposite page.*)

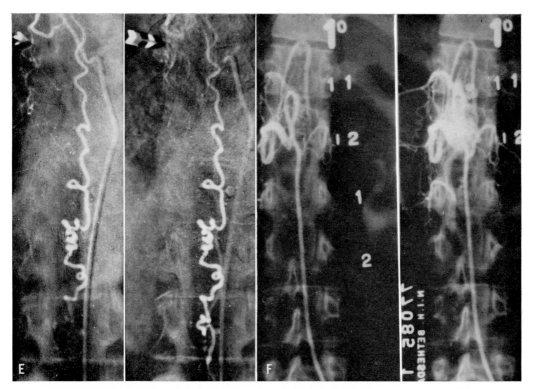

FIG. 453. *A*, A 56-year-old man with incontinence, saddle anesthesia and a sensory level at T10. A delay in the passage of Pantopaque is noted in the lower thoracic canal, with some widening of the cord and irregular, poorly defined channels highly suspicious of a vascular malformation. *B*, On caudad flow some of the Pantopaque did not descend, *C*. Another film 6 hours later revealed persistence of the Pantopaque at this site, now with clearly defined vascular shadows. *D*, At operation a large subarachnoid arteriovenous malformation is visible. The operative site is the same as *C*, and extension cephalad and caudad was prominent. *E*, Selective angiographic study of a middle-aged man with "single coiled vessel type" of arteriovenous malformation. *F*, Selective angiographic examination of an adolescent girl with the "juvenile type" of arteriovenous malformation with a "fast flow" type of circulation. (*E* and *F* courtesy of Giovanni Di Chiro and John J. Doppman.)

sate. Houdart, Djindjian and Hurth (1966) were of the opinion that the classical division of "arterial" and "venous" angiomas are exceptional, if they exist at all. The lesions they operated upon were all arteriovenous malformations. The abnormal vessels are not limited to the surface of the cord and the meninges, but extend into the medullary substance as well. These may bleed into the subarachnoid space as well as into the cord, resulting in arachnoiditis, intramedullary damage or both.

Small, and probably undiagnosable, intramedullary vascular malformations may rupture and cause intramedullary bleeding with sudden onset of pain and long tract signs.

If confined to the cord, this produces hematomyelia, and the cerebrospinal fluid remains clear. Should the lesion swell the cord, myelography may disclose a fusiform prominence like an intramedullary tumor.

X-ray examination of the spine in cases of intraspinal vascular abnormalities usually are normal. However, if a localized mass of sufficient size exists, there is evidence of local bone pressure atrophy. Widening of the spinal canal with an intradural hemangioma and aneurysm with calcification was described by Walker (1944) in his discussion of congenital anomalies of the spinal cord. The interpedicular spaces in this patient were widened, but no erosion was present,

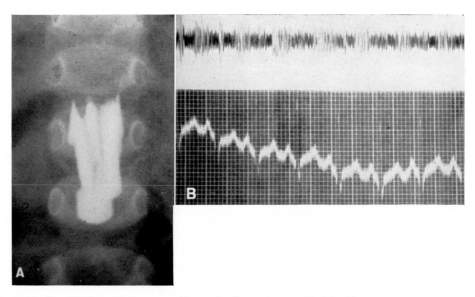

Fig. 454. Localized arteriovenous malformation in an 8-year-old girl with symptoms of a spinal cord tumor at the level of the twelfth thoracic vertebra. Myelography, *A*, disclosed a complete block at this level. On auscultation a murmur was heard at this site, confirmed by phonocardiogram, *B*, and at operation, when intramedullary hemorrhage was found. (Courtesy of Dr. Joseph A. Epstein, North Shore Hospital, Manhasset, N. Y.)

and it was assumed that the altered configuration of the spine was part of the congenital anomaly.

In the presence of spinal cord vascular malformations, myelography is of great diagnostic importance. Pressure of the dilated vascular channels in the Pantopaque column results in sinuous, radiolucent channels which are quite characteristic (Fig. 453). Their appearance varies, depending on the degree of filling at the time. If only a single focal lesion is present, the myelographic picture may be only a single defect in the Pantopaque column without any distinguishing characteristics (Fig. 454).

It is not possible to differentiate sharply between arterial, venous or arteriovenous malformations myelographically (Epstein, Beller and Cohen, 1949). It has been mentioned that there may be difficulty in differential diagnosis between vascular anomalies and adhesive arachnoiditis. In our experience, and from reviewing the published roentgenograms of others, the sinuous, smooth-walled channel-like structures of vascular dilatations are rarely simulated by

the more diffuse changes of arachnoiditis. Bassett, Peet and Holt (1949) pointed out that adhesive arachnoiditis might be superimposed on angiomatous malformations as a result of organized hemorrhage.

Höök and Lidvall (1958) and Matthews (1959) commented on the presence of a bruit over intraspinal vascular malformations. A similar observation is documented in Figure 454.

Arteriography is becoming increasingly important in the demonstration of intraspinal vascular malformations. In the cervical region visualization of the vertebral arteries is required, a procedure which can be accomplished either by direct injection (which I do not favor), by introduction of a catheter into the artery, or by retrograde brachial artery injection. Höök and Lidvall (1958) reported two such cases, and presented a phonocardiogram of the bruit in one.

The value of aortography by means of catheter placement in the aorta using the Seldinger technic was brought into the fore by the work of Djindjian and his colleagues, beautifully summarized and illustrated in their 1966 monograph. They pointed out that even though myelography demonstrated the lesion in about 75 per cent of cases, arteriography is essential in clearly demonstrating the lesion and the vessels leading into it. Placement of the catheter tip so that the artery of Adamkiewicz is opacified for demonstration of lesions in the lower spinal cord is important, and for visualization of higher levels the catheter tip has to be correspondingly situated to visualize the muscular branches. It is essential to avoid introducing the catheter into a major spinal artery directly to avoid toxic effects. The use of subtraction technics to bring out the vessels is helpful. Di Chiro, Doppman and Ommaya (1967) recommended "midstream aortography" by injection into the descending thoracic aorta as a preliminary step to selective angiography. On the initial examination they identified the approximate origin of the feeding vessels, and by using selective examinations they could delineate each arterial feeder to pinpoint the level of spinal entrance (Figs. 453E and F). The type of contrast material used is important in these examinations, because concentrated material should not be directly injected for selective studies. In the event of a possible high lesion they utilize an arch injection as the preliminary investigation. Subtraction technics do much to enhance the diagnostic elegance of vascular opacification within the spinal canal.

Spinal transosseous phlebography may opacify vertebral and epidural angiomas, but is not helpful in spinal cord arteriovenous and angiomatous lesions (Vogelsgang and Pia, 1965; Houdart, Djindjian and Hurth, 1966).

References

Antoni, N.: Spinal Vascular Malformations (Angiomas) and Myelomalacia, Neurology, 12, 795, 1962.

Baker, H. L., Love, J. G. and Layton, D. D.: Angiographic and Surgical Aspects of Spinal Cord Vascular Anomalies, Radiology, 88, 1078, 1967.

Bassett, R. C., Peet, M. M. and Holt, J. F.: Pial-Medullary Angiomas, Arch. Neurol. & Psychiat., 61, 558, 1949.

Berenbruch, K.: Ein Fall von multiplen angiolipomen Kombiniert mit einem Angiom des Ruckenmarks, Deutsch. Ztschr. f. Nervenh., 6, 127, 1895.

Cohen, I.: Extradural Varix Simulating Herniated Nucleus Pulposus, J. Mt. Sinai Hosp., 8, 136, 1941.

Craig, W. McK. and Horrax, G.: Hemangioblastomas (2 Cerebellar and 1 Spinal) in 3 Members of a Family, J. Neurosurg., 6, 518, 1949.

Cross, G. O.: Subarachnoid Cervical Angioma with Cutaneous Hemangioma of a Corresponding Metamere, Arch. Neurol. & Psychiat., 58, 359, 1948.

Di Chiro, G., Doppman, F. and Ommaya, A. K.: Selective Arteriography of Arteriovenous Aneurysms of Spinal Cord, Radiology, 88, 1065, 1967.

Djindjian, R., Fauré, C. and Hurth, M.: Explorations Artériographiques des Aneurysmes Artério-Veineux de la Moelle Epinière, Les Monographies des Anna les de Radiologie, Expansion Scientifique Francaise, 1966.

Epstein, B. S.: Low Back Pain Associated with Varices of Epidural Veins Simulating Herniation of Nucleus Pulposus, Am. J. Roentgenol., 57, 736, 1947.

Epstein, B. S. and Davidoff, L. M.: Roentgenologic Diagnosis of Dilatations of Spinal Cord Veins, Am. J. Roentgenol., 49, 476, 1943.

Epstein, J. A., Beller, A. J. and Cohen, I.: Arterial Anomalies of the Spinal Cord, J. Neurosurg., 6, 45, 1949.

Globus, J. H. and Doshay, L. J.: Venous Dilatations and Other Intraspinal Vessel Alterations, Including True Angiomata, with Signs and Symptoms of Cord Compression, Surg., Gynec. & Obst., 48, 345, 1929.

Goran, A., Carlson, D. J., and Fisher, R. G.: Successful Treatment of Intramedullary Angioma of the Cord, J. Neurosurg., 21, 311, 1964.

Gross, S. W. and Ralston, B. L.: Vascular Malformations of the Spinal Cord, Surg., Gynec. & Obst., 108, 673, 1959.

Hare, C. C. and Everts, W. H.: Calcified Subpial Lesions of Spinal Cord with Associated Varicose Veins, Bull. Neurol. Inst., New York, 6, 295, 1937.

Höök, O. and Lidvall, H.: Arteriovenous Aneurysms of the Spinal Cord. A Report of Two Cases Investigated by Vertebral Angiography, J. Neurosurg., 15, 84, 1958.

Houdart, R., Djindjian, R. and Hurth, M.: Vascular Malformations of the Spinal Cord. The Anatomic and Therapeutic Significance of Arteriography, J. Neurosurg., 24, 583, 1966.

Johnson, H. F.: Herniation of Intervertebral Disc with Referred Sciatic Symptoms, J. Bone & Joint Surg., 22, 708, 1940.

Karshner, R. G., Rand, C. W. and Reeves, D. L.: Epidural Hemangioma Associated with Hemangioma of the Vertebrae, Arch. Surg., 39, 942, 1939.

Kaydi: Quoted by Globus and Doshay, Surg., Gynec. & Obst., 48, 345, 1929.

Kendall, B. and Russell, J.: Haemangioblastoma of the Spinal Cord, Brit. J. Radiol., 39, 818, 1966.

Maltby, G. L. and Pendergrass, R. C.: Pantopaque Myelography, Radiology, *47*, 35, 1946.

Matthews, W. B.: The Spinal Bruit, Lancet, *2*, 1117, 1959.

Morris, L.: Angioma of the Cervical Spinal Cord, Radiology, *75*, 785, 1960.

Newman, M. J. D.: Racemose Angioma of the Spinal Cord, Quart. J. Med., *28*, 97, 1959.

Odom, G. L., Woodhall, B. and Margolis, G.: Spontaneous Hematomyelia and Angiomas of the Spinal Cord, J. Neurosurg., *14*, 192, 1957.

Otenasek, F. J. and Silver, M. L.: Spinal Hemangioma (Hemangioblastoma) in Lindau's Disease, J. Neurosurg., *18*, 295, 1961.

Richardson, J. C.: Spontaneous Hematomyelia, Brain, *61*, 17, 1938.

Teng, P. and Papatheodorou, C.: Myelographic Appearance of Vascular Anomalies of the Spinal Cord, Brit. J. Radiol., *37*, 358, 1964.

Teng, P. and Shapiro, M. J.: Arterial Anomalies of the Spinal Cord. Myelographic Diagnosis and Treatment by Section of Dentate Ligaments, Arch. Neurol. & Psychiat., *80*, 577, 1958.

Trupp, M. and Sachs, E.: Vascular Tumors of Brain and Spinal Cord, J. Neurosurg., *5*, 354, 1948.

Turner, O. A. and Kernohan, J. W.: Vascular Malformations and Tumors Involving the Spinal Cord, Arch. Neurol. & Psychiat., *46*, 444, 1941.

Vogelsgang, H. and Pia, H. W.: Bedeutung der Wirbelangiographie für die Diagnose spinale Angiome, Fortschr. Röntgenstr., *102*, 660, 1965.

Walker, A. E.: Dilatation of Vertebral Canal with Congenital Anomalies of Spinal Cord, Am. J. Roentgenol., *52*, 571, 1944.

Wyburn-Mason, R.: *The Vascular Abnormalities and Tumors of the Spinal Cord and its Membranes*, London, H. Kimpton, 1943.

Spinal Epidural Hematomas

Epidural bleeding in the spinal canal occurs from many causes, including strain or trauma (Mayer, 1963), vascular malformations (Dawson, 1963), anticoagulant therapy (Spurny and co-workers, 1964; Jacobson and co-workers, 1966), or spontaneously in normotensive or hypertensive individuals. Epidural hematomas appear in every age group from infancy to old age, and has no particular predilection for either sex. They appear anywhere in the spinal canal, most often in the thoracic region. The cervical canal is affected next in order, and the lumbar canal is least involved. The hematomas are situated on the dorsal aspect of the cord, and extend laterally to one side or both, but do not proceed anteriorly. The thickness of the clot varies from a few mm to over 1 cm. With recurrent bleeding the hematoma becomes partly organized and is covered by a membrane. Epidural hematomas vary in extent from a few to over 10 or 12 segments.

Symptoms appear suddenly, with severe pain in the affected area and associated radicular involvement. This may be followed by paraplegia or quadriplegia, depending on the localization of the clot. In some patients there may be no warning symptoms, and in others there are intermittent minor attacks of back pain with transient episodes reflecting nerve root involvement. These usually are disregarded until a major episode occurs. Neurologic signs appear within minutes or hours, but sometimes are delayed for a few days, with an intermittent pattern of pain. The cerebrospinal fluid is clear, xanthochromic or bloody, and the protein content varies from normal to values well over 300 mg per cent. Manometric determinations may or may not indicate a block. The presence of blood in the cerebrospinal fluid does not contraindicate myelography if an epidural hemorrhage is suspected (Markhan, Lynge and Stahlman, 1967). Indeed, prompt diagnosis and action is imperative if surgical relief is to be obtained.

Yaskin and Groff (1941) reported a case following slight trauma, with slowly progressive symptoms due to epidural hemorrhage in the upper thoracic region. The plain films of the spine were normal, but cerebrospinal fluid manometric measurements indicated a partial block. At operation a hematoma 4 cm long and from 1.5 to 2 cm thick was removed. VerBrugghen (1946) mentioned 8 cases from the literature, and described another in a 75-year-old man following indirect trauma. In this case the short progressive history with gradual onset of paraplegia and the absence of a bony lesion suggested an extradural hemorrhage. Svien, Adson and Dodge (1950) also reported a case following trauma in which the plain films were normal, but myelograms disclosed a block at the superior margin of the third lumbar vertebra which was diagnosed as a herniated disc. At operation a hard fibrous mass compressing the dural sac was encountered. When this was opened old blood exuded, and examination of the excised sac showed an old organized hematoma. This patient made an uneventful recovery. Schultz, Johnson, Brown and Mosberg (1953) collected 12 cases and reported 4 of their own. They also noted the association with mild trauma, and corroborated the clinical similarity with lumbar disc lesions.

Plain film roentgenograms of the spine rarely are helpful, except when a vertebral injury provides an indication of the lesion. Myelographic investigation is essential, disclosing a picture pf partial or complete extradural block which in itself is not indicative of the nature of the lesion. In the event of complete block it may be helpful to outline the upper aspect of the lesion by means of cisternal instillation of Pantopaque. However, this should not be done if the clinical picture indicates the necessity for rapid intervention. In some situations it may even be advisable to forego myelographic study (Jacobson and co-workers, 1966). When complete obstruction is present, the spreading of the cephalad aspect of the Pantopaque column suggests an intramedullary tumor (Fig. 455). However, a transverse pattern of block, or displacement of the column to one side or the other also can be seen. There may be difficulty in diagnosis in the absence of block, as occurred in 2 of the 24 cases reviewed by Lowrey (1959) and 3 out of the 33 reported by Markhan, Lynge and Stahlman (1967).

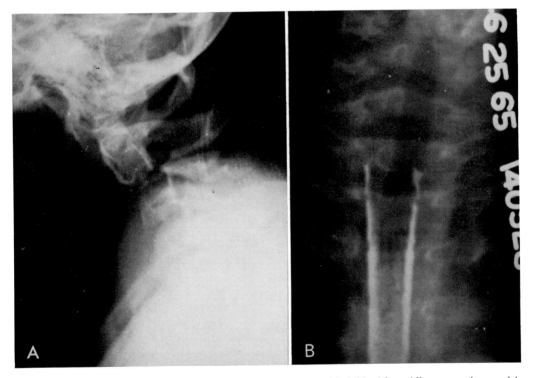

FIG. 455. A, Lateral cervical spine roentgenogram in a 6-year-old child with rapidly progressive quadriplegia after trauma. There is a fracture of the third cervical vertebral neural arch with anterior displacement of C3 on C4. B, Myelography, reveals a block at C7, with spreading of the lateral aspects of the column. At operation a large epidural hematoma was found practically filling the cervical spinal canal. Removal of the clot was followed by recovery. (Courtesy of J. A. Epstein, from the North Shore Hospital, Manhasset, N. Y.)

In differential diagnosis the possibility of spinal cord tumor, epidural abscess or infectious or granulomatous lesions of bone with epidural extension, spinal artery thrombosis and cord infarction, necrotizing myelitis, and various degenerative spinal cord diseases must be considered. When repeated episodes of pain after trauma or effort occur, the clinical picture in patients with spontaneous epidural hematomas may simulate discal herniation (Khatib and Cook, 1966).

References

Ainslie, J. P.: Paraplegia Due to Spontaneous Extradural or Subdural Hematoma, Brit. J. Surg., 45, 565, 1958.

Alderman, D. B.: Extradural Spinal-Cord Hematoma, New England J. Med., 255, 839, 1956.

Cooper, D. W.: Spontaneous Spinal Epidural Hematoma, J. Neurosurg., 26, 323, 1967.

Dawson, B. H.: Paraplegia Due to Spinal Epidural Haematoma, J. Neurol., Neurosurg. & Psychiat., 26, 171, 1963.

Gold, M. E.: Spontaneous Spinal Epidural Hematoma, Radiology, 80, 823, 1963.

Jackson, F. E.: Spontaneous Spinal Epidural Hematoma Coincident with Whooping Cough, J. Neurosurg., 20, 715, 1963.

Jacobson, I., Maccabe, J. J., Harris, P. and Dott, N. M.: Spontaneous Spinal Epidural Haemorrhage During Anticoagulant Therapy, Brit. Med. J., 1, 522, 1966.

Khatib, R. and Cook, A. W.: Spontaneous Spinal Epidural Hematoma, New York State J. Med., 66, 989, 1966.

Lowrey, J. J.: Spinal Epidural Hematomas, J. Neurosurg., 16, 508, 1959.

Markhan, J. W., Lynge, H. N. and Stahlman, G. E. B.: The Syndrome of Spontaneous Epidural Hematoma, J. Neurosurg., 26, 334, 1967.

Mayer, J. A.: Extradural Spinal Hemorrhage, Canadian M. A. J., 89, 1034, 1963.

Schultz, C. E., Johnson, A. C., Brown, C. A. and Mosberg, W. H., Jr.: Paraplegia Caused by Spontaneous Spinal Epidural Hemorrhage, J. Neurosurg., 10, 608, 1953.

Spurny, O. M., Rubin, S., Wolf, J. H. and Wu, W. Q.: Spinal Epidural Hematoma During Anticoagulant Therapy, Ann. Int. Med., 114, 103, 1964.

Svien, H. J., Adson, A. W. and Dodge, H. W., Jr.: Lumbar Extradural Hematoma, J. Neurosurg., 7, 587, 1950.

Svien, H. J. and Peserico, L.: Spontaneous Epidural Hematoma of the Cervical Region, Proc. Staff Meet., Mayo Clin., 34, 209, 1959.

ver Brugghen, A.: Extradural Spinal Hemorrhage Ann. Surg., 123, 154, 1946.

Winer, B. M., Horenstein, S. and Starr, A. M.: Spinal Epidural Hematoma During Anticoagulant Therapy, Circulation, 19, 735, 1959.

Yaskin, J. C. and Groff, R. A.: Spina Epidural Hemorrhage, Arch. Neurol. & Psychiat., 45, 756, 1941.

SPONTANEOUS SUBARACHNOID INTRASPINAL HEMORRHAGE

Spontaneous subarachnoid hemorrhage with intraspinal tumors may give rise to severe pain in the lumbar region extending down both legs, accompanied by violent headache. Abbot (1939) reported the case of a 16-year-old boy who experienced sharp pain in the lumbar region and both legs after attempting a high jump. Severe headache followed, with weakness and flexor spasm of the legs, nuchal rigidity, positive Kernig and Brudzinski signs, but no paralysis. Examination of the cerebrospinal fluid showed blood but no block. The patient recovered rapidly, but had over 25 similar attacks in the next 14 months. Myelography finally disclosed a block at the level of of the first lumbar vertebra. A large encapsulated ependymoma atttached to the filum terminale was found at operation, with an unusual amount of hemorrhage.

Fincher (1951) called attention to the similarity of spontaneous subarachnoid hemorrhage in intradural tumors with subarachnoid bleeding from other causes. He mentioned that if such a picture were associated with radicular pain of the lower limbs, a lumbar tumor should be considered. Early myelography was recommended for detecting such a lesion before compressive symptoms or destructive spinal cord and nerve root changes appeared. He reported 5 such cases, including 3 ependymomas, 1 neurofibroma and 1 neuroglioma. In 1 of his cases myelograms showed a complete block although repeated manometric studies had not indicated this condition.

Subarachnoid hemorrhage also appears with vascular malformations of the spinal cord (Newman, 1959) (Morris, 1960), extramedullary aneurysms (Hoplins, Wilkie and

Voris, 1966), and with blood dyscrasias, and vascular diseases such as polyarteritis nodosa (Henson and Croft, 1956).

References

Abbott, K. H.: Subarachnoid Hemorrhage from an Ependymoma Arising in the Fllum Terminale, Bull. Los Angeles Neurol. Soc., *4*, 127, 1939.

Fincher, E. F.: Spontaneous Subarachnoid Hemorrhage in Intradural Tumors of the Lumbar Sac, J. Neurosurg., *8*, 576, 1951.

Henson, R. A. and Croft, P. B.: Spontaneous Spinal Subarachnoid Hemorrhage, Quart. J. Med. (N.S.) *25*, 53, 1956.

Hoplins, C. A., Wilkie, F. L. and Voris, D. C.: Extramedullary Aneurysm of the Spinal Cord, J. Neurosurg., *24*, 1021, 1966.

Mendelsohn, R. A. and Mora, F.: Spontaneous Subarachnoid Hemorrhage Caused by Ependymoma of Filum Terminale, J. Neurosurg., *15*, 460, 1958.

Morris, L.: Angioma of the Cervical Spinal Cord, Radiology, *75*, 785, 1960.

Newman, M. J. D.: Racemose Angioma of the Spinal Cord, Quart. J. Med., *28*, 97, 1959.

Rader, J. P.: Chronic Subdural Hematoma of the Spinal Cord, New England J. Med., *253*, 374, 1955.

MYELITIS

Necrotizing transverse myelitis combined with optic neuritis is referred to as neuromyelitis optica or Devic's disease. Massive necrosis associated with secondary demyelinization involves both the gray and white matter, producing ascending and descending Wallerian degeneration much the same as seen with transection of the cord. The optic chiasm is demyelinized and extensive gliosis appears. These lesions appear generally in the cervical and upper thoracic regions. The resultant swelling of the cord produces a myelographic picture of spreading of the lateral aspects of the Pantopaque column indistinguishable from that observed with intramedullary tumors and syringomyelia. Other lesions producing cord swelling such as hematomyelia, abscess, infarction due to spinal artery thrombosis, the effects of radiation, and various extramedullary neoplastic and inflammatory lesions also require consideration in differential diagnosis. However, the history of associated cerebral or ocular dysfunction is important in identifying neuromyelitis optica.

Inflammation of the spinal cord involving the white and gray matter may be limited to one or two segments (transverse myelitis), or spread over a greater length, with ascending and descending degeneration. Myelitis is caused by infection, and often is incident to metastatic involvement from a pyogenic focus elsewhere. It may extend from adjacent bone infection, such as osteomyelitis or tuberculosis, or be syphilitic in origin, or caused by a penetrating wound. Vascular disease with infarction is a possible cause. Parasitic and fungal infections and viral diseases are other causes. and in some instances no known etiologic agent can be identified. Radiation therapy in excessive dosage is another cause.

Compressive changes affecting the upper cervical spinal cord incident to skeletal changes in that region appear with a variety of conditions, including congenital malformations affecting the cervical vertebrae and the craniovertebral articulation. These have been mentioned previously. Here I would like to reiterate the fact that the initial manifestations of these conditions can be neurologic. Michie and Clark (1968) and Wadia (1967) recently re-emphasized the coexistence of myelopathic changes with high cervical malformations and with atlantoaxial dislocations.

The spinal cord is infiltrated, edematous and contains areas of softening. When the meninges are involved the term "meningomyelitis" is used. With spread into the nerve roots the condition is termed "myeloradiculitis." Concomitant small vessel disease may cause multiple foci of infarction. If pus forms, it may be encapsulated, constituting an intramedullary abscess.

The clinical picture often is acute, with pain in the involved area, often associated with radicular distribution. Motor and sensory loss is related to the involved areas, and bladder and rectal deficiencies are present as well. The tendon reflexes are diminished. There may be intermittent periods of relief of pain, but the neurologic deficit does not alter and progresses. The cerebrospinal fluid usually reveals increased cellular content and elevated protein values. Manometric determinations indicate a partial block in the presence of sufficient cord swelling. When the cord is not engorged sufficiently, the manometric measurements are normal.

Plain film examinations of the spine are not helpful, except when there is evidence of osseous involvement. Myelographic examination usually is helpful in indicating the site of a partial or complete block, with spreading of the lateral aspects of the column such as is seen with intramedullary diseases. In some patients Pantopaque traverses the area, and once in a while persistence of Pantopaque over the involved segments is observed.

In a recent case we followed to necropsy, a 62-year-old woman had a 4-month history of progressive interscapular pain radiating to both sides of the chest, low back pain, paresthesias in both lower limbs which were intermittent. Prior to admission the pain became intense, and radiated down both legs. This was followed by inability to move her left leg and numbness of the right leg, increasing constipation and difficulty in urination. Within a week she had lost movement in both legs, but this ameliorated a few days later. Cerebrospinal fluid protein content was 28 mg per cent and manometric determinations were normal.

Plain film examinations of her spine were normal, as was a skeletal survey. On myelography it was noted that the column was spread at the level of the third to sixth thoracic vertebrae, and difficulty in getting Pantopaque above this level was encoun-

tered. There was a persistence of Pantopaque at the involved levels, revealed as a thin layer of contrast which did not change in position when the patient was placed erect or in the inverted position. Three ml of Pantopaque were instilled intracisternally, but the upper aspect of the lesion was not clearly identified.

At operation a diffuse swelling and congestion of the upper thoracic cord was revealed through a laminectomy involving the third to seventh thoracic segments. This portion of the cord was pulseless, and the vessels on its dorsal surface were tortuous and distended. Cephalad the cord was of normal size and pulsated, and caudad it resumed a normal configuration.

Following operation there was progressive deterioration in the patient's condition. She became paraplegic and completely bedridden, and died about 6 months later.

At necropsy it was found that the thoracic cord was shrunken from the level of T4 to T10. All landmarks were obliterated, and the cord was soft in consistency. Microscopic examination revealed extensive degeneration of the white matter, and gliosis of the anterior horns. Ascending and descending degeneration was found in the posterior and lateral columns.

References

Adams, R. D. and Merritt, H. H.: Meningeal and Vascular Disease of the Spinal Cord, Medicine, *23*, 181, 1944.

Greenfield, J. G. and Turner, J. W.: Acute and Subacute Necrotic Myelitis, Brain, *62*, 227, 1939.

Michie, I. and Clark, M.: Neurological Syndromes Associated with Cervical and Craniocervical Anomalies, Arch. neurol., *18*, 241, 1968.

Reagan, T. J., Thomas, J. E. and Colby, M. Y., Jr.: Chronic Progressive Radiation Myelography, J.A.M.A., *203*, 106, 1968.

Wadia, N. H.: Myelopathy Complicating Congenital Atlanto-Axial Dislocation, Brain, *90*, 449, 1967.

9

Diseases of the Hematopoietic, Collagen and Reticuloendothelial Systems

THE LEUKEMIAS

It is generally accepted that the leukemias are neoplastic diseases of the blood-forming organs, from which abnormal white cells of varying maturity and quantity are discharged into the peripheral circulation. A relationship between the leukemias and lymphomas has been indicated by hematologic and pathologic investigations. Willis (1952) regarded the leukemias as circulating tumors, and felt that heterotopic infiltrations and tumors were true metastatic growths arising from the blood-borne malignant leukocytes. No sharp differentiation can be made in the osseous radiologic manifestations of the various types of leukemia, except that in children, the acute leukemias are often accompanied by more marked osseous manifestations.

The osseous manifestations of the leukemias appear most frequently in the appendicular skeleton of children. Caffey (1967) regarded these as due most likely to malignant proliferation of bone marrow reticulum cells, rather than to malignant proliferation of reticulum cells transported from lymphatic structures. However, Willis (1952) concluded that the leukemias are malignant neoplasms with circulating metastases from a tumor originating in the blood-forming tissues. Hence the heterotopic infiltrations and tumors are true metastatic growths arising from blood-borne malignant leukocytes. In early stages the marrow cavity may be packed with leukemic cells, and pain follows such increased pressure. Bone changes usually are of a lytic nature. Occasionally there is evidence of osteosclerosis due to an increase in the density of the spongiosa rather than cortical thickening. At times subperiosteal new bone formation occurs when there has been perforation of the cortex by leukemic spongiosal infiltrations with subsequent elevation of the periosteum or subperiosteal hemorrhage and elevation of the periosteum without underlying cortical perforation.

In the long bones, the most characteristic change is a zone of rarefaction immediately proximal to the metaphyses. This was noted in 70 per cent of 43 cases of childhood leukemia reported by Baty and Vogt (1935), who postulated that infiltration and erosion of bone by masses of leukemic cells was important in the production of this rarefied metaphyseal zone. Silverman (1948), in a report of 103 infants and children with leukemia, mentioned that this was the most common change observed.

In a report of 168 cases, Craver and Copeland (1935) observed that there were 6 with demonstrable changes in the femurs, sternum, humerus, pelvis, skull, metacarpals and ulna and vertebrae, in that order of frequency. Baty and Vogt (1935) observed leukemic destructive changes in the spine and pelvis in children with osteoporosis, softening and compression of the vertebral bodies, similar to that observed with lympho-blastoma and neuroblastoma. Hildebrand (1950) stated that in pronounced cases the vertebrae assume a biconcave appearance, with osteoporosis or a wedge-shaped deformity of the involved bodies. These changes may precede clinical manifestations by several months. Uehlinger (1952) regarded these changes as nonspecific. He postulated that it was not the tumor cells alone that caused the osseous alterations but rather their effects upon the osteoblasts and osteoclasts, with destruction of the former and sparing of the latter.

Jaffe (1952) mentioned that from 50 to 60 per cent of leukemic children had skeletal manifestations, and that the most frequent change consisted of the narrowed transverse zone of radiolucency at the distal ends of the long bones. He, too, noted the occurrence of infractions and compression of the vertebrae. During remissions and while under treatment, the bony lesions may regress. The radiolucent zones are then replaced by dense bands such as those seen with heavy metal poisoning. However, the original lesions reappear when the disease is reactivated. Skeletal changes were observed in adults in from 8 to 10 per cent of cases, principally osteoporosis, osteolytic foci, periosteal new bone formation and fractures.

Windholz and Foster (1949) reported roentgenologic evidence of monostotic or polyostotic sclerosis in leukemia. This had no bearing on the clinical course, and suggested that the bone marrow was becoming fibrous and aplastic. Osteosclerosis of this type was more common in monocytic leukemia and in aleukemia lymphadenosis. One patient with lymphatic leukemia had panostotic sclerosis.

Leukemia also affects the meninges, appearing as epidural deposits or superficial infiltrations of the arachnoid and dura. In the former instance a clinical picture like that of an intraspinal tumor may be encountered (Fig. 456), while in the latter there is perivascular cuffing of the dura, the meninges, the brain and the spinal cord. Sub-

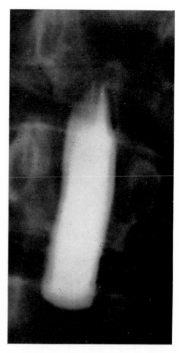

FIG. 456. Epidural mass of leukemic tissue causing a complete block in the lower thoracic spinal canal in a 16-year-old male, verified at operation.

dural, subarachnoid and cerebral hemorrhages ranging from petechial to massive are associated with this change. Increased intracranial pressure may be a presenting problem, and can be associated with intracranial as well as intraspinal meningeal involvement. Severe pain appears with no visible radiographic changes in these children.

Intense pain in the back also develops when retroperitoneal hematomas are incident to leukemia. These can gravitate into the pelvis, deforming the bladder, producing irritability and difficulty in urination. Large clusters of preaortic nodes also can be associated with back pain. These possibilities sometimes are suggested when there is obscuration of the psoas shadow on the left side. If this is suspected, it should be recalled that marked splenomegaly also may obscure the left psoas outline.

A case of extradural leukemic implants was reported by Mosberg (1951) in a 5-month-old child who became paraplegic within a period of 4 weeks. The plain films in this case showed dilatation of the spinal canal at the level of the twelfth thoracic and first lumbar vertebrae, and myelography revealed a complete block at the first lumbar interspace. This was reported as 1 of 23 cases of intraspinal tumors occurring during the first year of life.

The radiologic changes produced by leukemia in the vertebral column are more frequent than generally recognized, especially in infants and children. The usual change observed in younger patients is a diffuse demineralization of bone, loss of trabecular markings and a biconvex appearance of the vertebrae (Fig. 457). Anterior compression of the midthoracic vertebrae is relatively common. There appears to be a tendency for the anterior and posterior venous grooves to be persistent and rather prominent (Fig. 458). The use of steroid and chemotherapeutic measures influences the bony changes, and sometimes one cannot decide whether the bone loss is due to the leukemia or the effects of medication, especially steroids. At necropsy there is an actual absence of abnormal cells in the vertebrae of some children who received steroids and chemotherapy even though marked structural alteration are present, while in others with equally marked changes leukemic infiltrations are present (Fig. 459).

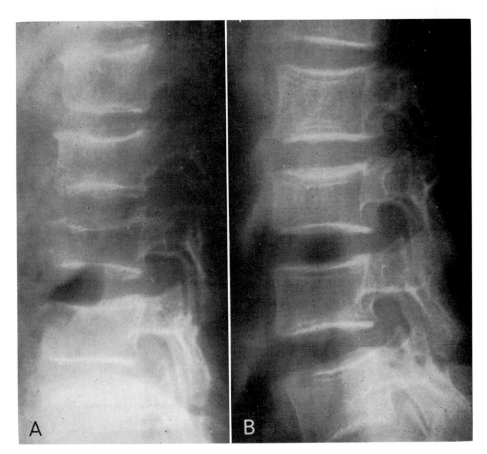

Fig. 457. *A*, Acute leukemia in a 10-year-old girl with moderate back pain. A partial collapse of the body of L3, and proportionate widening of the discs above and below is noted. Diffuse demineralization of the spine is present. *B*, Two years later lines of increased density indicate healing along the epiphyses of the vertebrae. The third lumbar vertebra has regained its usual configuration, but is still smaller than L2 and 4.

In children of from about 2 to 6 years of age the vertebral bodies also become demineralized, but the loss of bone is more prominent in the centrum of the vertebral body and in the epiphyseal zones at the superior and inferior aspects of the involved vertebrae. Zones of increased radiolucency appear at the cartilaginous-osseous junctions, comparable to those seen so frequently at the diaphyseal ends of the growing long bones. Occasionally one can identify one or two parallel lines of increased density between the demineralized epiphyseal zones and the centrum (Fig. 460). Frequently the verte-

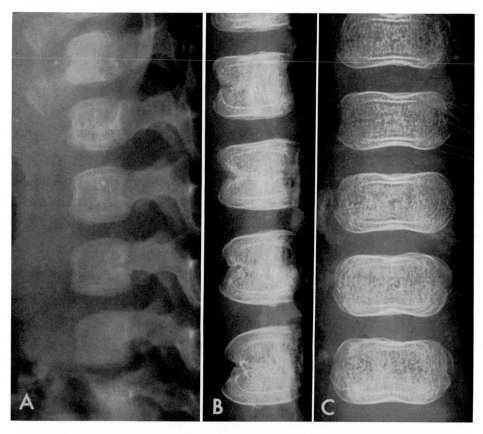

Fig. 458. *A*, Lateral spine film in a child with acute leukemia who had been under treatment with cortisone, mercaptopurine and amethopterin. The vertebrae are demineralized. The anterior vascular groove of L1 is prominent. Note the parallel linear streaks in the upper and lower aspect of the vertebral bodies. *B*, Specimen correlates the changes seen in *A*, lateral roentgenogram. *C*, AP roentgenogram of the specimen.

Fig. 459. *A*, A 3-year-old girl with acute lymphatic leukemia who had had intensive anti-leukemic treatment. At necropsy marked demineralization of bone with diffuse collapse of many vertebrae was found. There is a radiolucent zone parallel to the upper and lower surfaces of the vertebral bodies. At necropsy 3 months later, *B*, there was bulging of the cancellous bone as if under pressure. On gentle pressure it was possible to pop out the centra. On microscopic examination the marrow was packed with leukemic cells, especially at the growth zones. (From Epstein, B. S., Vertebral Changes in Childhood Leukemia, *Radiology, 68*, 65, 1957.) *C* and *D*, AP and lateral roentgenograms of spine specimen of a 4-year-old child with acute lymphatic leukemia who had been under intensive treatment. At necropsy the vertebrae were collapsed and the discs bulged prominently. Microscopic examination revealed almost complete cellular depletion.

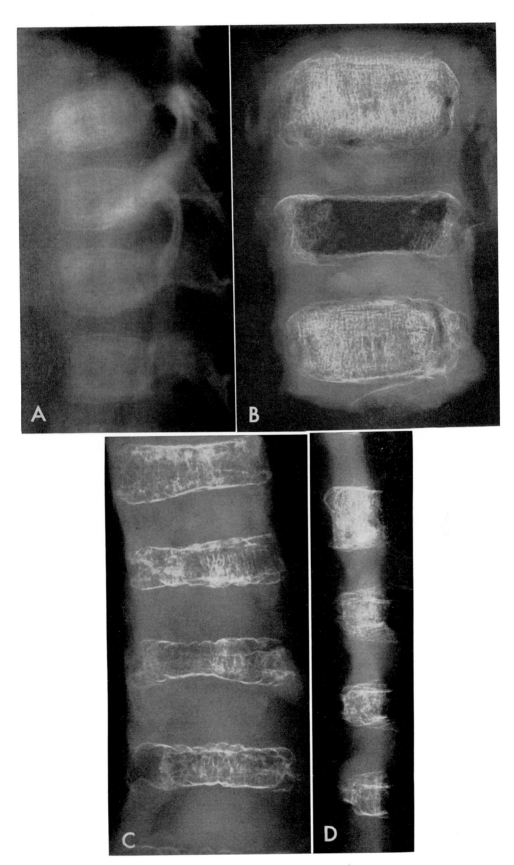

Fig. 459. (*Legend on opposite page.*)

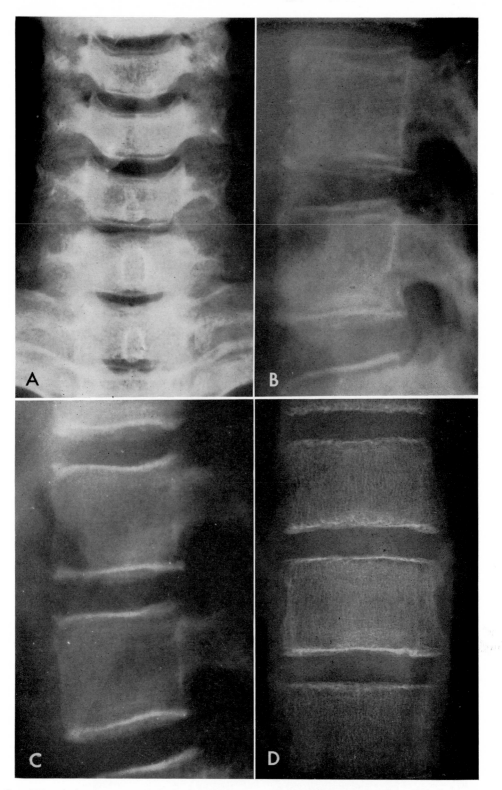

Fig. 460. *A*, Acute monocytic leukemia in a 14-year-old girl with multiple osseous lesions. Note the rarefied zones at the superior and inferior margins of the cervical and the lumbar vertebrae, *B*. *C*, a 14-year-old boy with acute leukemia. Diffuse demineralization of the lumbar vertebrae is present, with rarefied zones in the upper and lower subchondral plates. At necropsy, *D*, a roentgenogram of the specimen shows these lines.

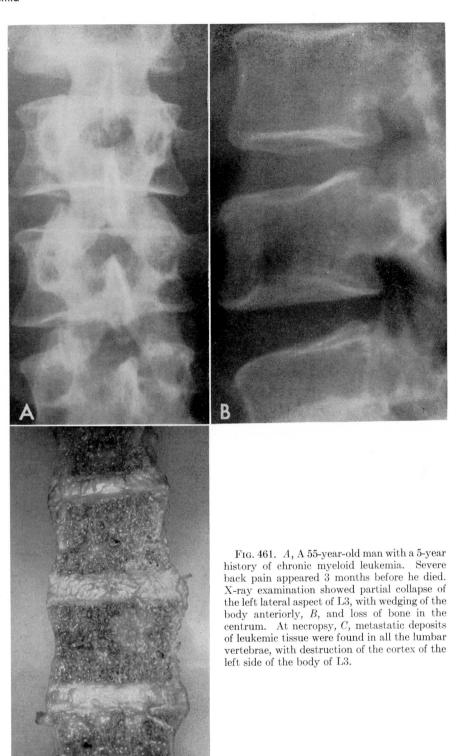

Fig. 461. *A*, A 55-year-old man with a 5-year history of chronic myeloid leukemia. Severe back pain appeared 3 months before he died. X-ray examination showed partial collapse of the left lateral aspect of L3, with wedging of the body anteriorly, *B*, and loss of bone in the centrum. At necropsy, *C*, metastatic deposits of leukemic tissue were found in all the lumbar vertebrae, with destruction of the cortex of the left side of the body of L3.

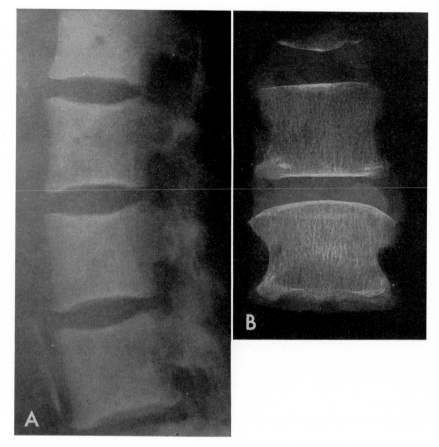

Fig. 462. *A*, Osteosclerosis as a terminal process in a 56-year-old woman with long-standing myelogenous leukema. *B*, Roentgenogram of the specimen.

bral bodies present rounded margins, or are diffusely and variably flattened. When healing and recurrences occur, lines of increased density may be found, as in the long bones (Fig. 457 and 458).

Changes in the growing ends of the vertebrae do not appear in patients past adolescence. Occasionally leukemic infiltrations in adults behave as do other locally invasive tumors, causing bone destruction and consequent partial collapse (Fig. 461). This is relatively infrequent, and cannot be distinguished from other metastatic lesions on the basis of radiologic changes alone. Osteoporosis in this group is likely to be exaggerated if they have been undergoing steroid treatment. Sclerotic changes in the vertebrae appear late in the disease. These

are caused by fibrotic changes in the cancellous bone, and render the vertebrae diffusely hazy in appearance in adults (Fig. 462). Similar changes appear in children who survive over a period of about a year. In these the sclerotic changes may be present in the periphery of the vertebral body, leaving a central rarefied area, or be more or less limited to the upper and lower aspects of the involved bodies (Fig. 463).

The clinical picture associated with leukemia of the spine is apt to be confusing. It is possible to observe rather pronounced changes, particularly in children, with no symptoms at all. However, in others, particularly if there is neural involvement, pain may be pronounced. If there is early vertebral involvement mild, and sometimes se-

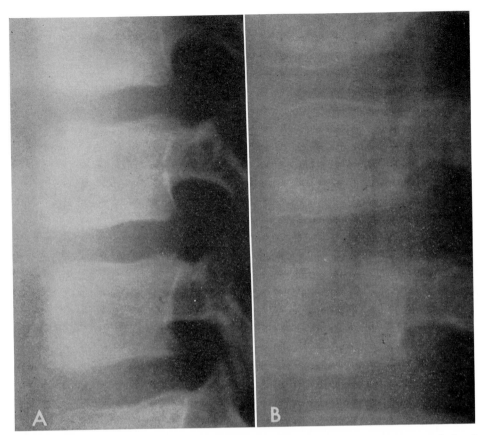

FIG. 463. *A*, Osteosclerosis as a terminal event in a 9-year-old patient with myelogenous leukemia and enormous hepatosplenomegaly. The sclerotic changes are more pronounced at the periphery of the vertebrae. *B*, A 3-year-old child with acute lymphatic leukemia who had been under treatment for 18 months. Osteosclerosis is present at the periphery of the vertebrae, the centra remaining porotic.

vere, back pain is present. In the event of tumorous meningeal implants the picture of an extradural mass may be present. Immediate investigation, including myelography, may be required in order to institute prompt and adequate treatment. In adults with bone destruction the symptoms observed with other metastatic bone deposits are present.

References

Baty, J. M. and Vogt, E. C.: Bone Changes of Leukemia in Children, Am. J. Roentgenol., *34*, 310, 1935.

Caffey, J.: *Pediatric X-ray Diagnosis*, 5th Ed., Chicago, The Year Book Medical Publishers, Inc., 1967.

Craver, L. F. and Copeland, M. M.: Changes of the Bones in Leukemias, Arch. Surg., *30*, 639, 1935.

Critchley, M. and Greenfield, J. G.: Spinal Symptoms in Chloroma and Leukemia, Brain, *53*, 11, 130.

Dale, J. H.: Leukemia in Childhood, J. Pediat., *34*, 421, 1949.

D'Angio, G. J., Evans, A. E. and Mitus, A.: Roentgen Therapy of Certain Complications of Acute Leukemia in Childhood, Am. J. Roentgenol., *82*, 541, 1959.

Epstein, B. S.: Vertebral Changes in Childhood Leukemia, Radiology, *68*, 65, 1957.

Eschenbach, C.: Über eine seltene Form der Wirbelsäulenbeteiligung an akuten Leukosen im Kindesalter, Monatschr. f. Kinderheilk., *113*, 68, 1965.

Hunt, W. E., Couroncle, B. A. and Meagher, J. N.: Neurologic Complications of Leukemias and Lymphomas, J. Neurosurg., *16*, 135, 1959.

Ibbott, J. W. and Whitelaw, D. M.: The Relation Between Lymphosarcoma and Leukemia, Canadian M.A.J., *94*, 517, 1966.

Jaffe, H. L.: Skeletal Manifestations of Leukemia and Malignant Lymphoma, Bull. Hosp. Joint Dis., *13*, 217, 1952.

Karpinski, F. E., Jr. and Martin, J. F.: The Skeletal Lesions of Leukemic Children Treated with Aminopterin, J. Pediat., *37*, 208, 1950.

Lyon, E.: Leukämie und Wirbelsäule, Acta radiol., *17*, 506, 1936.

Mazet, R., Jr.: Vertebral Manifestations of Malignant Lymphoma, Myeloid Leucemia and Multiple Myeloma, Surgery, *29*, 545, 1951.

Mosberg, W. H.: Spinal Tumors Diagnosed During 1st Year of Life, J. Neurosurg., *8*, 220, 1951.

Silverman, F. N.: Skeletal Lesions in Leukemia, Am. J. Roentgenol., *59*, 819, 1948.

Uehlinger, E.: Die skeletveränderungen bei leukamie, Fortschr. Röntgenstr., *77*, 263, 1952. Fortschr. Röntgenstr., *77*, 287, 1952.

Wilhydre, D. E., Jane, J. A. and Mullan, S.: Spinal Epidural Leukemia, Am. J. Med., *34*, 281, 1963.

Willis, R. A.: *The Spread of Tumours in the Human Body*, London, Butterworth & Co., Ltd., 1952.

Windholz, F. and Foster, S. E.: Bone Sclerosis in Leukemia and in Non-leukemic Myelosis, Am. J. Roentgenol., *61*, 61, 1949.

Myelosclerotic Anemia

Various names have been applied to this condition, including myelosclerosis, myelofibrosis, leukoerythroblastic anemia, myelophthysic anemia, nonleukemic myelosis, agnogenic myeloid metaplasia, and agnogenic splenomegaly. The disease may be classified as an atypical form of myelogenous leukemia, or a megakaryocytic leukemia because of an increase in megakaryocytes in the bone marrow or other organs. It is characterized by generalized fibrosis of the bone marrow with excessive proliferation of endosteal bone. The fibrosis may involve the marrow cavity alone, or extend to and elevate the periosteum. The patches of fibrosis within the marrow cavity are scattered or confluent, and vary greatly. The entire skeleton may be involved, particularly the blood-forming marrow as represented by the spinal column, the pelvis, the ribs and the proximal portions of the long bones. As a result of the replacement of the red marrow by fibrous tissue, compensatory hyperplasia appears in the remaining hematopoietic tissues, particularly the liver, the spleen, and occasionally the ovaries and adrenals, the mediastinum and retroperitoneal regions become active in extramedullary hematopoiesis (Lowman, Bloor and Newcomb, 1963).

Examination of the circulating blood reveals immature red blood cells and leukocytes which may lead to confusion with chronic myeloid leukemia. Anemia is frequent, although in the early stages of the disease a moderate polycythemia occurs. Splenomegaly becomes pronounced later in the disease, and is one of the factors adding confusion to the differential diagnosis. While a moderate polycythemia is not uncommon in early stages, anemia in these patients finally becomes progressive. Leukoblastic activity is heightened and death may follow leukemic invasion of the spleen and other organs, or bone marrow exhaustion with myelosclerosis. Windholz and Foster (1949) pointed out that either splenectomy or x-ray therapy might hasten death, commenting that many such patients may live comfortably for 30 years or more without treatment. Bastrup-Madsen (1952) emphasized the importance of differentiating myelosclerotic anemia from other diseases in which radiation therapy or splenectomy might be contemplated, inasmuch as these procedures might prove dangerous in myelosclerotic anemia. There is evidence, however, that x-ray therapy or splenectomy actually may be palliative when hypersplenism is pronounced (Linman and Bethell, 1957; Leigh, Corely, Huguley and Rogers, 1959).

The radiologic changes seen with myelosclerotic anemia, as indicated by the name, are predominantly sclerotic. In the vertebral column the splotchy confluent areas of increased density appear in the spongiosa as fairly uniformly distributed patches in the thoracic and lumbar vertebrae, and are less frequently seen in the cervical vertebrae (Fig. 464). No alterations are found in the configuration of the vertebrae or the intervertebral discs. Less frequently the bony changes are diffuse, giving rise to a relatively increased density of the vertebrae with loss of definition of the trabecular markings and replacement of these by a diffuse, almost ground-glass increase in osseous density (Fig. 465). The combination of hepatosplenomegaly with osteosclerotic changes in

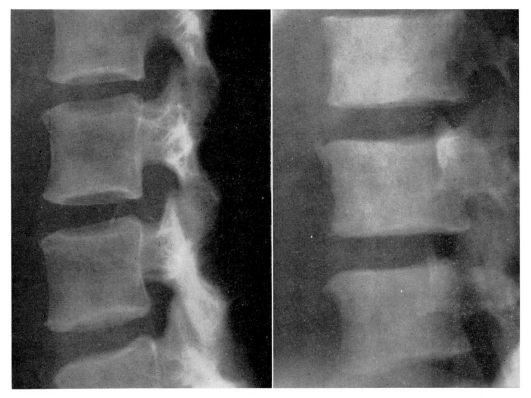

Fig. 464   Fig. 465

Fig. 464. A 42-year-old woman with osteosclerotic anemia known for 13 years. Patchy myelosclerosis is present, with no change in vertebral configuration.

Fig. 465. A 57-year-old man with myelosclerosis following polycythemia. On bone marrow aspiration the bone was found to be extremely hard. A diffuse osteosclerosis renders the vertebrae almost uniformly opaque except for small islands of denser calcification.

the vertebrae without alterations in their contours is regarded as a fairly reliable diagnostic point.

Microscopic examination of the diseased tissue reveals a diffuse or focal proliferation of endosteal bone, with prominent, large active osteoblasts. Osteoid tissue is minimal or absent, spicules composed of osseous tissue are found scattered through the medullary spaces and there is a distinct paucity of osteoclasts. This results in prominence and overgrowth of the trabeculae which become confluent in an irregular manner, producing scattered foci of denser bony spicules merging with the endosteum.

Secondary myelosclerosis may occur with other diseases of the osseous system, of which

metastatic prostatic carcinoma is the most common (Bersack and Feinstein, 1946). Diffuse endosteal sclerosis also is seen with widespread metastases from carcinoma of the breast, stomach or colon, or with chronic myelogenous leukemia. Reported elsewhere here are 2 cases of carcinoma of the stomach with widespread myelofibrosis secondary to metastatic disease in which the primary lesion was found at necropsy.

Osteosclerosis also occurs, although infrequently, with longstanding chronic renal insufficiency, and affects the lumbar vertebrae, the pelvis, the sacrum and less often the chest, skull and femurs. The cause for this is unknown, and the change is in interesting contrast with the more frequently observed resorptive changes resulting from the secondary hyperparathyroidi. m associated with uremia.

Myelosclerosis also occurs in Paget's disease, myeloma, terminal polycythemia vera (Fig. 465), tuberculosis and syphilis. Benzene, fluorine, lead, arsenic and phosphorus poisoning are also considered causative Bastrup-Madsen, 1952). Similar changes may also be part of the picture of metabolic disturbances such as Albright's disease, osteomalacia, osteitis fibrosa cystica and the various lipid dyscrasias (Erf and Herbut, 1944). One of the conditions which is frequently included as a cause of osteosclerotic anemia is Albers-Schönberg's disease, but this represents a defect in development of mesenchymatous elements rather than a fibroplastic reaction to a stimulus which also produces extramedullary hematopoiesis. Urticaria pigmentosa with bone involvement must also be distinguished.

References

Bastrup-Madsen, P.: Myelosclerotic Anemia, Acta radiol., *37*, 189, 1952.

Bersack, S. R. and Feinstein, H. R.: Secondary Myelofibrosis with Progressive Generalized Eburnation, Am. J. Roentgenol., *56*, 470, 1946.

Birkner, R. and Frey, J. G.: Über die röntgenologischen, hämatologischen und pathologischanatomischen Grundlagen der Anaemia leucoerythroblastica mid Myelosklerosis vom Typ Vaughan, Fortschr.Röntgenstr., *77*, 287, 1952.

Brookfield, R. W., Rubin, E. L. and Alexander, M. K.: Osteosclerosis in Renal Failure, J. Fac. Radiologists, *7*, 102, 1955.

Erf, L. A. and Herbut, P. A.: Primary and Secondary Myelofibrosis, Ann. Int. Med., *21*, 863, 1944.

Green, T. W., Donley, C. L., Ashburn, L. L. and Peters, H. R.: Splenectomy for Myeloid Metaplasia of Spleen, New England J. Med., *248*, 211, 1953.

Hickling, R. A.: Chronic Non-leukaemic Myelosis, Quart. J. Med., *6*, 253, 1937.

Jacobson, H. G., Fateh, H., Shapiro, J. H., Spaet, T. H. and Poppel, M. H.: Agnogenic Myeloid Metaplasia, Radiology, *72*, 716, 1959.

Jensen, W. N. and Lasser, E. C.: Urticaria Pigmentosa Associated with Wide-spread Sclerosis of the Spongiosa of Bone, Radiology, *71*, 826, 1958.

Kaye, M., Pritchard, J. E., Halpenny, G. W. and Light, W.: Bone Disease in Chronic Renal Failure with Particular Reference to Osteosclerosis, Medicine, *39*, 157, 1960.

Korst, D. R., Clatanoff, D. V. and Schilling, R. F.: On Myelofibrosis, Arch. Int. Med., *97*, 169, 1956.

Leigh, T. F., Corely, C. C., Jr., Huguley, C. M., Jr. and Rogers, J. V., Jr.: Myelofibrosis: The General and Radiologic Findings in 25 Proved Cases, Am. J. Roentgenol., *82*, 183, 1959.

Lewis, S. M. and Szur, L.: Malignant Myelosclerosis, Brit. Med. J., *2*, 472, 1963.

Linman, J. W. and Bethell, F. H.: Agnogenic Myeloid Metaplasia, Its Natural History and Present Day Management, Am. J. Med., *22*, 107, 1957.

Lowman, R. M., Bloor, C. M. and Newcomb, A. W.: Roentgen Manifestations of Thoracic Extramedullary Hematopoiesis, Dis. Chest, *44*, 154, 1963.

Mulcahy, R.: Bone Changes in Myelosclerosis, Proc. Royal Soc. Med., *50*, 100, 1957.

Rohr, K.: Myelofibrose und Osteomyelosklerose, Acta haemat., *15*, 209, 1956.

Rosenthal, N. and Erf, L. A.: Osteopetrosis and Myelofibrosis, Arch. Int. Med., *71*, 793, 1943.

Schorr, S., Sagher, F. and Liban, E.: Generalized Osteosclerosis in Urticaria Pigmentosa, Acta radiol., *46*, 576, 1956.

Sussman, M. L.: Myelosclerosis with Leukoerythroblastic Anemia, Am. J. Roentgenol., *57*, 313, 1947.

Windholz, F. and Foster, A. E.: Bone Sclerosis in Leukemia and in Nonleukemic Myelosis, Am. J. Roentgenol., *61*, 61, 1949.

Wolf, H. L. and Denko, J. V.: Osteosclerosis in Chronic Renal Disease, Am. J. Med. Sci., *235*, 33, 1958.

POLYCYTHEMIA VERA

This condition, characterized by a pronounced increase in the circulating red blood cells, presents with cyanosis, particularly of the face and mucous membranes, enlargement of the liver, and to a lesser degree, of the spleen. Other complaints are headaches, diffuse aches and pains over the limbs and trunk, easy fatiguability, dizziness, tinnitus, dyspnea on exertion and mental depression. The concomitance of polycythemia vera and peptic ulcer and various neurogenic diseases centering on the midbrain-pituitary area has been described. The association of polycythemia vera with leukemia is recognized, and it is believed that the disease is not limited to the erythropoietic system but rather involves the entire blood-forming apparatus. Polycythemia may be accompanied by a corresponding non-malignant proliferation in the leukoblastic portion of the bone marrow, as evidenced by the elevated white cell count not infrequently encountered. A high incidence of leukemia is noted in patients surviving more than 10 years.

Histologic examination of sections of the bone marrow from the sternum show hyperplastic marrow with replacement of fatty tissue by hematopoietic tissue. Hyperplasia of cells of the megakaryocytic, erythroid, and myeloid series and a tendency for the cells of the erythroblastic series to occur in small clusters was reported by Lawrence, Berline and Huff (1953). In 2 cases observed at necropsy hyperplastic bone marrow was found in the vertebrae. In 1935, Hirsch reported post-mortem observations in a male patient 55 years old who had polycythemia for 31 years. Examination of the lumbar vertebrae showed the marrow to be tan-red in color and reduced to approximately one-fifth of its usual volume. The bone trabeculae were markedly thickened and the dimensions of the marrow spaces were correspondingly reduced. Along the edges of the trabeculae were narrow layers of new bone. Hirsch concluded that the generalized osteosclerosis in this case was probably part of the picture of the advanced chronic stage of the disease. Stodmeister and Sandkühler (1952) also mentioned that patients with polycythemia vera who survived long enough developed myelofibrosis which ultimately might progress to osteomyelosclerosis.

The radiologic changes in the spine associated with polycythemia vera are minimal. In a review of 88 proved cases Hodgson, Good and Hall (1946) were unable to find any bone lesions attributable to the disease. However, in cases of extremely long duration such as that described by Hirsch (1935), radiographic examination of the spine might in occasional instances reveal sclerotic bone marrow changes (Fig. 465).

References

Hirsch, E. F.: Generalized Osteosclerosis with Chronic Polycythemia Vera, Arch. Path., *19*, 91, 1935.

Hodgson, J. R., Good, C. A. and Hall, B. E.: Roentgenographic Aspects of Polycythemia Vera, Proc. Staff Meet., Mayo Clin., *21*, 152, 1946.

Lawrence, J. H., Berline, N. I. and Huff, R. L.: Polycythemia, Medicine, *32*, 323, 1953.

Skversky, N., Mendell, T. H. and Frumin, A. M.: Polycythemia Vera Terminating in Acute Leukemia, Arch. Int. Med., *96*, 565, 1955.

Stodtmesiter, R. and Sandkühler, S.: Grundsatzliches zur röntgenologischen Beurteilung der Osteomyelosklerose, Fortschr. Röntgenstr., *77*, 283, 1952.

Wasserman, L. R.: Polycythemia Vera: Its Relation to Myeloid Metaplasia and Leukemia, Bull. New York Acad. Med., *30*, 343, 1954.

ACQUIRED HEMOLYTIC ANEMIA

This is a disease of unknown etiology in which the red blood cells are destroyed, presumably by an auto-agglutinin attached to the red cells and capable of reacting with normal human erythrocytes. It may appear in previously healthy persons or may develop in patients with primary atypical pneumonia, with lymphomas or with collagen

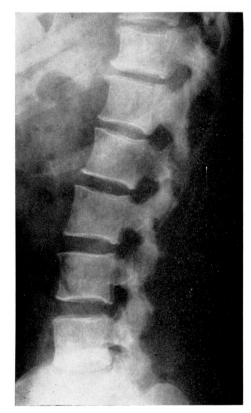

FIG. 466. Lateral lumbar spine of a 37-year-old male who had had a splenectomy 7 years before for acquired hemolytic anemia. There is diffuse and spotty osteosclerosis in the vertebral bodies.

disease. It occurs at any age, and is more frequent in females. The condition was reviewed by Sacks, Workman and Jahn (1952) who reported on 19 patients studied by them and 47 collected from the literature. No mention was made of skeletal changes.

In our material was one man 37 years old who had had a splenectomy for acquired hemolytic anemia 7 years before the present films were made. Spine roentgenograms revealed osteosclerotic changes, much the same in appearance as with osteosclerotic anemia (Fig. 466). Of interest in this patient is the fact that x-ray films of the lower femurs showed a flask-like appearance similar to that described in Gaucher's disease. Mild osteosclerotic changes were also present in the distal ends of the femurs and the upper ends of the tibias.

Reference

Sacks, M. E., Workman, J. B. and Jahn, E. F.: Diagnosis and Treatment of Acquired Hemolytic Anemia, J.A.M.A., *150*, 1556, 1952.

Sickle Cell Anemia

This condition is a hemolytic anemia occurring principally, but not exclusively in the Negro race. It is a chronic familial disease characterized by sickle-shaped red blood cells, attributed to a characteristic inherited type of pathologic hemoglobin which can be differentiated from normal by electrophoresis. The abnormal hemoglobin, designated as Hemoglobin S, is inherited as a dominant Mendelian characteristic. If this is received from both parents, a homozygous state results in sickle cell anemia. When the S factor comes from but one parent, a heterozygous state produces the sickle cell trait. Sickling then appears under stresses like exposure to cold, and symptoms appear only if thrombotic phenomena follow. Bony changes are rarely seen in patients with the sickle-cell trait. Another hemoglobin variant, hemoglobin C, also can interact with hemoglobin S to produce sickle cell

hemoglobin C disease, which is milder than the true sickle cell homozygous S/S disease.

In acute stages of S/S sickle cell disease vascular occlusive phenomena affecting all the organs of the body produce variously abdominal, central nervous system, bone and joint, urogenital and skin lesions. There are periods of exacerbation and remission. Anemia, leg ulcers, abdominal and joint pains, splenomegaly, cardiac murmurs, fever and leukocytosis occur in children. Bone and joint pains may predominate, and be sufficiently severe to simulate osteomyelitis. The joint pains may be migratory and associated with fever and leukocytosis, simulating rheumatic fever or rheumatoid arthritis. The widespread changes encountered in the various visceral organs are due to thromboses from the rigid sickle cells in the capillaries, which rapidly ascend to larger vessels, particularly on the arterial side. The crises of sickle cell anemia follow the widespread thromboses which appear as the capillaries are plugged. This may induce a widespread concomitant vasospasm. Hyperplasia of the bone marrow occurs in an effort to maintain the circulating blood. This takes place in the cancellous bone, and is most marked in the axial skeleton, the skull and the long bones.

Patients with sickle cell anemia of long duration present a fairly characteristic habitus in which the patient is underweight, thin, with narrow hips and shoulders and decreased stature. An increase in the upper dorsal spine curvature and lumbar lordosis is common. The neck and trunk are short, and an increase in the anteroposterior diameter of the chest often is present. The abdomen may protrude and the limbs remain thin. The hands are long, narrow and tapering. Margolies (1951) believed that the characteristic body habitus was probably due to anemia during the formative years, and to the frequent arteriolar thromboses. The decreased weight and stature was presumed to be due to changes in the anterior pituitary body, which in turn is accompanied by atrophy of the testes and other signs of hypogonadism in males.

Skeletal changes are observed frequently, principally in the skull, the spinal column, the femurs and the tibias and fibulae. Less commonly rarefied, trabeculated changes with patches of osteosclerosis appear in the small bones of the hands and feet and the long bones of the arms. The bony changes are produced by hyperplasia of the erythroblastic tissues in the bone marrow. As the marrow is increased in bulk there is a concomitant attempt to replace the marrow with osteoid tissue and new bone. In childhood, the predominant change is usually widening of the medullary canals and thinning of the cortex of the tubular bones. In a case reported by Henkin (1949) with col-

lapse of the vertebral bodies, examination of the bone marrow at necropsy in a 14-year-old Negro boy revealed great cellularity and congestion, with trabecular destruction and connective tissue replacement taking place in the erythropoietic portions of the cancellous bone. He believed that the process was a form of osteoporosis in which the osteoblasts do not lay down sufficient osseous matrix because of a numerical decrease in osteoblasts rather than a decrease in their activity. This process is intermittent, and probably associated with diminished circulation due to the thrombotic tendencies affecting the intraosseous circulation. This combination of intraosseous destruction of trabeculae, hyperplasia of the marrow and reparative processes is basically responsible

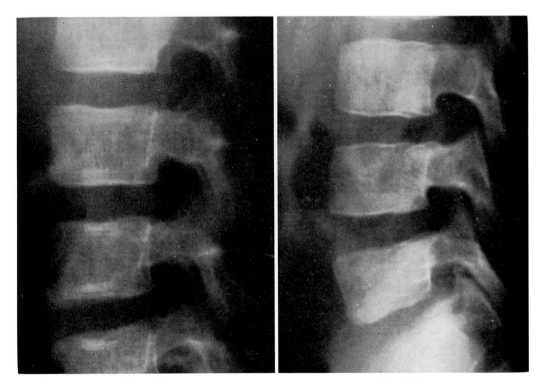

FIG. 467   FIG. 468

FIG. 467. A 6-year-old boy with sickle cell anemia. Diffuse rarefaction of the vertebrae with interlacing spans of cancellous bone is seen. There is no flattening of the bodies, but the discs are wide and beginning to indent the bodies.

FIG. 468. A 9-year-old patient with known sickle cell anemia, with diffuse demineralization of the vertebrae. The discs are widened. Radiolucent lines are present in the superior and inferior margins of L3 and 4, much the same as seen in some leukemic patients. The nature of these lines is not clear.

for the presence of patchy areas of demineralization and increased bone activity.

The early radiologic changes in the spine associated with sickle cell anemia are a diffuse osteoporosis and slight widening of the intervertebral discs. Later in the disease the vertebral bodies become flattened, and as reparative efforts occur, osteosclerotic foci become demonstrable as streaky interwoven filaments of increased bony density within the vertebral bodies. These changes occur either in the thoracic or in the lumbar vertebrae, the cervical spine usually remaining unchanged. In a report of 48 cases with examinations of the spine, Ehrenpreis and Schwinger (1952) reported that changes were found in 34. These were marked in 7 cases, moderate in 14 and minimal in the remaining 13.

The roentgenologic appearance of the vertebrae varies with the stage of the disease encountered at the time of examination. In young individuals in whom there has been relatively little in the way of occlusive phenomena and reparative effort, there may be no visible changes. When the occlusive phenomena are more advanced, and reparative efforts have taken place to an appreciable degree, the interlacing streaky appearance of the vertebral bodies become more prominent (Figs. 467 and 468). In later stages, particularly in adolescents, the efforts at repair may be pronounced, and the vertebral bodies assume a biconvex appearance together with patchy sclerotic areas. The opening of the anterior vertebral vein occasionally becomes prominent because of loss of adjacent bone (Fig. 469).

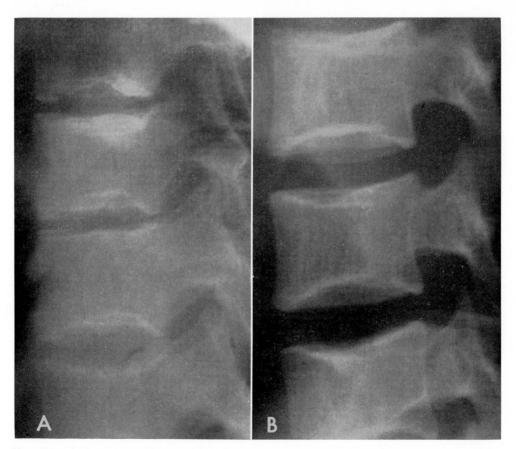

Fig. 469. *A*, An 18-year-old man with sickle cell anemia for 14 years. The thoracic vertebrae show indentations into the bodies, with slight adjacent bone condensation. Erosive changes are seen in the vicinity of the anterior vascular channels. The lumbar vertebrae, *B*, are diffusely porotic. The discs are biconvex and intrude into the bodies. Diffuse sclerotic changes are present in the cancellous bone.

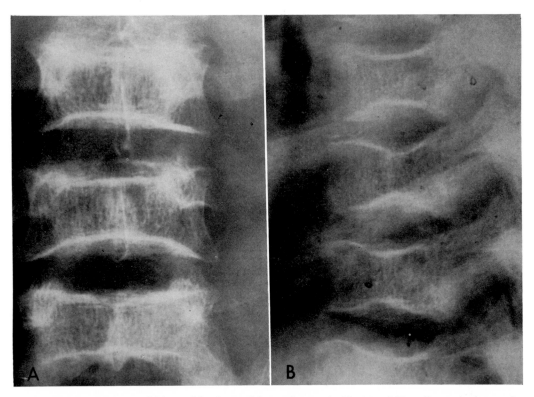

Fig. 470. *A*, A 15-year-old boy with advanced bony changes incident to sickle cell anemia, known for about 13 years. There is a diffuse flattening of the bodies with biconvex discs. Intermingled sclerotic and porotic changes are present. The indentations into the midportions of the vertebrae are prominent. *B*.

In older patients, at or past adolescence, the more advanced changes include flattening and broadening of the vertebrae, with pronounced biconvex alterations in the bodies of the thoracic and lumbar segments. The trabeculae are sclerotic, with prominence of the vertical components (Fig. 470). Reynolds (1966) regarded this appearance as produced more likely by local inhibition of bone growth as a result of regional ischemia rather than destruction and compression of bone as with osteoporosis. He pointed out that the end plates of the growing centra where the cupping takes place are functionally analogous to metaphyses, and that the regional vascular anatomy is such that only the central portion of the growth plate suffers damage when the circulation through branches of the nutrient arteries is impaired. The period during which the deformity evolves is related to the time when rapid bone growth occurs. He regards this cupping as virtually pathognomonic of the hemoglobinopathy.

The occurrence of vertebral changes incident to what was presumed to be a massive infarction was reported by Legant and Ball (1948). In one of their patients, a 39-year-old male, the lowermost two lumbar vertebrae presented an unusual appearance. They noted that 2 weeks after an abdominal crisis roentgenograms of the spine were normal. Eight weeks later areas of rarefaction appeared, with compression of the adjacent margins of the fourth and fifth lumbar vertebrae. Ten weeks later the bodies were further compressed with areas of rarefaction in the anterosuperior aspect of the fifth lumbar vertebra. Eight, 10 and 12 months thereafter there was restitution of the architecture of these vertebral bodies almost to normal, with a homogeneous increase in the density of both vertebrae and narrowing of the third and fourth intervertebral discs. Actual collapse of the vertebral bodies with sickle cell anemia is rare. Carrol and Evans (1949) stated that this had not been reported in the literature up until the time of their report. They described an 11-year-old patient in whom there was destruction and collapse of the bodies of the ninth and tenth thoracic vertebrae.

References

Barton, C. J. and Cockshott, W. P.: Bone Changes in Hemoglobin SC Disease, Am. J. Roentgenol., *88*, 523, 1962.

Becker, J. A.: Hemoblobin S-C Disease, Am. J. Roentgenol., *88*, 503, 1962.

Carrol, D. S. and Evans, J. W.: Roentgen Findings in Sickle-cell Anemia, Radiology, *53*, 834, 1949.

Cockshott, W. P.: Hemoglobin S-C Disease, J. Fac. Radiologists, *9*, 211, 1958.

Ehrenpreis, B. and Schwinger, H. N.: Sickle Cell Anemia, Am. J. Roentgenol., *68*, 28, 1952.

Golding, J. S. R., MacIver, J. E. and Went, L. N.: The Bone Changes in Sickle Cell Anemia and its Genetic Variants, J. Bone & Joint Surg., *41-B*, 711, 1959.

Hamburg, A. E.: Skeletal Changes in Sickle-cell Anemia, J. Bone & Joint Surg., *32-A*, 893, 1950.

Henkin, W. A.: Collapse of Vertebral Bodies in Sickle Cell Anemia, Am. J. Roentgenol., *62*, 395, 1949.

Kraft, E. and Bertel, G.: Sickle Cell Anemia, Am. J. Roentgenol., *57*, 224, 1947.

Kimmelstiel, P.: Vascular Occlusion and Ischemic Infarction in Sickle Cell Disease, Am. J. Med. Sci., *216*, 11, 1948.

Legant, O. and Ball, R. P.: Sickle-cell Anemia in Adults, Radiology, *51*, 665, 1948.

Macht, S. H. and Roman, P. W.: The Radiological Changes in Sickle Cell Anemia, Radiology, *51*, 697, 1948.

Margolies, M. P.: Sickle Cell Anemia, Medicine, *30*, 357, 1951.

Middlemiss, J. H.: Sickle-cell Anemia, J. Fac. Radiologists, *9*, 16, 1958.

Mosely, J. E.: Patterns of Bone Changes in the Sickle Cell States, J. Mt. Sinai Hosp., *26*, 424, 1959.

Ogden, M. A.: Sickle Cell Anemia in White Race, Arch. Int. Med., *71*, 164, 1943.

Patterson, R. H., Wilson, H. and Diggs, L. W.: Sickle-cell Anemia, Surgery, *28*, 393, 1950.

Reynolds, J.: A Re-Evaluation of the "Fish Vertebra" Sign in Sickle Cell Hemoglobinopathy, Am. J. Roentgenol., *97*, 693, 1966.

Winsor, T. and Burch, G. E.: Habitus of Patients with Active Sickle-Cell Anemia of Long Duration, Arch. Int. Med., *76*, 47, 1945.

THALASSEMIA

In 1925 Cooley and Lee described an unusual type of progressive anemia in childhood, with erythroblastosis, splenomegaly, hepatomegaly and peculiar osseous changes, called Mediterranean anemia, erythroblastic anemia, thalassemia, or target cell anemia. The patient is underdeveloped, pale and listless and the condition is associated with cardiac dilatation, edema and effusion into the serous cavities. The disease is familial, and while generally observed in people of Mediterranean origin, has been reported in others such as Chinese, Mexican, American Indian, Filipino and other non-Mediterranean people (Silver, 1950) (Minnich, Na-Nakorn, Chong-Chaveonsuk and Kochasini, 1954). Cooley's anemia may affect adolescents and adults in a less severe heterozygous form, with the patient unaware of his illness. The clinical differentiation between Cooley's anemia and Cooley's trait and their genetic relationships were discussed by Daland and Strauss (1948). The thalassemia gene also can combine with that of the sickle cell trait, resulting in sickle cell thalassemia disease (MacIver, Went and Cruickshank, 1958). Other combinations with abnormal hemoglobins, such as hemoglobin A, F and S, present a variety of clinical manifestations. Both thalassemia major and the variants associated with combined hemoglobinopathies are not entirely consistent in their manifestations, and the longevity of these patients is not predictable.

The milder forms of the disease may be associated with a mild or even absent anemia, increased reticulocytosis, absence of erythroblastosis and the presence of anisocytosis, poikilocytosis, target cells and basophilic stippling of the red cells in the peripheral blood. In the severe homozygous form anemia is pronounced, with hypochromic microcytic and nucleated red cells prominent in the peripheral smear. The blood shows signs of increased erythrocyte formation, with anisocytosis and poikilocytosis. In young children the leukocyte count may be increased, with an increased lymphocyte content. Myeloblasts and myelocytes also are found. Aspiration of the bone marrow reveals hyperplasia of red cells with a pronounced increase in normoblasts. The red cells are remarkably resistant to rupture in hypotonic saline solutions.

The osseous changes present with thalassemia are due primarily to over-activity and overgrowth of the bone marrow. Consequently the skeletal changes in infants and children reflect the disposition of red marrow. The characteristic osteoporosis, thinning of the cortex of the long bones, widening of the medullary canals and the heavy traversing cancellous interlacing web-like strands may be observed in all the bones except the skull, which has its own peculiar spreading of the tables, prominent frontal bones, small facial bones and hair-on-end picture. In patients surviving adolescence, regression of the bony changes takes place, particularly in the shafts of the long bones. Caffey (1951) followed 4 patients to their 28th, 26th, 18th and 14th birthdays respectively, and found that after puberty the optimal sites for demonstrating osseous x-ray changes were the skull, the spine and the pelvis. This reflected the sites of active bone marrow as the individuals grew into adult life. Premature fusion of the epiphyses occurs fairly often in patients over 10 years old (Currarino and Erlandson, 1964). Maturation of the epiphyses is delayed. Caminopetros (1938) reported bone changes of erythroblastic anemia in apparently healthy parents of patients

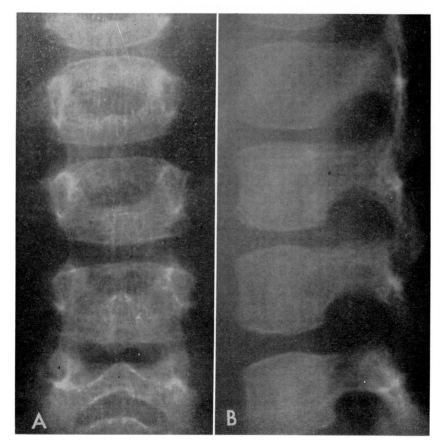

Fig. 471. *A*, Diffuse reticular changes in the vertebrae of a 7-year-old boy with Cooley's anemia. The entire skeleton was affected. The vertebral bodies are ovoid, and the reticular changes involve the neural arches. *B*, The intervertebral discs, are well maintained.

with this condition. March, Schlyen and Schwartz (1952) followed several patients in the 4th and 5th decades in the same family with characteristic changes in the bones including the vertebrae.

The earliest vertebral changes observed with Cooley's anemia include diffuse demineralization of the thoracolumbar spine. The upper and lower aspects of the bodies assume a rounded appearance, so that the intervertebral discs are slightly biconvex anteriorly. The anterior walls of the vertebrae are slightly indented, and occasionally the opening for the anterior spinal vein is prominent, particularly in the lower thoracic segments. As the condition progresses a

reticular increase in the trabeculae becomes apparent in the bodies and the neural arches, with no significant changes in alignment (Fig. 471). The youngest patient in whom this was observed was 20 months old. Later changes include continued loss of cortical bone, particularly in the anterior aspect of the vertebral bodies. The centra present moderate rarefaction of the core of some segments, with a relative increase in the density of the upper and lower portions (Fig. 472). At this stage a more pronounced concavity appears anteriorly in the bodies of the thoracolumbar segments (Fig. 473). Still later progression includes mild vertebral wedging in this region and in the midthoracic

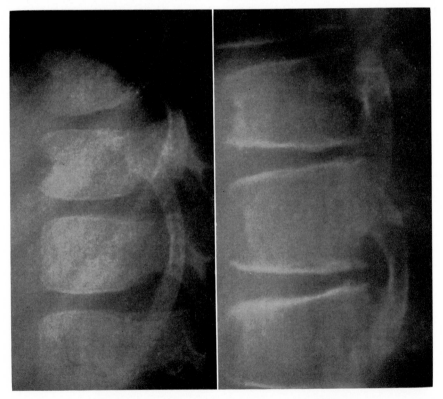

FIG. 472   FIG. 473

FIG. 472. A 5-year-old girl with Cooley's anemia for 20 months. The thoracolumbar vertebrae are diffusely involved with a sclerotic process together with loss of bone. The anterior vascular grooves at T10 and 11 are unusually prominent.

FIG. 473. A 9-year-old girl with known Cooley's anemia since the age of 7 months. Extensive skeletal changes are present. Compression of the anterior aspect of the lower thoracic and upper lumbar vertebrae is present, with widening of the anterior portions of the discs. A diffuse loss of bone of the anterior wall of several of the vertebrae is present as well.

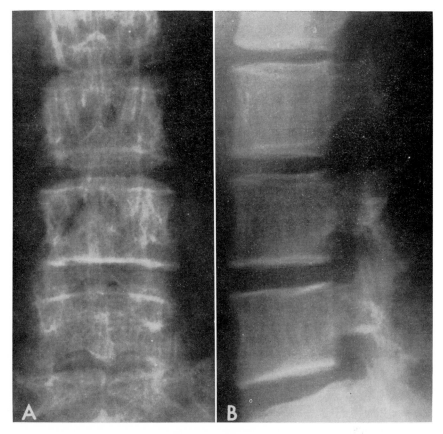

Fig. 474. *A*, A 15-year-old girl with known Cooley's anemia for 12 years. A widespread pattern of reticular bony thickening is evident. The discs are not disturbed. *B*, Some loss of bone in the anterior aspect of L2 is visible on the lateral study.

vertebrae. Flattening and cup-shaped deformities are not, as a rule, visible, nor do the intervertebral discs assume a biconvex appearance. In those who survive the vertebrae retain a rather square configuration, with persistence of the sclerotic changes in the cancellous portion (Fig. 474).

References

Baty, J. M., Blackfan, K. D. and Diamond, L. K.: Erythroblastic Anemia; Clinical and Pathologic Study, Am. J. Dis. Child., *43*, 667, 1932.

Caffey, J.: Cooley's Erythroblastic Anemia, Am. J. Roentgenol., *65*, 547, 1951.

———: Cooley's Anemia: A Review of the Roentgenographic Findings in the Skeleton, Am. J. Roentgenol., *78*, 381, 1957.

Caminopteros, J.: Recherches sur l'anémie Erythroblastique Infantile des Peuples de la Mediterranee Orientale, Ann. de Méd., *43*, 104, 1938.

Cooley, T. B. and Lee, P.: Erythroblastic Anemia, Am. J. Dis. Child., *43*, 705, 1932.

Cooley, T. B., Witwer, E. R. and Lee, P.: Anemia in Children with Splenomegaly and Peculiar Changes in the Bones, Am. J. Dis. Child., *34*, 347, 1927.

Currarino, G. and Erlandson, M. E.: Premature Fusion of Epiphyses in Cooley's Anemia, Radiology, *83*, 656, 1964.

Daland, G. A. and Strauss, M. D.: Genetic Relation and Clinical Differentiation of Cooley's Anemia and Cooley's Trait, Blood, *3*, 438, 1948.

MacIver, J. E., Went, L. N. and Cruickshank, E. K.: Sickle Cell-Thalassemia Disease in Jamaica, Blood, *13*, 359, 1958.

March, H. W., Schlyen, S. M. and Schwartz, S. E.: Mediterranean Hemopathic Syndromes (Cooley's Anemia) in Adults, Am. J. Med., *13*, 46, 1952.

Minnich, V., Na-Nakorn, S., Chong-Chareonsuk, S. and Kochaseni, S.: Mediterranean Anemia, Blood, *9*, 1, 1954.

Silver, H. K.: Mediterranean Anemia in Children of Non-Mediterranean Ancestry, Am. J. Dis. Child., *80*, 676, 1950.

Wintrobe, M. M., Mathews, E., Pollack, R. and Dobyno, B. M.: Familial Hemopoietic Disorder in Italian Adolescents and Adults Resembling Mediterranean Disease (Thalassemia), J.A.M.A., *114*, 1530, 1940.

Vertebral Changes with Cyanotic Heart Disease

Sclerotic changes appear infrequently in the vertebrae of patients with cyanotic heart disease of long standing. Nice, Daves and Wood (1964) reported 6 patients from 19 months to 42 years old who had been cyanotic from birth or childhood. Polycythemia was present in 5. The skull had thickened tables, wide diploe and hair-on-end appearance. Widening of the medullary cavities and thinning of the cortex was seen in the long bones. The trabecular pattern was coarse. In some periosteal deposition of bone was noted in the midportion or distal ends of the shafts of the long bones, as seen with pulmonary osteoarthropathy. These changes were rather similar to those with Cooley's anemia, congenital hemolytic anemia, polycythemia, iron deficiency anemia, myeloid metaplasia and sicklemia, and are attributed to the hypoxia of cyanotic congenital heart disease acting as a marrow stimulant. Only one such patient appears in our files.

Reference

Nice, C. M., Daves, M. L. and Wood, G. H.: Changes in Bone Associated with Cyanotic Congenital Cardiac Disease, Am. Heart J., *68*, 25, 1964.

Hemophilia

Hemophilia is a hereditary disease which is predominant in the male and recessive in the female. It does not occur in women, but is transmitted through them to their male offspring. The hereditary defects involve the thromboplastic activity of the plasma, thereby preventing normal clotting. The disease is characterized by hemorrhage which follows trauma or is spontaneous. The joints most frequently involved are those of the extremities, particularly the hips, knees and elbows. Characteristic defects with areas of destruction of bone due to necrosis following hemorrhage are quite frequent. Subperiosteal hemorrhages and resultant proliferative changes together with erosion of the underlying cortex have been reported by Echternacht (1943), who remarked that a hematoma, when organized and calcified, might produce an x-ray appearance resembling bone sarcoma.

Although considerable has been written concerning the bony changes in the appendicular skeleton, there is little concerning changes which may appear in the spine with hemophilia. Priest (1935) reported a case of spinal cord compression caused by epidural hemorrhage due to hemophilia. Changes in the sacrum in 1 case out of 44 were mentioned by Ghormley and Clegg (1948). In the cases seen by us the spinal roentgenograms were all normal.

References

Brinkhous, K. M.: Hemophilia, Bull. New York Acad. Med., *30*, 325, 1954.
Echternacht, A. P.: Pseudotumor of Bone in Hemophilia, Radiology, *41*, 565, 1943.
Ghormley, R. K. and Clegg, R. S.: Bone and Joint Changes in Hemophilia, J. Bone & Joint Surg., *30-A*, 589, 1948.
Priest, W. M.: Spinal Cord Compression Caused by Epidural Hemorrhage Due to Hemophilia, Lancet, *2*, 1289, 1935.
Stiris, G.: Bone and Joint Changes in Haemophiliacs, Acta radiol., *49*, 269, 1958.

Collagen Diseases

The collagen diseases include disseminated lupus erythematosus, systemic sclerosis (scleroderma), polyarteritis nodosa and dermatomyositis. Other disorders of the connective tissue system are regarded as collagen diseases, including, among others, rheumatic fever, rheumatoid arthritis, ankylosing spondylitis, Wegener's granulomatosis, temporal arteritis and Sjogren's syndrome. The origin of these is obscure, and transitional forms make precise classification difficult in some instances. The disease affects mainly the connective tissues, including the extracellular components of the collagen system and the ground substance. The process involves proliferation, degeneration and inflammation in the connective tissues with deposition of fibrinoid material in the ground substance. The regions mainly affected include the joints, particularly the synovial and capsular structures, the blood vessels, skin, muscle, heart and the reticulum of internal organs, especially the kidney. The morphologic similarities do not necessarily indicate a common pathogenetic mechanism.

Involvement of the spine in the various collagen disorders other than ankylosing spondylitis and rheumatoid arthritis is rare. A slight separation of the atlanto-odontoid articulation was observed in a series of 25 patients with systemic lupus erythematosus in 2 out of 3 instances in which there was marked joint deformities. In these two no odontoid erosions were seen, nor was there pain or limitation of motion (Noonan and co-workers, 1963).

Depositions of calcium in the soft tissues is observed fairly often in patients with systemic sclerosis. These may be in approximation to the spine in some instances. In a discussion of tumoral calcinosis, Barton and Reeves (1961) mentioned that in 40 per cent of cases scleroderma was present.

The neurologic aspects of lupus erythematosus were reported by Sedgwick and von Hagen (1948). They believed that the central nervous system symptoms might be explained by focal vascular disease resulting in hemorrhage or occlusion. Indirect central nervous system effects occur by reason of involvement of the kidneys or by hemorrhage due to thrombopenia. Piper (1953) found no cases of focal involvement of the spinal cord. He reported a case in a 19-year-old girl with vascular changes including thrombosis of the meningeal vessels resulting in ischemic necrosis of the lumbar cord. The patient had complained of numbness and tingling of the lower limbs which gradually extended upwards, with progressive weakness, marked diminution in motility and difficulty in urination. At necropsy focal swelling with infarction of the lumbar spinal cord was evident on reflection of the dura. This was due to vasculitis, with thrombosis of the vessels supplying the meningeal vessels to the lumbar spinal cord. Other cases have been reported in which the essential change was vasculitis with fibrinoid change in the involved vessels and an associated myelomalacia which might have given rise to an adhesive meningitis or chronic meningoencephalitis.

We observed a 19-year-old girl with lupus erythematosus who complained of pains in the mid-dorsal region associated with sensory disturbances referable to the same area. On myelographic investigation a hesitation in the passage of Pantopaque was noted at the seventh thoracic vertebra. This was rapidly followed by paraplegia and she presented a picture considered indicative of a transection of the spinal cord due to a vascular accident. Laminectomy was performed (Dr. A. J. Berman), and no mass lesion was encountered. Even though the coverings appeared to be normal, definite epidural venous dilatation was encountered. When the dura was opened, the cord appeared normal. Although this is not a confirmed case, the history and neurologic changes suggest that it might be included under the present category.

References

Barton, D. L. and Reeves, R. J.: Tumoral Calcinosis, Am. J. Roentgenol., *86*, 351, 1961.
DuBois, E. L. and Martel, S.: Discoid Lupus Erythematosus: An Analysis of its Systemic Manifestations, Ann. Int. Med., *44*, 482, 1956.
Kierland, R. R.: The Collagenoses: Transitional Forms of Lupus Erythematosus, Dermatomyositis and Scleroderma, Proc. Staff Meet., Mayo Clin., *39*, 53, 1964.
Noonan, C. D., Odone, D. T., Engleman, E. P. and Splitter, S. D.: Roentgenographic Manifestations of Joint Disease in Systemic Lupus Erythematosus, Radiology, *80*, 837, 1963.
Piper, P. G.: Disseminated Lupus Erythematosus with Involvement of the Spinal Cord, J.A.M.A., *153*, 215, 1953.

Sedgwick, R. P. and von Hagen, K. O.: Neurological Manifestations of Lupus Erythematosus and Periarteritis Nodosa, Bull. Los Angeles Neurological Soc., *13*, 129, 1948.

Sokoloff, L.: Some Aspects of the Pathology of Collagen Diseases, Bull. N. Y. Acad. Med., *32*, 760, 1956.

The Reticuloendothelioses

Gaucher's diseases is one of the storage diseases of lipoid metabolism. This condition is primarily a disturbance in which deposition of cerebrosides occurs in the reticuloendothelial cells, producing a typical mottled infiltration with foamy "Gaucher's cells." The disease is a simple dominant hereditary one which is especially frequent in persons of Jewish origin, but also occurs in others. The clinical picture is varied, and is found from childhood to old age. Symptoms appear as a rule during childhood and the progression of the disease may extend over many years.

Among the outstanding characteristics in the more common adult form of the disease are marked enlargement of the spleen and liver. The splenomegaly is responsible for the designation of the disease as splenic anemia. Involvement of the abdominal and intrathoracic lymph nodes and of the external lymph nodes is moderate or minimal. Brownish pigmentation of the exposed parts of the skin, wedge-shaped pingueculae, a hemorrhagic tendency with leukopenia and thrombocytopenia may appear. Some divide the condition into two forms designated as visceral and osseous types. In the first, enlargement of the spleen and liver and sometimes of the lymph nodes predominate, with relatively mild osseous involvement. In the osseous form the involvement of the skeleton is more marked, and the visceral changes are less pronounced. Anemia is usually more profound with the osseous form (Tennent, 1945). When the disease appears in infancy, it follows an acute course, with death occurring before 2 years of age.

The roentgenologic changes in the skeleton associated with Gaucher's disease is attributed to infiltration and replacement of the bone trabeculae by the cerebroside-containing reticulum cells. Infiltration of these cells around the small arteries and capillaries may produce aseptic necrosis (Schein and Arkin, 1942; Arkin and Schein, 1948). As a result of the infiltration of the marrow with Gaucher's cells minimal, moderate or extensive osteolysis may occur. Secondary changes such as bowing osseous collapse and pathologic fracture are not uncommon. In cases with bone involvement pain, stiffness and limping are the outstanding complaints (Welt, Rosenthal and Oppenheimer, 1929). In the acute stages swelling, bone tenderness, and occasionally redness and limitation of motion suggests the diagnosis of osteomyelitis.

The bones most frequently affected by Gaucher's disease include the long bones, particularly the humeri and the distal ends of the femurs, the spine, pelvis and hips and the hands. Sections through these bones reveal the spongiosa infiltrated with yellow or grey deposits of Gaucher's tissue infiltrating between and replacing the trabeculae. This is followed by thinning of the cortex from within, resulting in a scalloped, irregularly widened medullary canal.

Involvement of the spine is by infiltration of the spongiosa with Gaucher's cells. As a result the vertebral body is weakened and wedge-shaped deformities appear. If the disease is extensive, diffuse collapse of the vertebral bodies eventually results in flattening of the involved segments (Fig. 475). Reed and Sosman (1942) described areas of rarefaction intermingled with areas of sclerosis in the involved vertebral bodies, followed by compression and relatively intact intervertebral discs. Kyphotic deformities with Gaucher's disease were mentioned by Tennent (1945). Welt, Rosenthal and Oppenheimer (1929) mentioned that one of their cases presented a gibbus without deformity of the intervertebral discs. Schein and Arkin (1942) in their eighth case reported numerous collapsed vertebrae which at necropsy were infiltrated with Gaucher's cells.

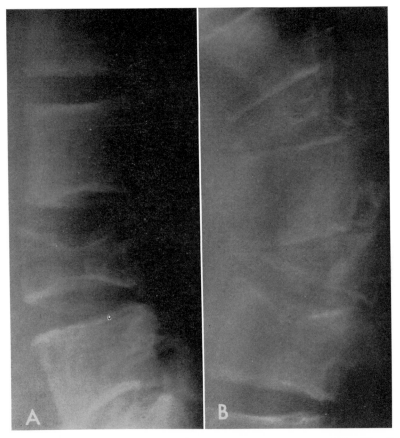

FIG. 475. *A*, Gaucher's disease in a 24-year-old man with partial collapse of L4. The discs above and below deeply intrude into the body. *B*, Two years later the patient had lost height and multiple collapsed vertebrae have appeared.

Windholz and Foster (1948) confirmed Pick's (1925) observation of sclerotic changes in the medullary canals of bones with Gaucher's disease, similar in appearance to regenerative ossification seen with inflammatory lesions. While the formation of osseous tissue as a rule was only slight, it pointed to an effort at repair, and occurred in parts of the medullary canal without bone destruction as well as in structures adjoining typical absorptive changes. They believed that roentgen signs of pathological ossification in Gaucher's disease may be of diagnostic significance, and pointed out that such ossification appeared after splenectomy. Spinal cord compression is rare (Raynor, 1962).

Included in our own material are cases of Gaucher's disease with roentgenograms of the spine. Of these, 5 had vertebral changes. The youngest patient was 4 years old, with an advanced hepatosplenomegaly and early changes in the long bones of the extremities. In this patient only a mild degree of osteoporosis of the lumbar vertebrae could be discerned. The intervertebral spaces were normal, and the usual lumbar lordotic curve was straightened, probably as a result of the hepatosplenomegaly. The marked increase in the soft tissue densities overlying the abdomen resulted in a peculiar haziness of the lumbar vertebrae as seen on anteroposterior films.

One 26-year-old patient was later reported in detail by Melamed and Chester (1938). The involvement of his spine was extensive, and it was during our period of observation that his height diminished perceptibly. The appearance of the spine was such that we described it as an "accordion spine" (Fig. 475). Wedge-like deformities of the vertebral bodies of both the thoracic and lumbar spine first developed and later the vertebral bodies were reduced to thin discs no more than 0.5 cm in height. The earliest change noted was a collapse of the superior aspect of the body of the first lumbar vertebra, with some anterior angulation of the twelfth thoracic vertebra. The inferior aspect of the body of the first lumbar vertebra remained normal, and the intervertebral spaces above and beneath

were not disturbed. Some increased density in the superior half of the compressed body of the first lumbar vertebra was observed initially, due to compression of bony structure weakened by infiltration with Gaucher's cells. This patient, who was first observed in 1928, when the film mentioned above was obtained, required splenectomy. He was again seen in 1932 with symptoms referable to multiple collapsed vertebrae and fracture of the sternum. At this time an enormous enlargement of the liver had appeared. The patient became mentally retarded and a generalized lymphadenopathy developed. The necropsy observations were included in the report by Melamed and Chester (1938).

Another woman, 42 years old, had a splenomegaly which was first noted 4 years

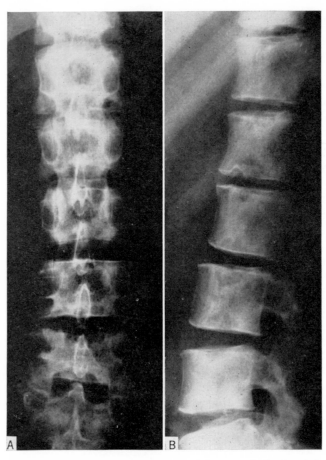

Fig. 476. Gaucher's disease in a 42-year-old woman with diffuse vertebral sclerosis involving mainly the cancellous bone. The cortical bone is thin, and nuclear intrusions are seen in the upper lumbar segments.

before she was seen by us. The diagnosis of Gaucher's disease was confirmed by positive splenic and bone marrow punctures. Her spine presented a most interesting appearance. The vertebral bodies were intact, but indentations of nuclear material into the bodies of the first and second lumbar vertebrae were seen on the lateral views. Slight narrowing of the intervertebral disc between these vertebrae was present. Particularly interesting was the presence of intermingled linear and slightly broader areas of bony increased density, indicating sclerosis in the spongiosa of the vertebral bodies (Fig. 476). Sclerotic changes could also be demonstrated in the lateral aspects of the sacro-iliac joints. This appearance was much the same as mentioned by Kulowski (1950), who described juxta-articular mottling in the sacroiliac joints with a tendency towards partial or complete obliteration of the joint spaces. A skeletal survey in this patient revealed characterisitc changes of the Erlenmeyer flask deformity in the lower femurs. Extensive sclerotic changes were present in both lower femurs and in the humeri. Similar changes of lesser degree were seen in the tibias and in the thoracic spine.

Included among the lipoid granulomas are Niemann-Pick's disease and xanthomatosis. Niemann-Pick's disease is a storage disturbance of phospholipids, and bony changes are rare, although patchy osteoporotic areas may appear. Xanthomatosis occurs sometimes in a symptomatic form with cholesterolemia, in which lipoid granulomas of foam cells filled with cholesterol are deposited in tendon sheaths, joints or viscera. Bony involvement is rare.

References

Arkin, A. M. and Schein, A. J.: Aseptic Necrosis in Gaucher's Disease, J. Bone & Joint Surg., 30-A, 631, 1948.

Kulowski, J.: Gaucher's Disease in Bone, Am. J. Roentgenol., 63, 840, 1950.

Levin, B.: Gaucher's Disease, Am. J. Roentgenol., 85, 685, 1961.

Melamed, S. and Chester, W.: Osseous Form of Gaucher's Disease, Arch. Int. Med., 61, 798, 1938.

Pick, L.: Zur Histiogenese der Gaucherzellen in der Milz, Virchow's Arch. f. path. Anat., 254, 782, 1925.

Raynor, R. B.: Spinal-Cord Compression Secondary to Gaucher's Disease, J. Neurosurg., 19, 902, 1962.

Reed, J. and Sosman, M. C.: Gaucher's Disease, Radiology, 38, 579, 1942.

Rourke, J. A. and Heslin, D. J.: Gaucher's Disease, Am. J. Roentgenol., 94, 621, 1965.

Schein, A. J. and Arkin, A. M.: Hip-joint Involvement in Gaucher's Disease, J. Bone & Joint Surg., 24, 396, 1942.

Strickland, B.: Skeletal Manifestations of Gaucher's Disease with Some Unusual Findings, Brit. J. Radiol., 31, 246, 1958.

Tennent, W.: Gaucher's Disease, Brit. J. Radiol., 18, 356, 1945.

Welt, S., Rosenthal, N. and Oppenheimer, B. S.: Gaucher's Splenomegaly, with Reference to Skeletal Changes, J.A.M.A., 92, 637, 1929.

Windholz, F. and Foster, S. E.: Sclerosis of Bones in Gaucher's Disease, Am. J. Roentgenol., 60, 246, 1948.

URTICARIA PIGMENTOSA

Urticaria pigmentosa is a systemic disease rather than one limited to the skin. Involvement of the lymph nodes, the spleen, liver, bone marrow and other organs have been reported. It is a proliferative disorder of tissue mast cells which affects mainly the reticuloendothelial system, and resembles the reticuloses in that the tissue mast cells originate from reticulum cells and fibroblasts. The disease is characterized by skin and mucous membrane single or multiple pigmented macules or nodules which, in adults, appear without known cause, and become confluent and irritated. The cutaneous changes become progressive, and the lesions are pigmented. Swelling and itching appear on rubbing. There is a hemorrhagic tendency, with prolonged bleeding time and increased coagulation time. The mast cells elaborate hyaluronic acid and serotonin, histamine and heparin. Symptoms of histamine release, including itching, flushing, weakness, dizziness and hypotension occur. At necropsy mast cells appear in almost all tissues, and in severe cases which approximate mast cell leukemia, there is malignant transformation.

The disease also appears in children, and differs from the adult form in that it disappears by adolescence and follows a benign course. The characteristic change is accumulations of mast cells in the dermis. However, the systemic type of the disease can occur in children.

The bone changes associated with urticaria pigmentosa are most prominent in the spine, the long bones and the pelvis. The lesions are characterized by bone resorption and proliferation, producing areas of interspersed radiolucency and increased density. No deformity of the bony architecture is observed. The vertebrae retain their normal contours, with a tendency to a square configuration with thin cortical margins. The upper and lower surfaces of the verte-

bral bodies occasionally present indentations from the intervertebral discs, but not to the same extent as seen with gross osteoporosis (Fig. 477). The interstitial proliferation of bone may be delicate or prominent, with a tendency towards exaggeration of the vertical cancellous trabeculae.

The lytic lesions are produced by resorption of bone by the mast cells which accumulate in the marrow spaces. Sometimes these areas coalesce, forming irregular localized or confluent cystic lesions.

The disease is readily recognized when the entire clinical picture is known. Radiologically it can be mistaken for osteosclerotic anemia, diffuse metastatic disease, lymphoma of bone, or other conditions resulting in diffuse osteosclerotic changes.

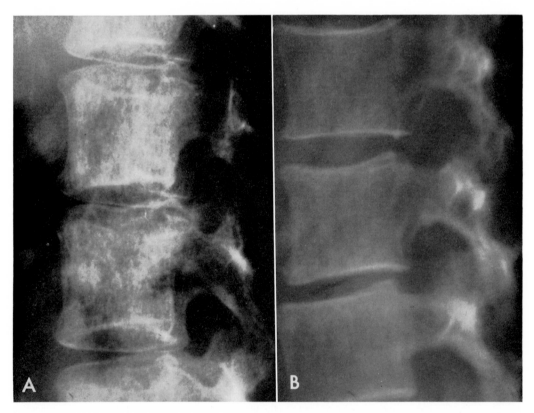

FIG. 477. A, Urticaria pigmentosa in a 70-year-old patient with myelofibrosis. A prominent diffuse reticular increase in the vertebrae appears in the cancellous bone. The vertebrae are intact. B, Another 70-year-old patient with urticaria pigmentosa. The bony changes are less prominent than in the former patient. Biopsy revealed mast cells nested among spicules of bone. (From Zak, F. G., Covey, J. A. and Snodgrass, J. J.: Osseous Lesions in Urticaria Pigmentosa, New England J. Med., *256*, 56, 1957.)

References

Barev, M., Peterson, L. F. A., Dahlin, D. C., Winkelmann, R. K. and Stewart, J. R.: Mastocytosis with Osseous Lesions Resembling Metastatic Malignant Lesions in Bone, J. Bone & Joint Surg., 50-A, 142, 1968.

Bendel, W. L., Jr. and Race, G. J.: Urticaria Pigmentosa with Bone Involvement, J. Bone & Joint Surg., 45-A, 1043, 1963.

Havard, C. W. H. and Scott, R. B.: Urticaria Pigmentosa with Visceral and Skeletal Lesions, Quart. J. Med., 28, 459, 1959.

Poppel, M. H., Gruber, W. F., Silber, R., Holder, A. K. and Christman, R. O.: The Roentgen Manifestations of Urticaria Pigmentosa (Mastocytosis), Am. J. Roentgenol., 82, 239, 1959.

Zak, F. G., Covey, J. A. and Snodgrass, J. J.: Osseous Lesions in Urticaria Pigmentosa, New England J. Med., 256, 56, 1957.

THE NON-LIPID RETICULOENDOTHELIOSES

This group includes Hand-Schüller-Christian's disease, eosinophilic granuloma of bone and acute disseminated reticuloendotheliosis (Letterer-Siwe's disease). Even though the clinical manifestations of these conditions differ, histologic evidence suggests a common origin for all three. The progress of one of the three into one or both of the remaining two has been cited as evidence for the underlying similarity. However, Otani (1957) and Siwe (1949) disagree with this concept, and consider them separate entities because of dissimilarities in their clinical and pathologic aspects. The name "Histiocytosis X" was suggested as a designation for this group of diseases by Lichtenstein (1953).

HAND-SCHULLER-CHRISTIAN DISEASE

This disease is characterized histologically by the presence of granulomatous tissue made up of large numbers of mononuclear cells, probably histiocytes, and a smaller number of leukocytes. Eosinophiles are present to a lesser degree. The cytoplasm of the histiocytes is finely or coarsely vacuolated. The granulomatous tissue contains varying amounts of foam cells and foreign body giant cells. These are observed more often in the spleen and lymph nodes than in the skeleton. The presence of foam cells may be minimal or absent in some cases, but in others they are widely and extensively present (Ponseti, 1948).

With Hand-Schüller-Christian disease there may be storage of cholesterol in the foam cells which later is replaced by spindle cells and connective tissue. In older lesions, therefore, foam cells are scant. The degree of eosinophilic infiltration also varies considerably. The opinion has been expressed that foam cells are commonly observed in the early stages of the disease, and disappear during the healing stage.

The triad associated with Hand-Schüller-Christian disease includes exophthalmos, diabetes insipidus and defects in the membranous bones. Concomitant with these are varying degrees of splenomegaly, pigmentation of the skin and evidences of endocrine dysfunction such as dystrophia adiposa genitalis and dwarfism. Polyuria, skin lesions and pulmonary manifestations are sometimes present (Currens and Popp, 1943; Hodgson, Kennedy and Camp, 1951).

The bony lesions are most extensive in the skull, the pelvis and the limbs. The lesions usually are circumscribed, rarefied, and present scalloped borders, sometimes with increased density of the margins of the scallops. Involvement of the vertebral column is infrequent. Troxler and Niemetz (1946) reported a 35-year-old man with an area of destruction involving the anterior aspect of the body of the first lumbar vertebra. Davies (1949) mentioned a female child, $2\frac{1}{2}$ years of age, in whom there was a flattening of the body of the ninth thoracic vertebra. Lateral body section roentgenograms of the cervical spine in this patient showed considerable destruction of the body of the fourth cervical vertebra and loss of the joint space between the fourth and fifth cervical segments. Further survey of the skeleton showed lesions in the pelvis and femurs, and a biopsy from the left iliac crest was reported as Hand-Schüller-Christian type of reticulosis. Hodgson, Kennedy and Camp (1951) mentioned that the vertebrae were involved in 3 out of 28 cases of reticulo-endotheliosis, including in their series patients with Hand-Schüller-Christian disease, eosinophilic granuloma and Letterer-Siwe's disease.

Eosinophilic Granuloma

The condition was first reported by Otani and Ehrlich (1940), who emphasized its granulomatous and benign nature, and the prominent eosinophilic infiltration occurring in bone. In their 7 cases, Otani and Ehrlich proposed the designation "solitary granuloma of bone." Jaffe and Lichtenstein (1944) described the lesion as radiolucent and sharply delimited. On pathologic study in an early phase, the lesion appeared grossly as a more or less hemorrhagic and cystic area from which only a relatively small amount of granulation tissue could be curetted. The tissue was not necrotic, and contained conspicuous numbers of histiocytes. Some showed phagocytic activity, and interspersed among these were large accumulations of eosinophiles.

The disease usually occurs in young people. Green and Farber (1942) observed that their 10 patients varied in age from 11 months to 10 years, 11 months. Gross and Jacox (1942), in a review of 60 cases, noted that all except three were younger than 21 years. The oldest patient seen by us was a male 58 years of age. Pain over the involved areas may be a prominent symptom. The regions involved most often include the skull, ribs and the long bones. Involvement of the spinal column is not uncommon. Green and Farber (1942) described a case in which the second and third lumbar vertebrae were involved, associated with paravertebral soft tissue swelling suggesting a tuberculous lesion. Another case showed a flattening of the ninth thoracic vertebra which remained unchanged over a 4-year period. Dundon, Williams and Laipply (1946) mentioned that out of 46 cases collected by them from the literature, including 5 of their own, there were 10 cases with multiple lesions, of which 9 had vertebral involvement. Ackerman

(1947) reported a 19-year-old male in whom there was a large area of destruction in the second cervical vertebra. The eleventh and twelfth dorsal vertebrae and all the lumbar vertebrae were markedly altered. The normal trabecular bony architecture was replaced by cystic areas of rarefaction involving the vertebral bodies and their processes. In addition there was some lateral wedging of the vertebrae. This patient also had involvement of the lungs and diaphragm with the eosinophilic granuloma. Walker (1952) mentioned a case involving destruction of the third lumbar vertebra and recalcification of after x-ray therapy. Osborne, Freis and Levin (1944) reported a 21-year-old patient with evidence of neurologic impairment. This patient had headache, giddiness, vomiting, deafness, tinnitus, vertigo and ear pain as his chief complaints. There was involvement of the skull by a solitary confluent polycystic lesion in the temporal bone and mandible. Of interest was the fact that the seventh cervical, the first and second thoracic and a fifth lumbar vertebrae also showed evidence of destruction. There was a favorable response to x-ray therapy in this patient. A case described by Weinstein, Francis and Sprofkin (1947) with headache associated with defects in the skull likewise complained of backache. Radiographic examination of the spine disclosed areas of destruction in the left iliac and pubic bones and the body of the third lumbar vertebra. This patient also presented radiologic evidence of pulmonary fine nodular infiltrations, and proof of the eosinophilic granulomatous nature of the lesion was obtained by biopsy from the involved left parietal bone. This patient also did quite well with x-ray therapy.

Involvement of the spine is considerably more common with eosinophilic granuloma than with Hand-Schüller-Christian disease or Letterer-Siwe's disease. Of the 8 cases of Hand-Schuller-Christian disease and 9 cases of eosinophilic granuloma seen by us, four of the latter had vertebral involvement. There were identified because of flattened middle thoracic vertebrae. Three were verified by vertebral biopsy and the other by gum biopsy.

In 1925 Calvé described a flattening of vertebral bodies which he considered similar to Legge-Calvé-Perthe's disease of the femoral heads and other osteochondritides. Buchman (1927) and Mezzari (1938), and later Massaro (1945) agreed that the etiology probably was an aseptic necrosis of the vertebral body resulting from diminution of the blood supply. Pathologic investigations disclosed fragmentation and collapse of the affected vertebral body. A propensity for regeneration of bone and gradual restoration of the vertebra to approximately its normal height was noted.

In 1954 Compere, Johnson and Coventry advanced the concept that Calvé's disease actually was due to eosinophilic granuloma

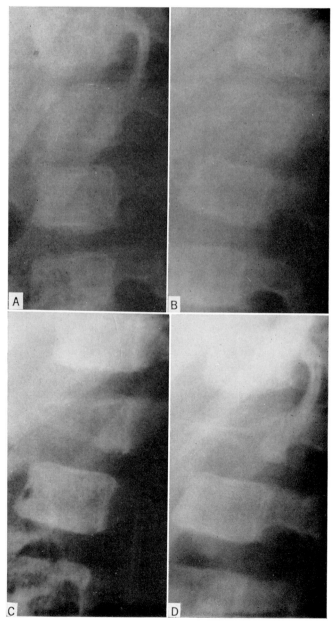

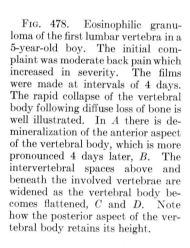

FIG. 478. Eosinophilic granuloma of the first lumbar vertebra in a 5-year-old boy. The initial complaint was moderate back pain which increased in severity. The films were made at intervals of 4 days. The rapid collapse of the vertebral body following diffuse loss of bone is well illustrated. In *A* there is demineralization of the anterior aspect of the vertebral body, which is more pronounced 4 days later, *B*. The intervertebral spaces above and beneath the involved vertebrae are widened as the vertebral body becomes flattened, *C* and *D*. Note how the posterior aspect of the vertebral body retains its height.

of the vertebral body, substantiating their impression with evidence obtained from vertebral body biopsy. This concept has gained general recognition, and the diagnosis of Calvé's disease has lost acceptance because of the frequency with which biopsy discloses the tissue characteristics of eosinophilic granuloma.

Vertebra plana due to eosinophilic granuloma occurs mainly in children from about 3 to 13 years of age. The associated symptoms may be only a mild backache and malaise, with some tenderness and spasm (Fig. 478). The lesion may be symptomless, and progress rapidly. A good response to x-ray therapy has been observed. Fripp (1958) reported that healing occurred spontaneously in four cases seen by him. Paraplegia due to compression by a solitary eosinophilic granuloma of a vertebral body was reported by Yabsley and Harris (1966).

As a rule vertebra plana in children can be differentiated from other conditions which produce a similar malformation. Included in this group are conditions as diverse as lymphoma, Gaucher's disease, osteogenesis imperfecta, and other osteoporotic disturbances.

LETTERER-SIWE'S DISEASE

This is another of the nonlipoid granulomatous diseases of the reticuloendothelial system. It occurs in infants, who rarely survive long enough to develop skeletal changes. The syndrome of Letterer-Siwe's disease is characterized by a diffuse, generalized hyperplasia of the reticuloendothelial system with splenomegaly, a hemorrhagic tendency, generalized lymphadenopathy, generalized tumors overlying the bones, secondary anemia and increase in nonlipoid containing macrophages. The disease is of relatively short duration, with a fatal outcome (Siwe, 1933; Abt and Denenholtz, 1936; Dennis and Rosahn, 1951). Microscopically, the eosinophiles and macrophages are numerous, but foam cells are absent or relatively scant. Reports of ver-

tebral extension of this disease are infrequent. Wallace (1949) encountered a collapsed first lumbar vertebra in a 4-year-old boy with Letterer-Siwe's disease.

References

Abt, A. F. and Denenholtz, E. J.: Letterer-Siwe's Disease, Am. J. Dis. Child., *51*, 499, 1936.

Ackermann, A. J.: Eosinophilic Granuloma of Bones Associated with Involvement of Lungs and Diaphragm, Am. J. Roentgenol., *58*, 733, 1947.

Batson, R., Shapiro, J., Christie, A. and Riley, H. D.: Acute Nonlipid Disseminated Reticulo-endotheliosis, Am. J. Dis. Child., *90*, 323, 1955.

Calhoun, J. D. and Thompson, S. B.: Vertebra Plana in Children Produced by Xanthomatous Disease, Am. J. Roentgenol., *82*, 482, 1959.

Calvé, J.: Localized Affection of Spine Suggesting Osteochondritis of Vertebral Body, J. Bone & Joint Surg., *7*, 41, 1925.

Davies, P. M.: Xanthomatosis Associated with Vertebra Plana, Brit. J. Radiol., *22*, 725, 1949.

Dennis, W. J. and Rosahn, P. D.: Primary Reticulo-Endothelial Granulomas, Am. J. Path., *27*, 627, 1951.

Dickey, L. E., Jr., Hobbs, R. J. W. and Sherrill, J. D.: Vertebra Plana and the Histiocytoses, J. Bone & Joint Surg., *37-A*, 1261, 1955.

Dundon, C. C., Williams, H. A. and Paipply, T. C.: Eosinophilic Granuloma of Bone, Radiology, *47*, 433, 1946.

Fawcitt, R.: Osteochondritis Vertebralis (Calvé) Associated with Pathologic Changes in Other Bones, Brit. J. Radiol., *13*, 172, 1940.

Fenyes, I. and Zoltan, L.: Calvé's Disease; Does It Exist? The Question of its Aetiology, Brit. J. Radiol., *32*, 394, 1959.

Fripp, A. T.: Vertebra Plana, J. Bone & Joint Surg., *40-B*, 378, 1958.

Green, W. T. and Farber, S. (with the assistance of McDermott, L. J.): Eosinophilic or Solitary Granuloma of Bone, J. Bone & Joint Surg., *24*, 499, 1942.

Gross, P. and Jacox, H. W.: Eosinophilic Granuloma and Certain Other Reticulo-Endothelial Hyperplasias of Bone, Am. J. Med. Sci., *203*, 673, 1942.

Hodgson, J. R., Kennedy, R. L. and Camp, J. D.: Reticulo-Endotheliosis (Hand-Schüller-Christian Disease), Radiology, *57*, 642, 1951.

Hunter, T.: Solitary Eosinophilic Granuloma of Bone, J. Bone & Joint Surg., *38-B*, 545, 1956.

Kelley, J. H. and McMillan, J. T.: Eosinophilic Granuloma of Bone, Ann. Surg., *156*, 147, 1962.

Leeser, F.: Relationship between Tuberculosis and Osteochonditis Vertebrae (Calvé), Am. J. Roentgenol., *57*, 744, 1947.

Lichtenstein, L.: Histiocytosis X: Integration of Eosinophilic Granuloma of Bone, "Letterer-Siwe's Disease," and "Schüller-Christian's Disease" as Related Manifestations of a Single Nosologic Entity, Arch. Path., *56*, 84, 1953.

Lichtenstein, L. and Jaffe, H. L.: Eosinophilic Granuloma of Bone with Report of a Case, Am. J. Path., *16*, 595, 1940.

Lichtenstein, L.: Histiocytosis X (Eosinophilic Granuloma of Bone, Letterer-Siwe Disease, and Schüller-Christian Disease), J. Bone & Joint Surg., *46-A*, 76, 1964.

Massaro, A. F.: Vertebra Plana (Calvé), Radiology, *45*, 284, 1945.

Mezzari, A.: Über die Calvésche Vertebra plana (Infantile pseudospondylitis), Fortschr. Röntgenstr., *57*, 275, 1938.

Mitchell, J.: Vertebral Osteochondritis, Arch. Surg., *25*, 544, 1932.

Otani, S.: A Discussion on Eosinophilic Granuloma of Bone, Letterer-Siwe's Disease and Schüller-Christian's Disease, J. Mt. Sinai Hosp., *24*, 1079, 1957.

Otani, S. and Ehrlich, J. C.: Solitary Granuloma of Bone Simulating a Neoplasm, Am. J. Path., *63*, 49, 1957.

Ponseti, I.: Bone Lesions in Eosinophilic Granuloma, Hand-Schüller-Christian's Disease and Letterer-Siwe's Disease, J. Bone & Joint Surg., *30-A*, 811, 1948.

Rosselet, E.: Contribution a l'Etude de la Vertebra Plana Osteonecrotica, Radiol. clin., *18*, 371, 1949.

Schulz, D. M., Hamilton, G. B. and Nay, L. B.: Nonlipid Reticuloendotheliosis in an Adult, Arch. Path., *63*, 49, 1940.

Siwe, S. A.: The Reticuloses in Children. In *Advances in Pediatrics*, New York, Interscience Publishers, 1949, Vol. 4, p. 117.

Sundt, H.: Vertebra plana-Calvé. Eine Übersich und zwei Kasuistiche Mitteilungen, Acta chirurg. scandinav., *76*, 501, 1935.

Troxler, E. R. and Niemetz, D.: Generalized Xanthomatosis with Pulmonary, Skeletal and Cerebral Manifestations, Ann. Int. Med., *25*, 960, 1946.

Walker, J. W.: Benign Bone Tumors in Pediatric Practice, Radiology, *58*, 662, 1952.

Wallace, W. S.: Reticulo-Endotheliosis, Am. J. Roentgenol., *62*, 189, 1949.

Weinstein, A., Francis, H. C. and Sprofkin, B. F.: Eosinophilic Granuloma of Bone, Arch. Neurol. & Psychiat., *51*, 452, 1944.

Yabsley, R. H. and Harris, W. R.: Solitary Eosinophilic Granuloma of a Vertebral Body Causing Paraplegia, J. Bone & Joint Surg., *48-A*, 1570, 1966.

10

Vascular Disorders

AORTIC ANEURYSMS

Aneurysms of the aorta usually are arteriosclerotic or syphilitic in origin. Those in the thoracic aorta are likely to be syphilitic, while abdominal aortic aneurysms are predominantly of the arteriosclerotic variety (Epstein, 1945). Arteriosclerotic aneurysms have a tendency to be of the diffuse fusiform type, while syphilitic aneurysms are more often of the sacculated and multiple variety. Other factors infrequently associated with aneurysms are trauma, contiguous extra-arterial disease with secondary injury to the vascular walls, inflammatory vascular lesions and rheumatic fever. An unusual form of aneurysmal dilatation of the abdominal aorta with communication with the abdominal venous circulation was described by Gordon, Aronson and Azulay (1952). This occurred in a 34-year-old male who had a Corrigan pulse without clinical signs of aortic insufficiency. Murmurs were heard in the lower vertebral and posterior pelvic regions. Radiographic examination disclosed numerous lytic lesions in the first lumbar vertebra and mixed lytic and blastic lesions in the left sacrum and ilium. The radiologic diagnosis was angiosarcoma resulting in arteriovenous fistulas. Necropsy revealed a large aneurysmal sac occupying most of the posterior pelvic cavity. Extending posteriorly were dilated vessels which entered the pelvic and vertebral bones to form loculated interconnected intraosseous vascular channels which were considered developmental anomalies. This patient died in cardiac failure.

Aneurysms of the ascending and transverse thoracic aorta are not accompanied by vertebral changes because of their anatomic positions. Aneurysms of the descending thoracic aorta may produce erosive changes in the anterolateral aspects of the vertebrae against which they impinge. This constant compressive and pulsatile trauma produces smooth, scalloped erosions which are deepest in the midportions of the involved vertebrae (Fig. 479). Such changes are more common in the lower thoracic vertebrae, but may occur at any level associated with aortic vertebral compression. They are usually multiple. The intervertebral discs, being avascular and relatively resilient, are resistant to erosive changes. Similar changes are produced in the upper lumbar vertebral bodies by abdominal aortic aneurysms.

Aortic aneurysms often can be identified on plain film thoracic examinations. Dilatation of the transverse and descending thoracic aorta is well demonstrated on both frontal and lateral chest roentgenograms. This is facilitated when calcifications appear within the intima of the diseased aorta, a change which in itself often is diagnostic. Visualization of the esophagus with barium paste is useful for identifying the anterior aspect of the aorta, and should be included in all examinations for thoracic aortic aneurysms. Abdominal aortic aneurysms often are lined with calcification, and can be identified on frontal and lateral roentgenograms. Body section examinations are useful when bowel markings obscure the outlines of the aorta. Determination of the

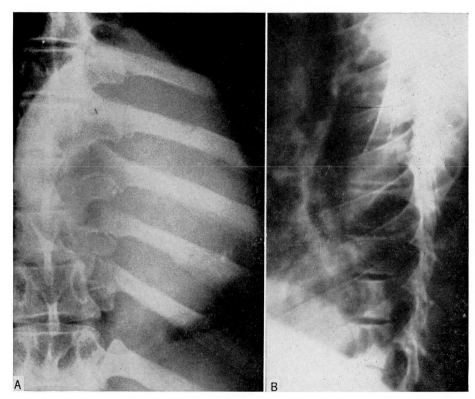

Fig. 479. Aneurysm of descending thoracic aorta eroding the left lateral aspect of the midthoracic vertebrae and adjacent rib heads, *A*. Erosion of the anterior aspects of the lower thoracic vertebrae, *B*, in another case. Note the scalloped edges of the eroded vertebrae. The intervertebral discs are well maintained.

presence of a clot and its thickness is best made on aortograms. Intravenous aortography often suffices for demonstration of acute aneurysms.

Abdominal aortic aneurysms may intrude into the stomach and duodenum, simulating a retroperitoneal mass or a gastric tumor. Death follows rupture of an aneurysm into the intestinal tract. A case of aneurysm perforating into the third portion of the duodenum and eroding adjacent vertebrae was reported as early as 1859 (Rottino, 1943). A large aneurysm with retropsoas extension was reported by Putts and Bacon (1935).

Renal Artery Aneurysms. Aneurysms of the renal artery are relatively uncommon, and as a rule are not in relation to the spine. They are identified on plain film examinations of the abdomen by a ring-shaped shadow with a dense periphery in the kidney pelvis region. The diagnosis is best established by means of aortography and renal angiography.

Dissecting Aneurysms. Dissectiong aneurysms of the aorta occur about once in every 400 to 500 autopsies (Moersch and Sayre, 1950). They appear more often in males of middle age. The usual clinical picture is one of sudden pain and progressive prostration. Death may occur suddenly, or the patient survive for a considerable time. Plain film examinations of the chest are important in identifying this lesion. The usual change which leads to the diagnosis is a widening of the aortic shadow, and an increased soft tissue depth as measured from a calcific plaque in the intima of the aorta is an important sign. A similar change may appear in the ascending aorta, and sudden increase in this area raises suspicion that the intimal break initiating the dissecting aneurysm is close to the aortic valve. Alteration in the paracardiac density and the paraspinal soft tissue shadows also are of diagnostic importance. Visible changes in the pulsatile activity of the aorta is another change which can be identified.

Dissecting aortic aneurysms may be associated with spinal cord ischemia and infarction, producing paralysis and sensory disturbances. Tuohy, Boman and Berde (1941) reported that spinal cord ischemia results from interruption of blood supply directly from the aorta. Moersch and Sayre (1950) ascribed the neurologic changes to impairment of the blood supply to the cord because of interference with the intercostal arteries, depriving the anterior spinal artery of its circulation. Scott and Sancetta (1949) gathered 28 cases of paraplegia and paraparesis resulting from dissecting aneurysm from the literature. They reported a 56-year-old male in whom the intercostal arteries had been severed, causing hemorrhagic infarction of the cord and subarachnoid hemorrhage. The plain film roentgenograms and myelography were normal.

With the advent of improved technics for the surgical correction of aortic aneurysms, neurologic complications after aortic surgery have been reported. Adams and van Geertruyden (1956) reported 24 instances of ischemia of the spinal cord associated with aortic surgery from the literature and their own experience. They found that cord lesions were localized to the lower spinal cord, and the variations of clinical manifestations resulted from differences in the extent and degree of ischemia. Hogan and Romanul (1966) commented on spinal cord infarction during aortic surgery.

Aortography has become almost routine in the investigation of aortic disease. Intravenous aortography often suffices for the diagnosis of aneurysmal dilatation, and sometimes affords adequate information in the investigation of dissecting aneurysms. The results usually are adequate when the heart is not dilated, so that a bolus large enough to opacify the aorta satisfactorily is possible. The use of a rapid changer and pressure injectors is required in obtaining adequate films. As a rule, it is not possible to get good visualization of the renal arteries, nor can satisfactory run-off studies for the pelvic and leg vessels be obtained. Opacification of the neck vessels is occasionally adequate, but filling of the intracranial circulation usually is inadequate in adults.

Aortography is accomplished mainly with the introduction of a catheter into a femoral artery, and advancing it to the desired level before making the injection under image intensification control. Serial films are obtained as desired. Following a "midstream injection" special examinations can be accomplished by selectively catheterizing the desired vessels for study of the celiac axis, the renal arteries, the bronchial arteries and the cephalobrachial vessels.

The possibility of an untoward reaction is less with intravenous aortography than with direct aortic injections. With improvement in the contrast materials available there has been a diminution in the number and the extent of complications due to toxicity of the substance used. The highest incidence of reactions occurred with sodium acetrizoate, which no longer is used. Today the diatrizoate and iothalamate preparations are favored, and even these have to be handled with care. Pressure injections used for midstream placement of the contrast material should be preceded by measures to make sure that the catheter tip is not in approximation to one of the major branches. Selective injections should be made with hand pressure, and a lesser concentration of the contrast solution should be utilized. For both midstream and selective examinations it is advisable to use the least quantity necessary to obtain a diagnostic study. Highly concentrated agents should be avoided, particularly for selective studies.

The translumbar approach to abdominal aortography is being superseded by forced pressure retrograde femoral or catheter injections. The possibility of extravasation or intramural injections of contrast material is thereby avoided.

The greatest incidence of spinal cord lesions complicating abdominal aortography followed translumbar injections of sodium acetrizoate. Paralysis of the lower extremities, loss of sphincter control and sensation, and later persistence or recession of symptoms were the predominant changes. Examination of the spinal cord in patients who came to necropsy disclosed myelomalacia, fatty degeneration and necrosis of the gray matter (Killen and Foster, 1966; Efsen, 1966).

References

Adams, H. D. and van Geertruyden, H. H.: Neurologic Complications of Aortic Surgery, Ann. Surg., 144, 574, 1956.

Efsen, F.: Spinal Cord Lesion as a Complication of Abdominal Aortography, Acta radiol., 4, 47, 1966.

Epstein, J. A.: Aneurysms of Abdominal Aorta, Ann. Int. Med., 22, 252, 1945.

Feigelson, H. H. and Ravin, H. A.: Transverse Myelitis Following Selective Bronchial Arteriography, Radiology, 85, 663, 1965.

Gordon, B. S., Aronson, S. M. and Azulay, A.: Multiple Arteriovenous Aneurysms of Soft Tissue and Bone (Pelvis and Vertebrae) Resulting in Cardiac Failure, Am. Heart J., 44, 51, 1952.

Hill, C. S. and Vasquez, J. M.: Massive Infarction of the Spinal Cord and Vertebral Bodies as a Complication of Dissecting Aneurysm of the Aorta, Circulation, 25, 99, 1962.

Hogan, E. L. and Romanul, F. C. A.: Spinal Cord Infarction Occurring During Insertion of Aortic Graft, Neurology, 16, 67, 1966.

Howard, H. H., Suby, H. I. and Harberson, J.: Aneurysm of the Renal Artery, J. Urol., 5, 51, 1941.

Killen, D. A. and Foster, J. H.: Spinal Cord Injury as a Complication of Contrast Angiography, Surgery, 59, 969, 1966.

Klinefelter, E. W.: Significance of Calcification for Roentgen Diagnosis of Aneurysm of Abdominal Aorta, Radiology, 47, 597, 1946.

Laufman, H., Berggren, R. E., Finley, T. and Anson, B. J.: Anatomical Studies of the Lumbar Arteries: With Reference to the Safety of Translumbar Aortography, Ann. Surg., 152, 621, 1960.

Moersch, F. P. and Sayre, G. P.: Neurologic Manifestations Associated with Dissecting Aneurysms of the Aorta, J.A.M.A., 144, 1141, 1950.

Putts, B. S. and Bacon, R. D.: Large Aneurysm of the Descending Thoracic Aorta with Retropsoas Extension, Am. J. Roentgenol., 35, 59, 1936.

Rottino, A.: Aneurysm of the Abdominal Aorta with Rupture into the Duodenum, Am. Heart, J., 25, 826, 1943.

Scott, R. W. and Sancetta, S. M.: Dissecting Aneurysm of Aorta with Hemorrhagic Infarction of the Spinal Cord and Complete Paraplegia, Am. Heart J., 38, 747, 1949.

Tarazi, A. K., Margolis G. and Grimson, K. S.: Spinal Cord Lesions Produced by Aortography in Dogs, Arch. Surg., 72, 38, 1956.

Tuohy, E. L., Boman, P. G. and Berdez, G. L.: Spinal Cord Ischaemia in Dissecting Aortic Aneurysm, Am. Heart J., 22, 305, 1941.

Uhle, C. A. W.: The Significance of Aneurysm of the Abdominal Aorta Masquerading as Primary Urologic Disease, J. Urol., 5, 13, 1941.

VERTEBRAL ARTERY DISEASE

Visualization of the vertebral arteries can be accomplished adequately by retrograde pressure injection of the brachial arteries. Right retrograde brachial angiograms opacify the right vertebral artery from its point of origin to and including the basilar artery. At the same time the carotid circulation is seen from its origin, with excellent portrayal of the bifurcation of the common carotid artery. In most patients reliable cerebral angiograms are obtained as well. For visualization of the left vertebral artery left brachial angiograms are required. This approach is used if visualization of the basilar artery and its branches are required, and when the supratentorial vessels are not in question. The vertebral arteries, particularly the left, can be readily catheterized from the femoral artery. Selective catheterization of the vessels from the aortic arch also can be accomplished from the brachial, axillary and subclavian arteries. Aortic arch injections provide information about the origins of the cephalobrachial vessels and the neck arteries. However, the visualization of the vessels distal to the bifurcation of the common carotid arteries and of the basilar artery is not as satisfactory. The intracranial vessels usually are not filled adequately.

Direct puncture examinations of the vertebral arteries have been highly recommended. Krayenbuhl and Yasargil (1966) reported a series of 1,035 vertebral angiograms using the percutaneous technic with good filling in 80 per cent of their cases. Complications were rare and minor, but one patient was lost because of accidental intrathecal injection of the contrast substance. On the other hand, complications such as arteriovenous fistulas and subarachnoid injections with consequent necrosis of the cord have been mentioned (Newton and Darrach, 1966; Lester, 1966; Ederli, Sassaroli and Spaccarelli, 1962; McCleery and Lewtas, 1966). The procedure is done under general anesthesia, and sometimes takes a considerable time to perform. While percutaneous needling may provide superior opacification of the vessel and particularly of the basilar artery and its branches, it seems reasonable that use of the retrograde brachial injection be considered, especially when the entire vessel is to be examined.

The vertebral arteries are subject to compression, particularly in patients with spondylosis. The symptoms of vertigo, hearing loss, ataxia and limb weakness is attributed to interference with the blood supply to the brain stem, the ear and the cervical spinal cord. Symptoms are transient, and may be precipitated by hyperextension of the neck, sudden forced rotary movements or turning the head laterally and upwards. Spondylotic intrusions into the lateral margins of the vertebral bodies become exaggerated in the presence of narrowed intervertebral discs and intervertebral foramina. Changes in the angulation of the transverse processes also may kink the enclosed vertebral artery. The principal site of compression is at the various intervertebral joints. However, the occurrence of significant vertebral artery compression is infrequent even with extensive spondylotic changes.

The radiologic diagnosis of vertebral artery insufficiency is based on angiographic evidence. This is difficult to evaluate, particularly in patients who have one hypoplastic vessel. There are reports in the literature regarding the arteriographic demonstration of vertebral artery insufficiency while the patient rotates and extends his neck.

In the evaluation of vertebral angiograms the possibility of congenital variations in caliber must be kept in mind. As a rule, the right side is smaller than the left when this occurs. On retrograde brachial injections the right vertebral artery may be slender, and taper off as it bends around the first and second cervical vertebrae so that its distal portion and the basilar artery are only faintly seen, or not at all. In these patients a left brachial angiogram usually discloses a normal vertebral and basilar artery.

Dilatation of one or both vertebral arteries appears in patients with arteriovenous malformations involving the posterior cranial fossa and the tentorium. In these patients it is occasionally possible to demonstrate widening of the foramen transversarium of the first or second cervical vertebrae, and widening of the notch on the superior aspect of the lamina of the atlas. This can be accomplished by inspecting base views of the skull for the transverse processes of the atlas. Oblique views of the neck reveal the foramen transversarium of the atlas. Erosive changes also appear in the lateral margins of the cervical vertebrae where tortuosity of the vessel causes impingement. This is demonstrable as concave indentations, and is best seen on body section examinations (Fig. 480).

Post-traumatic arteriovenous fistulas in the neck, such as those which follow gunshot wounds, knife wounds and percutaneous vertebral angiography, are readily visualized by means of brachial angiography. The identification of a bruit and a thrill in the neck, together with an appropriate history, makes this a diagnosis which can be verified accurately and quickly.

Occlusion of the subclavian artery proximal to the opening of the vertebral artery results in a shunting of blood from the opposite vertebral artery down the ipsilateral vessel. This condition is referred to as "subclavian steal." The symptoms are much the same as seen with vertebro-basilar insufficiency, consisting of vertigo, syncope,

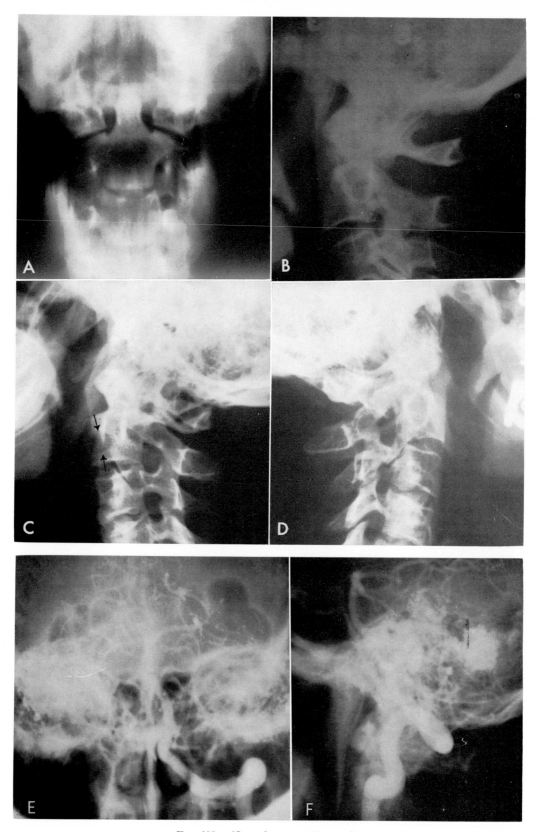

FIG. 480. (*Legend on opposite page.*)

headache, ataxia, blurred vision and tinnitus. The radial pulse on the affected side is diminished or absent, and the blood pressure in the involved arm is lowered. Ischemia of the upper limb may be present as well.

The diagnosis of a "subclavian steal" can be made on midstream injections into the ascending aorta. Demonstration of delayed visualization of the involved vertebral artery leading into the axillary artery is important, as is identification of the point of block proximal to the involved vertebral artery. The diagnosis can be made as well on retrograde brachial angiograms, injecting the artery on the normal side. Demonstration of the contrast material passing into the opposite vertebral artery and down the arm vessels is diagnostic (Fig. 481). Instances of bilateral steal have been reported (Agee, 1966). The presence of concomitant lesions in the carotid arteries and elsewhere is fairly frequent. In 8 patients with subclavian steal syndromes 5, in our experience, had carotid lesions, abdominal aortic lesions and femoral artery disease singly or in combination.

Aneurysms of the vertebral artery can be of a size sufficient to simulate high cervical tumors or tumors in the posterior fossa. Some of these lesions thrombose, but nevertheless leave the channel of the involved artery patent. On myelography they act like tumors of the cranio-vertebral junction (Fig. 482). and the diagnosis may be made first at operation. If the thrombosis extends to involve the artery and extends to the basilar artery, sudden death may ensue. Large vertebral artery aneurysms entirely within the posterior fossa simulate angle tumors.

References

Agee, O. F.: Two Unusual Cases of Subclavian Steal Syndrome. Bilateral Steal and Steal Secondary to Tumor Thrombus, Am. J. Roentgenol., 97, 447, 1966.

Aronson, N. I.: Traumatic Arteriovenous Fistula of the Vertebral Vessels, Neurology, 11, 817, 1961.

Brown, B. St. J. and Tatlow, W. F. T.: Radiographic Studies of the Vertebral Arteries in Cadavers, Radiology, 81, 80, 1963.

Bryant, L. R. and Spencer, F. C.: Occlusive Disease of Subclavian Artery, J.A.M.A., 196, 123, 1966.

Campbell, J. A. and Campbell, R. L.: Angiographic Diagnosis of Traumatic Head and Neck Lesions, J.A.M.A., 175, 761, 1961.

Ederli, A., Sassaroli, S. and Spaccarelli, G.: Vertebral Angiography as a Cause of Necrosis of the Cervical Spinal Cord, Brit. J. Radiol., 35, 261, 1962.

Hadley, L. A.: The Covertebral Articulations and Cervical Foramen Encroachment, J. Bone & Joint Surg., 39-A, 910, 1957.

————Tortuosity and Deflection of the Vertebral Artery, Am. J. Roentgenol., 80, 306, 1958.

Hardin, C. A.: Vertebral Artery Insufficiency Produced by Cervical Osteoarthritic Spurs, Arch. Surg., 90, 629, 1965.

Hardin, C. A., Williamson, W. P. and Steegman, A. T.: Vertebral Artery Insufficiency Produced by Cervical Osteoarthritic Spurs, Neurology, 10, 855, 1960.

Harzer, K. and Töndury, G.: Zum Verhalten der Arteria Vertebralis in der Alternden Halswirbelsäule, Fortschr. Röntgenstr., 104, 687, 1966.

Husni, E. A., Bell, H. S. and Storer, J.: Mechanical Occlusion of the Vertebral Artery, J.A.M.A., 196, 475, 1966.

Irvine, W. T., Luck, R. J. and Jacobey, J. A.: Reversed Blood-flow in the Vertebral Arteries Causing Recurrent Brain-stem Ischaemia, Lancet, 1, 994, 1965.

Krayenbühl, H. and Yasargil, M. G.: Percutaneous Vertebral Angiography, Acta radiol., 5, 263, 1965.

Lester, J.: Arteriovenous Fistula After Percutaneous Vertebral Angiography, Acta radiol., 5, 337, 1965.

McCleery, W. N. C. and Lewtas, N. A.: Subarachnoid Injection of Contrast Medium. A Complication of Vertebral Angiography, Brit. J. Radiol., 39, 112, 1966.

Newton, T. H. and Darroch, H. J.: Vertebral Arteriovenous Fistula Complicating Vertebral Angiography, Acta radiol., 5, 428, 1965.

Fig. 480. A, AP laminagram of the cervical spine in a 43-year-old man with posterior fossa bleeding and acute right facial pain. An erosive change is seen in the lateral aspect of the bodies of C1 and 2. On lateral examination, B, of the cervico-occipital region no change is seen other than a deepening of the notch for the vertebral artery in the left lamina of C1. C, On oblique studies the foramen transversarium of the second cervical vertebra on the left side (arrow) is expanded, while that on the right is hard to identify, D. A right brachial angiogram showed the right vertebral artery to be hypoplastic. A left brachial angiogram, E and F, reveals a dilated left vertebral artery feeding an arteriovenous malformation over the right cerebellum.

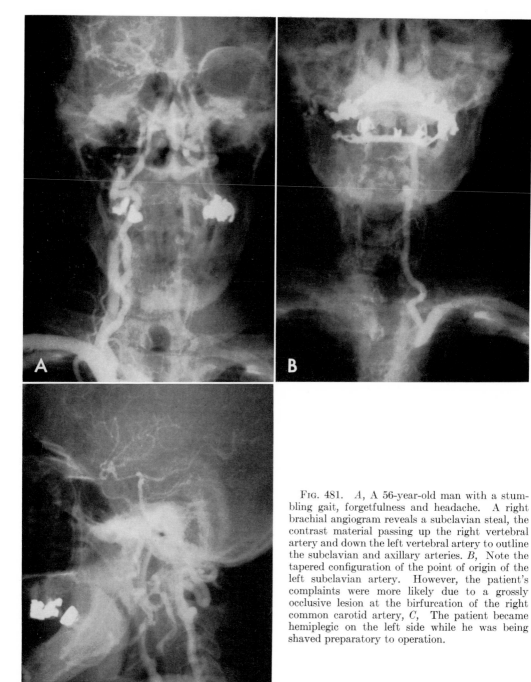

FIG. 481. *A,* A 56-year-old man with a stumbling gait, forgetfulness and headache. A right brachial angiogram reveals a subclavian steal, the contrast material passing up the right vertebral artery and down the left vertebral artery to outline the subclavian and axillary arteries. *B,* Note the tapered configuration of the point of origin of the left subclavian artery. However, the patient's complaints were more likely due to a grossly occlusive lesion at the birfurcation of the right common carotid artery, *C,* The patient became hemiplegic on the left side while he was being shaved preparatory to operation.

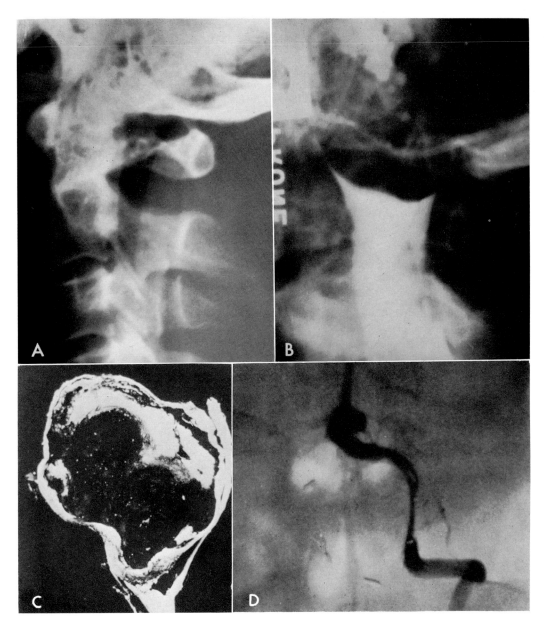

Fig. 482. *A*, Patient with symptoms referable to the cervico-occipital junction. Myelography with air showed the cord to be displaced dorsad. *B*, Myelographic examination reveals a complete block at C1. *C*, At operation a thrombosed aneurysm of the left vertebral artery was found, D. Subsequent angiogram reveals the vessel deformed but still patent. (Courtesy of T. Newton, University of California Medical School, San Francisco, California.)

Schneider, R. C. and Schemm, G. W.: Vertebral Artery Insufficiency in Acute and Chronic Spinal Trauma. With Special Reference to the Syndrome of Acute Central Cervical Spinal Cord Injury, J. Neurosurg., *18*, 348, 1961.

Sheehan, S., Bauer, R. B. and Meyer, J. S.: Vertebral Artery Compression in Cervical Spondylosis. Arteriographic Demonstration during Life of Vertebral Artery Insufficiency Due to Rotation and Extension of the Neck, Neurology, *10*, 968, 1960.

Slover, W. P. and Kiley, R. F.: Cervical Vertebral Erosion Caused by Tortuous Vertebral Artery, Radiology, *84*, 112, 1965.

Tatsumi, T. and Shenkin, H. A.: Occlusion of the Vertebral Artery, J. Neurol., Neurosurg. & Psychiat., *28*, 235, 1965.

Wilson, McC.: Angiography in Cerebrovascular Occlusive Disease, Am. J. Med. Sci., *250*, 554, 1965.

Yates, P. O. and Hutchinson, E. C.: Cerebral Infarction: the Role of Stenosis of the Extracranial Cerebral Arteries, Medical Research Council. Special Report Series No. 300, London, 1961.

Index